Target Organ Toxicology Series

Free Radical Toxicology

Target Organ Toxicology Series

Series Editors
A. Wallace Hayes, John A. Thomas, and Donald E. Garner

Target Organ Toxicology Series

Free Radical Toxicology

Edited by

Kendall B. Wallace
University of Minnesota, School of Medicine
Duluth, Minnesota

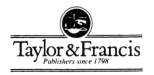

Taylor & Francis
Publishers since 1798

USA	Publishing Office:	Taylor & Francis 1101 Vermont Avenue, NW, Suite 200 Washington, DC 20005-3521 Tel: (202) 289-2174 Fax: (202) 289-3665
	Distribution Center:	Taylor & Francis 1900 Frost Road, Suite 101 Bristol, PA 19007-1598 Tel: (215) 785-5800 Fax: (215) 785-5515
UK		Taylor & Francis Ltd. 1 Gunpowder Square London EC4A 3DE Tel: 0171 583 0490 Fax: 0171 583 0581

FREE RADICAL TOXICOLOGY

1 2 3 4 5 6 7 8 9 0   B R B R   9 8 7

This book was set in Times Roman. The editors were Christine Williams and Elizabeth Dugger. Cover design by Michelle Fleitz.

A CIP catalog record for this book is available from the British Library.
♾ The paper in this publication meets the requirements of the ANSI Standard Z39.48-1984 (Permanence of Paper)

Library of Congress Cataloging-in-Publication Data

Free radical toxicology / edited by Kendall B. Wallace.
    p. cm.
  Includes index.

  1. Free radicals (Chemistry)—Pathophysiology. 2. Molecular
toxicology. I. Wallace, Kendall Bruce. II. Series.
  [DNLM: 1. Free Radicals—toxicity. 2. Free Radicals—metabolism.
QD 471 F8532 1997]
RB170.F69 1997
616.07—dc21
DNLM/DLC   96-37786
for Library of Congress   CIP

ISBN 1-56032-632-8 (case)

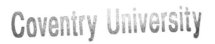

Contents

v

Contributing Authors

Stephen Bachowski, Ph.D. *Division of Toxicology, Department of Pharmacology and Toxicology, School of Medicine, Indiana University, Indianapolis, IN 46202-5196*

Barbara S. Berlett *National Heart, Lung, and Blood Institute, National Institutes of Health, Building 3, Room 222, Bethesda, MD 20892-0342*

Stephen C. Bondy, Ph.D. *Department of Community and Environmental Medicine, Center for Occupational and Environmental Health, University of California, Irvine, CA 92697-1825*

Enrique Cadenas, Ph.D. *Department of Molecular Pharmacology and Toxicology, School of Pharmacy, University of Southern California, Los Angeles, CA 90033*

John W. Eaton, Ph.D. *Department of Pediatrics, Baylor College of Medicine, One Baylor Plaza, Houston, TX 77030-3498*

Yvonne M. W. Janssen, Ph.D. *Department of Pathology, College of Medicine, University of Vermont, Burlington, VT 05405*

Jiazhong Jiang, M.D. *Division of Toxicology, Department of Pharmacology and Toxicology, School of Medicine, Indiana University, Indianapolis, IN 46202-5196*

George E. N. Kass, Ph.D. *School of Biological Sciences, University of Surrey, Guildford, Surrey GU2 5XH, United Kingdom*

James E. Klaunig, Ph.D. *Division of Toxicology, Department of Pharmacology and Toxicology, School of Medicine, Indiana University, 1001 Walnut St., Medical Facility 003, Indianapolis, IN 46202-5196*

W. H. Koppenol, D.Sc. *Laboratorium für Anorganische Chemie, Eidgenossische Technische Hochschule, CH-8092 Zürich, Switzerland*

Daniel C. Liebler, Ph.D. *Department of Pharmacology & Toxicology, College of Pharmacy, University of Arizona, Tucson, AZ 85721*

Ronald P. Mason, Ph.D.   *Laboratory of Molecular Biophysics, National Institute of Environmental Health Sciences, National Institutes of Health, Research Triangle Park, NC 27709*

Laurie McLeod   *Department of Molecular Pharmacology & Toxicology, School of Pharmacy, University of Southern California, 1985 Zonal Avenue, Los Angeles, CA 90033*

Brooke T. Mossman, Ph.D.   *Department of Pathology, College of Medicine, University of Vermont, Burlington, VT 05405*

Charles R. Myers, Ph.D.   *Department of Pharmacology and Toxicology, Medical College of Wisconsin, Milwaukee, WI 53226*

J. Fred Nagelkerke, Ph.D.   *Leiden/Amsterdam Center for Drug Research, Division of Toxicology, Leiden University, Sylvius Laboratory, P.O. Box 9503, 2300 RA Leiden, The Netherlands*

Gabriel L. Plaa, Ph.D.   *Département de pharmacologie, Faculté de médecine, Université de Montréal, C. P. 6128, succursale Centre-ville, Montréal, Québec H3C 3J7, Canada*

Donald J. Reed, Ph.D.   *Department of Biochemistry and Biophysics, Oregon State University, 2011 ALS, Corvallis, OR 97331*

Christoph Richter, Ph.D.   *Laboratorium fur Biochemie I (Laboratory of Biochemistry I), Eidgenossische Technische Hochschule (Swiss Federal Institute of Technology) (ETH), Universitatstr. 16, Zurich CH-8092, Switzerland*

Mark D. Scott, Ph.D.   *Division of Experimental Pathology, A-81, Department of Pathology and Laboratory Medicine, Albany Medical College, 47 New Scotland Avenue, Albany, NY 12208*

Alex Sevanian, Ph.D.   *Department of Molecular Pharmacology & Toxicology, School of Pharmacy, University of Southern California, 1985 Zonal Avenue, Los Angeles, CA 90033*

Martyn T. Smith, Ph.D.   *Division of Environmental Health Sciences, School of Public Health, University of California, Berkeley, CA 94720*

Earl R. Stadtman, Ph.D.   *National Heart, Lung, and Blood Institute, National Institutes of Health, Building 3, Room 222, Bethesda, MD 20892-0342*

Vangala V. Subrahmanyam, Ph.D.   *Department of Biotransformation, Division of Drug Safety and Metabolism, Wyeth Ayerst Research Laboratories, 9 Deer Park Drive, Monmouth Junction, NJ 08852*

Cynthia R. Timblin, Ph.D. *Department of Pathology, College of Medicine, University of Vermont, Burlington, VT 05405*

Bob van de Water, Ph.D. *Leiden/Amsterdam Center for Drug Research, Division of Toxicology, Leiden University, Sylvius Laboratory, P.O. Box 9503, 2300 RA Leiden, The Netherlands*

James Varani, Ph.D. *Department of Pathology, University of Michigan, 1301 Catherine Road, Box 0602, Ann Arbor, MI 48109-0602*

Kendall B. Wallace, Ph.D. *Department of Biochemistry and Molecular Biology, School of Medicine, University of Minnesota, Duluth, MN 55812*

Peter A. Ward, M.D. *University of Michigan Medical School, Medical Science I M5240/0602, 1301 Catherine Road, Ann Arbor, MI 48109-0602*

Hanspeter R. Witschi, M.D. *Institute of Toxicology and Environmental Health and Department of Molecular Biosciences, School of Veterinary Medicine, University of California, Davis, CA 95616*

Yong Xu, M.D. *Division of Toxicology, Department of Pharmacology and Toxicology, School of Medicine, Indiana University, Indianapolis, IN 46202-5196*

Preface

The field of free radical toxicology has its origins in the realization that for many redox reactions, especially those catalyzed by metalloenzymes, electrons are transferred sequentially rather than in parallel. Accordingly, there exists for a brief moment a highly reactive intermediate possessing an unpaired electron, which by definition constitutes a free radical. The brevity of the moment is determined by the stability of the unpaired electron and the availability of alternate electron acceptors or donors.

The past two decades have witnessed an explosion of interest and understanding of oxygen free radicals and their implication in assorted pathogenic processes. It has come to light that free radical intermediates are not foreign to the normal biology of the cell. Reactive oxygen species are byproducts of a number of metabolic processes and are formed deliberately as part of the normal inflammatory response. To accommodate this, tissues have developed elaborate antioxidant defense systems to hold in-check the potential for free-radical-mediated tissue damage. Since molecular oxygen is the most prevalent and ubiquitous biological electron acceptor, the majority of the antioxidants are tailored to defend against free radical intermediates of oxygen. It is when the rates of free radical generation exceed the finite capacity of the antioxidant defense systems that tissue damage occurs.

Because of the abundant and provocative sources of free radicals in biological systems, it is not an uncommon event when endogenous antioxidant defense systems are overwhelmed. In fact, oxygen free radicals are implicated in the pathogenesis of a number of disease processes, including ischemia/reperfusion, atherosclerosis, neurodegenerative disorders, rheumatoid arthritis, muscular dystrophy, and aging. The implication of oxygen free radicals in the etiology of various disease processes has been the subject of a number of excellent reviews.

An alternate cause for excessive free radical generation is in the presence of selected xenobiotics. There exists a rapidly growing list of chemicals which when added to biological systems stimulate several-fold increases in the rate of free radical generation. For the most part, the free radicals are generated either as byproducts of oxygen reduction during xenobiotic metabolism or are liberated as the result of the futile redox cycling of the chemical agent. Regardless, such free radical intermediates are widely invoked in mediating the biological response to chemical exposure, whether it be a therapeutic or toxic response. It is this xenobiotic-induced free radical-mediated toxic tissue injury that is the subject of this book. With the increasing implication of free radical-mediated and oxidative mechanisms of chemical-induced tissue injury, a treatise on this subject is both justified and timely. A better understanding of the mechanisms of free radical toxicity may yield valuable insight and opportunity to managing the risks associated with chemical exposures.

This monograph is divided into four thematic sections. The first two sections set the stage for the book. Section I describes the fundamentals of free radical chemistry and the theoretical basis for electron transfer reactions leading to free radical generation. Section II opens with a description of the various subcellular sources of free radicals followed by three chapters, each written by experts on the subject of the biological reactivity of free radicals with lipid, protein, and nucleic acids. The section concludes with chapters describing the physicochemical determinants of free radical-induced cell injury and the various antioxidant defense systems that guard against such damage. The third section of the book focuses on the theme of this series of monographs: Target Organ Toxicity. Each chapter describes morphological and biochemical nuances of individual tissues then gives examples of free radical-mediated toxicity to one of seven distinct target organ systems. The molecular biology of free-radical-mediated alterations in gene expression, signal transduction, and carcinogenesis is the subject of the final section of this monograph. The book concludes, appropriately so, with an overview of the evidence implicating free radicals in the etiology of various chemical toxicities, challenging the possibility of misguided use of biomarkers for oxidative damage. The authors lend their candid insight into the appropriate and inappropriate allegations of free radicals as causative intermediates in the forensics of toxic tissue injury.

This monograph represents the culmination of considerable thought and work on the part of many individuals. I wish to thank each author for their expert and generous contributions. I hope that each considers the experience both productive and rewarding. However, the ultimate goal of the book has yet to be measured; that it will provide the reader with a concise description and valuable insight into the involvement of free radicals in the pathogenesis of chemical-induced toxic tissue injury. Many of the concepts contained in this monograph will hopefully inspire strategies and create opportunities for the reader to advance their personal and professional interests in the subject of free radical-mediated target organ toxicity.

PART I

Free-Radical Chemistry

Free Radical Toxicology
Edited by K. B. Wallace
Copyright © 1997 Taylor & Francis

1

The Chemical Reactivity of Radicals

W. H. Koppenol*

*Laboratorium für Anorganische Chemie, Eidgenössische Technische Hochschule,
CH-8092 Zürich, Switzerland*

DEFINITION AND NOMENCLATURE OF RADICALS

A radical is an atom or group of atoms with one or more unpaired electrons (1). It may have positive, negative or zero charge.

The word "free" in front of "radical" should not be used. In the past the word "radical" was used to indicate a group, or substituent, like "methyl" in 2-methylbutane. To indicate a methyl radical by itself, the word "free" was added. Since currently a radical is an unattached particle, the word "free" in front of "radical" is considered unnecessary and obsolete: all radicals are "free" (2). If a radical is believed to be an intermediate in a chemical reaction, and is not able to escape to the bulk solvent, then a term like "bound" or "caged" should be added.

In a formula a radical is indicated by a superscript dot, which precedes any charge, e.g. $O_2^{\cdot-}$ (not $O_2^{-\cdot}$) and $PO_3^{\cdot 2-}$. It should be placed to the upper right of the chemical symbol, so as not to interfere with indications of mass number, atomic number or composition. In the case of diradicals, etc., the superscript dot is preceded by the appropriate superscript number, e.g. $O_2^{2\cdot}$ (1).

Ideally, the name of a radical, or for that matter, any chemical, should reveal its composition and structure. Presently, a number of trivial names are used that in that respect are less than helpful to the novice. As an example, the names nitric oxide and nitrous oxide for $NO^{\cdot}$ and N_2O, repectively, do not reveal the compositions of the respective compounds, which sometimes leads to confusion. There are essentially two systematic ways of naming compounds (1). One is called additive, and the other substitutive nomenclature. The first is used mostly for inorganic, and the other for organic compounds. Additive nomenclature is simpler: one gives the composition, as in nitrogen dioxide for NO_2. Substitutive nomenclature is based on names like methane, azane, oxidane, and silane for CH_4, NH_3, H_2O and SiH_4, respectively. Thus, CCl_4 is named tetrachloromethane according to substitutive nomenclature,

---

* Secretary (1994–1997), Commission for Nomenclature of Inorganic Chemistry, IUPAC

and carbon tetrachloride according to additive nomenclature. To return to the nitrogen oxides mentioned above, NO˙ is named nitrogen monoxide, and N_2O dinitrogen monoxide. The suffixes "-ic" and "-ous", as found in nitric and nitrous oxide refer to different oxygen contents, or oxidation states. Since nitric acid and nitric oxide have the same suffix, but different oxidation states, $+2$ and $+5$, respectively, confusion is possible. For that reason these suffixes are—since 1957—no longer recommended by IUPAC. For the present it is best to use names that are based on additive nomenclature for inorganic radicals, such as nitrogen monoxide for NO˙ and hydrogen dioxide for HO_2, and substitutive nomenclature for organic radicals, such as 1-hydroxyethane-1-yl for $CH_3C˙HOH$ (3). Please note that this compound is not named as an alcohol: the radical takes precedence over all functional groups (4). Old and venerable names, like superoxide radical for O_2^- and hydroxyl radical for HO˙, are still allowed. A number of examples are given in Table 1. As can be seen in that table, there exist no systematic names for certain inorganic radicals. However, new and self-consistent guidelines for inorganic radical nomenclature are in preparation by the Commission for the Nomenclature of Inorganic Chemistry, IUPAC.

TABLE 1. *Names of common radicals and parent compounds*

Radical	Additive name	Substitutive name	Allowed name
$C˙H_2OH$		hydroxymethyl	
$CH_3NH˙$		methanaminyl	
$CH_3O˙$		methoxyl	
$C˙Cl_3$		trichloromethyl	
CN˙			cyanyl
CO_2^-	dioxocarbonate(1−)		
$CH_3C˙HOH$		1-hydroxyethane-1-yl	
$C˙H_2CH_2OH$		2-hydroxyethane-1-yl	
$CH_3CH_2O˙$		ethanoxyl	
$CH_3CH_2CH(OO˙)CH_3$		butane-2-yldioxyl	
$C_6H_5O˙$		phenoxyl	
$C_6H_5S˙$		phenylsulfanyl	
ClO˙	chlorine monoxide	chlorooxidanyl	chlorosyl
ClO_2	chlorine dioxide		
HO˙		oxidanyl	hydroxyl
HO_2	hydrogen dioxide	dioxidanyl	hydroperoxyl
H_2O_2		dioxidane	hydrogen peroxide
NO^+			nitrosyl
NO˙	nitrogen monoxide		
NO^-	oxonitrate(1−)		
NO_2^+			nitryl
NO_2	nitrogen dioxide		
NO_2^-	dioxonitrate(1−)		nitrite
N_2O	dinitrogen monoxide		
$N_2O_2^-$	dioxodinitrate(1−)		
O–NOO˙		nitrosodioxidanyl	nitrosylperoxyl
O–NOO$^-$	oxoperoxonitrate(1−)		
O_2^-	dioxide(1−)	dioxidanidyl	superoxide
O_3^-	trioxide(1−)	trioxidanidyl	ozonide
HS˙		sulfanyl	

THERMODYNAMICS. GENERAL

With few exceptions, nitrogen monoxide being one of them, radicals either dispro-portionate or dimerize. Disproportionation (or dismutation) implies that thermodynamically the radical is both oxidizing and reducing. That is, they can react together to form the more stable oxidized and reduced forms. An example is shown in Equation 1.

$$2O_2^- + 2H^+ \rightarrow H_2O_2 + O_2 \qquad [1]$$

which is the sum of the following two half-reactions:

$$O_2^- + 2H^+ + e^- \rightarrow H_2O_2 \qquad [2]$$

$$O_2^- \qquad\qquad \rightarrow O_2 + e^- \qquad [3]$$

The reduction potentials of the couples O_2^-/H_2O_2 and O_2/O_2^- are 0.94 V and -0.16 V, respectively. The energetics are calculated by adding the potentials of a reduction reaction (Eq. 2) and that of an oxidation reaction (Eq. 3). Since Reaction 3 is written as an oxidation, one reverses the sign of the reduction potential and adds it to the value of that of the reduction reaction, reaction 2. One arrives at a value of 1.10 V, which via $\Delta G^{o'} = -nF\Delta E^{o'}$ results in -106 kJ/(2 mol superoxide). That the reaction as written (reaction 1) has a negligible rate constant (5) and takes place via the oxidation of superoxide by hydrogen dioxide is only of kinetic importance; it does not affect the energetics of the overall reaction.

Gibbs energies of formation of a number of radicals and parent compounds have been collected in Table 2. Taking, again, reaction 1 one calculates a Gibbs energy change of -106 kJ/(2 mol superoxide) with the help of the data listed in that Table.

The 1-hydroxyethane-1-yl radical, $CH_3CHOH^{\cdot}$, both disproportionates and dimer-izes, if left to itself (6). One cannot *a priori* say whether disproportionation or dimerization will take place. The dimerization reaction of two organic radicals is very favorable: the enthalpy of bond formation of a $C-C$ bond is negative by approximately 350 kJ/mol. A disproportionation is about equally favorable: A $C-H$ bond is formed, which is about 20 kcal more favorable than a $C-C$ bond, but also a $C=C$ bond, or in the case of the 1-hydroxyethane-1-yl, a $C=O$ bond, which are, respectively, about 20 kcal less than two single bonds, and the same as two single bonds. While the enthalpies are very similar, the disproportionation has an entropic advantage over the dimerization reaction, making it slightly more favourable when expressed in Gibbs energy. The T ΔS term is estimated at $+38$ kJ/(2 mol of radical).

The fact that most radicals are both oxidizing and reducing leads to a characteristic "saw-tooth" appearance of an oxidation state diagram, see Fig. 1 (7). In such diagrams the Gibbs energies of formation to make the radical and related compounds from the element and water are plotted as a function of the oxidation state of the element; it follows that lines joining compounds represent reduction potentials. Such diagrams have been constructed for oxygen (8,9), carbon (8), sulfur (10,11) and nitrogen (12,13). As an example, in Fig. 1 superoxide lies above a line joining its

TABLE 2. *Gibbs energies of formation of radicals and their parent species*

Compound	$\Delta_f G^{\circ\prime}$ (kJ/mol)[a]
HO·	+66
HOCl	−39.4
H_2O	−157.3
H_2O_2	−59.0
NO·	+102
NO^+	+219
NO^- (singlet)	+136
NO^- (triplet)	+64
NO_2	+63
NO_2^+	+218
NO_2^-	−32.2
NO_3	+131
NO_3^-	−108.7
N_2	+17.5
N_2O	+113.6
$N_2O_2^-$	+141[b]
N_2O_3	+147
ONOO·	+84
$ONOO^-$	+42
OCl^-	−36.8
O_2	+16.4
O_2 (singlet)	+112
O_2^-	+31.8

[a] The Gibbs energies of formation apply to 1 molal concentrations, even when gases are involved, and to pH 7, in the case of hydrogen containing compounds. Data were obtained from the literature (13,43–46). Modified after Ref. 47.
[b] From rate data (48), W. H. Koppenol, unpublished.

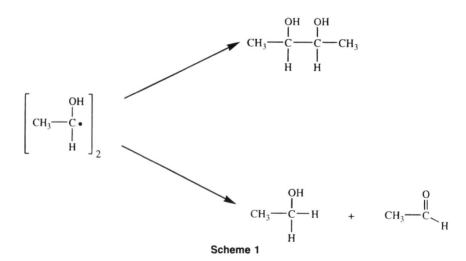

Scheme 1

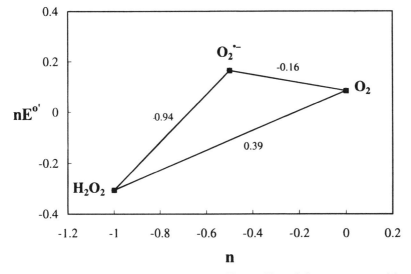

FIG. 1. Partial oxidation state diagram of oxygen. The position of dioxygen, superoxide and hydrogen peroxide along the x-axis represents the oxidation states (n) of 0, $-\frac{1}{2}$ and -1, respectively. The y-axis is the product of the oxidation state n and the reduction potential ($E^{o\prime}$), such that the slope of the line that connects dioxygen with superoxide represents the reduction potential O_2/O_2^-, -0.16 V. Dioxygen is not found at (0,0), while the reference state is 1 M O_2 in water: It costs 16.4 kJ to dissolve 1 mol of dioxygen (see Table 2).

neighbours, dioxygen and hydrogen peroxide, which shows that it is thermodynamically unstable with respect to disproportionation.

In Tables 3 and 4 one-electron reduction potentials of relevant couples have been collected from the literature. These are used to calculate Gibbs energies of radical reactions. The results of such calculations must be interpreted with caution, as shown below.

Reactions That Are Thermodynamically Possible and Do Occur

The one-electron reduction of hydrogen peroxide by an iron(II) complex, the Fenton reaction, has been cited innumerable times (See for review Refs. (9,14,15)) as the source of hydroxyl radicals *in vivo*, although until recently the bimolecular rate constants for physiologically relevant iron complexes were not known (16). Evidence has been presented that this reaction proceeds via a higher oxidation state of iron (14,17). The reduction potential of an iron(III)-/iron(II)-*atp* complex is probably close to that of the aminopolycarboxylate complexes, near $+0.1$ V. With this value one calculates the following energetics:

$$Fe^{2+}atp \rightarrow Fe^{3+}atp + e^- \qquad E^\circ = -0.1 \text{ V} \qquad [4]$$
$$H_2O_2 + e^- + H^+ \rightarrow HO^. + H_2O \qquad E^{o\prime} = +0.32 \text{ V} \qquad [5]$$

TABLE 3. *One-electron reduction potentials of biochemically relevant couples*

Couple	$E^{o\prime}$ (V)
ascorbyl($A^{\cdot-}$)/ascorbate(HA^-)	+0.282
dehydroascorbate(A)/ascorbyl($A^{\cdot-}$)	−0.174
$CH_2O/C^{\cdot}H_2OH$	−1.3
$C^{\cdot}H_2OH/CH_3OH$	+1.2
$CO_2/CO_2^{\cdot-}$	−1.8
$CO_2^{\cdot-}/HCO_2^-$	+1.1
$CH_3CHO/CH_3C^{\cdot}HOH$	−1.4
$CH_3C^{\cdot}HOH/CH_3CH_2OH$	+1.0
$HO^{\cdot}/H_2O$	+2.31
$HOCl/HO^{\cdot}$, Cl^-	+0.26
$HOBr/HO^{\cdot}$, Br^-	−0.05
$HO_2^{\cdot}/H_2O_2$	+1.07
$H_2O_2/HO^{\cdot}$, H_2O	+0.32
$NO^+/NO^{\cdot}$	+1.21
$NO^{\cdot}/NO^-$ (singlet)	−0.35
$NO^{\cdot}/NO^-$ (triplet)	+0.39
NO_2^+/NO_2	+1.6
$NO_2^{\cdot}/NO_2^-$	+0.99
$2NO^{\cdot}/N_2O_2^{2-}$	+0.65[a]
$N_2O_3/NO^{\cdot}$, NO_2^-	+0.8
$O=NOO^{\cdot}/O=NOO^-$	+0.4
$O=NOO^-/NO_2^{\cdot}$	+1.4
$^1O_2/O_2^{\cdot-}$	+0.83
$^3O_2/O_2^{\cdot-}$	−0.16
$O_2^{\cdot-}/H_2O_2$	+0.94

Note. All values refer to 1 molal concentrations and pH 7, where relevant. Data are taken from the literature (13,19,38,45–47,49,50).
[a] W. H. Koppenol, unpublished.

TABLE 4. *Reduction potentials of functional groups*

Couple	$E^{o\prime}$ (V)
allylic$^{\cdot}$/allylicH	+0.6
$RO^{\cdot}/ROH$	+1.6
$ROO^{\cdot}/ROOH$	+1.0
$PhenO^{\cdot}/PhenOH$	+0.9
$RS^{\cdot}/RSH$	+0.90
$RSNO/RSH$, $NO^{\cdot}$	−0.4[a]
$RSSR/RSSR^{\cdot-}$	−1.5

Note. Data apply to pH 7 and 1 molal concentrations. The uncertainties in these values are larger than those in Table 3. Data are from the literature (11,35,51,52).
[a] W. H. Koppenol, unpublished.

$$Fe^{2+}atp + H_2O_2 + H^+ \rightarrow Fe^{3+}atp + HO^{\cdot} + H_2O \qquad \Delta_{rxn}G^{\circ\prime} = -21 \text{ kJ/mol} \qquad [6]$$

Because the hydroxyl radical is a very oxidizing radical, nearly all its reactions have negative Gibbs energies. However, the hydroxyl radical can also add to a double bond, abstract a hydrogen, or combine with another radical. The Gibbs energy of such a combination reaction is also substantial:

$$NO^{\cdot} + HO^{\cdot} \rightarrow NO_2^- + H^+ \qquad \Delta_{rxn}G^{\circ\prime} = -200 \text{ kJ/mol} \qquad [7]$$

Please note that the nitrosyl cation, NO^+, is not formed. The value of 0.32 V at pH 7 for the $H_2O_2/HO^{\cdot}$, H_2O couple puts certain restrictions on what can reduce hydrogen peroxide and what cannot. No such thermodynamic restrictions exist for alkylhydroperoxides, due to the high value of 1.9 V of the $ROOH/RO^{\cdot}$, H_2O couple at pH 7.

Reactions That Are Thermodynamically Possible and Do Not Occur

Nitrogen monoxide does not react with hydrogen peroxide at pH 7, contrary to a recent report (18). However, a reaction with nitrogen dioxide and water as products is thermodynamically feasible (19):

$$NO^{\cdot} + H_2O_2 \rightarrow NO_2^{\cdot} + H_2O \qquad \Delta_{rxn}G^{\circ\prime} = -137 \text{ kJ/mol} \qquad [8]$$

At alkaline pH nitrogen monoxide is reported to react with HO_2^- to form $O{=}NOO^-$ (20), but the details of this reaction are unclear. Since more than one hydrogen peroxide was consumed per one oxoperoxonitrate($1-$) formed, it is possible that the following overall reaction took place:

$$NO^{\cdot} + 2H_2O_2 \rightarrow O{=}NOO^- + HO^{\cdot} + H_2O + H^+ \qquad \Delta_{rxn}G^{\circ\prime} = -73 \text{ kJ/mol} \qquad [9]$$

Reactions That Are Thermodynamically Not Possible and Do Occur

Reactions like that are more common than one would think, and can be found, for example, in the citric acid cycle. These reactions proceed because the products are removed in subsequent reactions. The same phenomenon is also observed in the reactions that are part of the superoxide sink hypothesis (21):

$$R^1R^2CHOO^{\cdot} + GSH \rightarrow R^1R^2CHOOH + GS^{\cdot} \qquad \Delta_{rxn}G^{\circ\prime} = -10 \text{ kJ/mol} \qquad [10]$$

$$GSH \rightarrow GS^- + H^+ \qquad \Delta_{rxn}G^{\circ\prime} = +9 \text{ kJ/mol} \qquad [11]$$

$$GS^{\cdot} + GS^- \rightarrow GSSG^{\cdot-} \qquad \Delta_{rxn}G^{\circ} = -18 \text{ kJ/mol} \qquad [12]$$

$$GSSG^{\cdot-} + O_2 \rightarrow GSSG + O_2^{\cdot-} \qquad \Delta_{rxn}G^{\circ} = -130 \text{ kJ/mol} \qquad [13]$$

The first reaction is the one-electron oxidation of glutathione by an oxidizing species. This reaction may, or may not, be favorable. The example given is only slightly favorable, and is not likely to go to completion. This is followed by reaction with another glutathione to form the diglutathione-disulfide anion radical, GSSG⁻⁻. This reaction does not go to completion either, because the cellular glutathione concentration is not high enough. What drives this sequence of reactions is the reduction of dioxygen, reaction 13 to superoxide, and the subsequent dismutation of this radical, reaction 1, which both are very favorable. This sequence of reactions makes it possible to "repair" radicals that have reduction potentials (R˙/RH) below that of the RS˙/RSH couple. As an example, the reduction of the acetaminophen phenoxyl radical by glutathione, which is unfavorable by 15 kJ/mol, proceeds to completion (22).

The lesson to be learned here is that reactions with positive Gibbs energies can occur when products are formed that disappear rapidly in subsequent reactions. This applies especially to radicals as products of unfavorable reactions. However, a large positive Gibbs energy, say >40 kJ, leads to a theoretical equilibrium concentration of radicals that is so small that subsequent reactions, even if their rate constants are diffusion controlled, proceed so slowly that an effective repair is not feasible.

Reactions That Are Thermodynamically Not Possible and Do Not Occur

Recently, it has been suggested that Reaction 14 is responsible for the initiation of oxyradical damage (16):

$$O_2^- + H_2O_2 + H^+ \rightarrow {}^1\Delta_gO_2 + HO^˙ + H_2O \qquad [14]$$

This reaction, with triplet dioxygen as a product, was first proposed in 1931 by Haber and Willstätter (23), and became known as the Haber-Weiss reaction in the seventies. Already in 1947 George carried out experiments that showed that this reaction has a very low rate constant, which led to a conflict with Weiss (24). In the seventies, unaware of George's result, several groups, including that of the author, measured the rate constant and came to the conclusion that the rate constant of this reaction is at most near 1 M^{-1} s^{-1}, and that this reaction can be neglected compared to the dismutation reaction of superoxide (25–31). The reaction with triplet dioxygen as a product is thermodynamically possible, but not with singlet dioxygen: $\Delta_{rxn}G° = +47$ kJ/mol. Thus, reaction 14 is insignificant for both kinetic and thermodynamic reasons.

INITIATION OF RADICAL DAMAGE

Generally, the Fenton reaction (reaction 6) is considered the initiator of radical damage, although the nature of the iron complexes and their concentrations *in vivo* is unknown. Another pathway to generate the hydroxyl radical involves the one electron reduction of hypochlorite by superoxide (32), or by an iron(II) complex (33,34):

$$O_2^- + HOCl \rightarrow HO^˙ + Cl^- + O_2 \qquad \Delta_{rxn}G° = -41 \text{ kJ/mol} \qquad [15]$$

$$Fe^{2+}atp + HOCl \rightarrow Fe^{3+}atp + HO^{\cdot} + Cl^{-} \quad \Delta_{rxn}G^{\circ\prime} = -15 \text{ kJ/mol} \quad [16]$$

Since the discovery of the formation of nitrogen monoxide *in vivo* it has become clear that another powerful (13) oxidizing agent is formed, namely oxoperoxonitrate($1-$). Many of the deleterious effects previously ascribed to the Fenton reaction may be caused by this molecule, because its formation is more likely than the occurrence of the Fenton reaction: superoxide reacts at a nearly diffusion-controlled rate with nitrogen monoxide, while the known rates of reduction of ferric complexes by superoxide is at least three orders of magnitude slower. While it is commonly assumed that O=NOOH undergoes homolysis, thermodynamic and kinetic arguments indicate that this is not the case. Instead, an intermediate in the isomerization to nitrate is believed to be the oxidizing agent (13).

Chain Reactions

The damage, caused by the initial reaction of an oxyradical with a biomolecule, is small. However, because a radical reaction begets another radical, there is the possibility of a cycle of reactions that amplifies the damage. A common example is lipid peroxidation. In the following two reactions RH stands for allylic H:

$$ROO^{\cdot} + RH \rightarrow ROOH + R^{\cdot} \quad \Delta_{rxn}G^{\circ} = -38 \text{ kJ/mol (35)} \quad [17]$$

$$R^{\cdot} + O_2 \rightarrow ROO^{\cdot} \quad \Delta_{rxn}G^{\circ} = -88 \text{ kJ/mol (35)} \quad [18]$$

Xanthine oxidase is a molybdoenzyme that produces superoxide (36). Aldehydic products of lipid oxidation are substrates for xanthine oxidase (37), which leads to more superoxide production, new radical chain reactions, and more damage. In such a case, a chain reaction has led to a cascade of radical reactions.

Transition metal complexes and redox-active organic compounds are well suited for the propagation of chain reactions. For instance, paraquat is toxic because it diverts electrons from the mitochondrial electron transport chain to dioxygen. Since the reduction potential of the paraquat couple is -0.45 V (38), the one-electron reduction of dioxygen, which has been studied by pulse radiolysis (39,40), is quite favorable:

$$Paraquat^{\cdot+} + O_2 \rightarrow Paraquat^{2+} + O_2^{\cdot-} \quad \Delta_{rxn}G^{\circ} = -28 \text{ kJ/mol} \quad [19]$$

Paraquat may also be toxic because the radical releases iron from ferritin by reduction (41). Such an event could start a metal-mediated chain of reactions that increases the damage. The reactions described above for paraquat are also relevant for antitumor quinones. Their activity as antitumor agents is based on their ability to generate oxyradicals and/or to alkylate DNA. Unfortunately, their toxicity, especially to the heart, also involves oxyradicals (42). The reduction potentials of the quinone/semiquinone couples are not far from that of the dioxygen/superoxide couple (38), such that electron transfer between the two couples is feasible. The semiquinone can reduce metal complexes, which then participate in a Fenton reaction.

Concluding Remarks

Thermodynamic and kinetic considerations are useful in that these can limit the number of possible mechanisms. While it is true that there are no thermodynamic standard conditions in the cell, one should consider that one always compares one standard Gibbs energy with another. By doing so the errors made in the assumption of the standard state often cancel. Concentration effects as they pertain to the hydron (H^+) were taken into account: all values given are for pH 7. One does not have to have 1 molal concentrations for other reactants either: If one considers the value of a reduction potential, one only needs equal concentrations of the oxidant and the reductant to obtain the standard value, whether these concentrations are in the micro- or nano-molar range. Thus, the time spent on thermodynamic considerations may be more than recouped in time not wasted in the laboratory!

ACKNOWLEDGMENT

I thank Dr. P.L. Bounds for helpful discussions during the preparation of this review.

REFERENCES

1. Leigh GJ, Ed. *Nomenclature of Inorganic Chemistry.* Oxford: Blackwell Scientific Publications; 1990.
2. Koppenol WH, Traynham JG. Say NO to nitric oxide. Nomenclature for nitrogen and oxygen containing compounds. *Meth. Enzymol.* 1996;268:3–7.
3. Powell WH, Ed. Revised Nomenclature for Radicals, Ions, Radical Ions and Related Species— Recommendations 1993. *Pure & Appl Chem.* 1993;65:1357–455.
4. Rigaudy J and Klesney SP, editors. *Nomenclature of Organic Chemistry. Sections A, B, C, D, E, F and H.* Oxford: Pergamon Press; 1979, p. 328.
5. Bielski BHJ. Re-evaluation of the spectral and kinetic properties of HO_2 and O_2^- free radicals. *Photochem. Photobiol.* 1978I28:645–9.
6. Taub IA, Dorfman LM. Pulse radiolysis studies. II. Transient spectra and rate processes in irradiated ethanol and aqueous ethanol solution. *J Am Chem Soc* 1962;84:4053–9.
7. Phillips CSG, Williams RJP. *Inorganic Chemistry.* Oxford: Clarendon Press; 1965;314–316.
8. Koppenol WH. The reduction potential of the couple O_3/O_3^-. *FEBS Lett.* 1982;140:169–72.
9. Koppenol WH. Chemistry of iron and copper in radical reactions. In: Rice-Evans CA, Burdon RH, eds. *Free Radical Damage and its Control.* Amsterdam: Elsevier Science B.V. 1994;3–24.
10. Koppenol WH. The paradox of oxygen: Thermodynamics *versus* Toxicity. In: King T, Mason HS, Morrison M, eds. *Oxidases and Related Redox Systems.* New York: A. Liss; 1988;93–109.
11. Koppenol WH. A thermodynamic appraisal of the radical sink theory. *Free Radical Biol. Med.* 1993;14:91–4.
12. Koppenol WH. Thermodynamic considerations on the generation of hydroxyl radicals from nitrous oxide—No laughing matter. *Free Radical Biol. Med.* 1991;10:85–7.
13. Koppenol WH, Moreno JJ, Pryor WA, Ischiropoulos H, Beckman JS. Peroxynitrite, a cloaked oxidant formed by nitric oxide and superoxide. *Chem. Res. Toxicol.* 1992;5:834–42.
14. Sutton HC, Winterbourn CC. On the participation of higher oxidation states of iron and copper in Fenton reactions. *Free Radical Biol. Med.* 1989;6:54–60.
15. Goldstein S, Meyerstein D, Czapski G. The Fenton reagents. *Free Radical Biol Med.* 1993;15:435–45.
16. Khan AU, Kasha M. Singlet molecular oxygen in the Haber-Weiss reaction. *Proc Natl Acad Sci USA* 1994;91:12365–7.
17. Rush JD, Maskos Z, Koppenol WH. Distinction between hydroxyl radical and ferryl species. In:

Packer L, Glazer AN, eds. *Methods in Enzymology, Vol. 186.* San Diego: Academic Press, 1990;148–56.

18. Stamler JS, Singel DJ, Loscalzo J. Biochemistry of nitric oxide and its redox-activated forms. *Science* 1992;258:1898–902.

19. Koppenol WH. Thermodynamic considerations on the formation of reactive species from hypochlorite, superoxide and nitrogen monoxide. Could nitrosyl chloride be produced by neutrophils and macrophages? *FEBS Lett.* 1994;347:5–8.

20. Petriconi GL, Papée HM. Aqueous solutions of "sodium pernitrite" from alkaline hydrogen peroxide and nitric oxide. *Can. J. Chem.* 1966;44:977–80.

21. Winterbourn CC. Superoxide as an intracellular radical sink. *Free Radical Biol. Med.* 1993;14:85–90.

22. Wardman P. Conjugation and oxidation of glutathione via thiyl free radicals. In: Sies H, Ketterer B, eds. *Glutathione Conjugation: Mechanisms and Biological Significance.* San Diego: Academic Press, 1988;43–72.

23. Haber F, Willstätter R. Unpaarigkeit und Radikalketten im Reaktionsmechanismus organischer und enzymatischer Vorgänge. *Ber deutschen chem Ges.* 1931;64:2844–56.

24. George P. Some experiments on the reactions of potassium superoxide in aqueous solutions. *Disc. Faraday Soc.* 1947;2:196–222.

25. Ferradini C, Seide C. Radiolyse de solutions acides et aerees de peroxyde d'hydrogene. *Int J Radiat Phys Chem.* 1969;1:219–24.

26. Melhuish WH, Sutton HC. Study of the Haber-Weiss reaction using a sensitive method for detection of OH radicals. *J.C.S. Chem. Commun.* 1978;970–1.

27. Koppenol WH, Butler J, van Leeuwen JW. The Haber-Weiss cycle. *Photochem. Photobiol.* 1978;28:655–60.

28. Czapski G, Ilan YA. On the generation of the hydroxylation agent from superoxide radical. Can the Haber-Weiss reaction be the source of OH radicals? *Photochem. Photobiol.* 1978;28:651–3.

29. Rigo A, Stevanato R, Finazzi-Agro A, Rotilio G. An attempt to evaluate the rate of the Haber Weiss reaction by using hydroxyl radical scavengers. *FEBS Lett.* 1977;80:130–2.

30. Weinstein J, Bielski BHJ. Kinetics of the interaction of HO_2 and O_2^- radicals with hydrogen peroxide; The Haber-Weiss reaction. *J Am Chem Soc.* 1979;101:58–62.

31. Bors W, Michel C, Saran M. Superoxide anions do not react with hydroperoxides. *FEBS Lett.* 1979;107:403–6.

32. Candeias LP, Patel KB, Stratford MRL, Wardman P. Free hydroxyl radicals are formed on reaction between the neutrophil-derived species superoxide anion and hypochlorous acid. *FEBS Lett.* 1993;333:151–3.

33. Fenton HJH. On a new reaction of tartaric acid. *Chem News* 1876;33:190.

34. Candeias LP, Stratford MRL, Wardman P. Formation of hydroxyl radicals on reaction of hypochlorous acid with ferrocyanide, a model iron(II) complex. *Free Radical Res. Commun.* 1994;20:241–9.

35. Koppenol WH. Oxyradical reactions: From bond-dissociation energies to reduction potentials. *FEBS Lett.* 1990;264:165–7.

36. Hodgson EK, Fridovich I. The accumulation of superoxide radical during the aerobic action of xanthine oxidase. A requiem for $H_2O_2^-$. *Biochem. Biophys. Acta.* 1976;430:182–8.

37. Bounds PL, Winston GW. The reaction of xanthine oxidase with aldehydic products of lipid peroxidation. *Free Radical Biol. Med.* 1991;11:447–53.

38. Wardman P. Reduction potentials of one-electron couples involving free radicals in aqueous solution. *J. Phys. Chem. Ref. Data* 1989;18:1637–755.

39. Farrington JA, Ebert M, Land EJ, Fletcher K. Bipyridylium quaternary salts and related compounds. V. Pulse radiolysis studies of the reaction of paraquat radical with oxygen. Implications for the mode of action of bipyridyl herbicides. *Biochim. Biophys. Acta.* 1990;314:372–81.

40. Patterson LK, Small RD, Scaiano JC. Reaction of paraquat radical cations with oxygen. A pulse radiolysis and laser photolysis study. *RR* 1990;72:218–25.

41. Thomas CE, Aust SD. Reductive release of iron from ferritin by cation free radicals of paraquat and other bipyridyls. *J. Biol. Chem.* 1986;261:13064–70.

42. Powis G. Free radical formation by antitumour quinones. *Free Radical Biol. Med.* 1989;6:63–101.

43. Williams MH, Yandell JK. Outer-sphere electron transfer reactions of ascorbate anions. *Aust. J. Chem.* 1982;35:1133–44.

44. Wagman DD, Evans WH, Parker VB, Schumm RH, Halow I, Bailey SM, Churney KL, Nuttal RL. Selected values for inorganic and C1 and C2 organic substances in SI units. *J. Phys. Chem. Ref. Data* 1982;11 (Suppl. 2):37–8.

45. Stanbury DM. Reduction potentials involving inorganic free radicals in aqueous solution. *Adv. Inorg. Chem.* 1989;33:69–138.
46. Koppenol WH. Generation and thermodynamic properties of oxyradicals. In: Vigo-Pelfrey C, ed. *Focus on Membrane Lipid Oxidation, Vol. I.* Boca Raton: CRC Press, 1989;1–13.
47. Koppenol WH. Thermodynamics of reactions involving nitrogen-oxygen compounds, *Meth. Enzymol.* 1996;268:7–12.
48. Seddon WA, Fletcher JW, Sopchyshyn FC. Pulse radiolysis of nitric oxide in aqueous solution. *Can. J. Chem.* 1973;51:1123–30.
49. Koppenol WH, Rush JD. The reduction potential of the couple CO_2/CO_2^-. A comparison with other C_1 radicals. *J. Phys. Chem.* 1987;91:4429–30.
50. Koppenol WH, Butler J. Energetics of interconversion reactions of oxyradicals. *Adv Free Radical Biol Med.* 1985;1:91–131.
51. Armstrong DA. Application of pulse radiolysis for the study of short-lived sulphur species. In: Asmus K-D, Chatgilialoglu C, eds. *Sulfur-Centered Reactive Intermediates in Chemistry and Biology.* New York: Plenum Press, 1990;121–33.
52. Surdhar PS, Armstrong DA. Reduction potentials and exchange reactions of thiyl radicals and disulfide anion radicals. *J. Phys. Chem.* 1987;91:6532–7.

Free Radical Toxicology
Edited by K. B. Wallace
Copyright © 1997 Taylor & Francis

2

Physical Chemical Determinants of Xenobiotic Free-Radical Generation—The Marcus Theory of Electron Transfer

Ronald P. Mason

Laboratory of Molecular Biophysics, National Institute of Environmental Health Sciences, National Institutes of Health, Research Triangle Park, NC 27709

A one-electron transfer results from an encounter between two species A (an *a*cceptor molecule) and D (a *d*onor molecule) in Equation 1. The exchange of an electron leads to the formation of two new species, $A^{\cdot-}$ and $D^{\cdot+}$.

$$A + B \xrightarrow{k_{et}} A^{-\cdot} + D^{\cdot+} \qquad [1]$$

If one of the starting components is a xenobiotic and the other is a redox enzyme, the xenobiotic's one-electron reduced or oxidized form is a free radical metabolite. For example, a neutral organic molecule (R) gives a radical anion upon one-electron reduction (Equation 2). A radical anion has the diverse reactivity of a nucleophile, a base,

$$R + e^- \rightarrow R^{\cdot-} \qquad [2]$$

and a radical and thus possesses high and non-selective reactivity toward other species. A living organism has available a host of different types of redox enzymes with standard potentials falling in a range of rather modest values from -0.42 V (versus the normal hydrogen electrode) for ferredoxin (1) to 0.94 V for compound I of peroxidase (2). Many xenobiotics are known to undergo electron transfer reactions to form free radical metabolites in a variety of biological systems (3,4).

The thermodynamics of electron-transfer reactions involving free-radical intermediates are characterized by the difference in reduction potentials between the electron donor and acceptor (Equation 1).

$$\Delta E_{et} = E(A/A^{\cdot-}) - E(D^{\cdot+}/D) \qquad [3]$$

15

$$\Delta E_{et}/V \sim 0.059 \log K_{et} \qquad [4]$$

However, only the position of equilibrium (equation 1) can be calculated from a knowledge of ΔE_{et} alone.

The rate constant k_{et} of Equation 1 can be related to the equilibrium constant K_{et} (i.e., ΔE_{et}) by the Marcus relationship (equation 5)

$$k_{et} = A \exp(-\Delta G_{et}/RT) \qquad [5]$$

where A is a collision number and ΔG_{et} is defined in its simplest form (one reactant uncharged) by:

$$\Delta G_{et} = (\lambda/4)(1 + \Delta G_{et}^0/\lambda)^2 \qquad [6]$$

where λ is a reorganization parameter for the molecules and their environment (5–7). Thus the general shape of $\log k_{et}$ versus ΔG_{et}^0 for an electron transfer reaction is a parabola. Since the ΔG_{et}^0 is defined by ΔE_{et}^0

$$\Delta G_{et}^0(\text{kJ mol}^{-1}) \sim -96.5(\Delta E_{et}^0 \ V) \qquad [7]$$

for a one-electron transfer reaction at 298 K, if the individual couples defined in equation 3 are known, then k_{et} as well as K_{et} can be predicted in principle.

One remarkable aspect of the Marcus parabola is the prediction that rate constants should decrease with increasing absolute value of ΔE_{et}^0 in both the exergonic and endergonic regions for a series of reactions with constant λ. The latter aspect that an energy requiring reaction becomes slower as ΔE_{et}^0 becomes more unfavorable is expected. However, the predicted rate decrease in the highly exergonic region is not obvious and reminds us that the Marcus electron transfer theory is quantum mechanical. Over small ranges in ΔE_{et}^0, $\log k_{et}$ will be approximately proportional to ΔE_{et}^0 as can be seen in the many examples of Eberson's highly recommended review (7).

Marcus' theory has been proposed as a sorting device for toxic compounds (7). Any xenobiotic species that possesses sufficient redox reactivity will undergo electron transfer in a rather nonselective manner to/from redox enzymes, thus creating a pathway for the generation of free radicals. These rates of formation for a vast number of xenobiotic free radical metabolites have been tabulated using a number of assumptions and guided by the experimental evidence of free radical metabolite formation (7).

To investigate a possible correlation between the one-electron reduction potentials of nitroaromatic compounds with the kinetic parameters of a nitroreductase enzyme as measured by the rate of oxygen consumption due to futile cycling, two nitroreductase enzymes were chosen for this study, ferredoxin:NADP$^+$ oxidoreductase and NADPH-cytochrome P-450 reductase (8). The former was chosen because of its potent nitroreductase activity, and the latter was chosen because it is ubiquitous in mammalian cells. K_m and V_{max} for the ferredoxin:NADP$^+$ oxidoreductase-nitroaromatic systems were determined from the rate of nitro anion-mediated oxygen consumption, taken as the initial slope, using a calibrated Clark electrode.

The enzyme kinetic parameters V_{max} and K_m were calculated utilizing the Lineweaver-Burk linearization (double-reciprocal plot) of the Michaelis-Menten equation (8). Although for nitrofurantoin there is a significant effect on the value of the K_m when catalase and superoxide dismutase are present, superoxide dismutase and catalase have little effect either on the V_{max} or K_m values of the other nitro compounds. Neither K_m, $\log K_m$, V_{max}, nor $\log V_{max}$ correlated well with the reduction potentials. On the other hand, the plot of $\log(V_{max}/K_m)$ versus the reduction potential of the nitro compound in the ferredoxin reductase system gives nearly perfect correlation (Figure 1). The V_{max}/K_m ratio is considered a measure of the enzyme-nitro substrate reactivity and of all consequent reactions that follow. In other words, the V_{max}/K_m value is a measure of the enzyme's commitment to catalyze nitro reduction. Notice that a tenth of a volt change in reduction potential causes over an order of magnitude change in V_{max}/K_m. Likewise, NADPH-cytochrome P-450 reductase gives a near perfect linear correlation of $\log V_{max}/K_m$ with the reduction potential of the nitro compound (Figure 2). The slope of the line defined by the equations in Figures 1 and 2 is analogous to the redox dependence of a simple chemical rate constant and

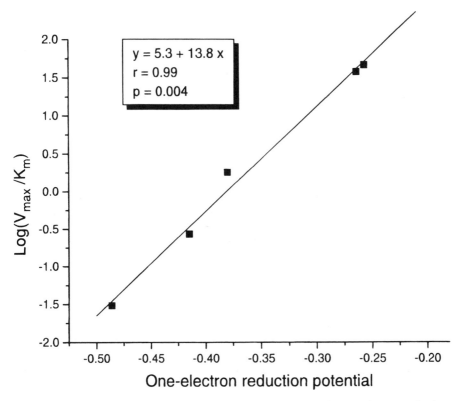

FIG. 1. Log (V_{max}/K_m) for ferredoxin:NADP$^+$ oxidoreductase versus the one-electron reduction potential of five nitro-compound substrates.

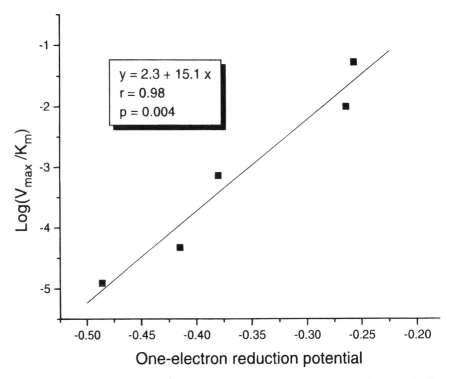

FIG. 2. Log (V_{max}/K_m) for NADPH-cytochrome P-450 reductase versus the one-electron reduction potential of five nitro-compound substrates.

can be taken as a measure of the redox dependence correlating biological reductions with ΔE_{et}^0 (9).

Clark et al. (10) studied the anaerobic reduction of 0.1 mM nitroimidazoles by xanthine-xanthine oxidase and demonstrated a linear dependence of the logarithm of the rate of anaerobic nitro reduction upon the one-electron reduction potential for 11 neutral nitroimidazoles. Initially, this result seems to be contradictory to those reported in this paper. How can the logs of the rate of reaction at a single, arbitrary substrate concentration and V_{max}/K_m both correlate with the reduction potential? The answer lies in the nature of Michaelis-Menten kinetics where if [RNO_2] $\ll K_m$, then the rate of reaction is [RNO_2] V_{max}/K_m. If the K_m values for the xanthine oxidase-catalyzed reduction of nitroimidazoles are much greater than the 0.1 mM substrate concentration used by Clark et al. (10), as they are for the nitroreductases we have studied, then a correlation will be found between the logs of the rates of reduction and reduction potential because the rates of reduction are proportional to V_{max}/K_m for all [RNO_2] $\ll K_m$. A K_m value of 3.6 mM for metronidazole reduction by hypoxanthine-xanthine oxidase is consistent with this assumption (11). Although the electron transfer theory of Marcus is the basis for our most successful correlation of V_{max}/K_m with the reduction potential of the nitro compounds, it is not obvious to us how Michaelis-Menten kinetics itself is compatible with Marcus electron transfer theory.

When asked to address this problem, Marcus wrote the following.[1] In the usual simplified reaction scheme we have

$$E_{red} + S_{ox} \xrightarrow{k_1} E_{red}S_{ox} \qquad [8]$$

$$\xleftarrow{}{k_2}$$

$$E_{red}S_{ox} \xrightarrow{k_{et}} E_{ox}S_{red} \qquad [9]$$

$$E_{ox}S_{red} \rightarrow E_{ox} + S_{red} \qquad [10]$$

where the red and ox are subscripts denoting the oxidized or reduced forms of the enzyme E and the substrate S. In this scheme k_1 and k_2 are associated with the complexing of E and S, and k_{et} is the rate constant of the elementary electron transfer step, reaction (9). When S_{ox} is a nitro compound, S_{red} is a nitro anion radical.

In a Michaelis-Menten scheme (12) for reactions 8 to 10, it is recalled that the initial reaction rate v depends on the substrate concentration S according to the equation

$$\frac{V_{max}}{v} = \frac{K_m}{S} + 1 \qquad [11]$$

where V_{max} is the limiting initial rate at high S concentrations and K_m is related to K_s, the dissociation constant for the enzyme-substrate complex $E_{red}S_{ox}$ by the relation

$$K_m = K_S + \frac{k_{et}}{k_1} \qquad [12]$$

It was pointed out (8), as is immediately seen from equation 11, that when the substrate concentration S is much less than K_m, the linear correlation of log V_{max}/K_m mentioned above is equivalent to the linear correlation observed for the logarithm of the initial rate v and the E_s^0 potential of the nitro compound S relative to the normal hydrogen electrode. In Equation 12, when $k_{et}/k_1 << 1$ we have $K_m \cong K_s$. It was noted that from the viewpoint of electron transfer reaction rate theory, the above correlation was not quite the theoretically based one (5–7), but nevertheless, a linear correlation was obtained. In the present note, we consider this aspect further, namely, what missing data are needed for a more detailed theoretical understanding and what approximations might be considered in the interim?

In the theory of electron transfer reactions, setting aside some details which are not important for the present purpose, the rate constant k_{et} of an elementary electron

---

[1] private communication

transfer step, such as reaction 9, is given upon rearrangement of Equations 5 and 6 (5, 6).

$$k_{et} = A \exp\left[-\left(\frac{\frac{1}{4}\lambda + \frac{1}{2}\Delta G_{et}^0}{4\lambda RT}\right)\right] \qquad [13]$$

Where ΔG_{et}^0 is the "standard" free energy of reaction at the typical separation distance (here the separation of E and S in the enzyme-substrate complex) and λ is a reorganization parameter, calculable if sufficient molecular structure and other data are available and obtained, otherwise, from the reaction rate data or from other sources (5,6). In particular, λ has an additivity property for each reactant that has been useful for the latter purpose. When $\Delta G_{et}^0 \ll \lambda$, equation 13 becomes

$$k_{et} \cong A \exp\left[-\left(\frac{\frac{1}{4}\lambda + \frac{1}{2}\Delta G_{et}^0}{RT}\right)\right] \qquad [14]$$

and the value of k_{et} can be obtained from the limiting rate V_{max} at high substrate concentrations (12),

$$k_{et} = V_{max}/E_{tot} \qquad [15]$$

where E_{tot} is the total concentration of E, bound to S and unbound. Thus, for a fixed concentration E_{tot}, a plot of $RT \ln V_{max}$ versus $-\Delta G_{et}^0$ would, on the basis of equation 14, be linear with a slope of $\frac{1}{2}$. We shall also need to consider in the analysis a quantity typically not measured, the equilibrium constant K_S^p, for the dissociation of the enzyme-substrate complex of the products of reaction 9:

$$E_{ox}S_{red} \rightleftarrows E_{ox} + S_{red}, \quad K_S^p \qquad [16]$$

The standard reduction potential of the enzyme relative to the normal hydrogen electrode is denoted by E_E^0. Some caution is needed here, since there can be more than one step, and since pH effects may also play a role. For the moment, we consider the simple case that E_{red} is a single species, and that the E-S separation distance is not part of the reaction coordinate in the transition state of reaction 9 (cf discussion later). The ΔG_{et}^0 in equation 13 is then given by

$$\Delta G_{et}^0 = -nF(E_S^0 - E_E^0) - RT \ln(K_S/K_S^p) \qquad [17]$$

where n is the number of electrons transferred in reaction 9 (one in the present instance) and F is the Faraday. The E_S^0 in Equation 17 is the one-electron reduction potential for the unprotonated nitro compound.

Experimentally, the K_m for the various nitro compounds studied by Orna and Mason (8) varied by about a factor of 200 for the ferrodoxin: NADP$^+$ oxidoreductase and by a factor of about 800 for the NADPH-cytochrome P-450 reductase. The V_{max}'s values varied by much smaller factors (10 and 30, respectively). Thus, in interpreting the V_{max}'s using equations 13 [or 14] and 15, the K_m and K_m^p can play a significant role.

From Equations 14 and 17 we have

$$\ln k_{et} \cong \frac{1}{2} \frac{E_S^0}{RT} + \frac{1}{2} \ln \frac{K_S}{K_S^p} + C \qquad [18]$$

where

$$C = \ln A - \frac{\lambda}{4RT} - \frac{1}{2} \frac{E_E^0}{RT} \qquad [19]$$

Even if K_S in Eq. 18 is approximated by K_m, the K_s and K_s^p are still needed, but the information on them appears to be absent.

One limiting situation exists, e.g., $K_s \gg K_m^p$, in which case Equations 15 and 18 would yield a linear plot of log V_{max} vs. E_s°, with a slope of $0.5/0.059 = 8.5$ at $25°C$.

Equation 17 for ΔG_{et}^0 presumes that the "binding coordinate" (the E-S separation distance) is not part of the reaction coordinate in the transition state of reaction 9. If, however, the change in E-S binding, and hence in K_m/K_m^p, were mainly due to one of the attractive terms for $E_{red}S_{ox}$ being replaced by a repulsive one for $E_{ox}S_{red}$, Equation 17 would have to be modified. One derivation, described elsewhere in a somewhat different context (the half-reaction being $e^- + RCl \rightarrow R^. + Cl^-$) yielded an expression in which the equivalent of the K_m^p term in Equation 17 has disappeared. In that reaction, the original attractive (bonding) interaction is replaced by the nonbonding (repulsive) interaction of the $(R^., Cl^-)$ pair. What is particularly needed, therefore, in the present case is a detailed understanding of the difference in bonding of E_{red} to RNO_2 and of E_{ox} to RNO_2^- and, in particular, of the origin of the relationship between K_m and E_S^0. If possible, an *in situ* determination of E_S^0 in the Michaelis enzyme-substrate ES compared with the E_S^0 in solution, would provide some insight.

Independently, O'Connor et al. (13) examined the effect of reduction potential on the rate of reduction of a series of nitro acridines by xanthine oxidase using Marcus electron-transfer theory. They have also chosen to plot $\log V_{max}/K_m$ versus the reduction potentials of their nitro compounds and have reported a correlation coefficient of $r = 0.800$ (Figure 3). They, like we, found that a plot of $\log V_{max}$ versus E_S^0 was fit more poorly by a straight line. In this case, K_m varied by a factor of 38 and V_{max} by a factor of 69.

More recently, the rates of reduction of 27 compounds (mainly nitro and quinone compounds) at 50 μM substrate concentration were found to be linearly correlated with their one-electron reduction potentials (14). It was stated that Marcus's theory will apply in the presence of Michaelis-Menten kinetics if there is a very weak association within the [ES] complex such that it readily dissociates back to [E] and [S], and/or the [ES] complex rapidly undergoes electron transfer and dissociates to the products. The first assumption is that $k_2 \gg k_1$ and the second is that k_{et} is large.

$$K_m = \frac{k_2 + k_{et}}{k_1}$$

This assumption is equivalent to assuming that $K_m = \infty$, i.e., that the reaction never

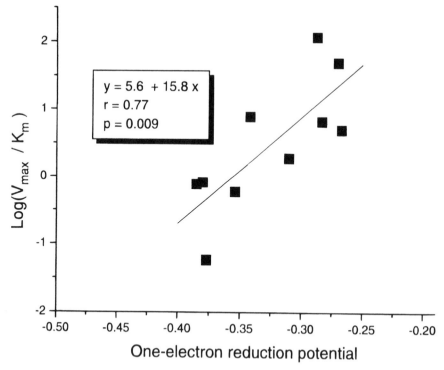

FIG. 3. Log (V_{max}/K_m) for xanthine oxidase versus the one-electron reduction potential of 10 nitroacridine substrates (data taken from reference 13).

saturates as the substrate concentration is increased. Therefore, these assumptions are incompatible with the observations of Michaelis-Menten kinetics.

Although the exact relationship of the linear correlation of $\log V_{max}/K_m$ with the substrate reduction potential to Marcus' theory remains unclear, ultimately the existence of such a correlation is what matters in the metabolic-dependent toxicity of redox active compounds. All of these studies support the proposal of a rate-determining single-electron transfer as the initial step in the reduction of nitro and quinone compounds by flavoenzymes. Wardman and Clarke (9) have summarized some of the numerous redox correlations for nitro compounds. Considering the diversity of these studies, the close quantitative agreement with redox dependencies around $10V^{-1}$ are striking. This coefficient defines an order of magnitude decrease in the concentration required to achieve a fixed response for an increase in the one-electron reduction potential of 0.1 V. Note that cytotoxicity or mutagenicity (Table 1) and the rate of reduction of nitro aromatic compounds (Table 2) have similar redox dependencies. With this in mind, it is not surprising that metronidazole, with the lowest reduction potential of any nitro drug, is also the safest nitro drug.

The traditional mechanism for cytotoxicity, mutagenicity, etc., of nitro compounds

TABLE 1. *Cytotoxicity and mutagenicity redox dependence of nitroaromatic compounds*

Toxicity	Redox dependence[a]
Cytotoxicity	
Bacteria	11.5
Anaerobic mammalian cells	10.1
Aerobic mammalian cells	8.7
Mutagenicity	
Aerobic bacteria	11.2
Aerobic mammalian cells	7.4
DNA synthesis	12.5
DNA strand breakage	9.8
DNA, release of dT	11

Note. Data taken from Wardman and Clarke (9).
[a] Mean of one to three studies.

TABLE 2. *Redox dependence of nitro aromatic compounds upon reduction by a variety of systems*

Reduction by	Redox dependence (V^{-1})[a]
Aerobic bacteria	8.2[b]
Anaerobic mammalian cells	10.7[b]
Anaerobic microsomes	10.5[b]
Reduced flavin mononucleotide	18.4[b]
Xanthine/xanthine oxidase	13.8[b], 15.8[c]
Ferredoxin:NADP$^+$ oxidoreductase	13.8[d]
NADPH-cytochrome P-450 reductase	15.1[d]

[a] $d(\log k)/d(\Delta E)$.
[b] Data taken from Wardman and Clarke (9).
[c] Data taken from O'Connor et al. (13).
[d] Data taken from Mason (15).

is that a reduction product such as the nitroso (the 2-electron reduction product) or hydroxylamine (the 4-electron reduction product) binds to DNA and/or proteins and leads ultimately to the biological response. Clearly, nitro anion formation is rate-limiting in the production of these damaging products, whatever they may be.

Under most aerobic conditions, futile metabolism of nitro compounds leads to the formation of superoxide instead of xenobiotic-derived products. Several investigations of this catalytic superoxide formation have shown that metabolite radical anion formation is also rate-determining for superoxide generation. The relative importance of superoxide and reactive metabolites of the redox-active compounds to toxicity depends on the specifics of each case, but clearly the one-electron reduction potential of these compounds is the primary determinant of toxicity.

REFERENCES

1. Aliverti, A, Hagen WR, Zanetti G. Direct electrochemistry and EPR spectroscopy of spinach ferredoxin mutants with modified electron transfer properties. *FEBS Letters* 1995;368:220–224.

2. Hayashi Y, Yamazaki I. The oxidation-reduction potentials of compound I/compound II and compound II/ferric couples of horseradish peroxidases A$_2$ and C. *J Biol Chem* 1979;254:9101–9106.
3. Mason RP. Free-radical intermediates in the metabolism of toxic chemicals. In: Pryor WA, ed. *Free Radicals in Biology, Vol. V.* New York: Academic Press, 1982;161–222.
4. Mason RP, Chignell CF. Free radicals in pharmacology and toxicology-selected topics. *Pharmacol Reviews.* 1982;33:189–211.
5. Marcus RA. Chemical and electrochemical electron-transfer theory. *Annu Rev Phys Chem* 1964;15:155–196.
6. Marcus RA, Sutin N. Electron transfers in chemistry and biology. *Biochim Biophys Acta* 1985;811:265–322.
7. Eberson L. The Marcus theory of electron transfer, a sorting device for toxic compounds. *Adv Free Radical Biol Med* 1985;1:19–90.
8. Orna MV, Mason RP. Correlation of kinetic parameters of nitroreductase enzymes with redox properties of nitroaromatic compounds. *J Biol Chem* 1989;264:12379–12384.
9. Wardman P, Clarke ED. Electron transfer and radical-addition in the radiosensitization and chemotherapy of hypoxic cells. In: Breccia A, Fowler JF, eds. *New Chemo and Radiosensitizing Drugs.* Bologna: Lo Scarabeo, 1985;21–38.
10. Clark ED, Goulding KH, Wardman P. Nitroimidazoles as anaerobic electron acceptors for xanthine oxidase. *Biochem Pharmacol* 1982;31:3237–3242.
11. Chrystal EJT, Koch RL, Goldman P. Metabolites from the reduction of metronidazole by xanthine oxidase. *Mol Pharmacol* 1980;18:105–111.
12. Lehninger AL. *Biochemistry* 2nd ed. New York: Worth Publishers, 1975.
13. O'Connor CJ, McLennan DJ, Sutton BM, Denny WA, Wilson, WR. Effect of reduction potential on the rate of reduction of nitroacridines by xanthine oxidase and by dihydroflavin mononucleotide. *J Chem Soc Perkin Trans 2* 1991;7:951–954.
14. Butler J, Hoey BM. The one-electron reduction potential of several substrates can be related to their reduction rates by cytochrome P-450 reductase. *Biochim Biophys Acta* 1993;1161:73–78.
15. Mason RP. Redox cycling of radical anion metabolites of toxic chemicals and drugs and the Marcus Theory of electron transfer. *Environ Health Perspect* 1990;87:237–243.

Free Radical Toxicology
Edited by K. B. Wallace
Copyright © 1997 Taylor & Francis

3

Subcellular Sites of Xenobiotic-Induced Free-Radical Generation

Charles R. Myers

*Department of Pharmacology and Toxicology, Medical College of Wisconsin,
Milwaukee, Wisconsin, USA*

A free radical may be broadly defined as any compound with one or more unpaired electrons; as such, free radicals are generally highly reactive. Because of their high degree of reactivity, it seems unlikely that many free radicals, or related active species, could travel long distances from their site of generation. Hence, in many instances, the site of their generation may also be the site where cellular damage is initiated. Therefore, knowledge of the subcellular site(s) of free-radical generation is fundamental to understanding the toxicity of a given radical species.

Some free radicals are generated by normal essential biologic processes. Examples include O_2-linked mitochondrial electron transport, the actions of lipoxygenase and cyclooxygenase in eicosanoid metabolism, the response of macrophages (phagocytes) against invading microorganisms, and the production of certain regulatory chemicals (e.g., nitric oxide). However, these sources are not emphasized here, except where they are known to be influenced by xenobiotics. Instead, this chapter emphasizes those free radicals that are generated as a result of exposure to xenobiotic compounds.

More specifically, the focus of this chapter is on the subcellular sites of free-radical generation, and the implications of these sites for potential toxic effects. Space limitations prevent a comprehensive treatise, and in some cases reviews are cited rather than original manuscripts. Hence, there are many worthwhile contributions that cannot be discussed or cited. Instead, representative examples are used to illustrate the major points. The enzymes or cellular chemicals responsible for generating free radicals at each subcellular site are briefly presented to clarify why and/or how a radical is generated at a certain site. The details of the mechanisms of free-radical generation, as well as a discussion of their potential toxicities, are left to other chapters in this book.

SUBCELLULAR SITES OF FREE-RADICAL GENERATION

Endoplasmic Reticulum

The endoplasmic reticulum contains numerous proteins that are involved in the metabolism of literally hundreds of foreign compounds. Relevant proteins include cytochromes P-450, NADPH:cytochrome P-450 reductase, cytochrome b_5, NADH:cytochrome b_5 reductase, flavin-containing monooxygenases (FMOs), and others. While the normal role of this microsomal mixed-function oxidase system is to detoxify various compounds, this system can activate some compounds to toxic species, some of which are free radicals. Because of the propensity of microsomal enzymes to interact with a wide variety of functional groups, it is not surprising that these enzymes can generate free radicals from a variety of compounds. Due to space limitations, only limited examples are cited.

NADPH:Cytochrome P-450 Reductase

The normal role of NADPH:cytochrome P-450 reductase, a microsomal flavoenzyme, is to transfer electrons from NADPH to the cytochromes P-450. It is well known, however, that this enzyme can also directly transfer electrons to a wide variety of xenobiotic compounds. Most frequently, this is a one-electron transfer in which the parent compound is reduced to a free radical. Some resulting free radicals can then donate their unpaired electron to O_2, generating superoxide (O_2^-), and regenerating the parent compound. This process, termed "redox cycling (Figure 1), is an example of indirect radical formation; that is, the free-radical product (O_2^-) is generated through the chemical reduction of O_2 by the parent compound radical. Because the parent compound is recycled, a small amount of parent can lead to the generation of a large amount of O_2^- (1). Via the Haber-Weiss reaction, hydroxyl radical ($\cdot$OH) could be generated from the resulting O_2^-.

Redox cycling is also associated with other reducing systems in the cell (2,3), which will be discussed below. However, P-450 reductase has a propensity to transfer electrons to a wide variety of compounds, and is therefore frequently associated with redox cycling. Some examples of compounds that are redox cycled via P-450 reductase include paraquat (4,5), diquat (4), menadione (5,6,7), duraquinone (7), aminochrome (8), nitrazepam (5), nitrofurantoin (6,7), nilutamide (9), alloxan (10), doxorubicin (adriamycin) (11,12), mitomycin C (13), benzo[a]pyrene diones (7), nitro-group-containing organics (e.g., nitrobenzene) (14), and naphthoquinone metabolites of 1-naphthol (15). While P-450 reductase-mediated redox cycling often occurs in the immediate vicinity of the microsomes, this is not always the case, particularly if the parent free radical is not highly reactive. For example, paraquat free radical is sufficiently stable so that some of it diffuses outside the cell before it reacts with O_2 to generate O_2^- (5).

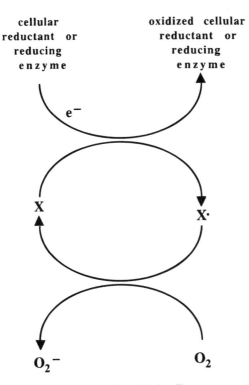

FIG. 1. Generic schematic of redox cycling of xenobiotics. The parent xenobiotic (X) accepts an electron and is thereby reduced to a radical species (X·). The free radical then donates an electron to O_2, generating superoxide (O_2^-) and regenerating the parent xenobiotic. Possible cellular reductants or reducing enzymes include ascorbate, GSH, NAD(P)H, NADPH:cytochrome P-450 reductase, glutathione reductase, cytochrome P-450, NADH:cytochrome b_5 reductase, mitochondrial NADH dehydrogenase, xanthine oxidase, peroxidase, ascorbate oxidase, prostaglandin endoperoxide synthetase, and nuclear NADPH:cytochrome P-450 reductase (2, 3).

It must be emphasized that, in addition to redox cycling, there are other potential fates for many of these free radicals (3): (a) they may abstract a hydrogen from a cellular molecule, thereby generating a cellular-derived radical; (b) they may covalently bind to cell components by radical addition; or (c) they may react with a cellular antioxidant (e.g., ascorbate, glutathione). For example, P-450 reductase mediates the reduction of nilutamide to a nitro anion free radical (9). While this free radical is redox cycled in the presence of O_2, it covalently binds to microsomal proteins in the absence of O_2 (9). Similarly, P-450 reductase reduces tirapazamine to a nitroxide free radical, which can directly damage DNA (16). It should also be emphasized that not all free radicals generated by P-450 reductase are capable of redox cycling. For instance, the main fate of phenyl radicals derived from the P-450 reductase-mediated reduction of iodonium diphenyl is to covalently bind to, and irreversibly inactivate, the P-450 reductase itself (17).

28   *FREE RADICAL TOXICOLOGY*

Cytochromes P-450

Many of the isozymes of the cytochrome P-450 superfamily are able to generate free radicals by various means. Even in the absence of inducers, xenobiotic substrates, or low-molecular-weight iron compounds, some P-450 isozymes are likely to generate reactive oxygen species (18), including O_2^- and hydrogen peroxide (H_2O_2) (19). The O_2^- is likely produced from the breakdown of the oxycytochrome P-450 complex, and the H_2O_2 from dismutation of O_2^- and decay of peroxygenated cytochrome P-450 complex (15,19,20,21). If ferric chelates are present, $\cdot$OH radicals are also formed (19). This shunting of electrons from P-450 to O_2, forming O_2^-, is referred to as "uncoupling" (14). Of the cytochrome P-450 isozymes examined to date, P-450s 2B and 2E1 exhibit the highest rates of uncoupling (14). The basal rate of uncoupling can be significantly enhanced by several xenobiotics, including pseudo-substrates (e.g., 1,1,1-trichloroethane, perfluoro-n-hexane), P-450 "uncouplers" (e.g., hexobarbital, benzphetamine, barbiturates), and the alkylating agent 2-bromo-4'-nitroacetophenone (14).

This P-450-associated rate of oxygen radical production can also be significantly increased by compounds that act to induce the expression of the P-450 isozymes. For example, P-450 2E1, which is highly induced by ethanol, appears to mediate significant production of oxygen radicals (22); chronic ethanol consumption therefore enhances the ability of microsomes to produce O_2^- and $\cdot$OH radicals (22). The resulting $\cdot$OH radicals could act to oxidize ethanol to 1-hydroxyethyl radicals (22). An even more significant source of ethanol radicals is probably via P-4502E1 (and other P-450 isozymes), involving perferryl iron complexes of the P-450 heme iron (22).

Cytochromes P-450 can also mediate the production of radicals from a variety of xenobiotics. For example, P-450s can activate methoxychlor to free-radical species that covalently bind to microsomal proteins, including the P-450s themselves (23). Various hydrazines are oxidized by cytochrome P-450 to yield reactive oxygen species and organic free radicals (24–26).

Cytochromes P-450 can also reductively metabolize a variety of xenobiotics to free radicals, especially under low O_2 tensions (14). One of the best-characterized examples is the P-450-mediated generation of trichloromethyl radical ($\cdot CCl_3$) from carbon tetrachloride (27); this highly reactive $\cdot CCl_3$ radical appears to damage the P-450, either by direct attack or by causing microsomal lipid peroxidation (27). The general anesthetic halothane can undergo both reductive and oxidative activation (14), and gentian violet and benzidines can be reduced to carbon-centered radicals (28). P-450s may also mediate free-radical production via reduction of certain metals (e.g., hexavalent chromium) (14,29–31) and azo dyes (e.g., dimethylaminoazobenzene) (14). Some of these P-450-mediated reductions may result in free radicals that can undergo redox cycling, including doxorubicin (11,14), mitomycin C (14), and some nitro-containing compounds (14).

Both cytochromes P-450 and NADPH:cytochrome P-450 reductase can also contribute to ADP-Fe^{3+}-linked lipid peroxidation (32). These enzymes can reduce ADP-

Fe^{3+} to ADP-Fe^{2+}, to which O_2 adds to form ADP-Fe^{3+}-O_2^-; ADP-Fe^{3+}-O_2^- can abstract a hydrogen from lipid, starting lipid peroxidation (32).

Other Microsomal Enzymes

While studies to date are limited, other microsomal enzymes can also mediate free-radical generation from various xenobiotics. For example, NADH:cytochrome b_5 reductase can reduce both mitomycin C and doxorubicin to their semiquinone free radicals, which are capable of redox cycling (14,33). Unidentified NADH-dependent microsomal enzymes can mediate the reduction of vanadium(V) to vanadium(IV), resulting in generation of ·OH radicals from O_2^- and H_2O_2 (34). Similarly, unidentified NADPH-dependent microsomal flavoenzymes can mediate the reduction of chromium(VI) to reactive forms (35).

Microsomal prostaglandin H synthase can generate radicals either by direct oxidation of xenobiotics, or indirectly by the generation of peroxyl radicals (36,37). For example, the peroxidase activity of prostaglandin H synthase couples the reduction of peroxides (e.g., H_2O_2, t-butyl hydroperoxide, 15-hydroperoxy-5,8,11,13-eicosatetraenoic acid) to the oxidation of aminopyrine, forming aminopyrine free radicals (36). Glutathione (GSH) can react with the aminopyrine radicals, generating thiyl radicals and regenerating aminopyrine (36). While this is not classical redox cycling, the concept is analogous in that the cycling of a small amount of aminopyrine can result in the consumption of large amounts of GSH. Similarly, benzidines can be oxidized to cation free-radical species by peroxidases, including microsomal prostaglandin synthase (38–41).

Endoplasmic Reticulum Overview

Overall, many enzymes of the endoplasmic reticulum can mediate the production of free radicals from a variety of xenobiotics. NADPH:cytochrome P-450 reductase, NADH:cytochrome b_5 reductase, and cytochromes P-450 can all mediate the one-electron reduction of various compounds to free radicals, some of which undergo redox cycling. Cytochromes P-450 can also generate radicals via oxidation of some xenobiotics, as can prostaglandin H synthase. In addition, several xenobiotics can enhance the generation of reactive oxygen species by some P-450 isozymes, either by enhancing the uncoupling process itself, or by inducing the expression of isoforms that exhibit high rates of uncoupling.

The levels of these enzymes can vary significantly from one tissue to another, and even within different cell populations in a given tissue, so their contribution to free-radical generation will likely vary considerably among various cell types. For example, cytochromes P-450 are apt to contribute more significantly to the generation of free radicals in hepatic cells than in other tissues with lower P-450 contents. Within human lung, NADPH:cytochrome P-450 reductase is localized most prominently in the bronchiolar epithelial cells (42), so these cells could possibly exhibit greater

P-450 reductase-mediated free-radical production than other lung cell types. Curiously, in both human lung and pancreas, the cellular P-450 reductase levels are by far the greatest in those cell types most commonly associated with tumor formation (42).

Mitochondria

Mitochondria are the sites of oxidative phosphorylation in cells. This process involves an electron transport chain comprised of numerous redox-active components (dehydrogenases, iron-sulfur proteins, quinones, cytochromes, etc.). Certain free radicals (e.g., O_2^-) are produced as minor products of normal mitochondrial electron transport (1). The most probable sources are NADH dehydrogenase and reduced ubisemiquinone radical (hydroquinone), the latter of which reacts with O_2 to form O_2^- (1). Acute ethanol exposure is associated with significant increases in liver mitochondrial O_2^- generation (22). One explanation for this is that the increased levels of NADH associated with the oxidation of ethanol by alcohol dehydrogenase would increase electron flow in the mitochondrial respiratory electron transport chain (22); this increase could be the cause of lipid peroxidative damage to mitochondria associated with acute ethanol exposure (22). In other instances, a partial inhibition of mitochondrial electron transport can lead to an increase in oxygen radical generation (43), probably because the electron transport chain cannot proceed to completion at a normal rate.

Redox cycling of certain xenobiotics, analogous to that just described, is also associated with mitochondria. For example, mitochondrial NADH dehydrogenase can mediate the redox cycling of doxorubicin (1,44), leading to the production of reactive oxygen species.

Mitochondria can also generate free radicals from organic peroxides. The addition of t-butyl hydroperoxide to nonrespiring mitochondria is associated with the production of methyl, alkoxyl, and peroxyl radicals, whereas respiring mitochondria generate mainly methyl radicals (45). One possible mechanism invokes a role for certain transition metals, such as copper (Cu) or iron (Fe). For example, mitochondrial electron transport complexes can reduce mitochondrial membrane-bound Cu^{2+} to Cu^+ (46). The resulting Cu^+ can then cleave the peroxide bond of organic peroxides (e.g., t-butyl hydroperoxide) to form both alkoxyl and methyl radicals (46). It is plausible that mitochondria could similarly generate radical species from lipid hydroperoxides (45); that is, mitochondria could generate new radical species from lipids damaged from previous free-radical exposure.

Mitochondria can also generate radicals through mechanisms other than their respiratory electron transport system. For example, monoamine oxidase (a flavoprotein located in the mitochondrial fraction of liver, brain, and kidney) can activate 1-methyl-4-phenyl-1,2,3,6-tetrahydropyridine (MPTP, a toxin causing neurological damage that closely resembles Parkinson's disease) to toxic pyridinium metabolites that stimulate dopamine efflux (47,48). The released dopamine is subject to iron-catalyzed autoxidation in the basal ganglia where dopamine and iron levels are high;

the net result is ·OH radical formation (47,48). In this instance, the mitochondria do not directly generate the radicals, but they are indirectly responsible for the dopamine release via the production of the pyridinium metabolites.

To summarize, mitochondria are capable of generating free radicals by various mechanisms. The generation of O_2^- during normal mitochondrial electron transport has received the most attention, and there are several xenobiotics that can enhance O_2^- generation by mitochondria. Mitochondria can also generate free radicals, either directly or indirectly, through metabolism of some foreign compounds, and some of the resulting radicals may undergo redox cycling. In addition, mitochondria have the capability of reducing certain transition metals to oxidation states that can catalyze the formation of radicals from various organic and lipid peroxides. Given the ubiquitous nature of mitochondria in various cell types, it seems likely that mitochondria could contribute to total free-radical production in essentially all cells.

Radicals That Can be Generated at Multiple Cell Sites

The production of free radicals can also be mediated by components that are widely distributed in cells. In some instances, these components are cytoplasmic. In other instances, they are associated with various membrane systems found throughout the cell, including nuclear, endoplasmic reticular, cellular, and mitochondrial membranes.

Nonenzymatic Reductants

Radicals can be generated by the reaction of xenobiotics with various cellular chemicals that are widely distributed throughout the cell, including NAD(P)H, GSH, cysteine, ascorbate, and hemoglobin. The latter is, of course, restricted to erythrocytes, whereas the others are essentially ubiquitous. For example, many nitroso compounds are reduced nonenzymatically to free-radical derivatives by NAD(P)H, GSH, cysteine, or hemoglobin (49,50).

In some instances, these nonenzymatic cellular reductants can mediate redox cycling of certain xenobiotics. An example is the reaction of NAD(P)H with nitrosobenzene and 2-nitrosotoluene to form phenylhydronitroxide and 2-methylphenylhydronitroxide free radicals, respectively (51). These nitroso free radicals can react with O_2 to form O_2^- (51). In addition to NAD(P)H, other cellular reductants (e.g., ascorbate, GSH) can also mediate redox cycling (2).

In addition to redox cycling, these same cellular reductants can mediate the formation of other types of radicals from a variety of organic xenobiotics. Sulfur-containing radicals, which are capable of inducing lipid peroxidation and DNA strand breaks, are generated by the reaction of nitrogen dioxide with cysteine or GSH (52,53). Similarly, both NADH and ascorbate can chemically reduce arene diazonium compounds, resulting in the formation of aryl radicals, which are known to damage DNA (54). The reaction of mucochloric acid with GSH can generate mutagenic mucochloric acid radicals (55), and ascorbate can mediate the formation of ethoxy radicals in the presence of ethanol (22,56). Cytosolic reductants can also mediate the formation of free radicals from various metals. The reaction of Cr(VI) with ascorbate generates carbon-based and ascorbyl radicals (57), which can directly damage DNA (58). Ascorbate, cysteine, and GSH can all reduce Cr(VI) to Cr(V) and/or Cr(IV) (58–62), and ascorbate can reduce vanadium(V) to V(IV) (63). These reduced metal species are highly reactive and can lead to the generation of other radicals. For example, V(IV) can mediate the formation of carboxylate radicals from small organics, and V(IV), Cr(V), and Cr(III) can all mediate the formation of lipid hydroperoxide-derived free radicals (62–64). Similarly, in the presence of H_2O_2, V(IV), Cr(V), and Cr(IV) can all mediate the production of ·OH radicals via Fenton-like reactions (58–63). In the presence of Fe and Cu ions, ascorbate can mediate the generation of cytotoxic oxygen radicals (65).

Thiyl radicals are also formed as a result of the reduction of Cr(VI) by cysteine or GSH (60,62,66). The reaction of selenite and selenocystine with GSH generates O_2^- and H_2O_2 (67). Other potentially carcinogenic metals, including nickel(II) and cobalt(II), can also generate DNA-damaging reactive oxygen species from H_2O_2 (68). Furthermore, in the presence of natural peptides (e.g., GSH, carnosine, homocarnosine, anserine, glycylglycylhistidine), nickel(II) interacts with lipid hydroperoxides to form peroxyl, alkoxyl, and alkyl radicals (69).

Nonenzymatic Autoxidation Reactions

Autoxidation reactions, which represent potentially significant sources of reactive oxygen species, can occur throughout the cell. Autoxidation involves the transfer of an electron from some chemical to O_2. For example, 6-aminodopamine and 6-hydroxydopamine autoxidize to form their respective semiquinone or semiquinone-imine free radicals, resulting in the generation of O_2^- from O_2 (70). Other examples of autoxidations include the oxidation of reduced flavins to form melanin plus O_2^-, and the oxidation of tetrahydropterin to form dihydropterin plus O_2^- (1). In many cases, autoxidations are associated with trace amounts of metals such as Fe and Cu, and in many cases the parent compound is regenerated by reducing agents (e.g., ascorbate) in a nonenzymatic redox cycle (3). Cu(II) and Fe(III) bound to cell components can be reduced to Cu(I) and Fe(II) by reductants (e.g., ascorbate, GSH, O_2^-), and these reduced metals can mediate free-radical formation, including the generation of ·OH radicals from O_2^- and H_2O_2 (1,71), and the generation of lipid hydroperoxide-derived free radicals from lipid hydroperoxides (72,73). Since the solubility of Cu and Fe are quite low, the Cu and Fe participating in these reactions are often complexed to cell components that can thus serve as centers for free-radical production (71). For example, Cu can form complexes with proteins, and Fe with nucleotide di- and triphosphates. Both Cu and Fe can complex to DNA, either at the phosphate backbone or at the purine/pyrimidine bases (71). Hence, such complexes may be widely distributed in many cells. A bound metal can undergo multiple cycles of reduction and reoxidation, generating a high concentration of ·OH radicals in a fixed locus (71,74). This could serve to concentrate free-radical damage, which would likely include damage to the metal-complexing species itself (71). Some organics can indirectly enhance the production of free radicals by these metal-associated processes. As an example, ethanol can cause a significant increase in non-heme Fe levels throughout the cell (mitochondrial, microsomal, and cytosolic fractions), which would be expected to enhance Fe-related free-radical generation (22). Several xenobiotics (e.g., paraquat, diquat, nitrofurantoin, doxorubicin) facilitate the release of Fe from ferritin (75), and may therefore represent another way in which some xenobiotics facilitate free-radical generation.

Cytoplasmic Enzymes

Several cytoplasmic enzymes have been implicated in free-radical generation. One of the most thoroughly studied is xanthine oxidase, which is primarily a cytosolic enzyme that normally behaves as a dehydrogenase (1). Xanthine oxidase catalyzes the conversion of hypoxanthine to xanthine to uric acid, during which O_2^- is produced (1,76). Xanthine oxidase can also directly generate ·OH radicals via reduction of H_2O_2 (77). While this process does not directly involve xenobiotics, the conversion to its oxidase function can be precipitated by oxidative stress as a result of xenobiotic-mediated generation of oxygen radicals by other processes or at other sites (1). Furthermore, acute ethanol exposure also favors the conversion of xanthine dehydrogenase to xanthine oxidase, possibly because of the increased NADH levels associated with the activity of alcohol dehydrogenase (22). Xanthine oxidase, therefore, represents an example where xenobiotics can induce free-radical generation via conversion of an enzyme to an alternate function. In addition, xanthine oxidase can directly mediate free-radical formation from some xenobiotics. For example, xanthine oxidase is capable of reducing nitro compounds (14), mitomycin C (13,14), and doxorubicin (14) to free radicals that are capable of redox cycling to generate O_2^-. Xanthine oxidase can also reduce iodonium diphenyl to phenyl radicals, which attack and irreversibly inhibit xanthine oxidase itself (17).

Aldehyde oxidase has also been associated with radical production (1). This enzyme oxidizes a wide variety of aldehydes, during which O_2^- can be produced as a by-product. There is also evidence that ethanol administration can further increase radical production by aldehyde oxidase (22). Aldehyde oxidase is also capable of reducing various xenobiotics, including azo dyes and nitro compounds (14), to free-radical species, some of which may redox cycle.

Similarly, DT-diaphorase (NADPH:quinone oxidoreductase) is also able to reduce azo dyes and nitro compounds to free-radical species capable of redox cycling (14). DT-diaphorase can also indirectly mediate free-radical production through two-electron reduction of quinones. As an example, DT-diaphorase catalyzes the two-electron reduction of 2-methyl-1,4-naphthoquinone (menadione), forming the hydroquinone product menadiol (5,78). Menadiol is slowly autoxidized to a semiquinone with the concomitant generation of O_2^- (5,78). This leads to chain propagation reactions that generate additional O_2^- (78). Ascorbate increases the rate of this redox cycling and hence the generation of free radicals, either by directly reducing the quinone or by reducing Fe(III) to enhance the autoxidation of menadiol (78).

The cytosolic enzyme glutathione reductase can also reduce certain compounds (e.g., diquat) to free radicals capable of redox cycling (2,79). The reduction of Cr(VI) to Cr(V) by glutathione reductase results in the production of ·OH radicals, probably via a Cr(V)-mediated Fenton-like reaction (80).

Soluble Factor Overview

There are many cytosolic components that have the capability of generating free radicals, including common cellular reductants (e.g., NAD(P)H, GSH, cysteine, ascorbate) and certain enzymes (xanthine oxidase, aldehyde oxidase, glutathione reductase). The number of potential xenobiotic substrates is large, both because there are so many cell components in this group, and because some of them (e.g., GSH, ascorbate) can react with a wide variety of functional groups. In many cases, the activation process is reductive in nature, with some of the free-radical products able to undergo redox cycling. In other cases, the radical products are highly reactive and therefore capable of causing damage to DNA, lipids, and other cell components. Some of these cytosolic components can also reduce certain metals to forms that catalyze various autoxidation reactions. For some of these cytosolic enzymes, xenobiotics may enhance their ability to generate reactive oxygen species, and, in the case of xanthine oxidase, the xenobiotics can induce the conversion of the enzyme to a form capable of free-radical generation.

IMPLICATIONS OF THE SITE OF RADICAL GENERATION FOR THE SITE OF DAMAGE

Given the high degree of reactivity of many radicals, many cell components are potential targets for free-radical attack. For the purposes of toxicity, key cellular targets could include DNA, lipids, and proteins. For chemical carcinogenesis, the key molecular event is likely to be the interaction of the chemical agent with DNA (81,82). Regardless of the mechanism of free-radical production, many chemicals associated with free-radical production are important in neoplastic transformation (81). In support of this, many chemical carcinogens are known to be metabolized via free-radical intermediates, and substances that inhibit free-radical production can inhibit the carcinogenic potential of many chemical carcinogens (81). There are several ways in which free radicals can negatively impact a key target such as DNA: (a) the free radical itself can directly attack the target, (b) the original free radical may lead to the production of other radicals that attack the target, (c) the free radical can activate a procarcinogen, or (d) following binding of the radical to the target, the adduct itself generates additional radicals in the immediate proximity of the target (81,83–85). Examples of the first three possibilities were presented earlier. An illustration of the last possibility is the association of cigarette tar species with DNA, which can be followed by the production of ·OH radical at that site (86); this process is referred to as site-specific damage to DNA (85).

To fully understand free-radical damage to key cellular targets (e.g., DNA, lipids), one must consider at least three relevant questions regarding the site of radical generation (81):

1. Are short-lived radicals generated close enough to the target so that damage to the target is likely?
2. Are normal cellular defense mechanisms (e.g., superoxide dismutase, catalase, peroxidase, β-carotene, α-tocopherol, ascorbic acid, GSH) at the site of radical generation sufficient to quench the radicals before the target is damaged?
3. How does the heterogeneous chemical nature of the cell affect free-radical production and damage at various cell sites?

While these questions can be posed individually, in some instances the issues are too interdependent to allow for separate consideration.

Free-Radical Reactivity and Proximity to Target

It seems unlikely that a short-lived free-radical or related active species could travel long distances from its site of generation (81). Hence, regarding the first question just given, the more reactive the radical, the closer the target must be to its site of generation for target damage to occur. This is because as the distance between the site of generation and the target increases, so does the likelihood that the radical will react with something else before it encounters the target. Perhaps the most extreme example of this is the ·OH radical, which is so reactive that it migrates less than 10 molecular diameters before it reacts (87). Direct damage is therefore likely to be very close to its site of generation. As an example, metals bound to DNA can generate significant amounts of ·OH radical, with the result being high concentrations of very deleterious double-strand breaks in localized regions of DNA (71).

In some cases, however, ·OH radicals can indirectly mediate damage quite distant from their site of generation. This involves the interaction of ·OH radicals with certain proteins, nucleotides, carbohydrates, and lipids to produce peroxyl radicals (1,84). Peroxyl radicals, which may also be generated via other processes (88), are relatively stable species with half-lives of seconds (87), and are therefore capable of diffusing to remote cell locations (84,88). It is possible that peroxyl radicals represent the bulk of oxygen-centered free radicals generated via oxygen activation, and, because of their relative stability, peroxyl radicals will be much more selective than ·OH radicals in their reactions with DNA and other potential cellular targets (84). They are capable of reacting directly with DNA or with other cell components that ultimately react with DNA (88). As an example, peroxyl radicals can react with benzo[a]pyrene to form its ultimate carcinogenic form, a dihydrodiol epoxide (88).

Alkoxyl radicals, displaying half-lives of 10^{-6} s, will also likely react very close to their site of generation (84). Certain alkyl radicals are also highly reactive. For example, phenyl radicals, produced reductively by P-450 reductase or xanthine oxidase, are so reactive that their primary target is the flavoenzyme that catalyzed their formation (17). Similarly, cytochrome P-450 2E1 is quickly inactivated, probably by direct attack of the trichloromethyl radical that it generates from carbon tetrachloride (14,89).

In comparison to ·OH radicals, O_2^- is not highly reactive and has a relatively long half-life (71). O_2^- can therefore migrate a fair distance from its site of generation (71). In metal-free systems, O_2^- probably does not often cause much damage on its own (71). However, in the presence of certain metals, it leads to the production of ·OH radicals, which are capable of causing extensive damage. Given the ability of O_2^- to migrate from its site of generation, however, the production of O_2^- at one site can ultimately be responsible for ·OH radical production at other sites.

In general, then, highly reactive radical species (e.g., ·OH, alkoxyl, alkyl) are likely to react very close to their site of generation and will be quite nonselective in what they attack. Conversely, less reactive radicals (e.g., peroxyl, O_2^-) will be able to migrate much further from their generation site, but will be much more selective in their reactivity. Through secondary reactions, however, it is possible for highly reactive species to mediate some damage distant from their site of generation, and for less reactive species to be converted to highly reactive ones after migration to a different subcellular site.

Cellular Defense Mechanisms at the Site of Radical Generation

Cells possess multiple protective agents that act to limit free-radical damage. These include both enzymatic (e.g., superoxide dismutase, catalase, peroxidase) and nonenzymatic species (GSH, ascorbate, β-carotene, α-tocopherol, retinoic acid) (90). To effectively quench free radicals, these protective factors must be both close to the site of generation and in sufficient concentration. Many cell types contain relative high levels of GSH and ascorbate (90), and since they are freely diffusible in the cytoplasm one would expect them to be relatively evenly distributed. In contrast, α-tocopherol is lipid-soluble and is therefore largely localized to membranes. Because of this, the ability of α-tocopherol to prevent membrane damage from free radicals depends on where the radicals are generated (91). When radicals are generated in the aqueous phase, α-tocopherol is not fully protective; that is, membrane proteins are attacked concurrently with α-tocopherol (91). In contrast, when radicals are generated within the lipid membrane, free-radical damage to membrane lipids and proteins does not occur until α-tocopherol falls below a critical level (91).

Superoxide dismutase (SOD) is generally widely distributed in cells, with mitochondria containing a manganese-based SOD and the cytosol a copper-zinc-based SOD (90). SOD catalyzes the dismutation of O_2^- to H_2O_2, and catalase can degrade

H_2O_2 to O_2 and H_2O. Alternatively, in the presence of certain metals, H_2O_2 can generate $\cdot OH$ radicals. In addition, the removal of O_2^- by SOD can further drive redox cycling; that is, product removal can shift the equilibrium in favor of enhanced redox cycling (3).

Protective factors are generally in much lower concentration in extracellular compartments. Therefore, free radicals generated outside the cell are less likely to be quickly quenched. Many such radicals could attack the cellular membrane and cause lipid peroxidation.

While these defense mechanisms are generally thought to serve protective roles, there are instances where the overall effect is not protective. Many examples were cited earlier in which reaction with GSH or ascorbate can lead to free-radical production. As another example, acetaminophen radicals react with either GSH or ascorbate, with the resulting formation of thiyl or ascorbyl radicals, respectively (92). While the glutathiyl radicals can be quenched by dimerizing to GSSG, they can also react with GSH to generate GSSG$^-$ radical, which can react with O_2 to generate O_2^- (92); this process is referred to as "thiol pumping" (92).

Overall, then, these cellular defense mechanisms will often act to quench free-radical damage, as long as they are present in sufficient concentration at the site of free-radical generation. There are instances, however, where their net effect will be an enhancement of free-radical production.

Cell Composition at the Site of Radical Generation

Since the cell is not structurally or functionally homogeneous, the site of radical generation will define the available targets for free-radical attack, and hence the nature of the toxic effects. For instance, radicals generated within or near membranes are likely to cause some damage to membrane proteins and lipids, including lipid peroxidation. There are many membrane systems within cells (cellular, nuclear, mitochondrial, endoplasmic reticular, etc.); especially for highly reactive radicals, the membrane closest to the site of free-radical generation will likely sustain the most damage. Furthermore, lipid peroxidation events can amplify free-radical processes; without quenching by an antioxidant, 4 to 10 propagation events can result from a single free-radical initiation (93). Free-radical membrane damage can lead to increased intracellular iron and subsequent increases in reactive oxygen species (94). In addition, lipid peroxidative events can profoundly influence normal cellular functions, and this influence strongly depends on which membrane is damaged. Lipid peroxidation of either cell membranes or membranes of the sarcoplasmic reticulum causes increased calcium permeability; this leads to increased cytoplasmic calcium, with dramatic consequences for calcium-dependent processes (94). In contrast, lipid peroxidation of mitochondrial membranes can increase proton permeability, resulting in energy depletion due to inefficiency of electron transport (94). Mitochondrial lipid peroxidation is also associated with mitochondrial swelling and loss of cytochrome *c* (94), and can lead to extensive damage to mitochondrial DNA (95).

Other evidence suggests a relationship between lipid peroxidation and genotoxicity as well as carcinogenesis and tumor promotion (84,96–99). Some DNA is juxtaposed to the nuclear membrane, and there are chromatin nuclear attachment sites (100), so lipid peroxidation of the nuclear membrane could directly interact with DNA. The nuclear membrane is also physically contiguous with some of the smooth endoplasmic reticulum, and free radicals generated by "microsomal" enzymes could therefore also damage DNA. In fact, some "microsomal" enzymes (e.g., NADPH:cytochrome P-450 reductase) are also present in the nuclear membrane (101). Not only can the radicals that initiate lipid peroxidation react with DNA (99), but DNA is also susceptible to damage by the lipid radicals themselves (99), as well as by nonradical products of lipid peroxidation (e.g., aldehydes, hydroxyacids, etc.) (99). Peroxyl radicals, which are formed by lipid peroxidation and through other means, can translocate damage from one membrane to another or from membrane to DNA. They are stable enough to diffuse to remote cellular locations, and they are capable of reacting directly with DNA or with other cell components that ultimately react with DNA (88). There are also varied nonradical mechanisms that can translate membrane damage into DNA alterations (102–104).

Furthermore, lipid peroxidative events are not necessarily confined to the membrane that sustained the initial damage. For example, extracellularly generated free radicals can attack the outer surface of the cell membrane leading to lipid peroxidation (81). While these membrane radicals would not likely travel to the nucleus and cause DNA damage, secondary radicals derived from their breakdown products can, through a second message system, cause clastogenic activity (83,103,105). For example, leukocytes that are stimulated by phorbol 12-myristate 13-acetate (PMA) can release diffusible clastogenic factors that can damage DNA in adjacent target cells (106–108). The formation of these lipophilic clastogenic factors is mediated by O_2^- radicals (107), which are thought to mediate the reduction of Fe(III) to Fe(II). The Fe(II) is thought to participate in a Fenton-type reaction involving the production of free radicals from arachidonic acid metabolites released by the PMA-exposed cells (102).

While specific proteins are often localized to specific organelles in the cell, proteins in general are widely distributed within cells and are therefore likely targets of attack by at least some free radicals. Depending on the nature of the free radical and protein, a radical-modified protein can possess either oxidizing or reducing groups, or both (109). Hydroperoxide oxidizing groups on proteins can consume ascorbate and GSH and therefore constitute additional oxidative stress within the cell (109), whereas reducing groups on proteins could reduce Cu or Fe, which can mediate radical production by Fenton-like reactions (109). Of key importance here, however, is that, in addition to altering or destroying the protein's normal function, both the reductive and oxidative protein moieties are long-lived, and may therefore diffuse far away from their site of formation (109). This, in essence, would allow for another mechanism whereby potentially damaging reactions are transferred to distant cellular sites.

The localization of other components can serve to focus free-radical damage at very specific sites. For example, as detailed earlier, metals bound to certain cell components can undergo multiple cycles of reduction and reoxidation, generating a high concentration of ·OH radicals in a fixed locus, which would concentrate the ·OH radical damage to the immediate vicinity of the complexed metal (71,74).

In total, the composition of the cell at the site of free-radical generation can markedly influence the nature and extent of free-radical generation and potential damage.

SUMMARY

Within cells, there are many xenobiotic compounds that can give rise to free radicals through the interaction of the compounds with specific cell machinery. As a whole, the cellular components capable of mediating free-radical generation are dispersed to sites throughout the cell, including the endoplasmic reticulum, mitochondria, and cytosol. Other components may be bound to various membranes, or even to DNA itself. However, specific components are often localized to specific subcellular compartments. Such components in the endoplasmic reticulum include NADPH:cytochrome P-450 reductase, cytochromes P-450, prostaglandin H synthase, and NADH:cytochrome b_5 reductase. Cytosolic components include xanthine oxidase, aldehyde oxidase, GSH reductase, DT-diaphorase, ascorbate, cysteine, and GSH. Mitochondrial components include the electron transport system. In some cases, the free radicals are derived directly from the xenobiotic itself. In other cases, xenobiotics enhance the ability of cell components to generate free radicals as by-products of normal processes.

Even though a given xenobiotic may gain access to many subcellular sites, it may not elicit free-radical generation at all of these sites. For example, the generation of free radicals from some compounds (e.g., paraquat, halothane, carbon tetrachloride) is largely associated with enzymes of the endoplasmic reticulum. For other compounds (e.g., doxorubicin, hexavalent chromium), there are numerous cellular components throughout the cell that can mediate free-radical generation. The important point here is that, especially with highly reactive radicals, much of the damage is likely to be close to the site of generation. Therefore, knowledge of the subcellular sites of free-radical generation is fundamental to understanding the potential toxicity of a given radical species. There are exceptions to this generalization, however, as less reactive free radicals can migrate to distant sites before mediating damage. In addition, there are various mechanisms by which damage from highly reactive radicals can be disseminated to sites distant from the initial site of radical generation.

For each subcellular site, there are adjunctive factors that can impact free-radical generation and potential damage. One of these is the nature and concentration of cellular defense mechanisms. If present in sufficient concentration at the site of generation, they will often act to quench at least some of the radicals. In other instances, however, these defense mechanisms can themselves generate radicals and thereby serve to enhance, rather than limit, free-radical production. The functional and structural heterogeneity of the cells further defines the available targets at various sites for free-radical attack, and thus the potential toxicity. If highly reactive radicals are generated close to key cellular targets (e.g., lipids, DNA), the resulting damage is likely to have more profound effects for the cell. The association of certain species (e.g., some metals) with key cellular targets can also serve to focus high concentrations of damage to very specific sites or targets.

Knowledge of the subcellular sites of free-radical generation is therefore one of the elements necessary to thoroughly understand free-radical toxicology. In and of itself, however, this knowledge will only provide a partial picture, as other factors will contribute to the ultimate toxic effects.

ACKNOWLEDGMENTS

The author was supported in part by grant 5-R21-50786-02 from the National Institute of General Medical Sciences and grant F49620-95-1-0200 from the Air Force Office of Scientific Research, Air Force Systems Command, U.S. Air Force. The U.S. government is authorized to reproduce and distribute reprints for governmental purposes.

REFERENCES

1. Grisham MB. *Reactive Metabolites of Oxygen and Nitrogen in Biology and Medicine*. Austin, TX: R.G. Landes, 1992.
2. Bhuyan KC, Bhuyan DK, Podos SM. Free radical enhancer xenobiotic is an inducer of cataract in rabbit. *Free Radical Res Commun* 1991;13:609–620.
3. Cohen GM, d'Arcy Doherty M. Free radical mediated cell toxicity by redox cycling chemicals. *Br J Cancer* 1987;55(Suppl. VIII):46–52.
4. DeGray JA, Rao DNR, Mason RP. Reduction of paraquat and related bipyridylium compounds to free radical metabolites by rat hepatocytes. *Arch Biochem Biophys* 1991;289:145–152.
5. Rosen GM, Hassett DJ, Yankaskas JR, Cohen MS. Detection of free radicals as a consequence of dog tracheal epithelial cellular xenobiotic metabolism. *Xenobiotica* 1989;19:635–643.
6. Lemaire P, Livingstone DR. Inhibition studies on the involvement of flavoprotein reductases in menadione- and nitrofurantoin-stimulated oxyradical production by hepatic microsomes of flounder (*Platichthys flesus*). *J Biochem Toxicol* 1994;9:87–95.
7. Lemaire P, Matthews A, Förlin L, Livingstone DR. Stimulation of oxyradical production of hepatic microsomes of flounder (*Platichthys flesus*) and perch (*Perca fluvatilis*) by model and pollutant xenobiotics. *Arch Environ Contam Toxicol* 1994;26:191–200.
8. Baez S, Linderson Y, Segura-Aguilar J. Superoxide dismutase and catalase enhance autoxidation during one-electron reduction of aminochrome by NADPH-cytochrome P-450 reductase. *Biochem Mol Med* 1995;54:12–18.
9. Berger V, Berson A, Wolf C, Chachaty C, Fan D, Fromenty B, Pessayre D. Generation of free radicals during the reductive metabolism of nilutamide by lung microsomes: Possible role in the development of lung lesions in patients treated with this anti-androgen. *Biochem Pharmacol* 1992;43:654–657.
10. Sakurai K, Ogiso T. Generation of alloxan radical in rat islet cells: Participation of NADPH: cytochrome P-450 reductase. *Biol Pharm Bull* 1994;17:1451–1455.
11. Goeptar AR, Te Koppele JM, Lamme EK, Piqué JM, Vermeulen NPE. Cytochrome P-450 2B1-mediated one-electron reduction of adriamycin: A study with rat liver microsomes and purified enzymes. *Mol Pharmacol* 1993;44:1267–1277.

12. Sinha BK, Mimnaugh EG, Rajagopalan S, Myers CE. Adriamycin activation and oxygen free radical formation in human breast tumor cells: Protective role of glutathione peroxidase in adriamycin resistance. *Cancer Res* 1989;49:3844–3848.

13. Pan S-S, Andrews PA, Glover CJ, Bachur NR. Reductive activation of mitomycin C and mitomycin C metabolites catalyzed by NADPH-cytochrome P-450 reductase and xanthine oxidase. *J Biol Chem* 1984;259:959–966.

14. Goeptar AR, Scheerens H, Vermeulen NPE. Oxygen and xenobiotic reductase activities of cytochrome P-450. *Crit Rev Toxicol* 1995;25:25–65.

15. Thornalley PJ, d'Arcy Doherty M, Smith MT, Bannister V, Cohen GM. The formation of active oxygen species following activation of 1-naphthol, 1,2- and 1,4-naphthoquinone by rat liver microsomes. *Chem-Biol Interact* 1984;48:195–206.

16. Fitzsimmons SA, Lewis AD, Riley RJ, Workman P. Reduction of 3-amino-1,2,4-benzotriazine-1,4-di-*N*-oxide (tirapazamine, WIN 59075, SR 4233) to a DNA-damaging species: A direct role for NADPH:cytochrome P-450 oxidoreductase. *Carcinogenesis* 1994;15:1503–1510.

17. O'Donnell VB, Smith GCM, Jones OTG. Involvement of phenyl radicals in iodonium compound inhibition of flavoenzymes. *Mol Pharmacol* 1994;46:778–785.

18. Bondy SC, Naderi S. Contribution of hepatic cytochrome P-450 systems to the generation of reactive oxygen species. *Biochem Pharmacol* 1994;48:155–159.

19. Rashba-Step J, Cederbaum AI. Generation of reactive oxygen intermediates by human liver microsomes in the presence of NADPH or NADH. *Mol Pharmacol* 1994;45:150–157.

20. Hildebrandt AG, Roots I. Reduced nicotinamide adenine dinucleotide phosphate (NADPH)-dependent formation and breakdown of hydrogen peroxide during mixed function oxidation reactions in liver microsomes. *Arch Biochem Biophys* 1975;171:385–397.

21. Kuthan H, Tsuji H, Graf H, Ullrich V, Werringloer J, Estabrook RW. Generation of superoxide anion as a source of hydrogen peroxide in a reconstituted monooxygenase system. *FEBS Lett* 1978;91:343–345.

22. Nordmann R, Ribière C, Rouach H. Implication of free radical mechanisms in ethanol-induced cellular injury. *Free Radical Biol Med* 1992;12:219–240.

23. Bulger WH, Kupfer D. Characteristics of monooxygenase-mediated covalent binding of methoxychlor in human and rat liver microsomes. *Drug Metab Dispos* 1989;17:487–494.

24. Muakkassah SF, Yang WCT. Mechanism of the inhibitory action of phenelzine on microsomal drug metabolism. *J Pharmacol Exp Ther* 1981;219:147–155.

25. Ortiz de Montellano PR, Augusto O, Viola F, Kunze KL. Carbon radicals in the metabolism of alkyl hydrazines. *J Biol Chem* 1983;258:8623–8629.

26. Ortiz de Montellano PR, Watanabe M. Free radical pathways in the *in vitro* hepatic metabolism of phenelzine. *Mol Pharmacol* 1987;31:213–219.

27. Noguchi T, Fong K-L, Lai EK, Alexander SS, King MM, Olson L, Payer JL, McCay PB. Specificity of a phenobarbital-induced cytochrome P-450 for metabolism of carbon tetrachloride to the trichloromethyl radical. *Biochem Pharmacol* 1982;31:615–624.

28. de Groot H, Sies H. Cytochrome P-450, reductive metabolism, and cell injury. *Drug Metab Rev* 1989;20:275–284.

29. Mikalsen A, Alexander J, Andersen RA, Daae H-L. Reduction of hexavalent chromium in a reconstituted system of cytochrome P-450 and cytochrome b_5. *Chem-Biol Interact* 1989;71:213–221.

30. Mikalsen A, Alexander J, Ryberg D. Microsomal metabolism of hexavalent chromium. Inhibitory effect of oxygen and involvement of cytochrome P-450. *Chem–Biol Interact* 1989;69:175–192.

31. Mikalsen A, Alexander J, Wallin H, Ingelman-Sundberg M, Andersen RA. Reductive metabolism and protein binding of chromium(VI) by P-450 protein enzymes. *Carcinogenesis* 1991;12:825–831.

32. Sevanian A, Nordenbrand K, Kim E, Ernster L, Hochstein P. Microsomal lipid peroxidation: the role of NADPH-cytochrome P-450 reductase and cytochrome P-450. *Free Radical Biol Med* 1990;8:145–152.

33. Hodnick WF, Sartorelli AC. Reductive activation of mitomycin C by NADH:cytochrome b_5 reductase. *Cancer Res* 1993;53:4907–4912.

34. Shi X, Dalal NS. Hydroxyl radical generation in the NADH/microsomal reduction of vanadate. *Free Radical Res Commun* 1992;17:369–376.

35. Pratt PF, Myers CR. Enzymatic reduction of chromium(VI) by human hepatic microsomes. *Carcinogenesis* 1993;14:2051–2057.

36. Eling TE, Mason RP, Sivarajah K. The formation of aminopyrine cation radical by the peroxidase

activity of prostaglandin H synthase and subsequent reactions of the radical. *J Biol Chem* 1985;260:1601–1607.

37. Smith BJ, Curtis JF, Eling TE. Bioactivation of xenobiotics by prostaglandin H synthase. *Chem-Biol Interact* 1991;79:245–264.

38. Josephy PD, Eling TE, Mason RP. An electron spin resonance study of the activation of benzidine by peroxidases. *Mol Pharmacol* 1983;23:766–770.

39. Josephy PD, Mason RP, Eling T. Cooxidation of the clinical reagent 3,5,3'5'-tetramethylbenzidine by prostaglandin synthase. *Cancer Res* 1982;42:2567–2570.

40. Zenser TV, Mattammal MB, Ambrecht HJ, Davis, BB. Benzidine binding to nucleic acids mediated by the peroxidative activity of prostaglandin endoperoxide synthetase. *Cancer Res* 1980;40:2839–2845.

41. Zenser TV, Mattammal MB, Davis BB. Cooxidation of benzidine by renal medullary prostaglandin cyclooxygenase. *J Pharmacol Exp Ther* 1979;211:460–464.

42. Hall P dela M, Stupans I, Burgess W, Birkett DJ, McManus ME. Immunohistochemical localization of NADPH-cytochrome P-450 reductase in human tissues. *Carcinogenesis* 1989;10:521–530.

43. Johnson JD, Conroy WG, Burris KD, Isom GE. Peroxidation of brain lipids following cyanide intoxication in mice. *Toxicology* 1987;46:21–28.

44. Davies KJA, Doroshow JH. Redox cycling of anthracyclines by cardiac mitochondria. I. Anthracycline radical formation by NADH dehydrogenase. *J Biol Chem* 1986;261:3060–3067.

45. Kennedy CH, Church DF, Winston GW, Pryor WA. *Tert*-butyl hydroperoxide-induced radical production in rat liver mitochondria. *Free Radical Biol Med* 1992;12:381–387.

46. Massa EM, Giulivi C. Alkoxyl and methyl radical formation during cleavage of *tert*-butyl hydroperoxide by a mitochondrial membrane-bound, redox active copper pool: An EPR study. *Free Radical Biol Med* 1993;14:559–565.

47. Chiueh CC, Huang S-J, Murphy DL. Enhanced hydroxyl radical generation by 2'-methyl analog of MPTP: Suppression by clorgyline and deprenyl. *Syanpse* 1992;11:346–348.

48. Chiueh CC, Huang S-J, Murphy DL. Suppression of hydroxyl radical formation by MAO inhibitors: A novel possible neuroprotective mechanism in dopaminergic neurotoxicity. *J Neural Transm* 1994;41(Suppl.):189–196.

49. Kalyanaraman B, Perez-Reyes E, Mason RP. The reduction of nitroso-spin traps in chemical and biological systems. *Tetrahedron Lett* 1979;50:4809–4812.

50. Takahashi N, Fischer V, Schreiber J, Mason RP. An ESR study of nonenzymatic reactions of nitroso compounds with biological reducing agents. *Free Radical Res Commun* 1988;4:351–358.

51. Fujii H, Koscielniak J, Kakinuma K, Berliner LJ. Biological reduction of aromatic nitroso compounds: evidence for the involvement of superoxide anions. *Free Radical Res* 1994;21:235–243.

52. Gorsdorf S, Appel KE, Engelholm C, Obe G. Nitrogen dioxide induces DNA single-strand breaks in cultured Chinese hamster cells. *Carcinogenesis* 1990;11:37–41.

53. Kikugawa K, Hiramoto K, Okamoto Y, Hasegawa Y-K. Enhancement of nitrogen dioxide-induced lipid peroxidation and DNA strand breaking by cysteine and glutathione. *Free Radical Res* 1994;21:399–408.

54. Reszka KJ, Chignell CF. One-electron reduction of arenediazonium compounds by physiological electron donors generates aryl radicals. An EPR and spin trapping investigation. *Chem-Biol Interact* 1995;96:223–234.

55. LaLonde RT, Xie S, Chamulitrat W, Mason RP. Oxidation and radical intermediates associated with the glutathione conjugation of mucochloric acid. *Chem Res Toxicol* 1994;7:482–486.

56. Ahmad FF, Cowan DL, Sun AY. Vitamin C mediates the formation of ethoxy radicals which damage biological membranes. In: Kuriyama K, Takada A, Ishii H, eds. *Biomedical and Social Aspects of Alcohol and Alcoholism*. Amsterdam: Excerpta Medica, 1988;681–684.

57. Stearns DM, Wetterhahn KE. Reaction of chromium(VI) with ascorbate produces chromium(V), chromium(IV), and carbon-based radicals. *Chem Res Toxicol* 1994;7:219–230.

58. Shi X, Mao Y, Knapton AD, Ding M, Rojanasakul Y, Gannett PM, Dalal N, Liu K. Reaction of Cr(VI) with ascorbate and hydrogen peroxide generates hydroxyl radicals and causes DNA damage: Role of a Cr(IV)-mediated Fenton-like reaction. *Carcinogenesis* 1994;15:2475–2478.

59. Aiyar J, Berkovits HJ, Floyd RA, Wetterhahn KE. Reaction of chromium (VI) with hydrogen peroxide in the presence of glutathione: Reactive intermediates and resulting DNA damage. *Chem Res Toxicol* 1990;3:595–603.

60. Aiyar J, Borges KM, Floyd RA, Wetterhahn KE. Role of chromium(V), glutathione thiyl radical

and hydroxyl radical intermediates in chromium(VI)-induced DNA damage. *Toxicol Environ Chem* 1989;22:135–148.

61. Shi X, Dalal NS. On the hydroxyl radical formation in the reaction between hydrogen peroxide and biologically generated chromium(V) species. *Arch Biochem Biophys* 1990;277:342–350.

62. Shi X, Dong Z, Dalal NS, Gannett PM. Chromate-mediated free-radical generation from cysteine, penicillamine, hydrogen peroxide, and lipid hydroperoxides. *Biochim Biophys Acta* 1994;1226:65–72.

63. Ding M, Gannett PM, Rojanasakul Y, Liu K, Shi X. One-electron reduction of vanadate by ascorbate and related free-radical generation at physiological pH. *J Inorg Biochem* 1994;55:101–112.

64. Shi X, Dalal NS, Kasprzak KS. Generation of free radicals from hydrogen peroxide and lipid hydroperoxides in the presence of Cr(III). *Arch Biochem Biophys* 1993;302:294–299.

65. Andersson M, Grankvist K. Ascorbate-induced free radical toxicity to isolated islet cells. *Int J Biochem Cell Biol* 1995;27:493–498.

66. Shi X, Dalal NS. On the mechanism of the chromate reduction by glutathione: ESR evidence for the glutathionyl radical and an insoluble Cr(V) intermediate. *Biochem Biophys Res Commun* 1988;156:137–142.

67. Yan L, Spallholz E. Generation of reactive oxygen species from the reaction of selenium compounds with thiols and mammary tumor cells. *Biochem Pharmacol* 1993;45:429–437.

68. Kawanishi S, Inoue S, Yamamoto K. Active oxygen species in DNA damage induced by carcinogenic metal compounds. *Environ Health Perspect* 1994;102(Suppl. 3):17–20.

69. Shi X, Dalal NS, Kasprzak KS. Generation of free radicals from lipid hydroperoxides by Ni^{2+} in the presence of oligopeptides. *Arch Biochem Biophys* 1992;299:154–162.

70. Perez-Reyes E, Mason RP. Electron spin resonance study of the autoxidation of 6-aminodopamine. *Mol Pharmacol* 1980;18:594–597.

71. Chevion M. A site-specific mechanism for free radical induced biological damage: The essential role of redox-active transition metals. *Free Radical Biol Med* 1988;5:27–37.

72. Davies MJ, Slater TF. Studies on the metal-ion and lipoxygenase-catalyzed breakdown of hydroperoxides using electron-spin-resonance spectroscopy. *Biochem J* 1987;245:167–173.

73. North JA, Spector AA, Buettner GR. Detection of lipid radicals by electron paramagnetic resonance spin trapping using intact cells enriched with polyunsaturated fatty acid. *J Biol Chem* 1992;267:5743–5746.

74. Stohs SJ, Bagchi D. Oxidative mechanisms in the toxicity of metal ions. *Free Radical Biol Med* 1995;18:321–336.

75. Ryan TP, Aust SD. The role of iron in oxygen-mediated toxicities. *Crit Rev Toxicol* 1992;22:119–141.

76. Pritsos CA, Gustafson DL. Xanthine dehydrogenase and its role in cancer chemotherapy. *Oncol Res* 1994;6:477–481.

77. Kuppusamy P, Zweier JL. Characterization of free-radical generation by xanthine oxidase. Evidence for hydroxyl radical generation. *J Biol Chem* 1989;264:9880–9884.

78. Jarabak R, Jarabak J. Effect of ascorbate on the DT-diaphorase-mediated redox cycling of 2-methyl-1,4-naphthoquinone. *Arch Biochem Biophys* 1995;318:418–423.

79. Pirie A, Rees JR, Holmberg NJ. Diquat cataract: Formation of the free radical and its reaction with constituents of the eye. *Exp Eye Res* 1970;9:204–218.

80. Coudray C, Faure P, Rachidi S, Jeunet A, Richard MJ, Roussel AM, Favier A. Hydroxyl radical formation and lipid peroxidation enhancement by chromium. *Biol Trace Elem Res* 1992;32:161–170.

81. Clemens MR. Free radicals in chemical carcinogenesis. *Klin Wochenschr* 1991;69:1123–1134.

82. Pitot HC. Principles of carcinogenesis: Chemical. In: DeVita VT Jr, Hellman S, Rosenberg SA, eds. *Cancer: Principles & Practice of Oncology*, 3rd ed. Philadelphia: JB Lippincott, 1989;116–135.

83. Emerit I. Clastogenic factors, a link between chronic inflammation and carcinogenesis. In: Cerutti PA, Nygaard OF, Simic MG, eds. *Anticarcinogenesis and Radiation Protection*. New York: Plenum Press, 1987;59–62.

84. Marnett LJ. Peroxyl free radicals: Potential mediators of tumor initiation and promotion. *Carcinogenesis* 1987;8:1365–1373.

85. Pryor WA. The involvement of free radicals in chemical carcinogenesis. In: Cerutti PA, Nygaard OF, Simic MG, eds. *Anticarcinogenesis and Radiation Protection*. New York: Plenum Press, 1987;1–9.

86. Pryor WA, Uehara K, Church DF. The chemistry and biochemistry of the radicals in cigarette smoke: ESR evidence for the binding of tar radical to DNA and polynucleotides. In: Bors W, Saran M, Tait D, eds. *Oxygen Radicals in Chemistry and Biology*. Berlin: Walter de Gruyter and Co., 1984;193–201.

87. Pryor WA. Oxy-radicals and related species: Their formation, lifetimes, and reactions. *Annu Rev Physiol* 1986;48:657–667.
88. Marnett LJ. The involvement of peroxyl free radicals in tumor initiation and promotion. In: Cerutti PA, Nygaard OF, Simic MG, eds. *Anticarcinogenesis and Radiation Protection*. New York: Plenum Press, 1987;71–80.
89. Kringstein P, Cederbaum AI. Boldine prevents human liver microsomal lipid peroxidation and inactivation of cytochrome P-4502E1. *Free Radical Biol Med* 1995;18:559–563.
90. Halliwell B, Gutteridge JMC. Oxygen radicals and the nervous system. *Trends Neurosci* 1985;8:22–26.
91. Takenaka Y, Miki M, Yasuda H, Mino M. The effect of α-tocopherol as an antioxidant on the oxidation of membrane protein thiols induced by free radicals generated in different sites. *Arch Biochem Biophys* 1991;285:344–350.
92. Rao DNR, Fischer V, Mason RP. Glutathione and ascorbate reduction of the acetaminophen radical formed by peroxidase. *J Biol Chem* 1990;265:844–847.
93. Reed DJ. Mechanisms of chemically induced cell injury and cellular protection mechanisms. In: Hodgson E, Levi PE, eds. *Introduction to Biochemical Toxicology*, 2nd ed. Norwalk, CT: Appleton and Lange, 1994;265–295.
94. Vladimirov YA. Free radical lipid peroxidation in biomembranes: Mechanism, regulation, and biological consequences. In: Johnson JE Jr, Walford R, Harman D, Miquel J, eds. *Free Radicals, Aging, and Degenerative Diseases*. New York: Alan R. Liss, Inc., 1986;141–195.
95. Hruszkewycz AM. Mitochondrial DNA damage during mitochondrial lipid peroxidation. In: Cerutti PA, Nygaard OF, Simic MG, eds. *Anticarcinogenesis and Radiation Protection*. New York: Plenum Press, 1987;103–108.
96. Ames BN, Hollstein MC, Cathcart R. Lipid peroxidation and oxidative damage to DNA. In: Yagi K, ed. *Lipid Peroxides in Biology and Medicine*. New York: Academic Press, 1982;339–351.
97. Cerutti PA. Prooxidant states and tumor promotion. *Science* 1985;227:375–381.
98. Kensler TW, Trush MA. Role of oxygen radicals in tumor promotion. *Environ Mutagen* 1984;6:593–616.
99. Vaca CE, Wilhelm J, Harms-Ringdahl M. Interaction of lipid peroxidation products with DNA. A review. *Mutat Res* 1988;195:137–149.
100. Franke WW, Scheer U. Structures and functions of the nuclear envelope. In: Busch H, ed. *The Cell Nucleus*. New York: Academic Press, 1974;219–347.
101. Cahill A, White INH. Reductive metabolism of 3-amino-1,2,4-benzotriazine-1,4-dioxide (SR 4233) and the induction of unscheduled DNA synthesis in rat and human derived cell lines. *Carcinogenesis* 1990;11:1407–1411.
102. Kozumbo W, Muehlematter D, Jörg A, Emerit I, Cerutti P. Phorbol ester-induced formation of clastogenic factor from human monocytes. *Carcinogenesis* 1987;8:521–526.
103. Kozumbo W, Muehlematter D, Ochi T, Cerutti P. The role of active oxygen and the metabolism of arachidonic acid in the formation of clastogenic factor by human monocytes. In: Cerutti PA, Nygaard OF, Simic MG, eds. *Anticarcinogenesis and Radiation Protection*. New York: Plenum Press, 1987;51–57.
104. McConkey DJ, Hartzell P, Duddy SK, Håkansson H, Orrenius S. 2,3,7,8-Tetrachlorodibenzo-*p*-dioxin kills immature thymocytes by Ca^{2+}-mediated endonuclease activation. *Science* 1988;242:256–259.
105. Demopoulos HB, Pietronigro DD, Flamm ES, Seligman ML. The possible role of free radical reactions in carcinogenesis. *J Environ Pathol Toxicol* 1980;3:273–303.
106. Birnboim HC. DNA strand breakage in human leukocytes exposed to a tumor promoter, phorbol myristate acetate. *Science* 1982;215:1247–1249.
107. Emerit I, Cerutti P. Clastogenic action of tumor promoter phorbol 12-myristate 13-acetate in mixed human leukocyte cultures. *Carcinogenesis* 1983;4:1313–1316.
108. Weitberg AB, Weitzman SA, Destrempes M, Latt SA, Stossel TP. Stimulated human phagocytes produce cytogenic changes in cultured mammalian cells. *N Engl J Med* 1983;308:26–30.
109. Simpson JA, Narita S, Gieseg S, Gebicki S, Gebicki JM, Dean RT. Long-lived reactive species on free-radical-damaged proteins. *Biochem J* 1992;282:621–624.

PART II

Biological Reactivity of Free Radicals

Free Radical Toxicology
Edited by K. B. Wallace
Copyright © 1997 Taylor & Francis

4

Formation and Biological Reactivity of Lipid Peroxidation Products

Alex Sevanian and Laurie McLeod

University of Southern California, Department of Molecular Pharmacology and Toxicology, School of Pharmacy, Los Angeles, California, USA

INTRODUCTION

The toxicity of a wide variety of xenobiotics appears to be related to their ability to induce oxidative stress, characterized by increased free radical production and/ or stimulation of cellular oxidant stress responses (1,2). If the insult is either sustained or of sufficient intensity to acutely overcome cell defenses, damage to macromolecules can accumulate, leading to loss of cell function, membrane damage, and ultimately, to cell death. The free radical species formed in cells by exogenous agents or endogenously generated responses can readily attack proteins, DNA, and unsaturated lipids, resulting in their loss of function and damage. Reactions with lipids are unique among cell constituents since the formation of lipid peroxidation products leads to the facile propagation of free radical reactions. The lipid peroxidation products contribute to cell injury by reacting with cells constituents similarly to the primary and initiating oxidants and free radical species. Further cell damage and death is manifested through disruption of membrane structure and/or composition, alteration or inactivation of membrane associated enzymes, and in some instances, activation of enzymes that respond to changes in cell redox status or to cell injury. The toxic effects of lipid peroxidation are considered to proceed through a sequence of oxidative reactions followed by metabolic changes to which antioxidants and related defenses may be ineffective.

Lipid peroxidation, a marker of cellular oxidative stress, has long been recognized as a potential contributor to the oxidative damage caused by xenobiotic compounds, as well as by inflammatory processes, ischemia/reperfusion injury, and chronic diseases such as atherosclerosis and cancer (3). Xenobiotic compounds, analogous to several pathological processes, are capable of inducing lipid peroxidation through a series of basic and well-described mechanisms. These include redox reactions generating reactive oxygen species, such as superoxide anion radical ($O_2^{-\cdot}$) and

H_2O_2, that are formed by redox cycling of compounds, as in the case of quinones and quinonoids (4), azo compounds (5), and furans (6). Other agents cause free radical production through mitochondrial electron transport activity (7) or by redox cycling during metabolism by mixed-function oxidases as in the case of nitrofuran-toin (6). Metabolic activation of xenobiotics to reactive intermediates has long been known to be accompanied by lipid peroxidation, either through P-450-mediated metabolism, other peroxidases, or xenobiotic radical intermediates (8). However, the extent to which lipid peroxidation resulting from these processes contributes to the pathology attributed to xenobiotic reactive intermediates remains uncertain. Although a number of compounds initiate lipid peroxidation through direct produc-tion of radical or reactive oxygen species, further peroxidation may take place by indirect processes involving enzyme activation where unsaturated lipids serve as substrates. Among the best examples are lipoxygenases, which are activated in response to disrupted membrane structure or composition (9), and utilize polyunsatu-rated lipids as cosubstrates for the metabolic activation of xenobiotics (10).

Details of mechanisms by which reactive oxygen species are produced via xenobi-otic reactions and metabolism are provided in the preceding chapters. We emphasize in this chapter selected mechanisms by which xenobiotics induce lipid peroxidation in biological systems. This review focuses on the biological reactions of lipid peroxidation and provides examples for the reaction of peroxidation products. Selected mechanisms by which cellular dysfunction and toxicity are manifested following exposure to oxidizing chemicals and amplified by lipid peroxidation are described.

OVERVIEW OF LIPID PEROXIDATION: RADICAL-MEDIATED REACTIONS AND PRODUCTS

As described in previous reviews, lipid peroxidation is evoked through one-electron reduction reactions where an initiating radical species combines with an unsaturated lipid and in turn with oxygen to form a lipid peroxyl radical. Redox-cycling xenobiotics are variably capable of generating O_2^- based on their redox potential (11), chemical environment (12), ability to interact with enzymatic systems that facilitate their reduction (e.g., flavoenzymes) (1), and metabolism of the resulting reactive oxygen species (13). Scheme 1 incorporates these reactions where a variety of xenobiotics can be envisioned as redox cycling to yield initiating reactive oxygen species. The scheme portrays the initial events during formation of a carbon-centered radical on a polyunsaturated fatty acid as would be found associated with a membrane phospholipid. Initiation reactions of this nature have been shown to arise from the generation of reactive oxygen species during the reduction and reoxidation of chemicals capable of undergoing facile one- or sequential two-electron redox cycling (14). Most commonly, this involves formation of O_2^- and its dismutation to H_2O_2, where the redox reactions are driven by a number of flavin-containing enzymes. Some xenobiotics, like quinones, continuously cycle between their radical and nonradical forms as long as reducing equivalents are available, as in the case of catalysis by flavin containing enzymes. In the case of many simple as well as substituted quinones, formation of O_2^- can be facilitated by reaction with nucleophiles such as glutathione (GSH), where the glutathionyl adduct experiences even more rapid reduction and reoxidation (4). In addition, certain enzymes have been shown to promote the production of O_2^- by forming the quinol, which, in some instances, experiences two-electron reoxidation to yield the quinone and H_2O_2, and where formation of the latter is enhanced. This applies to redox-labile hydroquinones in the presence of superoxide dismutase (4). A well-studied example is DT-diaphorase, which may function as either an antioxidant or a pro-oxidant depending on the types of hydroquinones formed during DT-diaphorase activity. A prooxidant effect is found following reduction of redox-labile hydroquinones that subsequently autoxidize with formation of reactive oxygen species (15). These redox reactions produce the components of the well known Haber-Weiss reaction which in turn yields hydroxyl radical, albeit at very slow rates (16). It has been widely held that the Haber-Weiss reaction may be catalyzed in the presence of transition metals (notably iron), in essence producing the reduced state of the metal which reacts with H_2O_2, according to the Fenton reaction, yielding hydroxyl radical (·OH) (16). The Fenton-catalyzed Haber-Weiss reaction, although clearly demonstrated chemi-

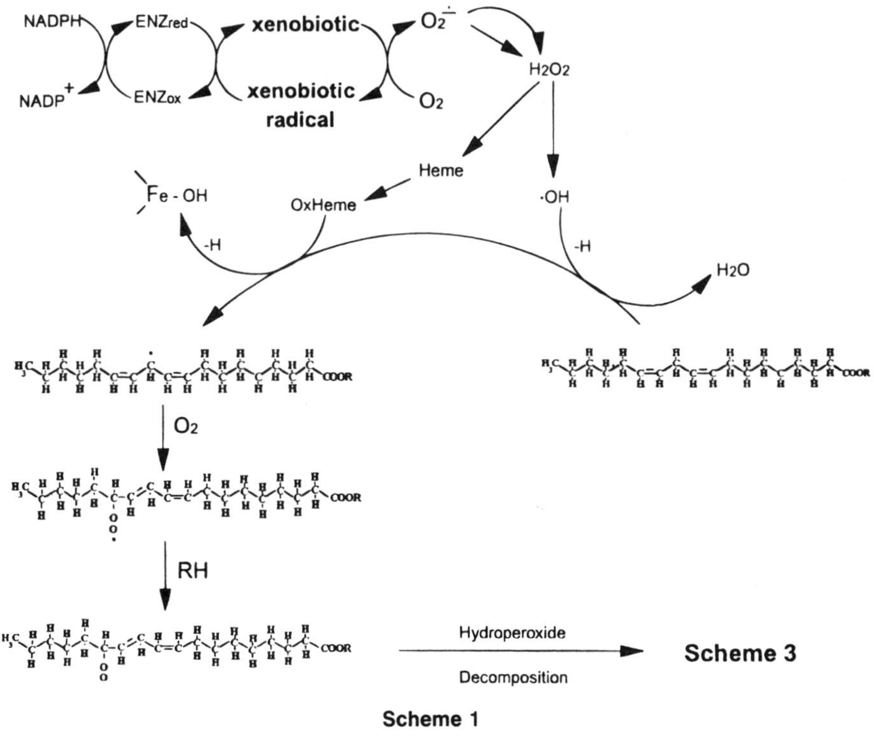

Scheme 1

cally to induce lipid peroxidation, may be of questionable importance in biological systems, although Fenton reactions may occur in lipid environments within membranes (17). It is likely that transition metals do not exist in normal tissues in the catalytic amounts (micromolar) required to produce ˙OH at rates sufficient to induce lipid peroxidation in cell systems. However, ˙OH may arise from chelated metal complexes, such as bleomycin (1), or from the homolytic scission ferryl hemoproteins such as ferryl-myoglobin (18). Other complex scenarios have been proposed involving protein-bound iron, which, especially when fully saturated (19), can release catalytic metals or catalyze lipid peroxidation as the metal-bound complex. Evidence for this has been recently offered for ceruloplasmin, implicating this copper transport protein in the oxidation of serum lipoproteins (20). Plausible mechanisms for initiating lipid peroxidation may also involve heme proteins, which have long been known to be converted to potent oxidants (21).

Peroxidation of lipids has been demonstrated in many studies following additions of heme proteins. The rapid oxidation of phospholipids in artificial membrane (22) and lipoproteins (23) was described with hemin as a model hemoprotein where the heme iron normally exists in the Fe^{3+} state and is oxidized by strong oxidants to higher valence states, usually in the form of an oxoheme ($O=Fe^{4+}$) (24). The autoxidation of hemoglobin or myoglobin represents a probable mechanism for lipid peroxidation involving heme normally in the Fe^{2+} state. Formation of H_2O_2 takes place by myoglobin oxidation in the presence of electron donors such as hydroquinones, nitrates, and aminophenols (14). This involves a concerted two-electron process where donation of an electron from the heme iron to oxygen forms a superoxoferrimyoglobin intermediate according to the reaction:

$$Mb-Fe^{2+}-O_2 + H^+ \rightarrow Mb-Fe^{3+}-O_2^- \qquad [1]$$

Donation of the second electron to O_2^- yields metmyoglobin and H_2O_2:

$$MbFe^{3+}-O_2^- + RH \rightarrow Mb-Fe^{3+} + H_2O_2 + R \qquad [2]$$

Aside from being a source of H_2O_2 and further oxyradical generation, metmyoglobin or methemoglobin can be oxidized by H_2O_2 to the ferryl state ($Mb-Fe^{4+}=O$), representing a concerted mechanism for oxidation where, in essence, the second electron resides on the protein as a transient radical (14). This higher oxidation state has been shown to initiate lipid peroxidation according to the reaction:

$$HX-Fe^{4+}=O + RH \rightarrow HX-Fe^{3+} + HO^- + R˙ \qquad [3]$$

Formation of H_2O_2 by cytochrome P-450 (25) and initiation of lipid peroxidation by ferryl intermediates formed on reaction with H_2O_2 have long been known (26). Provision of reducing equivalents via NADPH-cytochrome-P450 reductase, involving two electrons for O_2 reduction, was shown to catalyze propagation of lipid peroxidation (27). The involvement of cytochrome P-450 and cytochrome P-450 reductase is implicated together with complexed iron. The first electron appears to be used for the reduction of complexed iron and subsequent addition to O_2, forming the ferryl radical. This reacts with a polyunsaturated lipid to give a lipid radical, which in turn reacts with O_2 to produce the lipid peroxy radical. The second electron is thought to reduce the peroxy radical to the hydroperoxide. It was postulated that the second electron is also provided by the reductase (27); however, no direct proof for this exists. Moreover, redox-labile compounds, such as quinones, may provide an electron to the peroxy radical, generating the semiquinone. This represents a potentially important effect of redox-labile compounds on the propagation of lipid peroxidation. Scheme 2 includes an adaptation of a model proposed by Cadenas et al. (28) for the interaction of quinones with lipid peroxy radicals. Taking the redox potentials for various quinones as examples, that is, from -0.35 V for ubiquinone (UQ^-/UQH_2) to 0.473 V for benzoquinone (BQ^-/BQH_2), and assuming a redox potential of 1 V for $LOO^{\cdot}$/$LOOH$, thermodynamically favorable reactions are evident from the calculated ΔG ranging from -35.1 kcal/mol to -13.5 kcal/mol. This reaction is likely to be facilitated by the rapid reaction of the semiquinone with O_2 to give O_2^- (29) and elimination of O_2^- by superoxide dismutase (SOD). Scheme 2 also shows that this antioxidant-like reaction is similar to that described by reaction of lipid peroxy radicals with vitamin E. However, unlike vitamin E the facile redox cycling of quinones not only generates more reactive oxygen species but contradicts the required stabilization of the radical intermediate.

Since many phenolic compounds can be oxidatively metabolized to quinoid deriva-

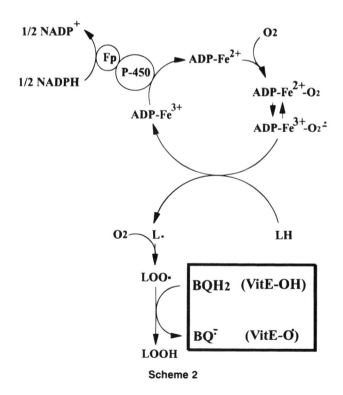

Scheme 2

tives by cytochrome P-450 monooxygenases, as well as by prostaglandin synthetase, myoglobin, or hemoglobin (30–32), the phenoxyl radical products may be toxic by reacting with nucleophilic compounds in the cell. This was recently demonstrated for etoposide, where radical scavenging activity was accompanied by reaction of the phenolic radical intermediate with intracellular thiols leading to glutathione depletion (32).

The reactive oxygen species and derived oxidants (e.g., H_2O_2) capable of initiating lipid peroxidation may arise during the metabolism of many xenobiotics, either by directly abstracting hydrogens from polyunsaturated fatty acids or by oxidizing heme (25). Chemicals that can redox cycle to yield O_2^- either provide two electrons required for direct lipid peroxidation or donate the second electron for peroxy radical reduction as described above. These enzymatically driven autoxidation reactions are analogous to the substrate-specific and stereospecific peroxidations catalyzed by cytochrome P-450 where arachidonic acid (33) or linoleic acid (34) is converted to biologically active peroxides, alcohols, and epoxides. Indeed, peroxidation reactions catalyzed by enzymes such as cytochrome P-450 and lipoxygenase represent a controlled stereospecific peroxidation of distinct fatty acids; however, these enzymes may be stimulated under pathological conditions to oxidize substrates excessively and eventually lipids that are normally not substrates. The rapid generation of hydroperoxides in a damaged tissue would likely facilitate extensive peroxidation reactions. These reactions and conditions that promote them are discussed later. The higher oxidation states of many heme proteins also react with formed lipid hydroperoxides in a *catalysis activation* reaction, resulting in the heterolytic decomposition of hydroperoxides to peroxyl radicals (35). The decomposition reactions for lipid hydroperoxides represent an important (possibly predominant) mechanism for peroxidation of biological lipids.

Some of the major routes for the decomposition of fatty acid hydroperoxides are presented in Scheme 3. A common initial reaction is homolytic scission to form an alkoxy and hydroxyl radical. This decomposition reaction is favored at elevated temperatures and in the presence of agents that readily donate electrons. Well known among such reactions is iron-catalyzed decomposition involving oxidation of a reduced transition metal:

$$Fe^{2+} + LOOH \rightarrow Fe^{3+} + LO^. \qquad [4]$$

The alkoxy radical, being highly reactive, undergoes a number of subsequent radical propagating or decomposition reactions depending on the availability of electron donors and environment (36). In unsaturated lipid systems alkoxyl radicals readily propagate lipid peroxidation by abstraction of a hydrogen from unsaturated lipids to initiate a new cycle of autoxidation. The peroxidation of lipids via decomposition of hydroperoxides to alkoxyl radicals represents a common mechanism for radical-mediated chain branching of lipid peroxidation. The following reactions are an elaboration of the radical chain branching resulting from homolysis of a hydroperoxide.

$$LOOH \rightarrow LO^. \qquad [5]$$

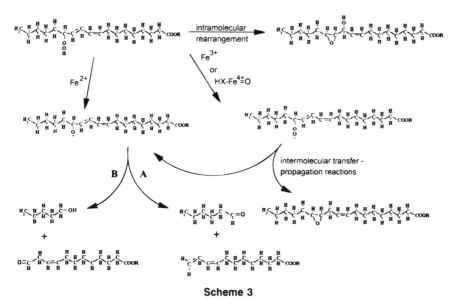

Scheme 3

$$LO' + LH \rightarrow LOH + L' \qquad [6]$$

$$L' + O_2 \rightarrow LOO' \qquad [7]$$

$$LOO' + LH \rightarrow LOOH + L' \qquad [8]$$

reactions (7) + (8) → propagation

Alternately, the alkoxyl radical may proceed via homolytic decomposition to form volatile and nonvolatile products. The breakdown of an unsaturated alkoxy radical proceeds thermally by radical elimination and β-scission of the carbon-carbon bonds adjacent to the oxygen-bearing carbon atom at either the olefin bond (Scheme 3, A) or the carbon-carbon bond away from the olefin (Scheme 3, B). Various carbonyl products arise from these decomposition reactions and are characterized as oxo-compounds and alkyl or alkenyl radicals. These chain-cleavage products are, in part, comprised of reactive aldehydes, which factor significantly in the biological effects of lipid peroxidation. Among the best studied are the α,β-unsaturated alde-hydes such as the volatile acrolein and nonvolatile 4-hydroxynonenal (4HNE) (37). These products appear to arise from linoleic and arachidonic acids according to a reaction mechanism described previously (38). Fragment products such as alkanes and alkenes derive via abstraction reactions proceeding from the alkyl or alkenyl radicals, whereas alcohols, ketones, furans, n-alkanals, 2,4-alkdienals, alktrienals, and 4-hydroxyalkenals arise as products of β-scission. The alkyl radicals derived from ω-3 and ω-6 fatty acids give rise to the volatile gases ethane and pentane frequently used as measures of lipid peroxidation (39,40). In the case of phospholip-ids, the cleavage reactions produce fragments arising from the methyl terminus of the acyl chain (free carbonyls) and alka(e)nes, and fragments remaining bound to the phospholipid (37). A reaction scheme depicting representative products is presented in Figure 1. These decomposition products, whether originating from the breakdown of free fatty acids or from the fatty acyl moieties of phospholipids, appear to have an array of biological effects that can be related to their reactivity with proteins, DNA, and thiol compounds, and, in the case of phospholipid aldehydes, to natural agonists via cell signaling pathways. Examples are presented later.

Transition metals and oxidized heme proteins catalyze propagation of lipid peroxidation by hydrogen atom abstraction. The transient radical states of hemoglobin or myoglobin have been proposed to propagate lipid peroxidation according to the reaction scheme:

$$\cdot Mb^{4+}(\cdot X-Fe^{4+}=O) + LH \rightarrow Mb^{4+}(HX-Fe^{4+}=O) + L\cdot \qquad [9]$$

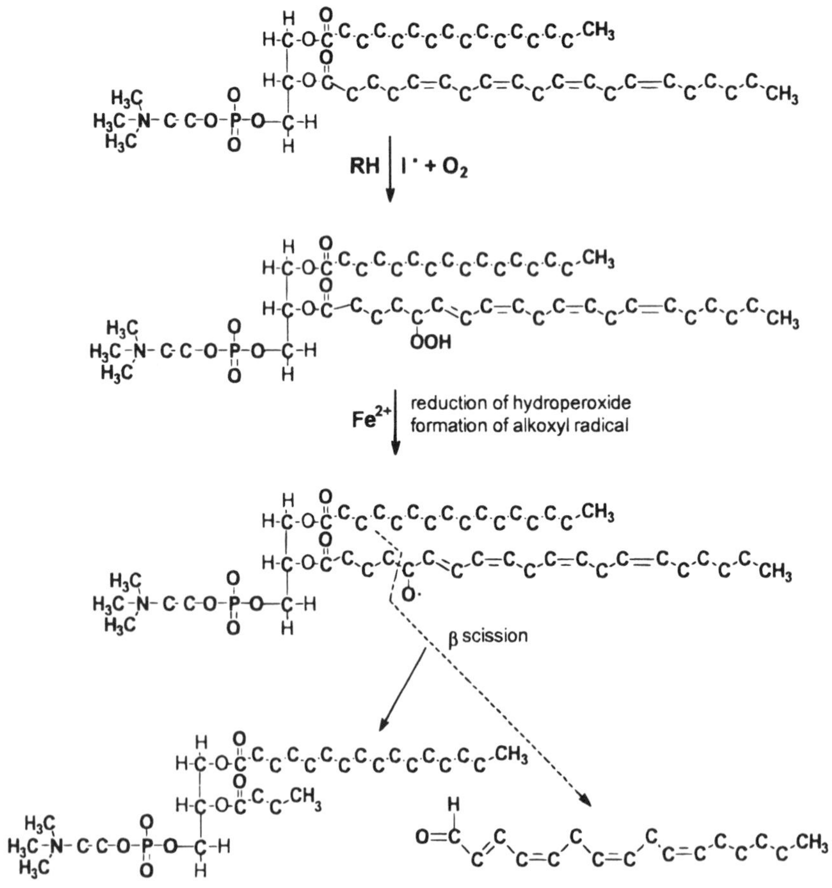

FIG. 1. A reaction scheme depicting representative products.

$$L^{\cdot} + O_2 \rightarrow LOO^{\cdot} \qquad [7]$$

$$LOO^{\cdot} + LH \rightarrow LOOH + L^{\cdot} \qquad [8]$$

Moreover, lipid peroxidation chain reactions may be initiated utilizing formed hydroperoxides by a "catalysis activation" reaction involving Mb^{3+} (41, 35) according to the reaction:

$$Mb^{3+}(HXFe^{3+}) + LOOH \rightarrow {}^{\cdot}Mb^{4+}({}^{\cdot}X-Fe^{4+}=O) + LO^{\cdot} \qquad [10]$$

where ${}^{\cdot}Mb^{4+}({}^{\cdot}X-Fe^{4+}=O)$ initiates new radical chain reactions. Similar reactions have been proposed for hematin or hemin (22, 23) and appear to require preexisting hydroperoxides. Studies utilizing model membrane and low-density lipoproteins indicate that peroxides at low micromolar concentrations may be sufficient for the radical propagation reactions to be sustained (42). Radical propagation through decomposition of hydroperoxides is facilitated by an initiating process known as molecule-assisted homolysis (38), in which a hydrogen bond donor such as an alcohol, acid, or hydroperoxide contributes to bond formation simultaneously with $O-O$ bond homolysis in order to lower the activation energy. Although the bond dissociation energy required to cleave the $O-O$ bond is low ($\sim$44 kcal mol^{-1}), some energy either in the form of heat or good hydrogen donors facilitates decomposition. Olefinic compounds accelerate this process by either a hydrogen atom transfer or by an attack of oxygen to form an olefin radical and a peroxyl radical or an alcohol radical and an alkoxy radical. As described later, heme proteins may play an important role in the amplification of acute tissue injury via rapid and extensive peroxidation of cell lipids utilizing initially small amounts of peroxidation products that arise enzymatically or by other "biological" processes. A good example of peroxide involvement in tissue injury and disease evolution is the development of atherosclerotic lesions. It has been hypothesized that heme proteins in the form of hemoglobin or methemoglobin might promote atherosclerosis by facilitating oxidation from low-density lipoprotein (LDL) containing trace levels of peroxides (43). This is supported by findings that free heme is released from injured cells in the areas of hemorrhagic plaques, iron accumulates in atherosclerotic lesions (44), and cells treated with heme induce the synthesis of heme oxygenase and ferritin as cytoprotectants (45). These lesioned areas also contain pronounced levels of oxidatively modified lipoproteins as measured by immunospecific staining techniques (46).

Hydroperoxides and alkoxyl radical forms of polyunsaturated fatty acids can, under appropriate circumstances (e.g., absence of metal catalysts), undergo intramolecular rearrangement reactions yielding epoxy-alcohols, diols, and ketones, while reactions subsequent to the rearrangement of alkoxy radicals can give rise to epoxyalcohols, ketones and alcohols (by radical disproportionation), and epoxy-ketones. These reactions are detailed by Gardner (36) and represent some of the major high-molecular-weight oxidation products of polyunsaturated fatty acids in food and membrane systems. It has been postulated that polyunsaturated fatty acid hydroperoxides found in membranes containing significant amounts of saturated fatty acids, as well as low levels of hydrogen donors, not only experience reduced rates of peroxidation, as expected, but undergo intramolecular oxygen transfer. The hydroperoxide rearranges to form epoxy-alcohols without involving an alkoxyl radical intermediate (47). Some of these epoxy-fatty acid products have been shown to have unique biological activities, as in the case of arachidonic acid epoxide formed by cytochrome P-450 (48). Similar products also arise from the intramolecular rearrangement of the alkoxy radical to an epoxyallylic radical:

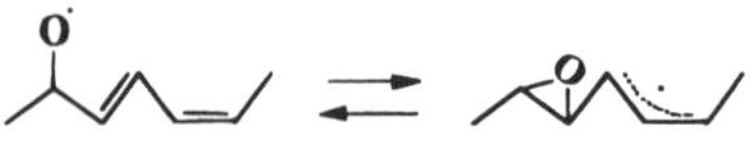

leading to further reactions of major importance based on isolable product yields (36). The epoxyallylic radical combines with oxygen, producing an epoxy-peroxy radical that can participate in further propagation reaction to form the epoxy-hydroperoxide. Decomposition or disproportionation to the alkoxyl radical leads to the formation of epoxyalcohols and epoxyketones:

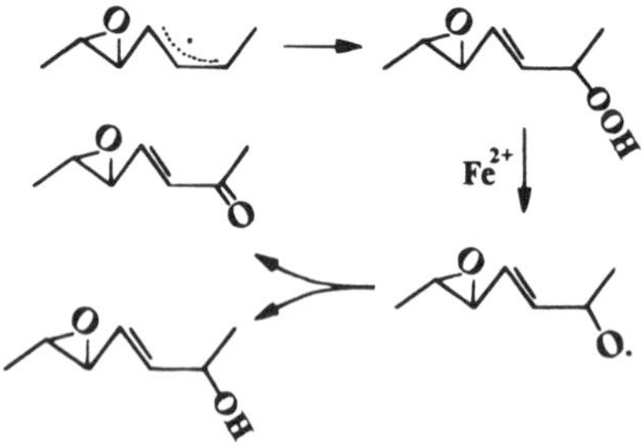

Intermolecular transfer reactions have also been found to be common for unsaturated fatty acid hydroperoxides in ordered systems (47). These reactions take place by intermolecular addition of hydroperoxide oxygen across the double bond of an adjacent fatty acid to yield an alkoxy radical and an epoxide. The former is likely to participate in further radical chain reactions and as such can be viewed as a component of hydroperoxide chain branching reactions. The latter is a commonly isolated product of lipid peroxidation in foods and biological membranes (49, 50, 51). Indeed, epoxides of fatty acids and cholesterol are thought to arise by hydroperoxide addition reactions in systems that contain polyunsaturated fatty acids and cholesterol (52). Nevertheless, one must be cautious in assuming that these products derive by autoxidation (metal or heme protein catalyzed) reactions (53), since some may also arise enzymatically (54). Hydroperoxide addition reactions are an important metabolic activation pathway for chemicals bearing olefinic or good electron donating groups. In many tissues containing low cytochrome P-450 monooxygenase activity this appears to be a primary mechanism by which chemical carcinogens are metabolically activated (30).

Recent attention has been given to bicyclic peroxides and related intermediates as markers of lipid peroxidation. Peroxides of fatty acids bearing three or more unsaturated bonds undergo intramolecular cyclization forming "prostaglandin-like" intermediates of the general structure:

The bicyclic peroxide intermediates of linolenic and arachidonic acids give rise to malondialdehyde (55), a commonly detected lipid peroxidation product that is found among a series of aldehydic products measured as thiobarbituric acid reacting substances (56). The radical intermediates of these fatty acids, as well as linoleic acid, can react with oxygen to form dioxans and dioxolanes (so-called diperoxides) bearing a variety of structures (57), or undergo elimination reactions analogous to that of prostaglandin synthetase to produce isoprostanes (58). An example is provided next for radical cyclization of linolenic acid. Formation of isoprostanes has recently been shown to be an important pathway for lipid peroxidation in vivo, as formation may be in amounts equal to, or even greater than, that of prostaglandins (58,59). Free radical generation of isoprostanes occurs by endocyclization to form bicyclic endoperoxides that derive from the four common positional isomers of arachidonic hydroperoxide. Thus, four isomers of F_2, D_2, and E_2 isoprostanes may arise from the corresponding parent arachidonic acid hydroperoxide (59, 60).

The F_2-isoprostanes (represented by the end product shown in the example) are most commonly encountered following in vivo lipid peroxidation and derive by reduction of the bicyclic endoperoxide (60). The D_2 and E_2 isoprostanes can also form in vivo by rearrangement of the endoperoxide intermediates (59). Various potent biological activities have been described that are analogous to the effects of prostaglandins (58), and thus, many of the prostaglandin-like effects of lipid peroxidation in tissues may be attributed to these products. One of these, 8-epi-prostaglandin $F_{2\alpha}$, is able to cause renal vasoconstriction and platelet aggregation through a site that is distinct from the related thromboxane A_2 receptor (58). An interesting aspect of isoprostane formation relates to the peroxidation of arachidonoyl acyl groups in membrane phospholipids (61). Recent studies indicate that F_2-isoprostanes form while esterified in phospholipids and are subsequently released (possibly by phospholipase A_2 action) into the circulation where they can be measured. This has been used to some advantage by commercial assay kits designed to measure in vivo lipid peroxidation; however, the reliability of these assays has yet to be established. As mentioned, several prostaglandin-like effects can be attributed to the biological effects of isoprostanes (58).

REACTIONS OF LIPID PEROXIDATION PRODUCTS

Formation of reactive oxygen species along with other excited-state products is found during peroxide decomposition reactions. Accumulation of lipid hydroperoxides with progressive lipid peroxidation leads to a series of decomposition, radical combination, and termination reactions that are described elsewhere (62). Well known among these is the Russell mechanism, where combination of two peroxy radicals forms a tetroxide intermediate.

$$ROO^{.} + ROO^{.} \rightarrow [ROOOOR] \rightarrow RO + ROH + O_2 \qquad [11a]$$

The tetroxide decays to form the expected triplet and singlet *excited-state products*, detected as singlet oxygen and excited carbonyls, and measured by formation of ketone and alcohol end products (63). Products may be generated in an electronically excited state during which part of the energy is concentrated in a ketone in the excited triplet state. Quenching of the triplet carbonyl by oxygen in a solvent cage is thought to support formation of singlet oxygen.

$$[ROOOOR] \rightarrow {}^3RO^* + ROH + O_2 \qquad [11b]$$

$$[{}^3RO^* + {}^3O_2]_{cage} \rightarrow RO + {}^1O_2 \qquad [11c]$$

These and other volatile and nonvolatile species are representative of the various stages of lipid peroxidation. In the course of peroxidation entailing the initiation, propagation, and termination reactions, formation of polymeric and carbonyl products indicates the prevalence of chain termination reactions. Accordingly, Figure 2 summarizes the stages of lipid peroxidation on the basis of the relative levels of major products.

Lipid hydroperoxides may react with proteins via a concerted mechanism involving addition of the peroxy radical to free amino groups, including those found in phosphatidylethanolamine (37). A concerted reaction of the hydroperoxide with protein has been proposed to involve release of $O_2^{-.}$ concurrent with the generation of the covalent linkage with protein, a reaction partially inhibited by SOD. The apparently metal-independent reaction may account for more of the fluorescent products found after LDL oxidation than is evidenced by reactions with aldehydic products (64). This reaction may take place in parallel with formation of Schiff bases as in the case of reactions with aldehydes. The spectrum for the fluorescent products of the concerted reaction with peroxyl radicals resembles the spectrum obtained for oxidized LDL, suggesting that similar reactions may occur during to the oxidation of lipoproteins in vivo. Evidence for the formation of $O_2^{-.}$ during the conjugate formation is consistent with previous findings describing $O_2^{-.}$ production during lipoxygenase-catalyzed peroxide decomposition (65). Lipoxygenase-mediated NADPH oxidation in the presence of linoleic acid has also been demonstrated (65). This is thought to occur by hydroperoxidase activity of lipoxygenase, generating LOO or LO from LOOH. LOO is able to propagate lipid peroxidation and to

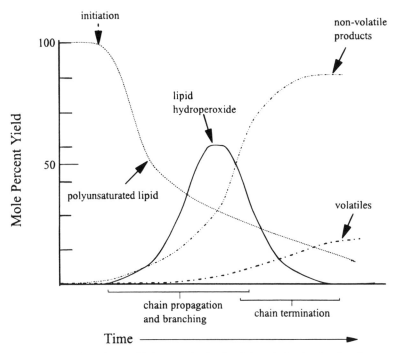

FIG. 2. The stages of lipid peroxidation on the basis of the relative levels of major products are summarized.

epoxidize olefinic moieties in a variety of chemicals (10, 30, 47), constituting a metabolic activation mechanism (66). LO· not only propagates lipid peroxidation but generates $O_2^{-·}$ after reaction with molecular oxygen (67). Activated species resulting from hydroperoxide decomposition are evidenced by the chemiluminescence measured directly or through the use of enhancers such as luminol (68). The kinetics of chemiluminescence signal emission suggest that formation and decomposition reactions are quite rapid in the presence of catalysts and can continue during the course of peroxide formation and accumulation. Ferric-catalyzed formation of peroxy radicals from hydroperoxides, and alkoxy radical formation utilizing ferrous iron, represent one-electron cleavage products (69) and can undergo concerted disproportionation reactions to produce chemiluminescent carbonyl fragments according to the Russell mechanism. Peroxidase activity involving the ferric and ferrous states of lipoxygenase gives rise to these hydroperoxide breakdown products through analogous transition-state intermediates (70). Alternate sources for excited carbonyls are described elsewhere (71).

Reactive aldehydes derived from lipid peroxidation have been extensively studied due to the relatively large quantities formed by the degradation of both ω-6 and ω-3 polyunsaturated fatty acids and also as products of liver mixed-function oxidase metabolism of certain alkaloids (37). 4-Hydroxynonenal (4HNE) attacks electrophilically the thiols and ϵ-amino moieties of proteins. Reactions with protein sulfhydryls are typified by the Michael addition forming a glutathionyl adduct:

Both reactions are reversible, although reaction products with thiols are more stable. Inactivation of enzymes by 4-HNE may account for some of the inhibitory effect of oxidized lipids on cells, particularly for enzymes with functional -SH groups; however, these enzymes can be reactivated in the presence of excess GSH, cysteine, and other thiols. The reaction with ϵ-amino moieties of lysine residues in apoB-100 of low-density lipoproteins (LDL) accompanies the generation of modified LDL, which are rapidly assimilated into atherosclerotic plaques (72). Similar reactions have been proposed for the inactivation of proteins following ischemia and reperfusion (73). Evidence that reactions of 4-HNE (74) and malondialdehyde (75) with apoB-100 involve lysine residues comes from detection of the modified lipoprotein using monoclonal antibodies raised against aldehyde-lysine conjugates. The accumulation of these conjugates appears to be highly dependent on the extent of lipid peroxidation. These adducts have been identified in modified LDL and in atherosclerotic lesions containing large numbers of macrophages (74, 76). Accumulation of the modified lipoproteins is mediated by rapid and unregulated uptake via the scavenger receptors in macrophages and endothelial cells, and the modified LDL becomes a better ligand for these receptors as it progressively oxidizes and accumulates the aldehyde-protein adducts. Detailed studies have shown that modifications at specific lysine-rich residues on the apoprotein B-100 (the receptor binding domain) are essential for the scavenger receptor-mediated uptake of LDL and that approximately 15% of the lysine groups must be modified before scavenger receptor uptake predominates (77). The role of lipid peroxidation is clearly central to the formation of these modified and atherogenic lipoproteins; however, these modifications go beyond effects involving the uptake and processing of lipoproteins. Recent studies show that the enhanced uptake and receptor-mediated delivery of the oxidized lipoproteins also provides a "targeted" means for delivering oxidized lipids and their decomposition products to intracellular sites, resulting in the signaling and expression of stress response genes (78, 79), cytokines, and adhesion molecules (80) and expression of enzymes regulating cholesterol homeostasis (81). These events may be evoked either directly or indirectly through the presence of lipid peroxidation products and, in a concerted manner, facilitate the development of an atherosclerotic lesion.

The association of increased atherosclerosis with exposures to dioxins (TCDD) has been formulated by implicating a role for lipid peroxidation and oxidant stress. The link between exposures to TCDD and atherosclerosis comes from a series of epidemiological studies, including accidental (82, 83) and occupational exposures (84). Studies with animals have shown that TCDD administration causes reductions in hepatic LDL binding, decrease in adipose lipoprotein lipase activity (85), and elevations in serum cholesterol, due to downregulation of lipoprotein receptors. Histological examination of the vessels showed evidence of preatherosclerotic lesions (85). Elevated levels of lipid peroxidation products were found after a 50 μg/kg dose of TCDD (86). Although a mechanism for TCDD induction of lipid peroxidation has not been firmly established, it is postulated that increased lipid deposition in the vascular intima may provide a pool of lipid susceptible to cell-mediated oxidation. Macrophages are suspected as mediators of oxidation due to the high infiltration seen after TCDD administration (85). Recent evidence indicates TCDD activates key protein kinases involved in signal transduction pathways for growth factors and for enzymes and receptors involved in lipoprotein metabolism, apparently by interaction with the Ah receptor (87). The extent to which this involves lipid peroxidation and the known effects of peroxidation products on cell signaling has yet to be clearly demonstrated.

EFFECTS ON CELL SIGNALING EVENTS

Lipid peroxidation products have been shown to participate in or perturb cell signaling events. Based on numerous examples where signal transduction processes are accompanied by oxidationreduction reactions, there are presently many studies examining the various redox signaling mediators. Among the most widely studied at present is nitric oxide, a radical species that interacts with heme-iron proteins, such as guanylyl cyclase or thiol groups, to initiate signaling events (88). However, other biological oxidants have been studied, especially H_2O_2 and lipid hydroperoxides or derived reactive aldehydes. The molecular events associated with peroxide-mediated signaling have been partly delineated, based largely on similarities to the signaling pathways described for biological agonists and cytokines.

H_2O_2 and organic peroxides are known to induce increases in intracellular calcium concentrations (89). Although part of the action of H_2O_2 appears to involve increases in intracellular calcium levels or calcium oscillations via a phosphoinositide (IP_3) mediated process, there is little evidence that this applies to organic peroxides (90,91). In the case of *tert*-butyl hydroperoxide, the increases in intracellular calcium may be due to oxidation of thiols forming mixed disulfides in calcium channels (92). Indeed, *tert*-butyl hydroperoxide appears to inhibit formation of IP_3 as elicited by agonists such as ADP (91). The suggestion that lipid peroxidation may also evoke similar responses comes from studies showing release of calcium from sarcoplasmic reticulum or intracellular membranes following treatments with oxygen radical-generating systems (91,93,94). Recently, Sweetman et al. (95) reported that influx of calcium as well as its release from intracellular stores could be induced after treatments with micromolar concentrations of linoleic acid hydroperoxide. The mechanism(s) by which peroxides or derived products cause the increase in intracellular calcium, and the sources of calcium, are not clear and remain an area for future study. There is evidence indicating formation of membrane pores or ionophore-like activity (96) and perturbations in ion pumps (97) that cause influx of calcium. Release from internal stores may include the mitochondria, possibly linked to oxidation of purine nucleotides (98), and release from other membrane stores (e.g., endoplasmic reticulum). This may take place through either agonist- or voltage-sensitive receptors (99) or inhibition of calcium sequestration enzymes (95). Rapid increases in intracellular calcium were accompanied by a stimulation of protein kinase C (PKC). This response resembles the reported activation of PKC following mild oxidation. It is postulated that oxidation of vicinal thiols and formation of disulfide bridges within the regulatory domain of PKC converts the enzyme to a state exhibiting calcium- and phospholipid-independent catalytic activity (100,101). Oxidation of amino acids is involved in PKC binding to the membrane, and this oxidation may take place via peroxidation of unsaturated fatty acids in proximity to specific amino acid residues of PKC. Further oxidation has been shown to inactivate PKC (100), indicating that the enzyme may undergo bimodal regulation based on the extent of oxidative modification. Accordingly, the redox status of the cell and the activities of reducing enzyme systems such as thioredoxin (102) or the presence of thiol agents can inhibit modification and regulate enzyme activity (103). The implication that PKC activity may be modulated by its redox state is far-reaching when one considers the mediating effects of peroxides on cell signaling via transcription factor activation.

Among the factors that allow cells to respond to stimuli by means of transcriptional activation of genes are the ubiquitous members of the NFkB/Rel family of transcription factors. These proteins are regulated at the transcriptional and posttranscriptional level, and the latter clearly facilitates activation, transduction to the nucleus, and binding to the promoter regions of cytokine genes (104). Maintenance of transcriptional activation requires continuous translocation of the activated form of NFkB to the nucleus. Activation of NFkB involves a dissociation of the inhibitory component, IkB, initiated by phosphorylation. NFkB appears to become activated by redox events in cells (105) and thus is regarded as an oxidative stress response factor. Baeuerle et al. (106) reported that peroxides, including lipid hydroperoxide, activated NFkB. Oxidatively modified LDLs also activate NFkB and induce NFkB controlled gene expression of proteins involved in the development of atheromatous lesions (107,108). The active components in modified LDL appear to be peroxidized lipids, based, in part, on evidence that linoleic acid hydroperoxide mimics the effects of modified LDL in terms of induction of proteins required for inflammatory cell migration and adhesion (109). Activation of NFkB by H_2O_2, the potentiation of phorbol ester activation of NFkB by H_2O_2, and the suppression of these effects by antioxidants (110) suggest that phorbol ester and peroxide signals converge into a common redox-sensitive pathway.

The ability to induce the expression of cytokine genes, along with a series of other acute response proteins in vascular cells, is shared by both oxidized LDL and fatty acid hydroperoxides. Treatment of endothelial cells with either "oxidant" results in the augmentation in their ability to express cytokine-mediated formation of adhesion molecules (VCAM-1 and ICAM-1) (109). Inhibition of these responses by antioxidants is taken as evidence that the effects occur through cellular oxidant stress involving redox-sensitive transcriptional or posttranscriptional factors (110).

Similarly, the induction of factors such as monocyte chemotactic peptide (MCP-1) is evoked by oxidized LDL and lipid peroxidation products by means of oxidant-sensitive transcriptional factors (111–113). In each of these cases the oxidant-sensitive/antioxidant-inhibitable mechanism involves activation of NFkB and binding to promoters of these genes sharing an NFkB enhancer motif (111, 113, 114). Although the precise signaling processes remain to be elucidated, the convergence of the pathways with those described for cytokines such as tumor necrosis factor α (TNFα) suggests a PKC-mediated phosphorylation and activation of NFkB (104). These peroxide signaling pathways have been methodically shown to stimulate chemotaxis and adhesion of inflammatory cells to vascular loci exhibiting enhanced levels of oxidant generation and lipid peroxidation, or to cells exposed to oxidants. These studies have focused on early atherogenesis; however, inflammatory cell signaling may follow parallel paths for other diseases where generation of oxidants can be demonstrated.

CELL INJURY AND ACTIVATION OF LIPOXYGENASE

The conversion of arachidonic and linoleic acids to eicosanoids, along with other polyunsaturated fatty acids, is in significant measure catalyzed by various mammalian lipoxygenases. Lipoxygenases comprise a family of nonheme proteins with stereospecific dioxygenase activity. The primary products of lipoxygenase are a series of isomeric hydroperoxides, each derived from a specific lipoxygenase (9). These hydroperoxides are converted to an array of biologically active products, referred to in general as eicosanoids. A salient feature of lipoxygenase activity is that the enzyme is converted from its resting (ferrous) state to the active (ferric) state by oxidation involving lipid hydroperoxide formed either by autoxidation or enzymatically (10). This activation may occur either directly, through gradual accumulation of hydroperoxides via the enzymes own action, by chemicals that stimulate lipid peroxidation, or by disruption of membranes from which lipoxygenase substrates are derived. Membrane phospholipid disruption represents a potentially important means by which lipid autoxidation is facilitated (115) and lipoxygenase activity potentially enhanced (116,117). The activation of lipoxygenase has been observed when membrane phospholipid structure becomes disordered, permitting the enzyme to oxidize unsaturated fatty acyl moieties in phospholipids directly (117) or attack substrates that are released through activation of phospholipases (118). Under these circumstances, very high rates of catalytic activity may be manifested as unlimited substrates become available and peroxide concentrations accumulate to levels where lipoxygenase is fully activated (119).

Disruption of the membrane bilayer is well known to stimulate a variety of phospholipases (120). Phospholipase activation may occur through signaling reactions leading to elevations in intracellular calcium (121) and enzyme phosphorylation mediated by activation of protein kinases (122). Stimulation of such signaling events by lipid peroxides and other reactive oxygen species was discussed earlier and appears to apply to the activation of high-molecular-weight phospholipase A$_2$ (95). Alternately, imposed structural transitions from bilayer to nonbilayer organization also activate phospholipase(s) A$_2$ without the apparent need for posttranscriptional modification. The biophysical basis for such activation is described elsewhere (120). Release of unsaturated fatty acids from phospholipids represents a potential mechanism for phospholipase A$_2$-mediated lipoxygenase activation.

A reverse situation for enzymatic peroxidation of membrane phospholipids followed by phospholipase-mediated degradation may also be manifested through activation of mammalian 15-lipoxygenase. This lipoxygenase has been shown to directly oxidize membrane phospholipids (9). The resulting hydroperoxide residues in phospholipids disrupt membrane structure (123), and the oxidized phospholipids are excellent substrates for phospholipase A$_2$ (118), which rapidly degrades membranes enriched in oxidized phospholipids (124). Recently, it was shown that antioxidant chemicals (e.g., probucol and butylated hydroxytoluene, BHT) can stimulate 15-lipoxygenase (117). The stimulation is accounted for by the physical disruption of membrane structure by these agents and oxidation is limited to lipoxygenase activity as these agents suppress the free radical-mediated oxidation of the membrane lipids. It is possible that other chemicals that disrupt membranes may also stimulate lipoxygenases, but it is also plausible that agents with little or no antioxidant activity may stimulate peroxidation by physical disruption of lipid structure.

The activation of 15-lipoxygenase appears to have a role in the maturation of cells such as erythrocytes, keratinocytes and lens epithelium (9). This activation appears to be part of the biologically programmed degradation of subcellular organelles. It is tempting to speculate that this programmed activity of lipoxygenases has evolutionary parallels in both the animal and plant kingdoms that are related on the basis of cellular differentiation and defense. In plants, lipoxygenases appear to be involved in seedling germination, seasonal blanching of leaf pigments, generation of wound/distress hormones, and formation of protective barriers against infestation (10,125). Mammalian examples have largely been identified in inflammatory cells and are represented by the leukotrienes and related eicosanoids (126). Evidence that such a diverse defense mechanism may go awry is best found in the various forms of tissue injury resulting from excessive production of lipoxygenase products. Examples include septic shock (127), ischemia/reperfusion, and atherosclerosis. Reperfusion of ischemic tissues has been shown to induce translocation of 5-lipoxygenase (128) leading to leukotriene production, but in addition, activation of 12-lipoxygenase (129) and 15-lipoxygenase (125) has been reported. Attenuation of ischemia/reperfusion injury by lipoxygenase inhibitors and antioxidants indicates the important role of lipoxygenase-mediated reactions in the common pathological condition. Similar observations have been made with respect to the formation of atherosclerotic lesions. The oxidation of LDL has been proposed to contribute to formation of atherosclerotic lesions (72), and although there are several possible sources for oxidants, activation of 15-lipoxygenase was found to trigger LDL oxidation with considerable facility (130). The immunological colocalization of 15-lipoxygenase and oxidized LDL in endothelial cells and the subendothelial space (46) and inhibition of LDL oxidation by lipoxygenase inhibitors (130, 131) provide evidence that lipoxygenase may serve as a trigger for progressive LDL oxidation. It is plausible that either specific stimuli or general tissue injury (132) can trigger lipoxygenase activity. In either case, enzymes alone or in conjunction with a range of oxidizing agents may account for the generation of lipid peroxidation products and the subsequent propagation of lipid peroxidation.

ACKNOWLEDGMENTS

Preparation of this chapter was made possible through a grant from the National Institutes of Health (HL45206), along with support from Astra/Merck and Pfizer Pharmaceuticals.

REFERENCES

1. Kappus H. Oxidative stress in chemical toxicity. *Arch Toxicol.* 1987;60:144–149.
2. Horton AA, Fairhurst S. Lipid peroxidation and mechanisms of toxicity. *CRC Crit Rev Toxicol* 1987;18:27–79.
3. Dargel R. Lipid peroxidationA common pathogenic mechanism? *Exp Toxicol Pathol* 1992; 44:169–181.
4. Brunmark A, Cadenas E. Redox and addition chemistry of quinoid compounds and its biological implications. *Free Radical Biol Med* 1989;7:435–477.
5. Kappus H. Overview of enzyme systems involved in bioreduction of drugs and in redox cycling. *Biochem Pharmacol* 1986;35:1–6.
6. Garcia-Martinez P, Winston GW, Metash-Dickey C, Ohara SC, Livingston DR. Nitrofurantoin-stimulated reactive oxygen species production and genotoxicity in digestive gland microsomes and cytosol of the common mussel (*Mytilus edulis* L.). *Toxicol Appl Pharmacol* 1995;131(2):332–341.
7. Bagchi M, Stohs SJ. In vitro induction of reactive oxygen species by 2,3,7,8-tetrachlorodibenzo-*p*-dioxin, endrin, and lindane in rat peritoneal macrophages, and hepatic mitochondria and microsomes. *Free Radical Biol Med* 1993;14(1):11–18.
8. Wendel A, Jaeschke H. Drug-induced lipid peroxidation in mice-III: Glutathione content of liver, kidney, and spleen after intravenous administration of free and liposomally entrappped glutathione. *Biochem Pharmacol* 1982;31(2):3607–3611.
9. Schewe T, Kuhn H. Do 15-lipoxygenases have a common biological role? *Trends Biochem Sci* 1991;16(10):369–373.
10. Naidu KA, Naidu KA, Kulkarni AP. Lipoxygenase: A nonspecific oxidative pathway for xenobiotic metabolism. *Prostaglandins, Leukotrienes, and Essential Fatty Acids* 1994;50:155–159.
11. Chambers, JQ. Electrochemistry of quinones. In: Patai S, ed. *The Chemistry of Quinonoid Compounds*. London: Wiley and Sons, 1974;737–791.
12. Mason R. Chapter 2, this volume.
13. Boveris A, Cadenas E. Production of superoxide radicals and hydrogen peroxide in mitochondria. In: Oberley LW, ed. *Superoxide Dismutase*, Vol. II. Boca Raton, FL: CRC Press, 1982;16–28.
14. Galaris D, Buffinton G, Hochstein P, Cadenas E. Role of ferryl myoglobin in lipid peroxidation and its reduction to met- or oxymyoglobin by glutathione, quinones, quinone thioether derivatives, and ascorbate. In: Vigo-Pelfrey C, ed. *Membrane Lipid Oxidation*, Vol. I. Boca Raton, FL: CRC Press, 1990;270–281.
15. Cadenas E. Antioxidant and prooxidant functions of DTdiaphorase in quinone metabolism. *Biochem Pharmacol* 1995;49:127–140.
16. Halliwell B, Gutteridge JMC. Metal ions in human disease: An overview. In: Packer L, Glazer, AN, eds. *Methods in Enzymology*, Vol. 186: *Oxygen Radicals in Biological Systems*. San Diego, California: Academic Press, 1990;1–85.
17. Schaich KM, Borg DC. Fenton reactions in lipid phases. *Lipids* 1988;23:570–579.

18. King KN, Winfield ME. The mechanism of metmyoglobin oxidation. *J Biol Chem* 1963; 238:1520–1528.
19. de Silva DM, Aust SD. Ferritin and ceruloplasmin in oxidative damage: Review and recent findings. *Can J Physiol Pharmacol* 1993;71(9):84322–84705.
20. Ehrenwald E, Chisholm GM, Fox PL. Intact human ceruloplasmin oxidatively modifies low density lipoprotein. *J. Clin Invest* 1994;93(4):1493–1501.
21. Tappel AL. Unsaturated lipid oxidation catalyzed by hematin compounds. *J Biol Chem* 1955;217:721–733.
22. Kim E, Sevanian A. Hematin and peroxide catalyzed peroxidation of phospholipid liposomes. *Arch Biochem Biophys* 1991;288:324–330.
23. Balla G, Jacob HS, Eaton JW, Belcher JD, Vercellotti GM. Hemin: A possible physiological mediator of low density lipoprotein oxidation and endothelial injury. *Arterioscler Thromb* 1991;11(6):1700–1711.
24. Giulivi C, Romero FJ, Cadenas E. The interaction of Trolox C, a water-soluble vitamin E analog, with ferrylmyoglobin: Reduction of the oxoferryl moiety. *Arch Biochem Biophys* 1992;299(2):302–312.
25. Estabrook RW, Werringloer J. Cytochrome P450: Its role in oxygen activation for drug metabolism. In: Donald MJ, Robert RG, eds. *Drug Metabolism Concepts*. Washington, DC: American Chemical Society, 1976;1.
26. Ernster L, Lind C, Nordenbrand K, Thor H, Orrenius S. NADPH-cytochrome P450 reductase as an oxygen-radical generator. In: Nozaki M, Yamamoto S, Ishimura Y, Coon MJ, Ernster L, Estabrook RW, eds. *Oxygenases and Oxygen Metabolism*. New York: Academic Press, 1982;357–370.
27. Sevanian A, Nordenbrand K, Kim E, Ernster L, Hochstein P. Microsomal lipid peroxidation: the role of NADPH-cytochrome P450 reductase and cytochrome P450. *Free Radical Biol Med* 1990;8:145–152.
28. Cadenas E, Hochstein P, Ernster L. Pro- and antioxidant functions of quinones and quinone reductases in mammalian cells. In: Meister A, ed. *Advances in Enzymology and Related Areas of Molecular Biology*, Vol. 65. New York: John Wiley and Sons, 1992;97–146.
29. Butler H, Hoey BM. The apparent inhibition of superoxide dismutase activity by quinones. *J Free Radical Biol Med* 1986;2(1):77–81.
30. Marnett LJ. Arachidonic acid metabolism and tumor initiation. In: Marnett LJ, ed. *Arachidonic Acid Metabolism and Tumor Initiation*. Boston: Nijhoff, 1985;39–82.
31. Sinha BK, Trush MA, Kalyanaraman B. Microsomal interactions and inhibition of lipid peroxidation by etoposide (VP-16): Implication for mode of action. *Biochem Pharmacol* 1985;34(11):2036–2040.
32. Tyurina YY, Tyurin VA, Yalowich JC, Quinn PJ, Claycamp HG, Schor NF, Pitt BR, Kagan VE. Phenoxy radicals of etoposide (VP-16) can directly oxidize intracellular thiols: Protective versus damaging effects of phenolic antioxidants. *Toxicol Appl. Pharmacol* 1995;131(2):277–288.
33. Capdevila J, Marnett LJ, Chacos N, Prough RA, Estabrook RW. Cytochrome P-450-dependent oxygenation of arachidonic acid to hydroxyicosatetraenoic acids. *Proc Natl Acad Sci USA* 1982;79(3):767–770.
34. Oliw EH, Brodowsky ID, Hornsten L, Hamberg M. Bis-allylic hydroxylation of polyunsaturated fatty acids by hepatic monoooxygenases and its relation to the enzymatic and nonenzymatic formation of conjugated hydroxy fatty acids. *Arch Biochem Biophys* 1993;300(1):434–439.
35. Kanner J, Harel S. Initiation of membranal lipid peroxidation by activated metmyoglobin and methemoglobin. *Arch Biochem Biophys* 1985;237(2):314–321.
36. Gardner HW. Reactions of hydroperoxide products of high molecular weight. In: Chan, HW-S, ed. *Autoxidation of Unsaturated Lipids*. Orlando, FL: Academic Press, 1987;51–94.
37. Esterbauer H, Schaur RJ, Zollner H. Chemistry and biochemistry of 4-hydroxynonenal, malonaldehyde, and related aldehydes. *Free Radical Biol Med* 1991;11:81–128.
38. Pryor WA. The role of free radical reactions in biological systems. In: Pryor WA, ed. *Free Radicals in Biology*. New York: Academic Press, 1976;1–50.
39. Thelen M, Wendel A. Drug induced lipid peroxidation in mice-V. Ethane production and glutathione release in the isolated liver upon perfusion with acetaminophen. *Biochem Pharmacol* 1983; 32(11):1701–1706.
40. Tappel AL, Dillard CJ. In vivo lipid peroxidation: Measurement via exhaled pentane and protection by vitamin E. *Fed Proc* 1981;40(2):174–178.
41. Galaris D, Mira D, Sevanian A, Cadenas E, Hochstein P. Co-oxidation of salicylate and cholesterol during the oxidation of myoglobin by H_2O_2. *Arch Biochem Biophys* 1988;262(1): 221–231.

42. Thomas JP, Kalyanaraman B, Girotti AW. Involvement of preexisting lipid hydroperoxides in Cu^{2+}-stimulated oxidation of low-density lipoprotein. *Arch Biochem Biophys* 1994;315(2):244–254.

43. Belcher JD, Balla J, Jacobs DR, Gross M, Jacob HS, Vercellotti GM. Vitamin E, LDL, and endothelium: Brief oral vitamin suppelmentation prevents oxidized LDL-mediated vascular injury in vitro. *Arterioscler Thromb* 1993;13:1779–1789.

44. Juckett MB, Balla J, Balla G, Burke B, Jacob HS, Vercellotti GM. Ferritin protects endothelial cells from oxidized low-density lipoprotein mediated cytotoxicity. *Clin Res* 1993;41:162A.

45. Balla J, Jacob HS, Balla G, Nath K, Eaton JW, Vercelloti GW. Endothelial cell heme uptake from heme proteins: induction of sensitization to oxidant damage. *Proc Natl Acad Sci USA* 1993;90:9285–9289.

46. Yla-Herttuala S, Rosenfield ME, Parthasarathy S, Glass CK, Sigal E, Witztum JL, Steinberg D. Colocalization of 15-lipoxygenase mRNA and protein with epitopes of oxidized low density lipoprotein in macrophage-rich areas of atherosclerotic regions. *Proc Natl Acad Sci USA* 1990; 87:6959–6963.

47. Mead JF, Wu GS, Stein RA, Gelmont D, Sevanian A, Sohlberg E, McElhaney RN. Mechanism of protection against membrane peroxidation. In: Yagi K, ed. *Lipid Peroxides in Biology and Medicine.* New York: Academic Press, 1982;161–178.

48. Sakairi Y, Jacobson HR, Noland TD, Capdevila JH, Falck JR, Breyer MD. 5,6-EET inhibits ion transport in collecting duct by stimulating endogenous prostaglandin synthesis. *Am J Physiol* 1995;268(5 Pt 2):F931–F939.

49. Sevanian A, Mead JF, Stein RA. Epoxides as products of lipid autoxidation in rat lungs. *Lipids* 1979;14(7):634–643.

50. Sessa DJ, Gardner HW, Kleiman R, Weisleder D. Oxygenated fatty acid constituents of soybean phosphatidylcholines. *Lipids* 1977;12:613–619.

51. Capdevila J, Pramanik B, Napoli JL, Manna S, Falck JR. Arachidonic acid epoxidation: epoxyeicosatrienoic acids are endogenous constituents of rat liver. *Arch Biochem Biophys* 1984;231(2):511–517.

52. Smith L. Cholesterol oxidation. In: Vigo-Pelfrey C, ed. *Membrane Lipid Oxidation*, Vol. I. Boca Raton, FL: CRC Press, 1990;130–154.

53. Hamberg M. A novel transformation of 13-LS-hydroperoxy-9,11-octadecadienoic acid. *Biochim Biophys Acta* 1983;752(2):191–197.

54. Egmond MR, Veldink GA, Vliegenthart JFG, Boldingh J. On the positional specificity of the oxygenation reaction catalyzed by soybean lipoxygenase 1. *Biochim Biophys Acta.* 1975; 409:399–401.

55. Pryor AW, Stanley PA. A suggested mechanism for the production of malonaldehyde during the autoxidation of polyunsaturated fatty acids. Nonenzymatic production of prostaglandin endoperoxides during autoxidation. *J Org Chem* 1975;40:3615–3617.

56. Martin RA, Richard C, Rousseau-Richard C. Oxidation of linoleic acid and related or similar compounds. In: Vigo-Pelfrey C, ed. *Membrane Lipid Oxidation*, Vol. I. Boca Raton, FL: CRC Press, 1990;63–99.

57. Chan HW-S, Coxon DT. Lipid hydroperoxides. In: Chan HW-S, ed. *Autoxidation of Unsaturated Lipids.* Orlando, FL: Academic Press, 1987;17–50.

58. Morrow JD, Hill KE, Burk RF, Nammour TM, Badr KF, Roberts LJ II. A series of prostaglandin F_2-like compounds are produced in vivo in humans by a non-cyclooxygenase, free-radical catalyzed mechanism. *Proc Natl Acad Sci USA* 1990;87:9383–9387.

59. Morrow JD, Minton TA, Mukundan CR, Campbell MD, Zackert WE, Daniel VC, Badr KF, Blair IA, Roberts LJ II. Free radical-induced generation of isoprostanes *in vivo*: Evidence for the formation of D-ring and E-ring isoprostanes. *J Biol Chem* 1994;269:4317–4326.

60. Awad JA, Morrow JD, Takahashi K, Roberts LJ II. Identification of non-cyclooxygenase-derived prostanoid(F_2-isoprostane) metabolites in human urine and plasma. *J Biol Chem* 1993; 263:4161–4169.

61. Morrow JD, Awad JA, Boss JJ, Blair IA, Roberts LJ II. Non-cyclooxygenase-derived prostanoids formed in situ on phospholipids. *Proc Natl Acad Sci USA* 1992;89:10721–10725.

62. Sevanian A, Hochstein P. Mechanisms and consequences of lipid peroxidation in biological systems. *Annu Rev Nutr* 1985;5:365–390.

63. Cadenas E. Lipid peroxidation during the oxidation of haemoproteins by hydroperoxides: Relation to electronically excited state formation. *J Biolumin Chemilumin* 1989;4:208–218.

64. Fruebis J, Parthasarathy S, Steinberg D. Evidence for a concerted reaction between lipid hydroperoxides and polypeptides. *Proc Natl Acad Sci USA* 1992;89:10588–10592.

65. Roy P, Roy SK, Mitra A,Kulkarni AP. Superoxide generation by lipoxygenase in the presence of NADH and NADPH. *Biochim Biophys Acta* 1994;1214:171–179.
66. Marnett LJ. Prostaglandin synthase-mediated metabolism of carcinogens and a potential role for peroxyl radicals as reactive intermediates. *Environ. Health Perspect.* 1990;88:5–12.
67. Chamulitrat W, Hughes MF, Eling TE, Mason RP. Superoxide and peroxyl radical generation from the reduction of polyunsaturated fatty acid hydroperoxides by soybean lipoxygenase. *Arch Biochem Biophys* 1991;290(1):153–159.
68. Vladimirov YA, Olenev VI, Suslova TB, Cheremisina ZP. Lipid peroxidation in mitochondrial membrane. *Adv Lipid Res* 1980;17:173–249.
69. Terao J. Reactions of lipid hydroperoxides. In: Vigo–Pelfrey C, ed. *Membrane Lipid Oxidation*, Vol. I. Boca Raton, FL: CRC Press, 1990;219–238.
70. Schulte-Herbruggen T, Sies H. The peroxidase/oxidase activity of soybean lipoxygenase—I. Triplet excited carbonyls from rhe reaction with isobutanal and the effect of glutathione. *Photochem. Photobiol.* 1989;49:697–704.
71. Cadenas E, Giulivi C, Ursini F, Boveris A. Electronically excited state formation during lipid peroxidation. In: Tyson CA, Frazier JM, eds. *Methods in Toxicology*. Orlando, FL: Academic Press. (in press).
72. Steinberg D, Parthasarathy S, Carew TE, Khoo JC, Witztum JL. Beyond cholesterol: modifications of low density lipoprotein that increase its atherogenicity. *N Engl J Med* 1989;320:915–924.
73. van Winkle WB, Snuggs M, Miller JC, Buja LM. Cytoskeletal alterations in cultured cardiomyocytes following exposure to the lipid peroxidation product, 4-nhydroxynonenal. *Cell Motil Cytoskeleton* 1994;28:119–134.
74. Rosenfeld ME, Palinski W, Yla-Herttuala S, Butler S, Witztum JL. Distribution of oxidation specific lipid-protein adducts and apolipoprotein B in atherosclerotic lesions of varying severity from WHHL rabbits. *Arteriosclerosis* 1990;10:336–349.
75. Haberland ME, Fong D, Cheng L. Malonaldehyde-altered protein occurs in atheroma of Watanabe heritable hyperlipidemic rabbits. *Science* 1988;241:215–218.
76. Hammer A, Kager G, Dohr G, Rabl H, Ghassempur I, Jurgens G. Generation, characterization, and histochemical application of monoclonal antibodies selectively recognizing oxidatively modified ApoB-containing serum lipoproteins. *Arterioscler Thromb Vasc Biol* 1995;15:704–713.
77. Haberland ME, Fogelman AM, Edwards PA. Specificity of receptor-mediated recognition of malondialdehyde-modified low density lipoproteins. *Proc Natl Acad Sci USA* 1982;79(6):1712–1716.
78. Berberian PA, Myers W, Tytell M, Challa V, Bond MG. Immunohistochemical localization of heat shock protein-70 in normal and atherosclerotic specimens of human arteries. *Am J Pathol.* 1990;136:71–80.
79. Johnson AD, Berberian PA, Tytell M, Bond MG. Differential distribution of 70-kD heat shock protein in atherosclerosis. Its potential role in arterial SMC survival. *Arterioscler Thromb Vasc Biol* 1995;15(1):27–36.
80. Khan BV, Parthasarathy SS, Alexander RW, Medford RM. Modified low density lipoprotein and its constituents augment cytokine–activated vascular cell adhesion molecule-1 gene expression in human vascular endothelial cells. *J Clin Invest* 1995;95(3):1262–1270.
81. Lechleitner M, Hoppichler F, Foger B, Patsch JR. Low-density lipoproteins of the prostprandial state induce cellular cholesteryl ester accumulation in macrophages. *Arterioscler Thromb* 1994; 14:1799–1807.
82. Bertazzi PA, Zocchetti C, Pesatori AC, Guercilena S, Sanarico M, Radice L. Ten-year mortality study of the population involved in the Seveso incident in 1976. *Am J Epidemiol* 1989;129:1187–1200.
83. Martin JV. Lipid abnormalities in workers exposed to dioxin. *Br J Ind Med* 1984;41:254–256.
84. Benner A, Edler L, Mayer K, Zober A. Untersuchungsprogramm "Dioxin" der Berufsgenossenschaft der Chemischen Industrie. Ergebnisbericht-Teil II. *Arbeitsmedizin Sozialmedizin Umweltmedizin* 1994;29:2–6.
85. Brewster DW, Bombick DW, Matsumura F. Rabbit serum hypertriglyceridemia after administration of 2,3,7,8-tetrachlorodibenzo-p-dioxin (TCDD). *J Toxicol Environ Health* 1988;25:495–507.
86. Pohjanvirta R, Sankari S, Kulju T, Naukkarinen A, Ylinen M, Tuomisto J. Studies on the role of lipid peroxidation in the acute toxicity of TCDD in rats. *Pharmacol Toxicol* 1990;66:399–408.
87. Matsumura F. Mechanism of action of dioxin-type chemicals, pesticides, and other xenobiotics affecting nutritional indexes. *Am J Clin Nutr* 1995;61(suppl):695S–701S.
88. Ignarro LJ. Signal transduction mechanisms involving nitric oxide. *Biochem Pharmacol* 199 1;41:485–490.

89. Elliot SJ, Meszaros G, Schilling WP. Effect of oxidant stress on calcium signalling in vascular endothelial cells. *Free Radical Biol Med* 1992;13:635–650.

90. Rooney TA, Renard DC, Sass EJ, Thomas AP. Oscillatory cytosolic calcium waves independent of stimulated inositol 1,4,5-triphosphate formation in hepatocytes. *J Biol Chem* 1991; 266(19):12272–12282.

91. Robison TW, Zhou H, Forman HJ. Modulation of ADP-stimulated inositol phosphate metabolism in rat liver alveolar macrophages by oxidative stress. *Arch Biochem Biophys* 1995;318(1):215–220.

92. Renard DC, Seitz MB, Thomas AP. Oxidized glutathione causes sensitization of calcium release to inositol 1,4,5-triphosphate in permeabilized hepatocytes. *Biochem J* 1992;284(2):507–512.

93. Stoyanovsky DA, Salama G, Kagan VE. Ascorbate/iron activates Ca^{2+}-release channels of skeletal sarcoplasmic reticulum vesicles reconstituted in lipid bilayers. *Arch Biochem Biophys* 1994; 308(1):214–221.

94. Kim RS, Sukhu B, LaBella FS. Lipoxygenase-induced lipid peroxidation of isolated cardiac microsomes modulates their calcium-transporting function. *Biochim Biophys Acta* 1988;961(2):270–277.

95. Sweetman LL, Zhang N, Peterson H, McLeod LL, Sevanian A. Effect of linoleic acid hydroperoxide on endothelial cell homeostasis and arachidonic acid release. *Arch Biochem Biophys* 1995; 323(1):97–107.

96. Kim RS, LaBella FS. The effect of linoleic and arachidonic derivatives on calcium transport in vesicles from cardiac sarcoplasmic reticulum. *J Cell Mol Cardiol* 1988;20(2):119–130.

97. Menshikova EV, Ritov VB, Shvedova AA, Elsayed N, Karol MH, Kagan VE. Pulmonary microsomes contain a Ca^{2+}-transport system sensitive to oxidative stress. *Biochim Biophys Acta* 1995; 1228(2–3):165–174.

98. Lotscher HR, Winterhalter KH, Carafoli E, Richter C. Hydroperoxides can modulate the redox state of pyridine nucleotides and the calcium balance in rat liver mitochondria. *Proc Natl Acad Sci USA* 1979;76:4340–4344.

99. Miyazaki S. Inositol triphosphate receptor mediated spatiotemporal calcium signalling. *Curr Opin Cell Biol* 1995;7(2):190–196.

100. Gopalakrishna R, Anderson WB. Ca^{2+}-and phospholipid-independent activation of protein kinase C by selective oxidative modification of the regulatory domain. *Proc Natl Acad Sci USA* 1989; 86(17):6758–6762.

101. Rippa M, Bellini T, Signorini M, Dallacchio F. Evidence for multiple pairs of vicinal thiols in some proteins. *J Biol Chem* 1981;256:451–455.

102. Holmgren A. Thioredoxin and glutaredoxin systems. *J Biol Chem* 1989;264(24):13963–13966.

103. Gopalakrishna R, Chen ZH, Gundimeda U. Irreversible oxidative activation of protein kinase C by photosensitive inhibitor calphostin C. *FEBS* 1992;314(2):149–154.

104. Offerman MK, Medford RM. Antioxidants and atherosclerosis: a molecular perspective. *Heart Dis Stroke* 1994;3:52–57.

105. Schreck R, Albermann K, Baeuerle PA. Nuclear factor kB: An oxidative stress–responsive transcription factor of eukaryotic cells (a review). *Free Radical Res Commun* 1992;17:221–237.

106. Baeuerle PA, Henkel T. Function and activation of NF-kappa-B in the immune system. *Annu. Rev. Immunol.* 1994;12:141–179.

107. Rajavashisth TB, Andalibi A, Territo MC, Berliner JA, Navab M, Fogelman AM, Lusis AJ. Induction of endothelial cell expression of granulocyte and macrophage colony-stimulating factors by modified low-density lipoproteins. *Nature* 1990;344:254–257.

108. Parhami F, Fang ZT, Fogelman AM, Andalibi A, Territo MC, Berliner JA. Minimally modified low density lipoprotein-induced inflammatory responses in endothelial cells are mediated by cyclic adenosine monophosphate. *J Clin Invest* 1993;92(1):471–478.

109. Khan BV, Parthasarathy SS, Alexander RW, Medford RM. Modified low density lipoprotein and its constituents augment cytokine-activated vascular cell adhesion molecule-1 gene expression in human vascular endothelial cells. *J Clin Invest* 1995;95(3):1262–1270.

110. Marui N, Offerman MK, Swerlick R, Kunsch C, Rosen CA, Ahmad M, Alexander RW, Medford RM. Vascular cell adhesion molecule-1 (VCAM-1) gene transcription and expression are regulated through an antioxidant-sensitive mechanism in human vascular endothelial cells. *J Clin Invest* 1993;92(4):1866–1874.

111. Berliner JA, Navab M, Fogelman AM, Frank JS, Demer LL, Edwards PA, Watson AD, Lusis AJ. Atherosclerosis: Basic mechanisms. *Oxidation Inflam Genet Circulation* 1995;91(9):2488–2496.

112. Watson AD, Navab M, Hama SY, Sevanian A, Prescott SM, Stafforini DM, McIntyre TM, Du

BN, Fogelman AM, Berliner JA. Effect of platelet activating factor-acetylhydrolase on the formation and action of minimally oxidized low density lipoprotein. *J Clin Invest* 1995;95(2):774–782.

113. Weyrich AS, McIntyre TM, McEver RP, Prescott SM, Zimmerman GA. Monocyte tethering by P-selectin regulates monocyte chemotactic protein-1 and tumor necrosis factor-alpha secretion. Signal integration and NF-kappa B translocation. *J Clin Invest* 1995;95(5):2297–2303.

114. Ahmad M, Marui N, Alexander RW, Medford RM. Cell type-specific transactivation of the VCAM-1 promoter through an NF-kappa B enhancer motif. *J Biol Chem* 1995;270(15):8976–8983.

115. Mowri H, Nojima S, Inoue K. Effect of lipid composition of liposomes on their sensitivity to peroxidation. *J Biochem* 1984;95:551–558.

116. Green FA. Generation and metabolism of lipoxygenase products in normal and membrane-damaged cultured human keratinocytes. *J Invest Dermatol* 1989;93:486–491.

117. Schnurr K, Kuhn H, Rapoport SM, Schewe T. 3,5-Di-t-butyl-4-hydroxytoluene (BHT) and probucol stimulate selectively the reaction of mammalian 15-lipoxygenase with biomembranes. *Biochim Biophys Acta* 1995;1254(1):66–72.

118. van Kuijk FJGM, Sevanian A, Handelman G, Dratz EA. A new role for phospholipase A_2. *TIBS* 1987;12:31–34.

119. Lands WE. Interactions of lipid hydroperoxides with eicosanoid biosynthesis. *J Free Radical Biol Med* 1985;1(2):97–101.

120. Burack WR, Biltonen RL. Lipid bilayer heterogeneities and modulation of phospholipase A_2 activity. *Chem Phys Lipids* 1994;73:209–222.

121. Dennis EA. Diversity of group types, regulation, and function of phospholipase A_2. *J Biol Chem* 1994;269(18):13057–13060.

122. Exton JH. Phosphatidylcholine breakdown and signal transduction. *Biochim Biophys Acta* 1994;1212:26–42.

123. Wratten ML, van Ginkel G, van't Veld AA, Bekker A, van Faassen E, Sevanian A. Structural and dynamic effects of oxidatively modified phospholipids in unsaturated lipid membranes. *Biochemistry* 1992;31:10901–10907.

124. Salgo MG, Corongiu FP, Sevanian A. Enhanced interfacial catalysis and hydrolytic specificity of phospholipase A_2 towards peroxidized phophatidylcholine. *Arch Biochem Biophys* 1993; 304:123–132.

125. Blee E. Oxygenated fatty acids and plant defenses. *Inform* 1995;6(7):852–861.

126. Rokach J, Fitzsimmons B. The lipoxins. *Int J Biochem* 1988;20(8):753–758.

127. Schade UF. The effect of endotoxin on the lipoxygenase-mediated conversion of exogenous and endogenous arachidonic acid in mouse peritoneal macrophages. *Prostaglandins* 1987; 34(3):385–400.

128. Ohtsuki T, Matsumoto M, Hayashi Y, Yamamoto K, Kitagawa K, Ogawa S, Yamamoto S, Kamada T. Reperfusion induces 5-lipoxygenase translocation and leukotriene C4 production in ischemic brain. *Am J Physiol* 1995;268(3):H1249–H1257.

129. Murphy E, Glasgow W, Fralix T, Steenbergen C. Role of lipoxygenase metabolites in ischemic preconditioning. *Circ Res* 1995;76(3):457–467.

130. Cathcart MK, McNally AK, Chisolm GM. Lipoxygenase-mediated transformation of human low density lipoprotein to an oxidized and cytotoxic complex. *J Lipid Res* 1991;32(1):63–70.

131. Rankin SM, Parthasarathy S, Steinberg D. Evidence for a dominant role of lipoxygenase(s) in the oxidation of LDL by mouse peritoneal macrophages. *J Lipid Res* 1991;32:449–456.

132. Spiteller G. Review: on the chemistry of oxidative stress. *J Lipid Mediat* 1993;7(3):199–221.

Free Radical Toxicology
Edited by K. B. Wallace
Copyright © 1997 Taylor & Francis

5

Free-Radical-Mediated Modification of Proteins

Earl R. Stadtman and Barbara S. Berlett

Laboratory of Biochemistry, National Heart, Lung, and Blood Institute, National Institutes of Health, Bethesda, Maryland, USA

REACTIVE OXYGEN SPECIES INVOLVED IN PROTEIN MODIFICATION

There is growing evidence that the modification of proteins by reactive oxygen species (ROS) is associated with aging (1–5) and a number of pathological conditions (reviewed in refs. 4–7). The ROS involved in these processes may be produced endogenously as unavoidable minor by-products of normal electron transport processes in metabolism (8,9), or may be generated during exposure to conditions of oxidative stress provided by metabolic disorders and/or environmental challenges, or may be produced by metal-catalyzed oxidation (MCO) systems (1,5,6). The ROS commonly implicated in protein modification include a number of free radical species-hydroxyl radical ($\cdot$OH), superoxide anion radical (O_2^-) thiyl radical (RS$\cdot$), and nitric oxide radical ($\cdot$NO)-as well as several nonradical species, such as hydrogen peroxide, alkyl peroxides, ozone, singlet oxygen, peroxynitrite ($ONOO^-$), nitronium ion (NO_2^+), and hypochlorous acid (HOCl). Of these, it is generally conceded that $\cdot$OH is the most damaging species. Hydroxyl radicals are produced: (a) by homolytic cleavage of water by ionizing radiation (x-rays, γ-rays) according to the overall reaction 1, in which aqueous electrons (e_{aq}^-), H_2O^+, and an excited state of water (H_2O^*) are intermediates (10); (b) by reactions of Fe(II) or Cu(I) with hydrogen peroxide, reaction 2 (9); (c) by homolytic cleavage of peroxynitrite, reaction 3 (11,12); and (d) by reaction of ozone with phenolics (PH), reaction 4 (13,14).

$$H_2 \rightarrow \cdot H + \cdot OH \tag{1}$$

$$H_2O_2 + Fe(II) \text{ or } Cu(I) \rightarrow \cdot OH + OH^- + Fe(III) \text{ or } Cu(II) \tag{2}$$

$$HONOO \rightarrow \cdot OH + \cdot NO_2 \tag{3}$$

$$PH + O_3 \rightarrow \cdot OH + P + O_2 \tag{4}$$

We are indebted to the pioneering studies of Garrison (15,16), Swallow (10), and Schuessler (17) and their colleagues for establishing the basic principles and reaction mechanisms involved in the modification of protein by 'OH. Results of their studies have contributed richly to an understanding of the mechanisms of action of other forms of ROS as well. It is now well established that exposure of proteins to ROS leads to modification of the side chains of amino acid residues, conversion of proteins to higher molecular weight forms (protein-protein cross-linking), and fragmentation of the polypeptide chain.

MODIFICATION OF AMINO ACID RESIDUE SIDE CHAINS

All amino acid residues of proteins are potential targets for attack by hydroxyl radicals produced by ionizing radiation (10,15). However, protein modification by other forms of ROS or by hydroxyl radicals produced by MCO systems exhibit a high degree of specificity (2,5,6,18). Even so, in only a few instances have the reaction products been identified. Table 1 lists some well-characterized modifications that are attributable to one or more kinds of ROS attack. For purposes of discussion, these are divided into three categories-namely, modification of the sulfur-containing amino acids, modification of the aromatic and heterocyclic amino acids, and modification of the aliphatic amino acids.

Modification of Sulfur-Containing Amino Acids

Cysteine residues of proteins are particularly sensitive to intra- or interprotein disulfide cross-linked derivatives, but also to mixed disulfide adducts of glutathione

TABLE 1. *ROS-mediated modification of amino acid residues*

Amino acid	Products	References
Cysteine	CyS-S-Cy, CyS-SG, CySOH, CySOOH, CySO$_2$H	10,15,19–21
Methionine	MeSOX; methionine sulfone	10,16,22–24
Tryptophan	2-, 4-, 5-, 6-, 7-Hydroxytryptophan formylkynurenine; 3-OH-kynurenine nitrotryptophan	25–31
Tyrosine	3,4-Dihydroxy phenylalanine tyr-tyr cross-links 3-nitrotyrosine	26,32–40
Phenylalanine	2-, 3-, 4-Hydroxyphenylalanine 2,3-dihydroxyphenylalanine	26,32,41–43
Histidine	2-Oxohistidine; 4-OH-glutamate; (aspartic acid): (asparagine)	44–48
Threonine	2-Amino-3-ketobutyric acid	49
Valine	3-OH-valine	15
Leucine	3-OH-leucine; 4-OH-leucine; 5-OH-leucine	15,50
Arginine	Glutamic semialdehyde	51,52
Lysine	α-Amino adipylsemialdehyde;	[a]
Proline	Glutamylsemialdehyde; 2-pyrrolidone; 4- and 5-OH-proline; pyroglutamic acid	51,53–55
Glutamic acid	Oxalic acid; pyruvyl adducts	15
Aspartic acid	Pyruvyl derivatives	15

[a] B. S. Berlett, D. G. Miller, L. Szweda, and E. R. Stadtman, unpublished data.

and, in some cases, to higher states of oxidation, namely, sulfinic, sulfenic, and sulfonic acid derivatives (15). When exposed to peroxynitrite, cysteine residues are converted to the *S*-nitrosothiol derivatives, which are thought to play an important role in the storage and/or transfer of NO equivalents (56–59).

Most forms of ROS are able to convert methionine residues of proteins to methionine sulfoxide (MeSOX) residues; sometimes low yields of methionine sulfone are also obtained (10,16,22–24). Significantly, the oxidation of cysteine residues to disulfides and the oxidation of methionine residues to MeSOX residues are the only ROS-mediated modifications of proteins that can be reversed. The regeneration of methionine and cysteine from their oxidized counterparts is mediated by the action of NADPH-dependent dehydrogenases. In the case of protein disulfides ($P-S-S-P$), reversal is catalyzed by various glutathione-dependent disulfide interchain reactions giving rise eventually to oxidized glutathione (GSSG):

$$P-S-S-P + 2\,GSH \rightarrow 2\,PSH + GSSG \qquad [5]$$

which is converted to GSH by glutathionine reduction:

$$GSSG + NADPH + H^+ \rightarrow NADP^+ + 2\,GSH \qquad [6]$$

The principal product of methionine oxidation, MeSOX, can be reduced to methionine by reaction 7, which is the sum of reaction 8 catalyzed by methionine sulfoxide reductase and reaction 9 catalyzed by thioredoxin reductase (22,60). In these reactions, $T(SH)_2$ and $T(S\text{-}S)$ represents the reduced and oxidized forms of thioredoxin, respectively.

$$MeSOX + NADPH + H^+ \rightarrow Methionine + H_2O + NAD^+ \qquad [7]$$

$$T(SH)_2 + MeSOX \rightarrow T(S-S) + Methionine + H_2O \qquad [8]$$

$$T(S-S) + NADPH + H^+ \rightarrow T(SH)_2 + NAD^+ \qquad [9]$$

The possibility that the conversion of methionine residues to MeSOX residues can have a profound effect on enzymes (proteins) involved in cell signaling pathways is underscored by the demonstration that the conversion of some methionine residues to MeSOX residues in *Escherichia coli* glutamine synthetase (GS) converts the enzyme to a form exhibiting regulatory characteristics similar to those obtained in vivo by enzyme-catalyzed adenylylation of a single tyrosine residue per subunit of the enzyme (B.S. Berlett and E.R. Stadtman, unpublished data).

Modification of Aromatic and Heterocyclic Amino Acids

As in the case of sulfur-containing amino acids, the aromatic amino acids and histidine are preferred targets of most ROS. Tryptophan residues are particularly sensitive to oxidation. Cleavage of the indole ring by most ROS leads to the formation of *N*-formylkyneurinine as a major product (25,26,29); however, the benzenoid ring is also attacked and, in the presence of ionizing radiation, this leads to hydroxylation of either the 4, 5, 6, or 7 carbon atoms (26,30,27). When proteins are exposed to ionizing radiation or to high concentrations of H_2O_2 and copper, the tyrosine residues are converted to 3,4-dihydroxyphenylalanine (36,37,39) and tyrosine—tyrosine cross-linkages may be formed (34,38,40,43). In the presence of peroxynitrite, tyrosine residues are converted to 3-nitrotyrosine derivative (35). It is noteworthy that nitration of one tyrosine residue per subunit of *E. coli* GS converts the enzyme to a form that is almost identical to that produced by enzyme-catalyzed adenylylation of one tyrosine per subunit; thus, nitration converts GS from a form that can utilize either Mg(II) or Mn(II) for activation of the γ-glutamyltranferase activity to a form that has an absolute requirement of Mn(II) for activity. Moreover, as in the case of adenylylated GS, the nitrated enzyme has lower affinity for substrate and is highly susceptible to feedback inhibition by multiple end products of glutamine metabolism (61). It was further established that the nitration of GS by peroxynitrite is absolutely dependent upon the presence of carbon dioxide (B.S. Berlett and E.R. Stadtman, unpublished data), consistent with the report that $ONOO^-$ reacts almost instantly with CO_2 to form the putative $ONOOCO_2^-$ adduct (62). The $ONOO^-$-dependent oxidation of methionine to methionine sulfoxide and the $ONOO^-$-promoted nitration of tyrosine residues are mutually exclusive processes, depending on the presence or absence of CO_2. In the presence of saturating levels of CO_2, the nitration of tyrosine is stimulated and the oxidation of methionine residues is completely blocked. Conversely, in the absence of CO_2, nitration of tyrosine is promoted but oxidation of methionine to MeSOX occurs readily (B.S. Berlett and E.R. Stadtman, unpublished results). It is therefore evident that different forms of ROS are intermediates in methionine oxidation and tyrosine nitration, as illustrated by the following scheme:

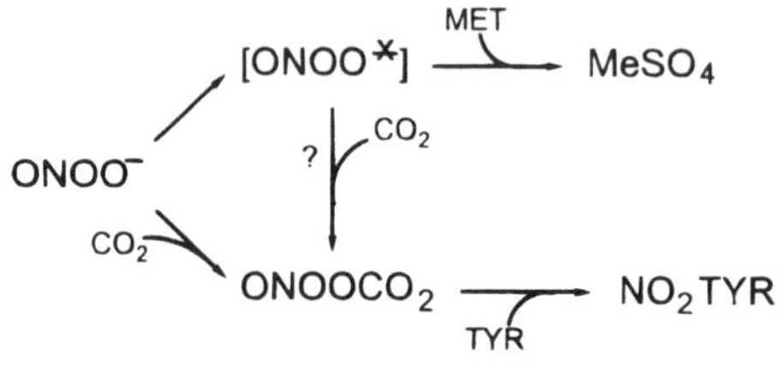

$$\text{ONOO}^- \nearrow [\text{ONOO}^*] \xrightarrow{\text{MET}} \text{MeSO}_4$$

This scheme takes into account the proposition of Pryor and Squadrito (24), based on kinetic considerations, that the peroxynitrite-mediated oxidation of methionine to MeSOX involves an activated intermediate [ONOO*] of unknown structure.

The oxidation of phenylalanine residues by various ROS can lead to the formation of 2-, 3-, or 4-hydroxy derivatives or 2,3-dihydroxyphenylalanine (26,37,39,42). The oxidation of histidine residues in proteins leads to the formation of 2-oxohistidine residues (44,45,48) and/or to compounds that, upon acid hydrolysis, are converted to aspartic acid (46). Oxidation of histidine residues in glutamine synthetase by the $O_2/Fe(III)/$ascorbate system is a highly site-specific process; only 2 of 15 histidine residues per subunit are oxidized (47,63). In contrast, the oxidation of histidine residues in GS by ozone is a more or less random process during which the histidine residues at the metal binding site are no more sensitive to oxidation than at least eight other histidine residues (46). Nevertheless, the rate of histidine oxidation by ozone does depend upon the primary, secondary, and quaternary structure of the protein. This is evident from the fact that the rate of oxidation of histidine residues in bovine serum albumin is two to three times greater than in *E. coli* glutamine synthetase, even though both proteins contain almost identical numbers of histidine residues per subunit (46).

Modification of Aliphatic Amino Acid Residues

The side chains of all aliphatic amino acid residues are potential targets for attack by hydroxyl radicals generated by high-energy radiolysis (10,15–17) or by reactions between high (nonphysiological) concentrations of transition metals and hydrogen peroxide (32,64). However, the susceptibility of amino acid residues to modification by ROS generated in the presence of the low intracellular concentrations of transition metals and hydrogen peroxide is mainly restricted to those amino acid residues at metal binding sites on proteins (5,18). Nevertheless, the products formed have been identified for only a few of the aliphatic amino acids. As shown in Table 1, lysine residues are converted to α-aminoadipylserine-aldehyde residues; arginine and proline residues are both converted to glutamyl semialdehyde, 4- and 5-hydroxyproline, and pyroglutamic acid; glutamyl residues are converted to oxalic acid and pyruvyl derivatives (15); threonine residues are converted to 2-amino-3-ketobutyric acid (49); and the hydrophobic amino acid residues, valine and leucine, are converted to 3-hydroxy and 3- and 4-hydroxy derivatives, respectively (15,50).

PEPTIDE BOND CLEAVAGE

The ·OH-mediated abstraction of the α-hydrogen atom from any one of the amino acid residues in a protein can initiate a series of reactions that, in the presence of oxygen, can lead to cleavage of the polypeptide chain by either of two pathways (15). As illustrated in Figure 1, abstraction of an α-hydrogen atom from the polypeptide backbone leads to the formation of a carbon-centered radical (reaction b), which upon reaction with O_2 gives rise to a peroxy radical adduct (reaction c). The peroxy radical derivative may lead ultimately to cleavage of the polypeptide chain by both iron-dependent (reactions e, g, I) and iron-independent (reactions d, f, h, o, q) pathways that involve the intermediate formation of protein peroxides (reactions d or e), protein alkoxy radicals (reactions o, g, or f), and hydroxyl derivatives (reactions h, or k and p) that undergo spontaneous cleavage of the polypeptide chain by either the α-amidation mechanism (reaction n) or the diamide pathway (reaction j). As illustrated in Figure 1, the C-terminal amino acid residue of fragment I, derived form the N-terminal portion of the protein, will be present as the amide derivative, and the N-terminal amino acid residue of fragment II, representing the C-terminal portion of the protein, is blocked by an α-ketoacyl group derived from the R^3-amino acid residue of the original protein. Accordingly, the occurrence of the α-amidation

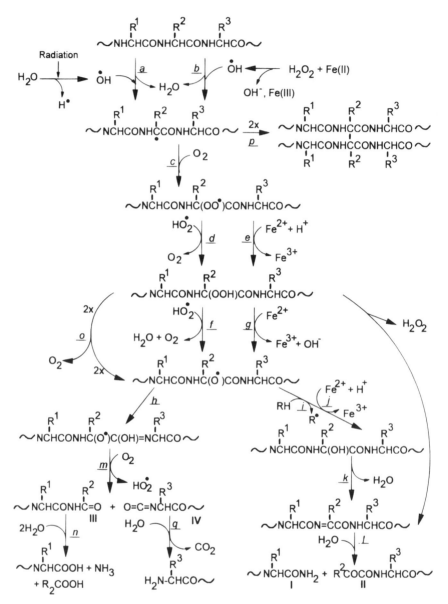

FIG. 1. Hydroxyl radical-mediated cleavage of the polypeptide chain. Based on reactions described by Garrison (15).

type of cleavage can be confirmed by conversion of the α-ketoacyl moiety of fragment II to its 2,4-dinitrophenyl hydrazone either before or after acid hydrolysis.

Fragments III and IV in Figure 1 represent the peptide fragments derived from the N-terminal and C-terminal portions, respectively, of the original protein, following cleavage by the diamide pathway. Fragment III possesses a diamide structure at the C-terminal end, whereas the N-terminal amino acid residue of fragment IV is blocked by an isocyanate group.

In addition to the more general, relatively non-site-specific modes of polypeptide cleavage illustrated in Figure 1, cleavage can occur also as a consequence of free radical attack of the glutamyl, prolyl, and aspartyl residues of proteins. Based on the consideration that tertiary amide bonds are more susceptible to oxidation than secondary amide bonds, and also the fact that the number of peptide fragments obtained when bovine serum albumin (BSA) is exposed to radiolysis is approximately equal to the number of protein residues in the protein, Schuessler and Schilling proposed (17) that the proline residues are preferred sites of free radical-mediated peptide bond cleavage. This proposition finds support from the studies of Uchida et al. (55) showing that the metal-catalyzed oxidation of proline residues in collagen and proline-containing peptides leads to the formation of 2-pyrrolidone residues and concomitant cleavage of the peptide bond (Figure 2).

Oxidation of the glutamyl side chains of proteins can lead ultimately to peptide

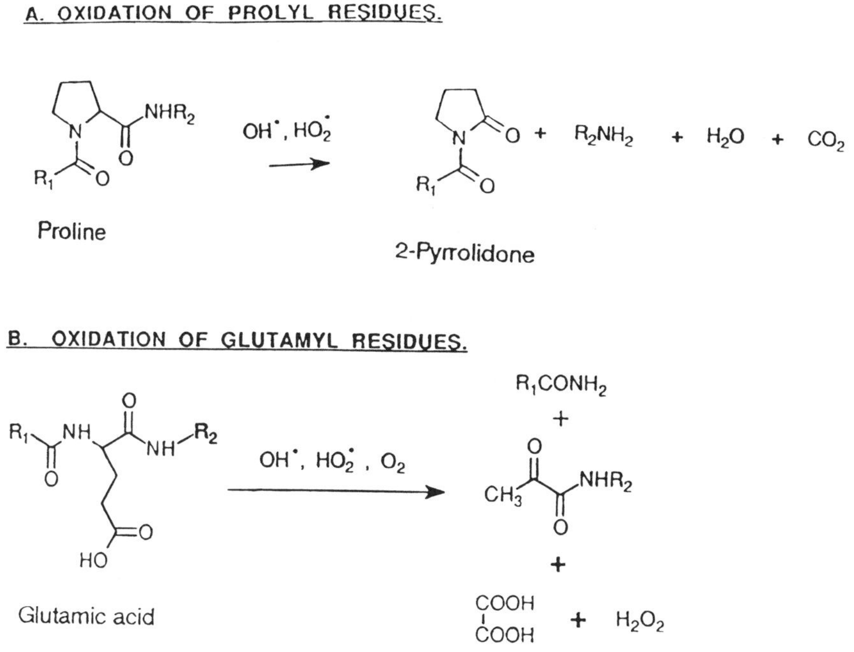

A. OXIDATION OF PROLYL RESIDUES.

Proline   2-Pyrrolidone

B. OXIDATION OF GLUTAMYL RESIDUES.

Glutamic acid

FIG. 2. Peptide bond cleavage by hydroxyl radical-mediated oxidation of proline or glutamate side chains. Based on reactions described by Garrison (15) and Uchida et al. (55).

bond cleavage and conversion of the glutamyl residue to a pyruvyl derivative of the N-terminal amino acid residue of the fragment obtained from the C-terminal portion of the proteins (Figure 2B). Garrison (15) proposes that this type of peptide bond cleavage can be explained by reactions involving the ˙OH-dependent abstraction of a hydrogen atom from the γ-carbon of the glutamyl side chain, followed by reactions with O_2 to yield peroxy-radical and alkoxy-radical intermediates. Analogous reactions of aspartyl residues can also lead to peptide bond cleavage (15).

The composition of the C- and N-terminal portions of peptide fragments generated by the various types of peptide cleavage reactions, together with the products formed upon hydrolysis of these fragments, is illustrated in Table 2. It is evident from an examination of Table 2 that the occurrence of the various modes of peptide cleavage can, at least in theory, be assessed by analysis of the hydrolysis products.

FORMATION OF PROTEIN CARBONYL GROUPS

As illustrated in Table 1, the metal-catalyzed oxidation of the side chains of lysine, arginine, proline, and threonine residues of proteins leads to the formation of protein carbonyl derivatives. Protein carbonyl derivatives are formed also by cleavage of the polypeptide chain by the α-amidation and glutamyl oxidation pathways (Figures 1 and 2 and Table 2). However, direct oxidation of the protein is not the only way that protein carbonyl derivatives can be formed. The introduction of carbonyl groups into proteins can occur also by interaction of functional groups of the protein with oxidation products of polyunsaturated fatty acids or by reaction with reducing sugars. As shown in Figure 3, α,β-unsaturated aldehydes, such as 4-hydroxy-2-nonenal (HNE), which are formed during the ROS-mediated oxidation of polyunsaturated fatty acids, can undergo Michael-type addition reactions with the ε-amino groups of lysyl residues, the imidazole groups of histidine residues, and the sulfhydryl groups of cysteinyl residues of proteins to form, respectively, the corresponding adducts with retention of the carbonyl function (65–67).

TABLE 2. *Hydroxyl-radical-mediated cleavage patterns*

Type of cleavage	C-terminal group of N-terminal fragment	N-terminal group of C-terminal fragment	Hydrolysis products
α-Amidation	$-CONH_2$	$RCOCONH-$	NH_3, $RCOCOOH$
Diamide	$-CONHCO$ $\|$ R	$O=C=N-$	CO_2, $RCOOH$, NH_3
Glutamate oxidation	$-CONH_2$	$CH_3COCONH-$	$CH_3COCOOH$, NH_3, $COOH$ $\|$ $COOH$
Proline oxidation	$-CON$	$HOCONH-$	$H_2NCH_2(CH_2)_2COOH$, CO_2

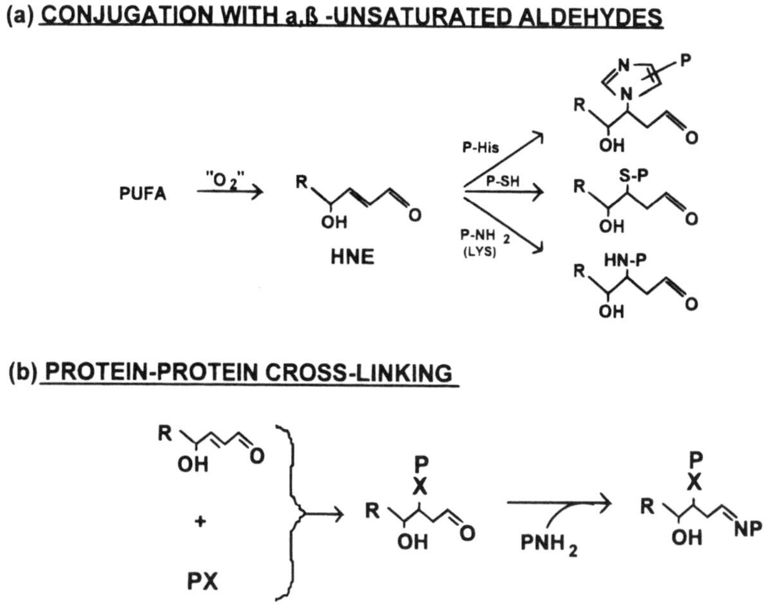

(a) CONJUGATION WITH a,ß -UNSATURATED ALDEHYDES

(b) PROTEIN-PROTEIN CROSS-LINKING

FIG. 3. Protein carbonyls derived from conjugates with 4-hydroxy-2-nonenal. After Uchida and Stadtman (66) and Shuenstein and Esterbauer (65).

Protein carbonyl derivatives are formed also by the interaction of proteins with reducing sugars or with carbohydrate oxidation products in a process referred to as glycation. Glycation involves reaction of the carbonyl group of sugars with the N-terminal amino group of proteins or the ϵ-amino group of lysyl residues to form Schiff base adducts that may subsequently undergo Amadori rearrangements to form ketoamines (Figure 4). The Amadori products are highly sensitive to metal-catalyzed oxidation (glycoxidation), leading eventually to N-carboxymethyl lysine residues, or, alternatively, they may react with arginine residues to form pentosidine protein cross-linked adducts (68,69). In addition, the primary Amadori products may undergo dehydration and oxidative fragmentation to yield deoxyosones that undergo further reactions to form highly fluorescent, pigmented cross-linked derivatives of ill-defined structures (68). These are collectively referred to as Maillard products or advanced glycosylation end products (AGEs) that accumulate during aging and are likely involved in the development of diabetes and some eye disorders (41,68). It is also claimed that some Maillard products can generate free radicals by metal-ion-independent mechanisms, and that they might be implicated in atherogenesis (70). The interaction of proteins with ketoaldehydes generated by metal-catalyzed oxidation of sugars provides another mechanism for the introduction of carbonyl groups into proteins (71). For a more thorough review of the role of glycation in aging and disease, the reader is referred to an excellent review by Kristal and Yu (72). Though undoubtedly involved, the quantitative contribution of adducts formed by reactions

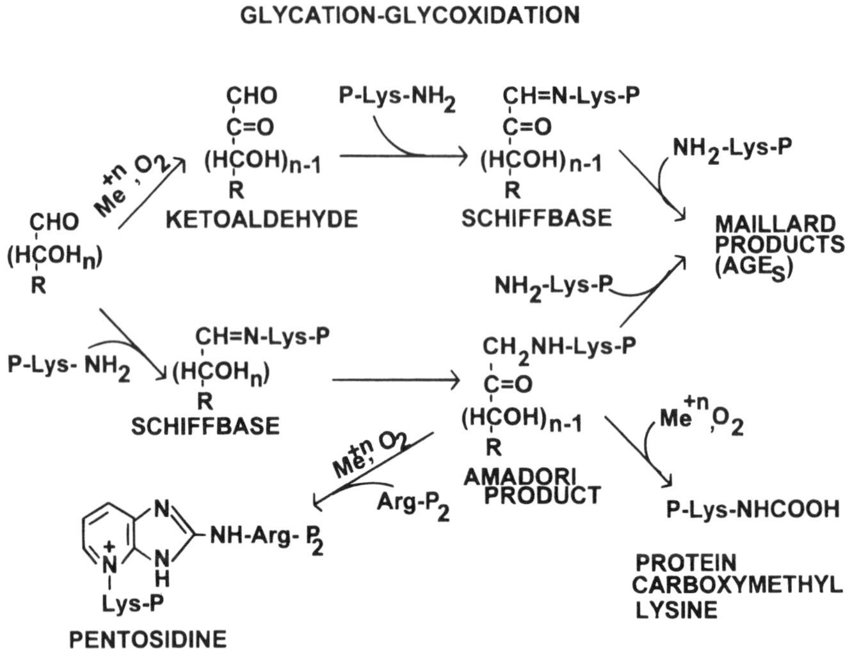

GLYCATION-GLYCOXIDATION

FIG. 4. Glycation and glycoxidation of proteins. Based on report of Monnier (68) and Wolf and Dean (71).

of proteins with oxidation products of PUFAs and carbohydrates to the total pool of protein carbonyl groups remains to be established.

PROTEIN CARBONYLS ARE MARKERS OF OXIDATIVE STRESS

In view of the fact that carbonyl derivatives of proteins are formed as a result of oxidative modification of amino acid side chains, ROS-mediated peptide cleavage reactions, and reactions with lipid and carbohydrate oxidation products, it is evident that the presence of carbonyl groups in proteins indicates that the proteins have been subjected to oxidative damage. This conclusion is supported by the results of studies summarized in Table 3, in which it has been demonstrated that the exposure of animals and/or cultured cells to various conditions of oxidative stress leads to an increase in the protein carbonyl content. Thus, exposures to either hyperoxia, x-irradiation, enforced chronic exercise, cigarette smoke, ischemia-reperfusion, magnesium deficiency, activated neutrophils, paraquat toxicity, ozone, MCO (metal catalyzed oxidation) systems, or peroxynitrite all lead to an increase in protein carbonyl content. These results, and the further demonstration that an increase in protein carbonyl content of tissues is associated with a number of pathological disorders, including rheumatoid arthritis (93), muscular dystrophy (94), amyotrophic lateral

TABLE 3. *Generation of protein carbonyls by oxidative stress*

Stress condition	Tissue or cells analyzed	References
Hyperoxia	Rat hepatocytes	73
	Houseflies	74
	Rat lung	75
Exercise	Rat hind leg muscle	76
	Houseflies	74
	Rat skeletal muscle	77
Ischemia-reperfusion	Gerbil brain	78
	Dog brain	81
	Rat heart	79
	Rat lung	33
		80
Neutrophil activation	Neutrophil proteins	82
		83
Rapid correction of hyponatremia	Rat brain	84
Paraquat toxicity	Hamster	75
Magnesium deficiency	Rat kidney, brain	85
Cigarette smoke	Human plasma	86
Xanthine/xanthine oxidase	Endothelial cells	83
MCO system	Human plasma	87
Ozone	Human plasma	88
	Rat heart	89
MCO system	Rat neurofilament	90
Peroxynitrite	Rat lung	33
X-irradiation	Housefly flight muscle mitochondria	91
	Housefly protein	92

sclerosis (95), Alzheimer's disease (96,97), cataractogenesis (98), respiratory distress syndrome (99), aging (2,3), iron nitrolotriacetate-induced renal carcinogenesis (100), and very likely Parkinson's disease (101) and atherosclerosis (102), serve notice that free-radical-mediated protein damage is involved in either the etiology or manifestation of various diseases.

PROTEIN-PROTEIN CROSS-LINKING

In addition to the fragmentation of proteins, ROS can also provoke the formation of higher molecular weight forms by facilitating the generation of covalent protein—protein cross-linkages. Six different kinds of cross-linking reactions are illustrated in Table 4. They involve: (i) formation of disulfide bridges between protein molecules as a result of the oxidation of cysteine residues; (ii) the secondary interaction of the aldehyde moiety of the Michael addition HNE conjugate (HNE-CHO) of one protein molecule with the lysine residue of another protein molecule (Figure 3); (iii) interaction of the carbonyl group of glycation derived carbonyl groups (G-CHO) in one protein with the lysine residue of another; (iv) the Schiff base coupling of lysine residues in two different protein molecules by their interaction with a dialdehyde (e.g., malondialdehyde formed in the oxidation of polyunsaturated fatty

TABLE 4. *Protein–protein cross-linking reaction types*

(i) $\quad$ P^{1}SH + P^{2}SH $\xrightarrow{[O]}$ P^{1}SSP^2 + H$_2$O

(ii) $\quad$ P^1–HNE–CHO + P^{2}NH$_2$ → P^1–HNE–CH=NP^2 + H$_2$O

(iii) $\quad$ P^1–CHO + P^{2}NH$_2$ → P^{1}C=NP^2 + H$_2$O

(iv) $\quad$ P^{1}NH$_2$ + P^{2}NH$_2$ + CH$_2$(CHO)$_2$ → P^{1}N=CHCH$_2$CH=NP^2 + H$_2$O

(v) $\quad$ P^{1}C(R)CHO + P^{2}NH$_2$ → P^{1}C(R)=NP^2 + H$_2$O

(vi)
$$P^1-\overset{\bullet}{\underset{R_1}{C}} + P^2-\overset{\bullet}{\underset{R_4}{C}} \longrightarrow P^1-\overset{R^1}{\underset{R_4}{C}}-\overset{R^2}{\underset{R_4}{C}}-P^2$$

Note. Formation of protein–protein cross-linkages. Based on studies by Friguet et al. (67), Stadtman (5), Garrison (15), Monnier (68), and Wolf and Dean (71). Abbreviations: PSH, protein sulfhydryls; P-HNE-CHO, protein hydroxynonenal adducts; PNH$_2$, N-terminal amino groups of ϵ-amino group of lysine residues on proteins; PC(R)CHO, carbonyl derivatives of oxidized lysine, arginine, or proline side chains of proteins, or carbonyl groups generated in peptide cleavage reactions; P, protein; P-CHO, carbonyl groups formed as a consequence of glycation reactions.

acids); (v) the reaction of the ROS-derived carbonyl group of an amino acid residue side chain in one protein molecule with the lysine residue of another; and (vi) formation of carbon–carbon covalent bonds by the interaction of a carbon-centered free radical of another protein.

Cross-linked adducts obtained as a result of Schiff base formation (mechanisms ii-v) may undergo secondary reactions leading to polymeric aggregates of undefined structure (67). Significantly, the higher molecular weight forms of some of these are not readily degraded by proteases that preferentially degrade the oxidized forms of monomeric substrates (67). In particular, the dimeric derivatives obtained by interaction of HNE with protein are not only poor substrates for degradation by the multicatalytic protease (proteosome), but they inhibit the ability of the protease to degrade the oxidized forms of other proteins, and thereby may contribute to the accumulation of oxidized forms of proteins as occurs during aging and some pathologies (67,103). It is noteworthy that little, if any, protein cross-linking by the interaction of carbon-centered radicals (mechanism vi, Table 4) occurs under aerobic conditions. This is likely due to the fact that in the presence of oxygen the reaction of carbon-centered radicals with O2 to form protein peroxy-radical derivatives (reaction c, Figure 1) is favored (15–17).

The 2,2′-biphenyl derivatives obtained by the covalent dimerization of tyrosine residues exhibit strong fluorescence at 410 nm when excited by light at 325 nm. This property is the basis of a widely used method for determination of protein tyr-tyr cross-linkages. However, estimates of the dityrosine content of proteins based on other compounds with similar fluorescence characteristics [e.g., conversion of tryptophan residues to N-formylkyneurenine (27), conjugation of HNE with lysine residues (67), and the binding of retinoic acid adducts with proteins (104)]. Indeed, the content of dityrosine in eye lens proteins as determined by a highly specific technique was less than 1% of that calculated from fluorescence measurements (41). In any case, the assumption that protein-protein cross-linking is due mainly to the formation of dityrosine cross-linkages is probably not valid. In fact, covalent cross-links can involve interactions of carbon-centered radicals of any two identical or nonidentical amino acid residues in the same or in two different protein molecules (15).

REFERENCES

1. Oliver CN, Fulks R, Levine RL, Fucci L, Rivett, AJ, Roseman JE, Stadtman, ER. Oxidative inactivation of key metabolic enzymes during aging. In: Roy AK, Chatterjee B, eds. *Molecular Basis of Aging.* New York: Academic Press, 1984:235–262.
2. Stadtman ER. Protein oxidation and aging. *Science* 1992;257:1220–1224.
3. Stadtman ER. The status of oxidatively modified proteins as a marker of aging. In: Esser K, Martin GM, eds. *Molecular Aspects of Aging.* New York: John Wiley & Sons, 1995:130–143.
4. Levine RL, Stadtman ER. Oxidation of proteins during aging. *Generations* 1992;14:39–42.
5. Stadtman ER. Metal ion-catalyzed oxidation of proteins: Biochemical mechanism and biological consequences. *Free Radical Biol Med* 1990;9:315–325.
6. Stadtman ER, Oliver CN. Metal-catalyzed oxidaiton of proteins. *J Biol Chem* 1991;266:2005–2008.
7. Halliwell B, Gutteridge JMC. Role of free radicals and catalytic metal ions in human disease: An overview. *Methods Enzymol* 1990;186:1–85.
8. Bovaris A, Oshino N, Chance B. The cellular production of hydrogen peroxide. *Biochem J* 1972;128:617–630.
9. Halliwell B, Gutteridge JMC, eds. *Free Radicals in Biology and Medicine.* Oxford: Clarendon Press, 1989.
10. Swallow AJ. Effect of ionizing radiation on proteins, RCO groups, peptide bond cleavage, inactivation, -SH oxidation. In: Swallow AJ, ed. *Radiation Chemistry of Organic Compounds.* New York: John Wiley & Sons, 1960:211–224.
11. Beckman JS, Beckman TW, Chen J, Marshall PA, Freeman B. Apparent hydroxyl radical production by peroxynitrite: Implications for endothelial injury from nitric oxide and superoxide. *Proc Natl Acad Sci USA* 1990;87:1620–1624.
12. van der Vliet A, O'Neill CA, Halliwell B, Cross CE, Kaur H. Aromatic hydroxylation and nitration of phenylalanine and tyrosine by peroxynitrite. Evidence for hydroxyl radical production from peroxynitrite. *FEBS Lett* 1994;339:89–92.
13. Grimes HD, Perkins KK, Boss WF. Ozone degrades into hydroxyl radical under physiological conditions. *Plant Physiol* 1983;72:1016–1020.
14. Pryor WA. Mechanisms of radical formation from reactions of ozone with target molecules in the lung. *Free Radical Biol Med* 1994;17:451–465.
15. Garrison WM. Reaction mechanisms in radiolysis of peptides, polypeptides, and proteins. *Chem Rev* 1987;87:381–398.
16. Garrison WM, Jayko ME, Bennett W. Radiation-induced oxidation of proteins in aqueous solution. *Radiat Res* 1962;16:487–502.
17. Schuessler H, Schilling K. Oxygen effect in radiolysis of proteins. Part 2. Bovine serum albumin. *Int J Radiat Biol* 1984;45:267–281.
18. Chevion M. A site specific mechanism for free radical induced biological damage: The essential role of redox-active transition metals. *Free Radical Biol Med* 1988;5:27–37.
19. Zhou JQ, Gafni A. Exposure of rat muscle phosphoglycerate kinase to a nonenzymatic MFO system generates the old form of enzyme. *J Gerontol* 1991;46:B217–B221.
20. Brodie E, Reed DJ. Cellular recovery of glyceraldehyde-3-phosphate dehydrogenase activity and thiol status after exposure to hydroperoxide. *Arch Biochem Biophys* 1990;276:210–218.
21. Takahashi R, Goto S. Alteration of aminoacyl-tRNA synthetase with age: Heat labilization of the enzyme by oxidative damage. *Arch Biochem Biophys* 1990;277:228–233.
22. Vogt W. Oxidation of methionine residues in proteins: Tools, targets, and reversal. *Free Radical Biol Med* 1995;18:93–105.

23. Pryor WA, Squadrito GL. The chemistry of peroxynitrite: A product from the reaction of nitric oxide with superoxide. *Am J Physiol* 1995;268:L699–L722.
24. Pryor WA, Jin X, Squadrito GL. One- and two-electron oxidations of methionine by peroxynitrite. *Proc Natl Acad Sci USA* 1994;91:11173–11177.
25. Armstrong RC, Swallow AJ. Pulse- and gamma-radiolysis of aqueous solutions of tryptophan. *Radiat Res* 1969;41:563–579.
26. Maskos Z, Rush JD, Koppenol WH. The hydroxylation of tryptophan. *Arch Biochem Biophys* 1992;296:514–520.
27. Guptasarma P, Balasubramanian D, Matsugo S, Saito I. Hydroxyl radical mediated damage to proteins, with special reference to the crystallins. *Biochemistry* 1992;31:4296–4302.
28. Winchester RV, Lynn KR. X- and γ-radiolysis of some tryptophan dipeptides. *Int J Radiat Biol* 1970;17:541–549.
29. Pryor WA, Uppu RM. A kinetic model for the competitive reactions of ozone with amino acid residues in proteins in reverse micelles. *J Biol Chem* 1993;268:3120–3126.
30. Solar S. Reactions of OH with phenylalanine in neutral aqueous solutions. *Radiat Phys Chem* 1985;26:103–108.
31. Kikugawa K, Kato T, Okamoto Y. Damage of amino acids and proteins induced by nitrogen dioxide, a free radical toxin in air. *Free Radical Biol Med* 1994;16:373–382.
32. Huggins TG, Wells-Knecht MC, Detorie NA, Baynes JW, Thorpe SR. Formation of o-tyrosine in proteins during radiolytic and metal-catalyzed oxidation. *J Biol Chem* 1993;268:12341–12347.
33. Ischiropoulos H, Al-Mehdi AB. Peroxynitrite-mediated oxidative protein modifications. *FEBS Lett* 1995;364:279–282.
34. Giulivi C, Davies KJA. Dityrosine and tyrosine oxidation products are endogenous markers for the selective proteolysis of oxidatively modified red blood cell hemoglobin by (the 19S) proteosome. *J Biol Chem* 1993;268:8752–8759.
35. Beckman JS, Ischiropoulos H, Zhu L, Van der Woerd M, Smith C, Chen J, Harrison J, Mautin JC, Tsai M. Kinetics of superoxide dismutase- and iron-catalyzed nitration of phenolics by peroxynitrite. *Arch Biochem Biophys* 1992;298:438–445.
36. Fletcher GL, Okada S. Radiation induced formation of dihydroxy phenylalanine from tyrosine and tyrosine-containing peptides in aqueous solution. *Radiat Res* 1961;15:349–351.
37. Gieseg SP, Simpson JA, Charlton TS, Duncan MW, Dean RT. Protein-bound 3,4-dihydroxyphenlyalanine is a major reductant formed during hydroxyl radical damage to proteins. *Biochemistry* 1993;32:4780–4786.
38. Davies KJA, Delsignore ME, Lin SW. Protein damage by oxygen radicals. II. Modification of amino acids. *J Biol Chem* 1987;262:9902–9907.
39. Dean RT, Gieseg S, Davies MJ. Reactive species and their accumulation on radical-damaged proteins. *Trends Biochem Sci* 1993;18:437–441.
40. Heinecke JW, Li W, Daehnke III HL, Goldstein JA. Dityrosine, a specific marker of oxidation, is synthesized by the myeloperoxidase-hydrogen peroxide system of human neutrophils and macrophages. *J Biol Chem* 1993;268:4069–4077.
41. Wells-Knecht MC, Huggins TG, Dyer DG, Thorpe SR, Baynes JW. Oxidized amino acids in lens protein with age. Measurement of o-tyrosine and dityrosine in aging human lens. *J Biol Chem* 1993;269:12348–12352.
42. Maskos Z, Rush JD, Koppenol WH. The hydroxylation of phenylalanine and tyrosine: A comparison with salicylate and tryptophan. *Arch Biochem Biophys* 1992;296:521–529.
43. van der Vliet A, Eiserich JP, O'Neill CA, Halliwell B, Cross CE. Tyrosine modification by reactive nitrogen species. A closer look. *Arch Biochem Biophys* 1995;319:341–349.
44. Uchida K, Kawakishi S. 2-Oxohistidine as a novel biological marker for oxidatively modified proteins. *FEBS Lett* 1993;332:208–210.
45. Uchida K, Kawakishi S. Identification of oxidized histidine generated at the active site of Cu,Zn-superoxide dismutase exposed to H_2O_2. *J Biol Chem* 1994;269:2405–2410.
46. Berlett BS, Levine RL, Stadtman ER. A comparison of the effects of ozone on the modification of amino acid residues in glutamine synthetase and bovine serum albumin. *J Biol Chem* 1996;271:4177–4182.
47. Farber JM, Levine RL. Sequence of a peptide susceptible to mixed-function oxidation: Probable cation binding site in glutamine synthetase. *J Biol Chem* 1986;261:4574–4578.
48. Lewisch SA, Levine RL. Determination of 2-oxohistidine by amino acid analysis. *Anal Biochem* 1995;231:440–446.

49. Taborsky G. Oxidative modification of proteins in the presence of ferrous iron and air. Effect of ionic constituents of the reaction medium on the nature of the oxidation products. *Biochemistry* 1973;12:1341–1348.

50. Kopoldova J, Liebsier J. The mechanism of radiation chemical degradation of amino acids V. *Int J Appl Radiation Isotopes* 1963;14:493–498.

51. Amici A, Tsai L, Levine RL, Stadtman ER. Conversion of amino acid residues in proteins and amino acid homopolymers to carbonyl derivatives by metal-catalyzed reactions. *J Biol Chem* 1989;264:3341–3346.

52. Climent I, Tsai L, Levine RL. Derivatization of γ-glutamyl semialdehyde residues in oxidized proteins by fluoresceinamine. *Anal Biochem* 1989;182:226–232.

53. Creeth JM, Cooper B, Donald ASR, Clamp JR. Studies of the limited degradation of mucous glycoproteins. *Biochem J* 1983;211:323–332.

54. Poston JM. Detection of oxidized amino acid residues using *p*-aminobenzoic acid adducts. *Fed Proc* 1979;46:1979 (Abstract)

55. Uchida K, Kato Y, Kawakishi S. A novel mechanism for oxidative damage of prolyl peptides induced by hydroxyl radicals. *Biochem Biophys Res Commun* 1990;169:265–271.

56. Mohr S, Stamler JS, Brüne B. Mechanism of covalent modification of glyceraldehyde-3-phosphate dehydrogenase at its active site thiol by nitric oxide, peroxynitrite, and related nitrosating agents. *FEBS Lett* 1994;348:223–227.

57. Rubbo H, Denicola A, Radi R. Peroxynitrite inactivates thiol-containing enzymes of *Trypanosoma cruzi* energetic metabolism and inhibits cell respiration. *Arch Biochem Biophys* 1994;308:96–102.

58. DeMaster EG, Quast BJ, Redfern B, Nagasawa HT. Reaction of nitric oxide with free sulfhydryl group of serum albumin yields a sulfonic acid and nitric oxide. *Biochemistry* 1995;34:11494–11499.

59. Wink DA, Nims RW, Darbyshire JF, Christodoulou D, Hanbauer I, Cox GW, Laval F, Laval J, Cook JA, Krishna MC, DeGaff WG, Mitchel JB. Reaction kinetics for nitrosation of cysteine and glutathione in aerobic nitric oxide solutions at neutral pH. Insights into the fate and physiological effecs of intermediates generated in NO/O₂ reaction. *Chem Res Tech* 1994;7:519–582.

60. Brot N, Weissbach H. Biochemistry and physiological role of methionine sulfoxide reductase in proteins. *Arch Biochem Biophys* 1983;223:271–281.

61. Stadtman ER, Ginsburg A. The glutamine synthetase of *Escherichia coli* structure and control. In: Boyer PD, ed. *The Enzymes.* New York: Academic Press, 1974:755–807.

62. Lymar SV, Hurst JK. Rapid reaction between peroxynitrite ion and carbon dioxide: Implication for biological activity. *J Am Chem Soc* 1995;117:8867–8868.

63. Apffel A, Sahakian J, Levine RL. Investigation of protein modification with electrospray LC/MS and Edmond sequencing techniques. *Protein Sci* 1994;3:99 (Abstract)

64. Neuzil J, Gebiki JM, Stocker R. Radical-induced chain oxidation of proteins and its inhibition by chain-breaking antioxidants. *Biochem J* 1993;293:601–606.

65. Schuenstein E, Esterbauer H. Formation and preparation of reactive aldehydes. In: *Submolecular biology of cancer,* CIBA Foundation Series 67. Amsterdam: Excerpta Medica/Elsevier, 1979:225–234.

66. Uchida K, Stadtman ER. Covalent modification of 4-hydroxynonenal to glyceraldehyde-3-phosphate. *J Biol Chem* 1993;268:6388–6393.

67. Friguet B, Stadtman ER, Szweda L. Modification of glucose-6-phosphate dehydrogenase by 4-hydroxy-2-nonenal. *J Biol Chem* 1994;269:21639–21643.

68. Monnier V. The Maillard reaction in the aging process. *J Gerontol* 1990;45:B105–B111.

69. Monnier V, Gerhardinger C, Marion MS, Taneda S. Novel approaches toward inhibition of the Maillard reaction *in vivo*: Search, isolation, and characterization of prokaryotic enzymes which degrade glycated substrates. In: Cuttler RG, Packer L, Bertram J, Mori A, eds. *Oxidative Stress and Aging.* Basel: Birkhauser Verlag, 1995:141–149.

70. Mularky CJ, Edelstein D, Brownlee M. Free radical generation by early glycation products. A mechanism for accelerated atherogenesis in diabetes. *Biochem Biophys Res Commun* 1990;173:932–939.

71. Wolf SP, Dean RT. Glucose autooxidation and protein modification. *Biochem J* 1987;245:243–250.

72. Kristal BS, Yu BP. An emerging hypothesis: Synergistic induction of aging by free radicals and Maillard reactions. *J Gerontol* 1992;47:B104–B107.

73. Starke-Reed PE, Oliver CN. Protein oxidation and proteolysis during aging and oxidative stress. *Arch Biochem Biophys* 1989;275:559–567.

74. Sohal RS, Agarwal S, Dubey A, Orr WC. Protein oxidative damage is associated with life expectancy of houseflies. *Proc Natl Acad Sci USA* 1993;90:7255–7259.
75. Winter ML, Liehr JG. Free radical-induced carbonyl content in protein of estrogen-treated hamsters assayed by sodium boro[³H]hydride reduction. *J Biol Chem* 1991;266:14446–14450.
76. Witt EH, Reznick AZ, Viguie CA, Starke-Reed PE, Packer L. Exercise, oxidative damage, and effects of antioxidant manipulation. *J Nutr* 1992;122:766–773.
77. Reznick AZ, Witt E, Matsumoto M, Packer L. Vitamin E inhibits protein oxidation in skeletal muscle of resting and exercised rats. *Biochem Biophys Res Commun* 1992;189:801–806.
78. Oliver CN, Starke-Reed PE, Stadtman ER, Liu GJ, Carney JM, Floyd RA. Oxidative damage to brain proteins, loss of glutamine synthetase activity, and production of free radicals during ischemia-reperfusion-induced injury to gerbil brain. *Proc Natl Acad Sci USA* 1990;87:5144–5147.
79. Poston JM, Parenteau GL. Biochemical effects of ischemia on isolated perfused rat heart tissues. *Arch Biochem Biophys* 1992;295:35–41.
80. Ayene IS, Al-Medi AB, Fisher AB. Inhibition of lung tissue oxidation during ischemia/reperfusion by 2-mercaptopropionyl glycine. *Arch Biochem Biophys* 1993;303:307–312.
81. Liu Y, Rosenthal RE, Starke-Reed PE, Fiskum G. Inhibition of post cardiac arrest brain protein oxidation by acetyl-L-carnitine. *Free Radical Biol Med* 1993;15:667–670.
82. Oliver CN. Inactivation of enzymes and oxidative modification of proteins by stimulated neutrophils. *Arch Biochem Biophys* 1987;253:62–72.
83. Krsek-Staples JA, Webster RO. Ceruloplasmin inhibits carbonyl formation in endogeneous cell proteins. *Free Radical Biol Med* 1993;14:115–125.
84. Mickel HS, Oliver CN, Starke-Reed PE. Protein oxidation and myelinolysis occur in brain following rapid correction of hyponatremia. *Biochem Biophys Res Commun* 1990;172:92–97.
85. Stafford RE, Mak TM, Kramer JH, Weglicki WB. Protein oxidation in magnesium deficient rat brains and kidneys. *Biochem Biophys Res Commun* 1993;196:596–600.
86. Reznick AZ, Cross CE, Hu M-L, Suzuki YJ, Khovaja S, Safadl, A, Motchnik PA, Packer L, Halliwell B. Modification of plasma proteins by cigarette smoke as measured by protein carbonyl formation. *Biochem J* 1992;286:607–611.
87. Shacter E, Williams JA, Lim M, Levine RL. Differential susceptibility of plasma proteins to oxidative modification: Examination by Western blot immunoassay. *Free Radical Biol Med* 1994;17:429–437.
88. Cross CE, Reznick AZ, Packer L, Davis PA, Suzuki YJ, Halliwell B. Oxidative damage to human plasma proteins by ozone. *Free Radical Res Commun* 1992;15:347–352.
89. Kelley FJ, Birch S. Ozone exposure-inhibits cardiac protein synthesis in the mouse. *Free Radical Biol Med* 1993;14:443–446.
90. Troncoso JC, Costello AC, Kim JH, Johnson GVW. Metal-catalyzed oxidation of bovine neurofilaments *in vitro*. *Free Radical Biol Med* 1995;18:891–899.
91. Sohal RS, Dubey A. Mitochondrial oxidative damage, hydrogen peroxide release, and aging. *Free Radical Biol Med* 1994;16:621–626.
92. Sohal RS, Ku H-H, Agarwal S. Biochemical correlates of longevity in two closely related rodent species. *Arch Biochem Biophys*;196:7–11.
93. Chapman ML, Rubin BR, Gracy RW. Increased carbonyl content of proteins in synovial fluid from patients with rheumatoid arthritis. *J Rheumatol* 1989;16:15–19.
94. Murphy ME, Kherer JP. Oxidation state of tissue thiol groups and content of protein carbonyl groups in chickens with inherited muscular dystrophy. *Biochem J* 1989;260:359–364.
95. Bowling AC, Schultz JB, Brown RH Jr., Beal MF. *J Neurochem* 1993;61:2322–2325.
96. Smith CD, Carney JM, Starke-Reed PE, Oliver CN, Stadtman ER, Floyd RA. Excess brain protein oxidation and enzyme dysfunction in normal and Alzheimer's disease. *Proc Natl Acad Sci USA* 1991;88:10540–10543.
97. Smith CD, Carney JM, Tatsuno T, Stadtman ER, Floyd RA, Markesbery WR. Protein oxidation in aging brain. In: Franceschi C, Cerpaldi G, Cristofalo VG, Vijg J, eds. *Aging and Cellular Defense Mechanisms*. New York: New York Academy of Science, 1996:110–119.
98. Garland D, Russell P, Zigler JS. Oxidative modification of lens proteins. In: Simic MG, Taylor KS, Ward JF, von Sontag V, eds. *Oxygen Radicals in Biology and Medicine*. New York: Plenum, 1988:347–353.
99. Gladstone IM, Levine RL. Oxidation of proteins in neonatal lungs. *Pediatrics* 1994;93:764–768.
100. Uchida K, Fukuda A, Kawakishi S, Hiai H, Toyokuni S. A renal carcinogen ferric nitriloacetate mediates a temporary accumulation of aldehyde-modified proteins within cytosolic compartment of rat kidney. *Arch Biochem Biophys* 1995;317:405–411.

101. Yoritaka A, Hattori N, Uchida K, Tanaka M, Stadtman ER, Mizuno Y. Immunochemical detection of 4-hydroxynonenal protein adducts in Parkinson's disease. *Proc Natl Acad Sci USA* 1996;93:2696–2701.
102. Uchida K, Toyokuni S, Kishikawa S, Oda H, Hiai H, Stadtman ER. Michael addition-type 4-hydroxy-2-nonenal adducts in modified low density lipoproteins: Markers for atherosclerosis. *Biochemistry* 1994;33:12487–12494.
103. Friguet B, Szweda L, Stadtman ER. Susceptibility of glucose-6-phosphate dehydrogenase modified by 4-hydroxy-2-nonenal and metal-catalyzed oxidation to proteolysis by the multicatalytic protease. *Arch Biochem Biophys* 1994;311:168–173.
104. Szweda L. Age-related increase in liver retinyl palmitate. Relationship to lipofuscin. *J Biol Chem* 1994;269:8712–8715.

Free Radical Toxicology
Edited by K. B. Wallace
Copyright © 1997 Taylor & Francis

6

Free-Radical-Mediated DNA Oxidation

Christoph Richter

Laboratory of Biochemistry I, Swiss Federal Institute of Technology (ETH), Zürich, Switzerland

INTRODUCTION

Eukaryotic cells harbor most of their DNA in the nucleus. A small percentage of cellular DNA is also present in mitochondria and chloroplasts, the semiautonomous organelles of prokaryotic descent. Nuclear DNA (nDNA) and mitochondrial DNA (mtDNA) are known to experience considerable oxidative damage, whereas no studies on chloroplast DNA oxidation have been reported to date. DNA oxidation and mutations resulting from it are implicated in the etiology of diseases and in natural aging. Much has recently been learned about the role of mtDNA, mutations of which are linked to myopathies, encephalomyopathies, heart diseases, late-onset diabetes, Parkinson's, Huntington's, and Alzheimer's disease, and to aging. This subject has been extensively reviewed (1–6).

The causal relationship between oxidative DNA modifications and diseases, cancer, and aging is rarely directly documented. Even for mtDNA, where the link between a defined mutation and a disease is often established, there is only one case in which the mutation was shown experimentally to be caused by oxidative insult to DNA (7). However, there is convincing indirect evidence that oxidative damage to nDNA causes or contributes to inflammation, neurodegenerative diseases, apoptosis, cancer, and aging (8–11). For example, oxidative mutagenesis contributes to cancer initiation, promotion, and progression (8), and overexpression of antioxidative enzymes results in decreased nDNA damage and increased longevity (11). The threat that oxidants impose on nDNA is also documented by the fact that all nucleated cells have repair endonucleases for oxidative DNA modifications in the nucleus, and that defects in repair enzymes are a major risk factor for cells (12). Thus, it can be safely assumed that oxidative DNA damage is not simply an epiphenomenon of but contributes importantly to diseases, cancer, and aging.

This chapter focuses on oxidation of nDNA. It selectively describes the types of oxidative modifications, which reactive oxygen and nitrogen species induce them, how the modifications can be detected, to what an extent they are formed, and the main groups of chemicals and physical agents which induce them. The important aspects of DNA repair and the relationship between oxidative DNA damage, diseases, and aging are not covered or are only briefly touched on because these aspects have been excellently reviewed in recent years (13–16).

ROS, RNS, AND OTHER OXIDANTS

Reactive oxygen species (ROS) are products of normal metabolism. The term ROS comprises oxygen radicals (superoxide, O_2^-; hydroxyl radical, OH˙; peroxyl radical, RO_2; alkoxyl radical, RO˙) as well as other particular oxidants, some of which may be converted to radicals (ozone, O_3; singlet oxygen, $^1O_2$; hydrogen peroxide, H_2O_2; hypochlorite, HOCl; peroxynitrite, $ONOO^-$). ROS are physiological reactants; some of them act, for example, as signaling molecules, but overproduction of ROS causes damage. ROS production can be increased by various compounds, such as so-called redox cyclers, by physical agents or manipulations (e.g., light or sonication), or by certain pathological states, for example, hypoxia alone or in combination with reoxygenation. RNS are NO˙, the nitrogen monoxide radical, commonly called nitric oxide; NO_2, the nitrogen dioxide radical; peroxynitrite, $ONOO^-$, and other compounds formed when NO˙ reacts with ROS. Like ROS, RNS are physiological reactants and participate in cell signaling, enzyme regulation, and killing of bacteria. When produced excessively, they are potentially dangerous. The dichotomy of RNS is also in part due to nitric oxide redox species with distinctive properties and reactivities, namely, NO^+, NO˙, and NO^- (reviewed in refs. 17 and 18), and to the ability of NO˙ to combine with O_2^- to yield $ONOO^-$ (19).

TYPES OF ROS- AND RNS-INDUCED MODIFICATIONS

ROS and RNS cause base modifications (oxidation and deamination), base loss (apurinic, AP sites), single- and double-strand breaks, and cross-links in DNA. Around 100 oxidative DNA modifications have been identified (20–22). The mechanisms of reaction between several oxygen-centered radicals and DNA, and the chemistry of DNA damage are well understood (reviewed in refs. 23 and 24), whereas much more has to be learned about the details of the reactions between RNS and DNA. It should also be noted that ROS (and presumably RNS) not only damage DNA but may also inhibit repair activities (25).

As could be expected from the different reactivities of ROS species, the pattern of DNA modifications depends on the nature of the ROS under consideration. Thus, O_2^- and H_2O_2 do not readily react with DNA but are important reactants in the metal-catalyzed formation of OH˙ (discussed later). The hydroxyl radical reacts with all four DNA bases and generates a large number of characteristic products, among them 8-hydroxyguanine (8-OHG). This modified base is also formed by the selective reaction of $^1O_2$ with DNA. Nitric oxide and its congeners cause mainly DNA deaminations, but in the form of $ONOO^-$ also lead to a pattern of damage similar to that induced by OH. The DNA damage profile induced by RNS needs to be determined further and is likely to be complex.

The chemistry of DNA modifications by ROS has been reviewed comprehensively (20–24). "Free" hydroxyl radicals are studied extensively. When produced by pulse radiolysis they preferentially react with DNA bases rather than with sugars. The former reaction leads to modified bases, and the latter reaction to cleavage of the sugar-phosphate backbone of the DNA.

Probably the most frequent base modification is 8-OHG, which is formed when DNA reacts with OH, $^1O_2$, excited photosensitizers, and ONOO$^-$. This modification is sensitively and easily measured by high-performance liquid chromatography (HPLC) in combination with electrochemical detection (discussed later). 8-Hydroxy-guanine mispairs with adenine during replication and causes G:C $\rightarrow$ T:A transversions. 8-Hydroxyguanine and its corresponding nucleoside (8-hydroxydeoxy-guanosine, 8-OHdG) can be removed from DNA by cellular repair enzymes and are present, as a consequence, in urine, where they serve as convenient in vivo markers for oxidative DNA damage. Other modified bases produced by OH attack on DNA, albeit in smaller amounts, are 8-hydroxyadenine, 2-hydroxyadenine, and formamidopyrimidines (Fapy lesions). Additional examples of oxidative base modifications are thymine glycols, 5-hydroxymethyluracil, and 5,6-dihydroxycytosines. Figure 1 shows examples of oxidatively modified DNA bases found in biological samples.

Apurinic/apyrimidinic sites (AP sites) can be formed by normal spontaneous hydrolysis and by oxidation due to attack at carbons 1, 2, or 4 of the sugar residues (see Figure 2). AP sites are noninstructive lesions, block DNA replication, and frequently result in deletions, presumably because they are easily transformed to strand breaks. Single-strand breaks are not very dangerous because they can easily be repaired, whereas double-strand breaks are very critical and seem to be responsible for chromosomal aberrations.

Hydroxyl radicals can be generated by reduction of H_2O_2 with reduced heavy metal ions such as Fe(II) or Cu(I) (Fenton reaction). Since O_2^- can dismutate to H_2O_2 and also reduce metal ions O_2^- and heavy metal ions are a potential source of OH. Some metal chelators prevent the formation of OH, apparently by blocking coordination sites important for OH formation, whereas others facilitate OH formation by keeping the reduced metal ions in solution or by changing their reduction potential. Hydroxyl radicals are also formed by photoinduced decomposition of hydroperoxides and *N*-oxides (see ref. 26).

Flavins and porphyrins excited by visible light or UV irradiation can transfer energy to ground-state molecular oxygen and thereby produce $^1O_2$.

METHODS TO DETECT OXIDATIVE DNA DAMAGE

Oxidative DNA base damage is principally measured either by determining the steady-state damage in DNA, which reflects the balance between damage and repair,

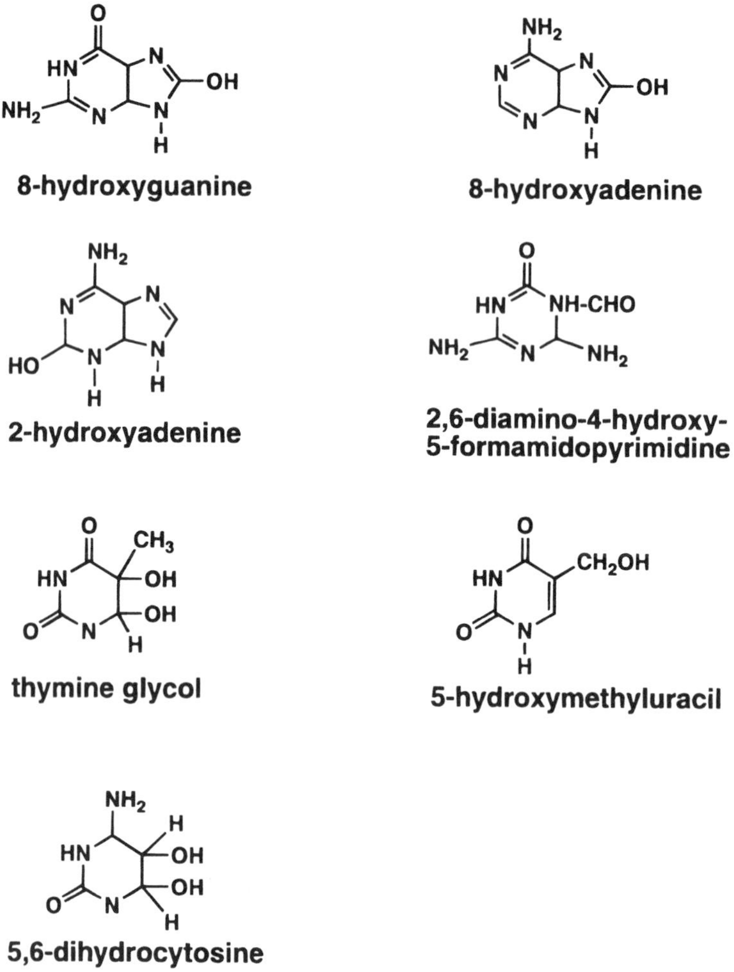

8-hydroxyguanine

8-hydroxyadenine

2-hydroxyadenine

**2,6-diamino-4-hydroxy-
5-formamidopyrimidine**

thymine glycol

5-hydroxymethyluracil

5,6-dihydrocytosine

FIG. 1. Structure of some oxidized base derivatives typically found in DNA.

or by monitoring nucleosides or bases released from DNA due to spontaneous or enzyme-catalyzed hydrolysis. There are four major techniques by which oxidative base modifications are detected: HPLC in combination with electrochemical detection (HPLC/EC) (27), gas chromatography in combination with mass spectrometry (GC/MS) (28), labeling of isolated DNA-derived material such as nucleosides or bases with appropriate reporter groups ("postlabeling") (29), and specific enzymatic removal of modified bases (30) with subsequent analysis by any of the preceding techniques or by analysis of the remaining DNA for strand breaks. Strand breaks, induced either directly by ROS or RNS or indirectly by spontaneous or enzyme-catalyzed hydrolysis, are usually analyzed by following the denaturation of double-

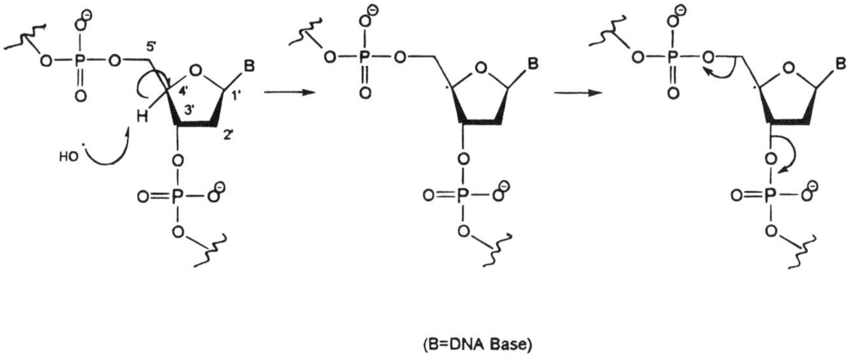

(B=DNA Base)

FIG. 2. Reaction of the hydroxyl radical (OH˙) with the ribose moiety of DNA. The hydroxyl radical abstracts a hydrogen atom from deoxyribose of DNA, the first step in DNA cleavage. In the example shown, hydrogen abstraction occurs at C-4′ of DNA, but attack at C-1′ or C-2′ is also possible. B, DNA base.

stranded DNA. This is determined via fluorescence analysis or filter binding under alkaline conditions (31,32). When fragmentation is extensive it can also be followed by pulsed-field or conventional agarose gel electrophoresis with ethidium bromide staining. Some of these techniques require isolation of the DNA under investigation, whereas others can detect oxidized bases or nucleosides liberated from DNA by repair enzymes in biological fluids, such as in urine. To date, a rigorous comparison and evaluation of all these various techniques has not been performed but is highly desirable.

HPLC/EC is the most frequently used technique to measure steady-state damage in DNA and modified bases in biological fluids. Only few types of oxidative modifications are detected by this technique. In pioneering studies the determination of 8-OHdG, the most common base modification detectable, gave important information about oxidative damage to DNA in cells and organisms (see ref. 33). The method has been used extensively for the determination of steady-state damage and of 8-OHdG in urine (27,34). The availability of monoclonal antibodies has greatly facilitated the latter. A drawback of the technique is the possibility that the removal of 8-OHdG from DNA prior to the analysis may not be complete, which would lead to an underestimation of the damage. An alternative to HPLC/EC is GC/MS, particularly when combined with selected ion monitoring (GC/MS/SIM), which allows the determination of many different modified (oxidized, deaminated) DNA bases, as well as DNA-protein adducts. GC/MS may overestimate damage because of the relatively harsh treatment of the samples during derivatization (35–37). This problem may be overcome by stable isotope dilution assays (38). The expense of the equipment prevents a widespread use of this technique. "Postlabeling" is a highly sensitive and relatively inexpensive technique. One possibility is to label nucleotides derived from DNA with ^{32}P (29). Because each nucleotide has to be prepared and concentrated separately before postlabeling with different kinases, the method is somewhat tedious. An alternative to ^{32}P is nonenzymatic acetylation of the oxidized nucleosides with [^{3}H]Ac$_2$O (acetic anhydride) (39). The use of repair endonucleases allows the determination of several types of base modifications as well as AP sites in DNA (30). The DNA strand breaks introduced by the enzymes are detected by alkaline elution assays (or relaxation assays in the case of supercoiled DNA). Drawbacks of this technique are the poorly understood substrate specificities of some repair enzymes and the limited access to them.

ESTIMATION OF THE EXTENT OF OXIDATIVE DAMAGE

Knowledge of the extent of oxidative DNA damage is important because damaged DNA may alter the flow of information from DNA to proteins. A large part of nDNA does not code for proteins but may still have important biological functions. At the moment it is not clear whether oxidative damage is evenly distributed over coding and noncoding regions of nDNA. It is, however, clear that proteins bound to DNA generally protect it from damage (40), and there is evidence that cell proliferation, such as in regenerating liver, renders DNA more susceptible to oxidative damage (41). Even if the damage were irrelevant for information storage and flow, analysis of the extent of damage would give useful information about the oxidative load in cells.

Our knowledge of the extent of oxidative DNA damage is, of course, largely dependent on the quality of the experimental analyses. From measurements of oxidized bases and nucleosides in urine it was estimated that on the average nDNA in each cell of a human or rat receives about 10,000 or 100,000, respectively, oxidative hits per day (42). The validity of these numbers was questioned on theoretical grounds (43). Using HPLC/EC to measure 8-OHdG it was found that its content in nDNA and mtDNA of liver isolated from 3-mo-old rats was 0.025 and 0.41 pmol/µg of DNA, respectively (44). These numbers were confirmed by subsequent HPLC/EC measurements (see refs. 4 and 26 for reviews). In the total DNA of cultured human lymphoblasts, the level of 8-OHdG measured by GC/MS/SIM was 0.1 pmol/µg of DNA (45). It should be noted that 10 fmol 8-OHdG/mg of DNA roughly corresponds to 1 8-OHdG/10^5 guanine residues in DNA. It should also be remembered that 8-OHdG is only one of many modifications produced in DNA by ROS and RNS.

Values of 8-OHdG obtained by GC/MS/SIM may be too high (46), and values obtained with repair enzyme analysis (47) are about one order of magnitude lower than that obtained with HPLC/EC. The reason for these discrepancies is not clear. Besides the harsh derivatization procedure for GC/MS, DNA workup for HPLC with phenol (48) may cause oxidative damage but can be excluded from responsibility for the observed level of 8-OHdG, at least in the case of mtDNA (Suter and Richter, unpublished manuscript). The low level of 8-OHdG observed with the enzymes may be due to incomplete removal of 8-OHdG from DNA from highly oxidized DNA stretches.

AGENTS AND MANIPULATIONS THAT MODIFY
OXIDATIVE DNA DAMAGE

Metals

Oxidative deterioration of biological macromolecules induced by transition metal ions is widespread and affects lipids, proteins, and nucleic acids. The role of ROS in metal toxicity has recently been reviewed (49). Iron, copper, chromium, and vanadium undergo redox cycling and thereby form ROS directly, whereas cadmium, mercury, lead, and nickel deplete cellular glutathione (GSH) and other sulhydryl compounds and thereby indirectly act as prooxidants. Although most studies point to the importance of Fenton-type mechanism(s) causing DNA damage, there are indications that metal-[hydrazines plus Mn(II)] induced DNA damage may also occur through non-Fenton-type reactions (50). Two modes of action seem to predominate in metal genotoxicity: the induction of oxidative DNA damage, best established for chromium compounds, and the interaction with enzymatic repair processes, as found with Cd(II), Ni(II), Co(II), Pb(II) and As(III) (reviewed in ref. 51; see also 52).

An important mechanistic study was done early with isolated DNA and an enzymatic source of superoxide (53). Using GC/MS it was shown that various modified bases are formed, and that stabilizing iron ions with ethylenediamine tetraacetic acid (EDTA) as chelator greatly augmented the damage. It was concluded that OH⁻ would modify several bases, and that 8-OHG was one of the major oxidation products. The study was then extended to include copper ions, chromatin, and nonenzymatic sources of ROS (54–56). A complex damage pattern was also found with carcinogenic metal compounds [Cr(VI), Fe(III) nitrilotriacetate (Fe-NTA, see also later discussion), Co(II), and Ni(II)], which induced the formation of various oxygen radical species in the presence of H_2O_2 (57,58). These oxygen radicals gave different kinds of site-specific DNA damage including 8-OHdG. In addition, using pulsed-field gel electrophoresis nickel sulfide was shown to induce oxidative DNA cleavage in cultured cells. More recent experiments revealed that factors like uptake and intracellular distribution of metals are important for the extent of DNA damage (59).

Acute iron overload in vivo resulted in a significant increase in 8-OHdG in rat testes DNA within 20 h, as measured by HPLC/EC (60). Iron also stimulated synergistically with the polychlorinated biphenyl mixture Aroclor 1254 in vivo 8-OHdG formation (61). In vivo administration of cobalt or nickel resulted in multiple base damage and DNA-protein cross-linking, as detected by GC/MS and alkaline elution (62–64). Damage was enhanced by the presence of L-histidine (63), in line with earlier in vitro investigations (65). Mammalian cells cultured in the presence of iron ions experience damage at all four DNA bases by reactions involving OH⁻ (66). Metals, particularly iron, are responsible for the ROS-induced DNA damage caused by asbestos and silica. Early studies reported asbestos-induced damage of isolated DNA in the presence of H_2O_2 (67,68). Crocidolite asbestos, which contains iron and is the most carcinogenic form of asbestos, increased, in an iron chelator-sensitive manner, 8-OHdG levels in isolated DNA (69), in DNA of cells kept in culture (70), in vivo in rats (71), and was mutagenic in a *Salmonella* tester strain (69). Nitric oxide participates in the formation of 8-OHdG stimulated by crocidolite (72). Iron also induced DNA unwinding in isolated rat liver nuclei, as measured by fluorometry (73). Asbestos-exposed workers have increased urinary 8-OHdG levels (74), as do industrial art glass workers (75). A DNA strand-break assay showed that probably OH˙ formed by iron in a Fenton-type reaction was responsible for silica-induced DNA damage (76). Tungsten oxide fibers form 8-OHdG in cultured human lung cells (77). Zinc fingers are important elements in DNA-binding transcription elements, which contain highly conserved cysteine residues; iron can replace zinc in zinc fingers and, in the presence of H_2O_2 and ascorbate, thereby induces the formation of OH˙ and DNA strand breaks (78). The way iron is complexed is important for its reactivity (see also the next paragraph), as very recently shown with cultured lung cells (79). Thus, iron bound to 8-hydroxy-quinoline (8HQ) caused extensive DNA strand breaks, whereas iron bound to EDTA or nitriloacetate (NTA) caused considerable hydroxylation of guanine residues. It was suggested that in cells the iron-8HQ complex acted through metal-bound oxyl radicals rather than OH˙.

Important contributions to the understanding of iron-mediated oxidative DNA damage came from the group of Linn. Exposure of *E. coli* to H_2O_2 leads to two kinetically distinguishable modes of cell killing: Mode I killing is maximal at 2 mM H_2O_2 and is decreased at higher concentrations, while mode II killing is independent of H_2O_2 up to 20 mM (80). A major portion of H_2O_2 toxicity seems to be caused by an iron-mediated Fenton-type reaction. The sites in DNA to which iron binds apparently determines the mode by which the cells are killed (81).

Copper can induce base-specific damage in DNA and is highly mutagenic, causing predominantly single-base substitutions (82). Cu(II) binds preferentially to guanine residues, as shown by x-ray diffraction analysis (83), and induces in combination with H_2O_2 oxidative damage at sites of two or more adjacent guanine residues (84). Copper is a rather selective catalyst of 8-OHdG formation in DNA in the presence of L-DOPA and H_2O_2, being much more effective than iron ions (85), findings relevant to several neurodegenerative diseases. Long-Evans cinnamon rats suffer from abnormal copper accumulation in the liver, which leads to hepatitis and hepato-cellular carcinoma; cinnamon rats accumulate 8-OHdG in the DNA of various organs (86). The amount of 8-OHdG in livers of such rats could be decreased by treatment with the copper chelator D-penicillamine (87). Copper was also investigated as inducer of oxidative DNA damage in conjunction with GSH. When the ratio of GSH to Cu(II) is low, damage as measured by 8-OHdG accumulation of DNA is promoted in vitro, but GSH becomes protective when the ratio of GSH to Cu(II) is high (88). The protective effect of GSH may be attributable to its stabilization of copper in the Cu(I) oxidation state (89). Glutathione did not enhance the Cr(VI)- and Cr(V)-induced formation of 8-OHdG in isolated DNA, which occurred via a Fenton-type mechanism (90). Finally, plutonium (^{242}Pu) catalyzed in a manner resembling that of iron the H_2O_2 and ascorbate-induced formation of 8-OHdG in the absence of significant α-particle irradiation (91).

Peroxisome Proliferators

Peroxisomes are an important intracellular source of H_2O_2. Peroxisome proliferators comprise a wide range of structurally dissimilar compounds such as clofibrate, a hypolipidemic drug, or plasticizers such as di(2-ethylhexyl)phthalate, and cause an increase in the number of peroxisomes when given to rats in vivo. Peroxisome proliferation and oxidative DNA damage have been associated with hepatocarcinogenesis (92). Indeed, since the first description of DNA oxidation induced by peroxisome proliferators (93) ample evidence has been accumulated that peroxisome proliferators can cause cellular DNA damage. Organ specificity and mtDNA contributions to the observed damage are presently of particular interest in this area of research.

In most studies with peroxisome proliferators 8-OHdG was chosen as indicator for oxidative DNA damage. A notable exception is the analysis of 5-hydroxymethyluracil, formed by the reaction of thymine with $OH^{\cdot}$, after in vivo labeling of DNA with [^{3}H]thymidine. This modified base was formed during peroxisome proliferation (94). 8-Hydroxydeoxyguanosine was reported to increase after treatment of rats with peroxisome proliferators, sometimes in an organ-specific manner, by several (95–98) but not all (99) research groups using comparable experimental setups. An intriguing finding that may shed light on some of the apparent discrepancies is the report that mitochondrial alterations (their amount, and extent of mtDNA damage) are crucial contributors to the observed overall DNA changes (100).

2-Nitropropane, Acetoxime, Nitrilotriacetate, and Bromate

Several industrially important carcinogenic compounds have been studied as inducers of oxidative DNA damage. This was mostly analyzed by measuring 8-OHdG by HPLC/EC but also with repair enzymes, GC/MS, and postlabeling.

2-Nitropropane is a widely used industrial chemical that is a mutagen in bacteria and a powerful hepatocarcinogen in rats. This compound, as well as the structurally related carcinogen acetoxime, induces 8-OHG in liver DNA (and RNA) of male rats (101–103). Consistent with the notion that these chemicals are weaker carcinogens in female rats, it was found that less 8-OHdG was induced in females than in males (104). Iron-deficiency renders rats more sensitive to 2-nitropropane (105). Nitrilotriacetate, a metal chelator used in detergents, in the form of the ferric chelate, Fe-NTA, is nephrotoxic and carcinogenic in rats; oxidative DNA damage was detected by HPLC/EC measurements of 8-OHdG in the kidneys of rats after administration of Fe-NTA (106). Administration of GSH and cysteine suppressed 8-OHdG formation (107). Oxidative DNA damage induced by Fe-NTA in male rats was also detected by postlabeling with ^{32}P (108), and by following the formation of base modifications and DNA-protein cross-linking by GC/MS (109,110). The damage in kidney DNA induced by Fe-NTA can be specifically repaired (111). Potassium bromate, a food additive, induces renal-cell tumors; it was the first chemical carcinogen for which a significant increase of 8-OHdG in kidney (the target organ) DNA, but not in liver (a nontarget organ) DNA after administration to rats was found (112; see also 113). Antioxidants such as GSH prevented in vivo KBrO$_3$-induced 8-OHdG formation, whereas diethylmaleate, a depletor of cellular GSH, elevated 8-OHdG (114). Potassium bromate may not directly form 8-OHdG but indirectly via induction of lipid peroxides (115). Oxidative DNA damage induced by KBrO$_3$ in cultured mammalian cells and cell-free systems was also studied with repair endonucleases (116). The predominant modification found was 8-OHdG. The damage profile and the effect of various inhibitors or ROS scavengers led to the conclusion that bromine radicals are reactants important for the induction of damage.

Aromatic Compounds, Redox Cyclers, and Carcinogens

Menadione is a compound that, depending on its subcellular localization, may or may not act as a redox cycler (117). Menadione administered to rats led to an increase in hepatic 8-OHdG levels but not to initiation of carcinogenesis (118). In hepatocytes, however, menadione caused DNA nicking in the absence of 8-OHdG induction (119). This suggests that in hepatocytes events other than ROS formation, possibly Ca^{2+} mobilization (117) followed by endonuclease activation, are stimulated by menadione. The phenolic food antioxidant butylated hydroxyanisole is a carcinogen, possibly because of its oxidative biotransformation in vivo; its metabolite 2-*tert*-butyl(1,4)hydroquinone (TBHQ), is a strong inducer of oxidative DNA damage (120). Butylated hydroxyanisole given to rats increased the level of 8-OHdG in a process that apparently involved prostaglandin H synthase (121). Butylated hydroxyanisole and TBHQ were also studied in human lymphocytes (122). The latter, but not the former, induced 8-OHdG in DNA, and again the involvement of prostaglandin H synthase was indicated. The carcinogen 4-nitroquinoline *N*-oxide induces oxidative stress in *E. coli*, where it acts as potent redox cycler (123). This compound causes 8-OHG formation in Ehrlich ascites cells (124) and strand breaks in human leukocyte DNA (125). 4-Hydroxyaminoquinoline-1-oxide stimulates after in vivo administration to rats 8-OHdG formation specifically in pancreatic DNA (126). Benzene, a leukemogenic component of fuel, increases 8-OHdG in cell culture and bone marrow (127) and in the urine of filling-station attendants (128,129). Benzene also causes DNA strand breaks in leukocytes (129). The polycyclic aromatic hydrocarbons benzo[α]pyrene and 1,6-dinitropyrene also cause base oxidation, as determined by 8-OHdG and thymine glycol measurements and postlabeling with ^{32}P (130–132). 8-Hydroxydeoxyguanosine levels are increased by redox cycling 3-amino-1,2,4-benzotriazine-1,4-dioxide and nitrogen mustard *N*-oxide (133), by aflatoxin B$_1$ (134), tetrachloro-*p*-hydroquinone (135) [which also induces single-strand breaks in DNA (136)], phenylhydroquinone (137), and diesel exhaust particles

(138). Low levels of 8-OHdG are found after treating fish intramuscularly with nitrofurantoin (139).

The teratogenic compound phenytoin induces 8-OHdG in a murine embryo culture model; superoxide dismutase and catalase virtually eliminate 8-OHdG induction and counteract dysmorphological anomalies (140), providing evidence that ROS-mediated damage is critical for phenytoin teratogenesis. Along this line it is interesting to note that a previous study showed DNA strand breaks to be induced by 2,3,7,8-tetrachlorodibenzo-*p*-dioxin in rats (141). Finally, the fungal metabolite gliotoxin, which is characterized by a epipolythiodioxopiperazine ring and causes light-induced facial eczemas in ruminants, is in the presence of NADH or reduced thiols a potent redox cycler able to introduce ROS-dependent DNA strand breaks (142).

Tumor Promoters

Initiation and promotion are major stages in the multistage carcinogenesis process. It is well established that the tumor-initiating properties are related to the formation of DNA base adducts. There is also evidence that ROS participate in at least one stage of tumor promotion (see 143 for review of early work). The group of Frenkel has recently provided more evidence for the conjecture that oxidative DNA damage is involved in tumor promotion. Using mice sensitive (SENCAR) or resistant (C57BL/6J) to tumor-promoting phorbol esters it was found that topically applied phorbol esters cause an increase in oxidized DNA derivatives, measured by $[^3H]Ac_2O$ postlabeling, in the epidermis (144). Oxidative DNA damage is paralleled by H_2O_2 formation and can be suppressed by antioxidants (145). At low doses of tumor promoter, tumor promoter-resistant mice formed much less H_2O_2 and oxidized DNA bases than promoter-sensitive mice (146), suggesting that oxidative events and DNA modifications are at least in part responsible for the strain-dependent sensitivity to tumor promotion. Also 7,12-dimethylbenz[a]anthracene, a carcinogen that requires oxidative metabolism for its activity, caused H_2O_2 and oxidized DNA base formation in SENCAR mice (147). In dimethyl sulfoxide-differentiated promyelocytic leukemia cells, which have characteristics similar to those of human neutrophils, phorbol ester-type (148) and non-phorbol ester-type tumor promotors (in combination with O_2^-) (149) stimulated 8-OHdG formation.

Anticancer Quinones

The relationship between free radical-mediated DNA damage, characterized mainly by double-strand breaks, and antitumor antibiotics such as bleomycin, neocarzinostatin, and calicheamicin has been thoroughly investigated and comprehensively reviewed (150,151). Its discussion is beyond the scope of the present overview. Particularly the reaction between the neocarzinostatin chromophor and the deoxyribose moiety of DNA is characterized in great detail. Antitumor quinones are typical redox cyclers, and generation of OH· is an important precondition for the manifestation of antitumor activity (152), but DNA is also cleaved by a quinone-oxo-iron ion complex (153). There is also evidence that antitumor quinones cause 8-OHdG formation in DNA (154,155).

Fecapentaenes and Aminolevulinic Acid

Fecapentaenes are unsaturated, ether-linked fecal lipids of potent genotoxicity in mammalian cells. They may play an initiating role in colon carcinogenesis. The genotoxicity of fecapentaenes is augmented by prostaglandin H synthase (156). Peroxidized fecapentaenes form ROS, as shown by spin trapping (157), but oxidative DNA damage may only be of minor importance for the genotoxic potential of fecapentaenes (158).

5-Aminolevulinic acid (ALA), a heme precursor accumulated in chemical-induced and inborn porphyrias, may be an endogenous prooxidant. In chronically ALA-treated rats 8-OHdG in liver DNA was 4.5 times higher than in nontreated rats. In vitro exposure of calf thymus DNA to ALA in the presence of Fe(II) caused the formation of 8-OHdG (159). The data support the hypothesis that ALA-generated ROS can oxidize DNA and may be involved in the development of primary liver-cell carcinoma during symptomatic acute intermittent porphyria.

Singlet Oxygen and Irradiation

Singlet oxygen can be generated with and without light. So-called photosensitizers absorb visible light, become thereby excited, and transfer their energy to ground state molecular oxygen with the formation of $^1O_2$ (type II reaction). Excited photosensitizers can also directly react with DNA without the participation of $^1O_2$ (type I reaction) (160). Singlet oxygen sources independent of light excitation are peroxy radicals, or hypochlorite and peroxynitrite plus H_2O_2 (26). Light of the appropriate wavelength can also directly modify DNA (161).

Photosensitized riboflavin induces 8-OHdG in cultured cells (162,163). The products formed from deoxyguanosine upon photosensitization of riboflavin (or methylene blue) are characterized (164,165). In combination with light, proflavine or meso-substituted porphyrin, cationic photosensitizers with high affinity for DNA, oxidized guanine residues and generated single-strand breaks (166,167). The porphyrin did not generate $^1O_2$, and damaged DNA at bases and strands by distinct mechanisms. Photosensitizers can also be used as convenient sources of OH· (168–170) without simultaneous generation of other ROS. Melanins are natural photosensitizers and can both quench and produce ROS. Melanotic and hypomelanotic, but not carcinoma, cells formed thymine glycols as oxidized DNA base products upon ultraviolet (UV) irradiation (171). In a detailed study with bacteriophage and plasmid DNA the mutagenic consequences of OH· and $^1O_2$ were analyzed (172). Also with plasmid DNA it was shown that $^1O_2$, with the aid of reduced thiol compounds, induces strand breaks (173) and 8-OHdG (174), with the latter modification leading selectively to breaks at guanine residues. Singlet oxygen-induced lesions interrupt DNA synthesis (175). The alkaline elution assay in combination with specific repair enzymes was used to investigate visible light-induced DNA damage in cells (176). Damage comprised predominantly 8-OHdG, and fewer strand breaks plus AP sites. The ratio of the various modifications indicated that damage resulted from type I and type II reactions and was not mediated by OH. The same study demonstrated rapid repair ($t_{1/2}$ about 1 h at 37°C) of 8-OHdG. Near-UV light caused induction followed by repair of 8-OHdG in the epidermis of hairless mice (177), and the formation of three novel products in DNA in aqueous solution (178). All four DNA bases of hepatic chromatin in mice are oxidized by ionizing radiation (179). The structures of γ-irradiation- and $^1O_2$-derived deoxyadenosine and deoxyguanosine decomposition products have recently been worked out (180–182).

Excited triplet carbonyl compounds appear to form 8-OHG directly without involvement of ROS (183).

Reactive Nitrogen Species

Early studies showed that nitric oxide and its congeners can deaminate DNA bases and are genotoxic (184–186). Nitric oxide provides significant protection to mammalian cells against the cytotoxic effect of H_2O_2 (187) but potentiates H_2O_2-induced killing of *E. coli*, where it induces double-strand breaks (188). In cells nitric oxide seems to react with DNA directly in an OH-like fashion, and indirectly by mobilizing iron to ultimately cause Fenton-type reactions (189). Nitric oxide cleaves DNA preferentially at GC sequences, as shown with plasmid DNA (190). In more complex systems NO may often act through ONOO⁻, which can cause 8-OHdG formation and DNA cleavage in isolated (191) and cellular (192) DNA. Peroxynitrite- and/or NO-induced DNA damage may result in apoptosis (193,194), and ONOO⁻ causes base oxidation in nucleosides and isolated DNA (195) and adduct formation when reacting with 2'-deoxyguanosine (196).

Diets, Exercise, and Stress

The impact of life-style and diet on longevity and cancer incidence is of great practical and theoretical importance (197). In humans, low-fat diet decreased oxidative DNA damage in nucleated peripheral blood cells (198). In rats, there was an increase of 8-OHdG upon feeding a diet enriched with unsaturated fatty acids (199). Betel-quid ingredients cause ROS production, 8-OHdG formation in isolated DNA, and micronucleated cells in Syrian golden hamsters and Indian betel-quid chewers (200). Diets deficient in choline alone or deficient in choline and amino acids cause hepatocellular carcinomas; choline deficiency increases the liver 8-OHdG content of rats (201), as does the combined deficiency of choline and amino acids (202) or chronic feeding of ethanol to rats (203). 8-Hydroxydeoxyguanosine could not be lowered by simultaneous feeding of the doubly deficient diet and the antioxidants N,N'-diphenyl-p-phenylenediamine or butylated hydroxytoluene (204). Caloric restriction suppresses the urinary output of oxidized bases in humans (205) and the steady-state oxidation level in DNA of rat (206,207) and mouse (208) tissues. However, a more recent study with humans detected no significant difference in urinary 8-OHdG excretion between restricted and nonrestricted individuals (209). The impact of exercise on DNA oxidation is incompletely understood. Oxygen consumption correlates with urinary 8-OHdG excretion in humans (210). In swimmers and distance runners there is a remarkable decrease in cellular and urinary base oxidation levels (211), possibly due to augmented DNA repair processes, but uncertainties with respect to proper sampling times after exercise warrant further studies. Thus, 10 h after a marathon run urinary 8-OHdG was increased 130% (212). In rats exposed to psychological stress 8-OHdG of liver DNA increased (213).

Tobacco Smoking and Air Pollution

About 3800 chemicals have been identified in cigarette smoke, with a large number of them being mutagenic and carcinogenic. Tobacco smoking increases the urinary output of 8-OHdG by up to 50% (210,211,214,215), and 8-OHdG in human peripheral leukocytes (128,216,217) within minutes (218). Cigarette smoke causes DNA strand breaks in cultured human lung cells (219). Nitrosamines, constituents of cigarette smoke, increases 8-OHdG levels particularly in lung, somewhat in liver, but not in kidney of mice and rats (220). Hydroquinone, another major constituent of tobacco smoke, causes dose-dependent H_2O_2 formation and 8-OHdG increases in isolated DNA (221), and strand breaks and 8-OHdG in cultured human epithelial lung cells (222). DNA in such cells is damaged at all four bases by ROS and RNS when exposed to gas-phase cigarette smoke (223). Inhalation of heavily polluted urban air increases urinary 8-OHG within 3 h (224).

Protection

Protection against oxidative DNA damage by a number of nonenzymatic antioxidants has been shown at various levels of complexity. With isolated DNA exposed to either UV light or a Fenton-type ROS generator the three compounds GSH, ascorbate, and 5-aminosalicylic acid proved protective against light-induced damage, but in the presence of iron they acted at high concentrations as prooxidants (225). Thus, the antioxidant dose should be carefully chosen. Spermine at 0.1 mM protected isolated DNA, but not free deoxyguanosine, against ROS-mediated damage (226). Human lymphocytes were protected by α-tocopherol against iron/ascorbate induced unscheduled DNA synthesis (227). *Escherichia coli* treated with H_2O_2 were protected against DNA scission and cell killing by cyclic stable nitroxide free radicals with superoxide dismutase-like activity (228). Protection was also seen under hypoxia, and it was suggested that the nitroxide may interfere with iron of a Fenton-type reaction. Endogenous chromatin is a very effective natural protector against damage caused by such reactions (229), but its protein and DNA can be cross-linked in the course of this reaction (230). Glutathione, ascorbate, and 5-aminosalicylic acid (see also earlier discussion) protected Chinese hamster cells from light-induced DNA damage (231).

Importantly, attempts were also made to protect animals and humans against DNA damage with antioxidants. Protection provided by GSH against Fe-NTA and $KBrO_3$ has already been pointed out (see refs. 107 and 114). Two successful studies and one negative outcome are known for humans. Dietary ascorbate protected against endogenous oxidative DNA damage in human sperm (232), and a diet rich in Brussels sprouts (300 g/d) decreased the urinary output of 8-OHdG (233). Male smokers, however, were not protected by β-carotene against oxidative DNA damage (234).

PERSPECTIVES

Oxidative DNA damage is induced by many natural and industrial agents and by several manipulations, as shown by in vitro and in vivo studies at various levels of complexity. There is considerable circumstantial evidence that oxidative DNA damage contributes to diseases, cancer, and aging. Important questions to be addressed in the future are: What is the true extent of oxidative damage? What is the causal relationship between oxidative damage and diseases, cancer, and aging? Can antioxidative interventions prevent damage and its consequences? How important are RNS for oxidative DNA damage? A combination of refined and comparative methodologies, the use of transgenic animals, and more nutritional studies will answer these questions.

ACKNOWLEDGMENTS

The work done in my laboratory was generously supported over the years by the Schweizerische Nationalfonds, and partly by the Eidgenössische Technische Hochschule Zürich. I am grateful to a number of colleagues for supplying unpublished material, and to those who forgive me for not having quoted their published work. I thank Patrick Walter for critically reading the manuscript.

REFERENCES

1. Bandy B, Davison AJ. Mitochondrial mutations may increase oxidative stress: Implications for carcinogenesis and aging? *Free Radical Biol Med* 1990;18:523–539.
2. Richter C. Reactive oxygen and DNA damage in mitochondria. *Mutat Res* 1992;275:249–255.
3. Richter C. Oxidative damage to mitochondrial DNA and its relationship to aging. In: Esser K, Martin GM, eds. *Dahlem Konferenz 74 Molecular Aspects of Aging*. Chichester: John Wiley & Sons, 1995;99–108.

4. Richter C. Oxidative damage to mitochondrial DNA and its relationship to ageing. *Int J Biochem Cell Biol* 1995;27:647–653.
5. Wallace DC, Richter C, Bohr VA, Cortopassi G, Kadenbach B, Linn S, Linnane AW, Shay JW. The role of bioenergetics and mitochondrial DNA in aging and age-related diseases. In: Esser K, Martin GM, eds. *Dahlem Konferenz 74 Molecular aspects of aging.* Chichester: John Wiley & Sons, 1995;199–225.
6. Richter C, Schweizer M. Oxidative stress in mitochondria. In: Scandalios J, ed. *Oxidative Stress and the Molecular Biology of Antioxidant Defenses.* Cold Spring Harbor, NY: Cold Spring Harbor Laboratory Press, 1997;169–200.
7. Adachi K, Fujiura Y Mayumi F, Nozuhara A, Sugiu Y, Sakanashi T, Hidaka T, Toshima H. A deletion of mitochondrial DNA in murine doxorubicin-induced cardiotoxicity. *Biochem Biophys Res Commun* 1993;195:945–951.
8. Wiseman G, Halliwell B. Damage to DNA by reactive oxygen and nitrogen species: Role in inflammatory disease and progression to cancer. *Biochem J* 1996;313:17–29.
9. Halliwell B. Free radicals, antioxidants, and human diseases: Curiosity, cause, or consequence? *Lancet* 1994;344:721–724.
10. Ames BN. Dietary carcinogens and anticarcinogens. Oxygen radicals and degenerative diseases. *Science* 1983;221:1256–1264.
11. Orr WC, Sohal RS. Extension of life-span by overexpression of superoxide dismutase and catalase in *Drosophila Melanogaster. Science* 1994;263:1128–1130.
12. Michaels ML, Cruz C, Grollman AP, Miller JH. Evidence that MutY and MutM combine to prevent mutations by an oxidative damaged form of guanine. *Proc Natl Acad Sci USA* 1992;89:7022–7025.
13. Sancar A. DNA repair in humans. *Annu Rev Genetics* 1995;29:69–105.
14. Demple B, Harrison L. Repair of oxidative damage to DNA: Enzymology and biology. *Annu Rev Biochem* 1994;63:915–948.
15. Halliwell B, Gutteridge JM. *Free Radicals in Biology and Medicine.* 2nd ed. Oxford: University Press, 1989.
16. Ames BN. Endogenous oxidative DNA damage, aging, and cancer. *Free Radical Res Commun* 1989;7:121–128.
17. Stamler JS, Singel DJ, Loscalzo J. Biochemistry of nitric oxide and its redox-activated forms. *Science* 1992;258:1898–1902.
18. Stamler JS. Redox signaling: Nitrosylation and related target interactions of nitric oxide. *Cell* 1994;78:931–936.
19. Beckman JS, Beckman TW, Chen J, Marshall PA, Freeman BA. Apparent hydroxyl radical production by peroxynitrite: Implications for endothelial injury from nitric oxide and superoxide. *Proc Natl Acad Sci USA* 1990;87:1620–1624.
20. von Sonntag C. *The Chemical Basis of Radiation Biology.* London: Taylor and Francis, 1989.
21. Dizdaroglu M. Oxidative damage to DNA in mammalian chromatin. *Mutat Res* 1992;275:331–342.
22. Cadet J. DNA damage caused by oxidation, deamination, ultraviolet radiation and photoexcited psoralens. In: Hemminki K, Dipple A, Shuker DEG, Kadlubar FF, Segerbäck D, Bartsch H, eds. *DNA Adducts: Identification and Biological Significance.* Lyon: International Agency for Research on Cancer, 1994;245–276.
23. Breen AP, Murphy JA. Reactions of oxyl radicals with DNA. *Free Radical Biol Med* 1995; 18:1033–1077.
24. Halliwell B, Aruoma OI, eds. *DNA and Free Radicals.* Chichester: Ellis Horwood, 1993.
25. Hu JJ, Dubin N, Kurland D, Ma BL, Roush GC. The effects of hydrogen peroxide on DNA repair activities. *Mutat Res* 1995;336:193–201.
26. Epe B. DNA damage profiles induced by oxidizing agents. In: Grunicke H, Schweiger M, eds. *Rev Physiol Biochem Pharmacol Vol 127.* Heidelberg: Springer Verlag, 1995;223–249.
27. Shigenaga MK, Aboujaoude EN, Chen Q, Ames BN. Assays of oxidative DNA damage biomarkers. 8-Oxo-2′-deoxyguanosine and 8-oxoguanine in nuclear DNA and biological fluids by high-performance liquid chromatography with electrochemical detection. *Methods Enzymol* 1994;234:16–33.
28. Dizdaroglu M. Chemical determination of oxidative DNA damage by gas chromatography-mass spectrometry. *Methods Enzymol* 1994;234:3–16.
29. Phillips DH, Castegnaro M, Bartsch H, eds. *Postlabeling Methods for Detection of DNA Adducts.* Lyon: International Agency for Research on Cancer, 1993.
30. Epe B, Hegler J. Oxidative DNA damage: Endonuclease fingerprinting. *Methods Enzymol* 1994;234:122–131.

31. Baumstark-Kahn C. Alkaline elution versus fluorescence analysis of DNA unwinding. *Methods Enzymol* 1994;234:88–102.
32. Leanderson P, Wennerberg K, Tagesson C. DNA microfiltration assay: A simple technique for detecting DNA damage in mammalian cells. *Carcinogenesis* 1994;15:137–139.
33. Halliwell B, Aruoma OI. DNA damage by oxygen-derived species. Its mechanism and measurement in mammalian systems. *FEBS Lett* 1991;281:9–19.
34. Loft S, Fischer-Nielsen A, Jeding IB, Vistisen K, Poulsen HE. 8-Hydroxydeoxyguanosine as a urinary biomarker of oxidative DNA damage. *J Toxicol Environ Health* 1993;40:391–404.
35. Hamberg M, Zhang LY. Quantitative determination of 8-hydroxyguanine and guanine by isotope dilution mass spectrometry. *Anal Biochem* 1995;229:336–344.
36. Halliwell B, Dizdaroglu M. The measurement of oxidative damage to DNA by HPLC and GC/MS techniques. *Free Radical Res Commun* 1992;16:75–87.
37. Douki T, Delatour T, Bianchini F, Cadet J. Observation and prevention of an artefactual formation of oxidized DNA bases and nucleosides in the GC-EIMS method. *Carcinogenesis* 1996;17:347–353.
38. Dizdaroglu M. Quantitative determination of oxidative base damage in DNA by stable isotope-dilution mass spectroscopy. *FEBS Lett* 1993;315:1–6.
39. Frenkel K, Zhong Z, Wei H, Karkoszka J, Patel U, Rashid K, Georgescu M, Solomon JJ. Quantitative high-performance liquid chromatography analysis of DNA oxidized in vitro and in vivo. *Anal Biochem* 1991;196:126–136.
40. Tullius TD. Chemical snapshot of DNA: Using the hydroxyl radical to study the structure of DNA and DNA-protein complexes. *Trends Biochem Sci* 1987;12:297–300.
41. Adachi S, Kawamura K, Takemoto K. Increased susceptibility to oxidative DNA damage in regenerating liver. *Carcinogenesis* 1994;15:539–543.
42. Fraga C, Shigenaga MK, Park J-W, Deagan P, Ames BN. Oxidative damage to DNA during aging: 8-Hydroxy-2'-deoxyguanosine in rat organ DNA and urine. *Proc Natl Acad Sci USA* 1990; 87:4533–4537.
43. Lindahl T. Instability and decay of the primary structure of DNA. *Nature* 1993;362:709–715.
44. Richter C, Park J-W, Ames BN. Normal oxidative damage to mitochondrial and nuclear DNA is extensive. *Proc Natl Acad Sci USA* 1988;85:6465–6467.
45. Jaruga P, Dizdaroglu M. Repair of products of oxidative DNA base damage in human cells. *Nucleic Acids Res* 1996;24:1389–1394.
46. Ravanat J-L, Turesky RJ, Gremaud E, Trudel LJ, Stadler RH. Determination of 8-oxoguanine in DNA by gas chromatography-mass spectrometry and HPLC-electrochemical detection: Overestimation of the background level of the oxidized base by the gas chromatography-mass spectrometry assay. *Chem Res Toxicol* 1995;8:1039–1045.
47. Pflaum M, Boiteux S, Epe B. Visible light generates oxidative DNA base modifications in high excess of strand breaks in mammalian cells. *Carcinogenesis* 1994;15:297–300.
48. Claycamp HG. Phenol sensitization of DNA to subsequent oxidative damage in 8-hydroxyguanine assays. *Carcinogenesis* 1992;13:1289–1292.
49. Stohs SJ, Bagchi D. Oxidative mechanisms in the toxicity of metal ions. *Free Radical Biol Med* 1995;18:321–336.
50. Ito K, Yamamoto K, Kawanishi S. Manganese-mediated oxidative damage of cellular and isolated DNA by isoniazid and related hydrazines: Non-Fenton-type hydroxyl radical formation. *Biochemistry* 1992;31:11606–11613.
51. Hartwig A. Current aspects in metal genotoxicity. *Biometals* 1995;8:3–11.
52. Hartwig A, Schlepegrell R, Dally H, Hartmann M. Interaction of carcinogenic metal compounds with deoxyribonucleic acid repair processes. *Annals Clin Lab Sci* 1996;26:31–38.
53. Aruoma OI, Halliwell B, Dizdaroglu M. Iron ion-dependent modification of bases in DNA by the superoxide radical-generating system hypoxanthine/xanthine oxidase. *J Biol Chem* 1989; 264:13024–1308.
54. Dizdaroglu M, Aruoma OI, Halliwell B. Modification of bases in DNA by copper ion–1,10-phenanthroline complexes. *Biochemistry* 1990;29:8447–8451.
55. Dizdaroglu M, Rao G, Halliwell B, Gajewski E. Damage to the DNA bases in mammalian chromatin by hydrogen peroxide in the presence of ferric and cupric ions. *Arch Biochem Biophys* 1991;285:317–324.
56. Aruoma OI, Halliwell B, Gajewski E, Dizdaroglu M. Copper-ion-dependent damage to the bases in DNA in the presence of hydrogen peroxide. *Biochem J* 1991;273:601–604.

57. Kawanishi S, Inoue S, Sano S. Mechanism of DNA cleavage induced by sodium chromate(VI) in the presence of hydrogen peroxide. *J Biol Chem* 1986;261:5952–5958.

58. Kawanishi S, Inoue S, Yamamoto K. Active oxygen species in DNA damage induced by carcinogenic metal compounds. *Environ Health Perspect* 1994;102:17–20.

59. Hartwig A, Schlepegrell R, Beyersmann D. Analysis of metal-induced oxidative damage in cultured mammalian cells. *Fresenius J Anal Chem* 1996;354:606–608.

60. Lucesoli F, Fraga GC. Oxidative damage to lipids and DNA concurrent with decrease of antioxidants in rat testes after acute iron intoxication. *Arch Biochem Biophys* 1995;316:567–571.

61. Faux SP, Francis JE, Smith AG. Chipman JK. Induction of 8-hydroxydeoxyguanosine in Ah-responsive mouse liver by iron and Aroclor 1254. *Carcinogenesis* 1992;13:247–250.

62. Kasprzak KS, Zastawny TH, North SL, Riggs CW, Diwan BA, Rice JM, Dizdaroglu M. Oxidative DNA base damage in renal, hepatic, and pulmonary chromatin of rats after intraperitoneal injection of cobalt(II) acetate. *Chem Res Toxicol* 1994;7:329–335.

63. Misra M, Olinsky R, Dizdaroglu M, Kasprzak KS. Enhancement by L-histidine of nickel-induced DNA–protein cross-linking and oxidative DNA base damage in the rat kidney. *Chem Res Toxicol* 1993;6:33–37.

64. Kasprzak KS, Diwan BA, Rice JM, Misra M, Riggs CW, Olinsky R, Dizdaroglu M. Nickel(II)-mediated oxidative DNA base damage in renal and hepatic chromatin of pregnant rats and their fetuses. Possible relevance to carcinogenesis. *Chem Res Toxicol* 1992;7:809–815.

65. Takagi A, Sai K, Hasegawa R, Kurokawa Y. Enhancing effect of L-histidine on the formation of 8-hydroxydeoxyguanosine induced by hydrogen peroxide in vitro. *Eisei Shikinjo Hokoku* 1991;109:113–115.

66. Zastawny TH, Altman SA, Randers-Eichhorn L, Madurawe R, Lumpkin JA, Dizdaroglu M, Rao G. DNA base modifications and membrane damage in cultured mammalian cells treated with iron ions. *Free Radical Biol Med* 1995;18:1013–1022.

67. Kasai H, Nishimura S. DNA damage induced by asbestos in the presence of hydrogen peroxide. *Gann* 1984;75:841–844.

68. Adachi S, Kawamura K, Yoshida S, Takemoto K. Oxidative damage on DNA induced by asbestos and man-made fibers in vitro. *Int Arch Occup Environ Health* 1992;63:553–557.

69. Faux SP, Howden PJ, Levy LS. Iron-dependent formation of 8-hydroxydeoxyguanosine in isolated DNA and mutagenicity in *Salmonella typhimurum* TA 102 induced by crocidolite. *Carcinogenesis* 1994;15:1749–1751.

70. Takeuchi T, Morimoto K. Crocidolite asbestos increased 8-hydroxydeoxyguanosine levels in cellular DNA of a human promyolytic leukemia cell line, HL 60. *Carcinogenesis* 1994;15:635–639.

71. Adachi S, Yoshida S, Kawamura K, Takahashi M, Uchida H, Odagiri Y, Takemoto K. Inductions of oxidative DNA damage and mesothelioma by crocidolite, with special reference to the presence of iron inside and outside of asbestos fiber. *Carcinogenesis* 1994;15:753–758.

72. Chao C-C, Park S-H, Aust AE. Participation of nitric oxide and iron in the oxidation of DNA in asbestos-treated human lung epithelial cells. *Arch Biochem Biophys* 1996;326:152–157.

73. Sahu SC, Washington MC. Iron-mediated oxidative DNA damage detected by fluorometric analysis of DNA unwinding in isolated rat liver nuclei. *Biomed Environ Sci* 1991;4:232–241.

74. Tagesson C, Chabiuk D, Axelson O, Baranski B, Palus J, Wyszynska K. Increased urinary excretion of the oxidative DNA adduct, 8-hydroxydeoxyguanosine, as a possible early indicator of occupational cancer hazards in the asbestos, rubber, and azo-dye industries. *Polish J Occup Med Environ Health* 1993;6:357–368.

75. Tagesson C, Källberg M, Wingren G. Urinary malondialdehyde and 8-hydroxydeoxyguanosine as potential markers of oxidative stress in industrial art glass workers. *Int Arch Occup Environ Health* 1996;69:5–13.

76. Daniel LN, Mao Y, Saffiotti U. Oxidative DNA damage by crystalline silica. *Free Radical Biol Med* 1993;14:463–472.

77. Leanderson P, Sahle W. Formation of hydroxyl radicals and toxicity of tungsten oxide fibres. *Toxicol In Vitro* 1995;9:175–183.

78. Conte D, Narindrasorasak S, Sarkar B. In vivo and in vitro iron-replaced zinc finger generates free radicals and causes DNA damage. *J Biol Chem* 1996;271:5125–5130.

79. Leanderson P, Tagesson C. Iron bound to the lipophilic iron chelator, 8-hydroxyquinoline, causes DNA strand breakage in cultured lung cells. *Carcinogenesis* 1996;17:545–550.

80. Imlay JA, Linn S. DNA damage and oxygen radical toxicity. *Science* 1988;240:1302–1309.

81. Luo Y, Han Z, Chin SM, Linn S. Three chemically distinct types of oxidants formed by iron-mediated Fenton reactions in the presence of DNA. *Proc Natl Acad Sci USA* 1994;91:12438–12442.

82. Tkeshelashvili LK, McBride T, Spence K, Loeb LA. Mutation spectrum of copper-induced DNA damage. *J Biol Chem* 1991;266:6401–6406.

83. Geierstanger BH, Kagawa TF, Chen SL, Quigley GJ, Ho PS. Base-specific binding of copper(II) to Z-DNA. The 1.3-A single crystal structure of d(m5CGUAm5CG) in the presence of $CuCl_2$. *J Biol Chem* 1991;266:20185–20191.

84. Sagripanti JL, Kraemer KH. Site-specific oxidative DNA damage at polyguanosines produced by copper plus hydrogen peroxide. *J Biol Chem* 1989;264:1729–1734.

85. Spencer JP, Jenner A, Aruoma OI, Evans PJ, Kaur H, Dexter DT, Jenner P, Lees AJ, Marsden DC, Halliwell B. Intense oxidative DNA damage promoted by L-dopa and its metabolites. Implications for neurodegenerative disease. *FEBS Lett* 1994;353:246–50.

86. Yamamoto F, Kasai H, Togashi Y, Takeichi N, Hori T, Nishimura S. Elevated level of 8-hydroxydeoxyguanosine in DNA of liver, kidney, and brain of Long-Evans cinnamon rats. *Jpn J Cancer Res* 1993;84:508–511.

87. Jong-Hon K, Togashi Y, Kasai H, Hosokawa M, Takeichi N. Prevention of spontaneous hepatocellular carcinoma in Long-Evans cinnamon rats with hereditary hepatitis by the administration of D-penicillamine. *Hepatology* 1993;18:614–620.

88. Spear N, Aust SD. Hydroxylation of deoxyguanosine in DNA by copper and thiols. *Arch Biochem Biophys* 1995;317:142–148.

89. Milne L, Nicotera P, Orrenius S, Burkitt MJ. Effects of glutathione and chelating agents on copper-mediated DNA oxidation: Prooxidant and antioxidant properties of glutathione. *Arch Biochem Biophys* 1993;304:102–109.

90. Faux SP, Gao M, Chipman JK, Levy LS. Production of 8-hydroxydeoxyguanosine in isolated DNA by chromium(VI) and chromium(V). *Carcinogenesis* 1992;13:1667–1669.

91. Claycamp HG, Luo D. Plutonium-catalyzed oxidative DNA damage in the absence of significant α-particle decay. *Radiat Res* 1994;137:114–117.

92. Reddy JK, Rao MS. Oxidative DNA damage caused by persistent peroxisome proliferation: Its role in hepatocarcinogenesis. *Mutat Res* 1989;214:63–68.

93. Kasai H, Okada Y, Nishimura S, Rao MS, Reddy JK. Formation of 8-hydroxydeoxyguanosine in liver DNA of rats following long-term exposure to a peroxisome proliferator. *Cancer Res* 1989;49:2603–2605.

94. Srinivasan S, Glauert HP. Formation of 5-hydroxymethyl-2'-deoxyuridine in hepatic DNA of rats treated with γ-irradiation, diethylnitrosamine, 2-acetylaminofluorene or the peroxisome proliferator ciprofibrate. *Carcinogenesis* 1990;11:2021–2024.

95. Huang CY, Wilson MW, Lay LT, Chow CK, Robertson LW, Glauert HP. Increased 8-hydroxydeoxyguanosine in hepatic DNA of rats treated with the peroxisome proliferators ciprofibrate and perfluorodecanoic acid. *Cancer Lett* 1994;87:223–228.

96. Cattley RC, Glover SE. Elevated 8-hydroxydeoxyguanosine in hepatic DNA of rats following exposure to peroxisome proliferators: Relationship to carcinogenesis and nuclear localization. *Carcinogenesis* 1993;14:2495–2499.

97. Takagi A, Sai K, Umemura T, Hasegawa R, Kurokawa Y. Relationship between hepatic peroxisome proliferation and 8-hydroxydeoxyguanosine formation in liver DNA of rats following long-term exposure to three peroxisome proliferators; di(2-ethylhexyl) phthalate, aluminium clofibrate and simfibrate. *Cancer Lett* 1990;53:33–8.

98. Takagi A, Sai K, Umemura T, Hasegawa R, Kurokawa Y. Short-term exposure to the peroxisome proliferators, perfluorooctanoic acid and perfluorodecanoic acid, causes significant increase of 8-hydroxydeoxyguanosine in liver DNA of rats. *Cancer Lett* 1991;57:55–60.

99. Hayashi F, Tamura H, Yamada J, Kasai H, Suga T. Characteristics of the hepatocarcinogenesis caused by dehydroepiandrosterone, a peroxisome proliferator, in male F-344 rats. *Carcinogenesis* 1994;15:2215–2219.

100. Sausen PJ, Lee DC, Rose ML, Cattley RC. Elevated 8-hydroxydeoxyguanosine in hepatic DNA of rats following exposure to peroxisome proliferators: Relationship to mitochondrial alterations. *Carcinogenesis* 1995;16:1795–1801.

101. Fiala ES, Conaway CC, Mathis JE. Oxidative DNA and RNA damage in the livers of Sprague-Dawley rats treated with the hepatocarcinogen 2-nitropropane. *Cancer Res* 1989;49:5518–5522.

102. Hussain NS, Conaway CC, Guo N, Asaad W, Fiala ES. Oxidative DNA and RNA damage in rat liver due to acetoxime: Similarity to effects of 2-nitropropane. *Carcinogenesis* 1990;11:1013–1016.

103. Dahlhaus M, Appel KE. *N*-Nitrosodimethylamine, *N*-nitrosodiethylamine, and *N*-nitrosomorpholine fail to generate 8-hydroxy-2'-deoxyguanosine in liver DNA of male F344 rats. *Mutat Res* 1993;285:295–302.

104. Guo N, Conaway CC, Hussain NS, Fiala ES. Sex and organ differences in oxidative DNA and RNA damage due to treatment of Sprague-Dawley rats with acetoxime or 2-nitropropane. *Carcinogenesis* 1990;11:1659–1662.

105. Adachi S, Takemoto K, Hirosue T, Hosogai Y. Spontaneous and 2-nitropropane induced levels of 8-hydroxy-2'-deoxyguanosine in liver DNA of rats fed iron-deficient or manganese- and copper-deficient diets. *Carcinogenesis* 1993;14:265–268.

106. Umemura T, Sai K, Takagi A, Hasegawa, R, Kurokawa Y. Oxidative DNA damage, lipid peroxidation and nephrotoxicity induced in the rat kidney after ferric nitrilotriacetate administration. *Cancer Lett* 1990;54:95–100.

107. Umemura T, Sai K, Takagi A, Hasegawa R, Kurokawa Y. The effects of exogenous glutathione and cysteine on oxidative stress induced by ferric nitrilotriacetate. *Cancer Lett* 1991;58:49–56.

108. Randerath E, Watson WP, Zhou GD, Chang J, Randerath K. Intensification and depletion of specific bulky renal DNA adducts (I-compounds) following exposure of male F344 rats to the renal carcinogen ferric nitrilotriacetate (Fe-NTA). *Mutat Res* 1995;341:265–279.

109. Toyokuni S, Mori T, Dizdaroglu M. DNA base modifications in renal chromatin of Wistar rats treated with a renal carcinogen, ferric nitrilotriacetate. *Int J Cancer* 1994;57:123–128.

110. Toyokuni S, Mori T, Hiai H, Dizdaroglu M. Treatment of Wistar rats with a renal carcinogen, ferric nitrilotriacetate, causes DNA-protein cross-linking between thymine and tyrosine in their renal chromatin. *Int J Cancer* 1995;62:309–313.

111. Yamaguchi R, Hirano T, Asami S, Sugita A, Kasai H. Increase in the 8-hydroxyguanine repair activity in the rat kidney after the administration of a renal carcinogen, ferric nitriloacetate. *Environ Health Perspect* 1996; 104 Suppl:651–653.

112. Kasai H, Nishimura S, Kurokawa Y, Hayashi Y. Oral administration of the renal carcinogen, potassium bromate, specifically produces 8-hydroxydeoxyguanosine in rat target organ DNA. *Carcinogenesis* 1987;8:1959–1961.

113. Cho DH, Hong JT, Chin K, Cho TS, Lee BM. Organotropic formation and disappearance of 8-hydroxydeoxyguanosine in the kidney of Sprague-Dawley rats exposed to adriamycin and $KBrO_3$. *Cancer Lett* 1993;74:141–145.

114. Sai K, Umemura T, Takagi A, Hasegawa R, Kurokawa Y. The protective role of glutathione, cysteine and vitamin C against oxidative DNA damage induced in rat kidney by potassium bromate. *Jpn J Cancer Res* 1992;83:45–51.

115. Sai K, Tyson CA, Thomas DW, Dabbs JE, Hasegawa R, Kurokawa Y. Oxidative DNA damage induced by potassium bromate in isolated rat renal proximal tubules and renal nuclei. *Cancer Lett* 1994;87:1–7.

116. Ballmaier D, Epe B. Oxidative DNA damage induced by potassium bromate under cell-free conditions and in mammalian cells. *Carcinogenesis* 1995;16:335–342.

117. Frei B, Winterhalter KH, Richter C. Menadione (2-methyl-1,4-naphthoquinone)-dependent enzymatic redox cycling and calcium release by mitochondria. *Biochemistry* 1986;25:4438–4443.

118. Denda A, Sai KM, Tang Q, Tsujiuchi T, Tsutsumi M, Amanuma T, Murata Y, Nakae D, Maruyama H, Kurokawa Y, Konishi Y. Induction of 8-hydroxydeoxyguanosine but not initiation of carcinogenesis by redox enzyme modulations with or without menadione in rat liver. *Carcinogenesis* 1991;12:719–726.

119. Fischer-Nielsen A, Corcoran GB, Poulsen HE, Kamendulis LM, Loft S. Menadione-induced DNA fragmentation without 8-oxo-2'-deoxyguanosine formation in isolated rat hepatocytes. *Biochem Pharmacol* 1995;49:1469–1474.

120. Schilderman PA, van Maanen JM, ten Vaarwerk FJ, Lafleur MV, Westmijze EJ, ten Hoor F, Kleinjans JC. The role of prostaglandin H synthase-mediated metabolism in the induction of oxidative DNA damage by BHA metabolites. *Carcinogenesis* 1993;14:1297–1302.

121. Schilderman PA, ten Vaarwerk FJ, Lutgerink JT, Van der Wurff A, ten Hoor F, Kleinjans JC. Induction of oxidative DNA damage and early lesions in rat gastro-intestinal epithelium in relation to prostaglandin H synthase-mediated metabolism of butylated hydroxyanisolee. *Food Chem Toxicol* 1995;33:99–109.

122. Schilderman PA, Rhijnsburger E, Zwingmann I, Kleinjans JC. Induction of oxidative DNA damages and enhancement of cell proliferation in human lymphocytes in vitro by butylated hydroxyanisole. *Carcinogenesis* 1995;16:507–512.

123. Nunoshiba T, Demple B. Potent intracellular oxidative stress exerted by the carcinogen 4-nitroquino-line-N-oxide. *Cancer Res* 1993;53:3250–3252.

124. Kohda K, Tada M, Kasai H, Nishimura S, Kawazoe Y. Formation of 8-hydroxyguanine residues in cellular DNA exposed to the carcinogen 4-nitroquinoline 1-oxide. *Biochem Biophys Res Commun* 1986;139:626–632.

125. Pero RW, Anderso MW, Doyle GA, Anna CH, Romagna F, Markovitz M, Bryngelsson C. Oxidative stress induces DNA damage and inhibits the repair of DNA lesions induced by *N*-acetoxy-2-acetylaminofluorene in human peripheral mononuclear leukocytes. *Cancer Res* 1990;50:4619–4625.

126. Nakae D, Andoh N, Mizumoto Y, Endoh T, Shimoji N, Horiguchi K, Shiraiwa K, Tamura K, Denda A, Konishi Y. Selective 8-hydroxyguanine formation in pancreatic DNA due to a single intravenous administration of 4-hydroxyaminoquinoline 1-oxide in rats. *Cancer Lett* 1994; 83:97–103.

127. Kolachana P, Subrahmanyam VV, Meyer KB, Zhang L, Smith MT. Benzene and its phenolic metabolites produce oxidative DNA damage in HL60 cells in vitro and in the bone marrow in vivo. *Cancer Res* 1993;53:1023–1026.

128. Lagorio S, Tagesson C, Forastiere F, Axelson O, Carere A. Exposure to benzene and urinary concentrations of 8-hydroxydeoxyguanosine, a biological marker of oxidative damage to DNA. *Occup Environ Med* 1994;51:739–743.

129. Nilsson RI, Nordlinder RG, Tagesson C, Walles S, Järvholm BG. Genotoxic effects in workers exposed to low levels of benzene from gasoline. *Am J Ind Med* 1996;30:317–324.

130. Mauthe RJ, Cook VM, Coffing SL, Baird WM. Exposure of mammalian cell cultures to benzo[α]pyrene and light results in oxidative DNA damage as measured by 8-hydroxydeoxyguanosine formation. *Carcinogenesis* 1995;16:133–137.

131. Leadon SA, Stampfer MR, Bartley J. Production of oxidative DNA damage during the metabolic activation of benzo[α]pyrene in human mammary epithelial cells correlates with cell killing. *Proc Natl Acad Sci USA* 1988;85:4365–4368.

132. Djuric Z, Potter DW, Culp SJ, Luongo DA, Beland FA. Formation of DNA adducts and oxidative DNA damage in rats treated with 1,6-dinitropyrene. *Cancer Lett* 1993;71:51–56.

133. Cahill A, Jenkins TC, Pickering P, White IN. Genotoxic effects of 3-amino-1,2,4-benzotriazine-1,4-dioxide (SR 4233) and nitrogen mustard-*N*-oxide (nitromin) in Walker carcinoma cells under aerobic and hypoxic conditions. *Chem Biol Interact* 1995;95:97–107.

134. Shen HM, Ong CN, Lee BL, Shi CY. Aflatoxin B$_1$-induced 8-hydroxydeoxyguanosine formation in rat hepatic DNA. *Carcinogenesis* 1995;16:419–422.

135. Dahlhaus M, Almstadt E, Appel KE. The pentachlorophenol metabolite tetrachloro-*p*-hydroquinone induces the formation of 8-hydroxy-2-deoxyguanosine in liver DNA of male B6C3F1 mice. *Toxicol Lett* 1994;74:265–74.

136. Dahlhaus M, Almstadt E, Henschke P, Luttgert S, Appel KE. Induction of 8-hydroxy-2-deoxyguanosine and single-strand breaks in DNA of V79 cells by tetrachloro-*p*-hydroquinone. *Mutat Res* 1995;329:29–36.

137. Nagai F, Ushiyama K, Satoh K, Kasai H, Kano I. Formation of 8-hydroxydeoxyguanosine in calf thymus DNA treated in vitro with phenylhydroquinone, the major metabolite of *O*-phenylphenol. *Carcinogenesis* 1995;16:837–840.

138. Nagashima M, Kasai H, Yokota J, Nagamachi Y, Ichinose T, Sagai M. Formation of an oxidative DNA damage, 8-hydroxydeoxyguanosine, in mouse lung DNA after intratracheal instillation of diesel exhaust particles and effects of high dietary fat and β-carotene on this process. *Carcinogenesis* 1995;16:1441–1445.

139. Nishimoto M, Roubal WT, Stein JE, Varanasi U. Oxidative DNA damage in tissues of English sole (*Parophrys vetulus*) exposed to nitrofurantoin. *Chem Biol Interact* 1991;80:317–326.

140. Winn LM, Wells PG. Phenytoin-initiated DNA oxidation in murine embryo culture, and embryo protection by the antioxidative enzymes superoxide dismutase and catalase: Evidence for reactive oxygen species-mediated DNA oxidation in the molecular mechanism of phenytoin teratogenicity. *Mol Pharmacol* 1995;48:112–120.

141. Stohs SJ, Shara MA, Alsharif NZ, Wahba ZZ, Al-Bayati ZAF. 2,3,7,8-Tetrachlorodibenzo-*p*-dioxin-induced oxidative stress in female rats. *Toxicol Appl Pharmacol* 1990;106:126–135.

142. Eichner RD, Waring P, Geue AM, Braithwaite AW, Müllbacher A. Gliotoxin causes oxidative damage to plasmid and cellular DNA. *J Biol Chem* 1988;263:3772–3777.

143. Frenkel K. Oxidation of DNA bases by tumor promoter-activated processes. *Environ Health Perspect* 1989;81:45–54.

144. Wei H, Frenkel K. In vivo formation of oxidized DNA bases in tumor promoter-treated mouse skin. *Cancer Res* 1991;51:4443–4449.
145. Wei H, Frenkel K. Relationship of oxidative events and DNA oxidation in SENCAR mice to in vivo promoting activity of phorbol ester-type tumor promoters. *Carcinogenesis* 1993;14:1195–1201.
146. Wei H, Frenkel K. Sensitivity to tumor promotion of SENCAR and C57BL/6J mice correlates with oxidative events and DNA damage. *Carcinogenesis* 1993;14:841–847.
147. Frenkel K, Wei L, Wei H. 7,12-Dimethylbenz[α]anthracene induces oxidative DNA modification in vivo. *Free Radical Biol Med* 1995;19:373–380.
148. Takeuchi T, Nakajima M, Morimoto K. Establishment of a human system that generates O_2^- and induces 8-hydroxydeoxyguanosine, typical of oxidative DNA damage, by a tumor promotor. *Cancer Res* 1994;54:5837–5840.
149. Takeuchi T, Nakajima M, Morimoto K. Calyculin A, a non-phorbol ester type tumor promotor, induced oxidative DNA damage in stimulated human neutrophil-like cells. *Biochem Biophys Res Commun* 1994;205:1803–1807.
150. Dedon PC, Goldberg IH. Free radical mechanisms involved in the formation of sequence-dependent bistranded DNA lesions by the antitumor antibiotics bleomycin, neocarzinostatin, and calicheamycin. *Chem Res Toxicol* 1992;5:311–332.
151. Goldberg IH, Kappen LS. Neocarzinostatin: Chemical and biological basis of oxidative DNA damage. In: Borders DB, Doyle TW, eds. *Enediyne Antibiotics as Antitumor Agents.* New York: Marcel Dekker, 1995;327–362.
152. Weiner LM. Oxygen radicals generation and DNA scission by anticancer and synthetic quinones. *Methods Enzymol* 1994;233:92–105.
153. Gajewski E, Aruoma OI, Dizdaroglu M, Halliwell B. Bleomycin-dependent damage to the bases in DNA is a minor side reaction. *Biochemistry* 1991;30:2444–2448.
154. Cho DH, Hong JT, Chin K, Cho TS, Lee BM. Organotropic formation and disappearance of 8-hydroxydeoxyguanosine in the kidney of Sprague-Dawley rats exposed to adriamycin and $KBrO_3$. *Cancer Lett* 1993;74:141–145.
155. Maccubbin AE, Ersing N, Budzinski EE, Box HC, Gurtoo HL. Formation of 8-hydroxyguanine in DNA during mitomycin C activation. *Cancer Biochem Biophys* 1994;14:183–191.
156. Plummer SM, Hall M, Faux SP. Oxidation and genotoxicity of fecapentaene-12 are potentiated by prostaglandin H synthase. *Carcinogenesis* 1995;16:1023–1028.
157. de Kok TM, van Maanen JM, Lankelma J, ten Hoor F, Kleinjans JC. Electron spin resonance spectroscopy of oxygen radicals generated by synthetic fecapentaene-12 and reduction of fecapentaene mutagenicity to *Salmonella typhimurium* by hydroxyl radical scavenging. *Carcinogenesis* 1992;13:1249–1255.
158. de Kok TM, Pachen DM, van Maanen JM, Lafleur MV, Westmijze EJ, ten Hoor F, Kleinjans JC. Role of oxidative DNA damage in the mechanism of fecapentaene-12 genotoxicity. *Carcinogenesis* 1994;15:2559–2565.
159. Fraga CG, Onuki J, Lucesoli F, Bechara EJ, Di Mascio P. 5-Aminolevulinic acid mediates the in vivo and in vitro formation of 8-hydroxy-2'-deoxyguanosine in DNA. *Carcinogenesis* 1994; 15:2241–2244.
160. Epe B, Pflaum M, Boiteux S. DNA damage induced by photosensitizers in cellular and cell-free systems. *Mutat Res* 1993;299:135–145.
161. Doetsch PW, Zastawny TH, Martin AM, Dizdaroglu M. Monomeric base damage products from adenine, guanine and thymine induced by exposure to ultraviolet radiation. *Biochemistry* 1995;34:737–742.
162. Yamamoto F, Nishimura S, Kasai H. Photosensitized formation of 8-hydroxydeoxyguanosine in cellular DNA by riboflavin. *Biochem Biophys Res Commun* 1992;187:809–813.
163. Bessho T, Tano K, Nishimura S, Kasai H. Induction of mutations in mouse FM3A cells by treatment with riboflavin plus visible light and its possible relation with formation of 8-hydroxyguanine (7,8-dihydro-8-oxoguanine) in DNA. *Carcinogenesis* 1993;14:1069–1071.
164. Buchko GW, Cadet J, Morin B, Weinfeld M. Photooxidation of d(TpG) by riboflavin and methylene blue. Isolation and characterization of thimidylyl-(3',5')-2-amino-5-[(2-deoxy-β-D-*erythro*-pentofuranosyl)amino]-4*H*-imidazol-4-one and its primary decomposition product thymidylyl-(3',5')-2,2-diamino-4-[(2-deoxy-β-D-*erythro*-pentofuranosyl)amino]-5(2*H*)-oxazolone. *Nucleic Acid Res* 1995;23:3954–3961.
165. Buchko GW, Wagner JR, Cadet J, Raoul S, Weinfeld M. Methylene blue-mediated photooxidation of 7,8-dihydro-8-oxo-2'-deoxyguanosine. *Biochim Biophys Acta* 1995;1263:17–24.

166. Legrand-Poels S, Bours V, Piret B, Pflaum M, Epe B, Rentier B, Piette J. Transcription factor NF-κ B is activated by photosensitization generating oxidative DNA damages. *J Biol Chem* 1995;270:6925–6934.
167. Nicotera TM, Munson BR, Fiel RJ. Photosensitized formation of 8-hydroxy-2'-deoxyguanosine and DNA strand breakage by a cationic meso-substituted porphyrin. *Photochem Photobiol* 1994;60:295–300.
168. Epe B, Häring M, Ramaiah D, Stopper H, Abou-Elzahab MM, Adam W, Saha-Möller CR. DNA damage induced by furocoumarin hydroperoxides plus UV (360 nm). *Carcinogenesis* 1993; 14:2271–2276.
169. Adam W, Cadet J, Dall'Aqua F, Epe B, Ramaiah D, Saha-Möller CR. Photosensitized formation of 8-hydroxy-2'-deoxyguanosine in salmon testes DNA by furocoumarin hydroperoxides: A novel, intercalating "photo-Fenton" reagent for oxidative DNA damage. *Angew Chem Int Ed Engl* 1995;34:107–110.
170. Epe B, Ballmaier D, Adam W, Grimm GN, Saha-Möller CR. Photolysis of *N*-hydroxypyridinethiones: A new source of hydroxyl radicals for the direct damage of cell-free and cellular DNA. *Nucleic Acids Res* 1996;24:1625–1631.
171. Huselton CA, Hill HZ. Melanin photosensitizes ultraviolet light (UVC) DNA damage in pigmented cells. *Environ Mol Mutagen* 1990;16:37–43.
172. Retel J, Hoebee B, Braun JE, Lutgerink JT, van den Akker E, Wanamarta AH, Joenje H, Lafleur MV. Mutational specificity of oxidative DNA damage. *Mutat Res* 1993;299:165–182.
173. Devasagayam TPA, Di Mascio P, Kaiser S, Sies H. Singlet oxygen induced single-strand breaks in plasmid pBR322 DNA: The enhancing effect of thiols. *FEBS Lett* 1991;1088:409–412.
174. Devasagayam TPA, Steenken S, Obendorf MSW, Schulz WA, Sies H. Formation of 8-hydroxy(deoxy)guanosine and generation of strand breaks at guanine residues in DNA by singlet oxygen. *Biochemistry* 1991;30:6283–6289.
175. Ribeiro DT, Bourre F, Sarasin A, Di Mascio P, Menck CFM. DNA synthesis blocking lesions induced by singlet oxygen are targeted to deoxyguanosines. *Nucleic Acids Res* 1992;20:2465–2469.
176. Pflaum M, Boiteux S, Epe B. Visible light generates oxidative DNA base modifications in high excess of strand breaks in mammalian cells. *Carcinogenesis* 1994;15:297–300.
177. Hattori-Nakakuki Y, Nishigori C, Okamoto K, Imamura S, Hiai H, Toyokuni S. Formation of 8-hydroxy-2'-deoxyguanosine in epidermis of hairless mice exposed to near-UV. *Biochem Biophys Res Commun* 1994;201:1132–1139.
178. Doetsch PW, Zasatawny TH, Martin AM, Dizdaroglu M. Monomeric base damage products from adenine, guanine, and thymine induced by exposure of DNA to ultraviolet radiation. *Biochemistry* 1995;34:737–742.
179. Mori T, Hori Y, Dizdaroglu M. DNA base damage generated in vivo in hepatic chromatin of mice upon whole body γ-irradiation. *Int J Radiat Biol* 1993;64:645–650.
180. Raoul S, Bardet M, Cadet J. γ Irradiation of 2'-deoxyadenosine in oxygen-free aqueous solutions: Identification and conformational features of formamidinopyrimidine nucleoside derivatives. *Chem Res Toxicol* 1995;8:924–933.
181. Ravanat J-L, Cadet J. Reaction of singlet oxygen with 2'-deoxyguanosine and DNA. Isolation and characterization of the main oxidation products. *Chem Res Toxicol* 1995;8:379–388.
182. Raoul S, Cadet J. Photosensitized reaction of 8-oxo-7,8-dihydro-2'-deoxyguanosine: Identification of 1-(2-deoxy-β-D-*erythro*-pentofuranosyl)cyanuric acid as the major singlet oxygen oxidation product. *J Am Chem Soc* 1996;118:1892–1898.
183. Epe B, Henzl H, Adam W, Saha-Möller CR. Endonuclease-sensitive DNA modifications induced by acetone and acetophenone as photosensitizers. *Nucleic Acids Res* 1993;21:863–869.
184. Wink DA, Kasprzak KS, Maragos CM, Elespuru RK, Misra M, Dunams TM, Cebula TA, Koch WH, Andrews AW, Allen JS. DNA deaminating ability and genotoxicity of nitric oxide and its progenitors. *Science* 1991;254:1001–1003.
185. Ngyen T, Brunson D, Crespi CL, Penman BW, Wishnok JS, Tannenbaum SR. DNA damage and mutation in human cells exposed to nitric oxide in vitro. *Proc Natl Acad Sci USA* 1992;89:3030–3034.
186. Routledge MN, Wink DA, Keefer LK, Dipple A. Mutations induced by saturated aqueous nitric oxide in the pSP189 *supF* gene in human Ad293 and *E. coli* MBM7070 cells. *Carcinogenesis* 1993;14:1251–1254.
187. Wink DA, Hanbauer I, Krishna MC, DeGraff W, Gamson J, Mitchell JB. Nitric oxide protects against cellular damage and cytotoxicity from reactive oxygen species. *Proc Natl Acad Sci USA* 1993;90:9813–9817.

188. Pacelli R, Wink DA, Cook JA, Krishna MC, DeGraff W, Friedman N, Tsokos M, Samuni A, Mitchell JB. Nitric oxide potentiates hydrogen peroxide-induced killing of *Escherichia coli. J Exp Med* 1995;182:1469–1479.

189. deRojas-Walker T, Tamir S, Ji H, Wishnok JS, Tannenbaum SR. Nitric oxide induces oxidative damage in addition to deamination in macrophage DNA. *Chem Res Toxicol* 1995;8:473–477.

190. Sugiura Y, Matsumoto T. Nucleotide-selective cleavage of duplex DNA by nitric oxide. *Biochem Biophys Res Commun* 1995;211:748–753.

191. Inoue S, Kawanishi S. Oxidative DNA damage induced by simultaneous generation of nitric oxide and superoxide. *FEBS Lett* 1995;371:86–88.

192. Szabo C, Zingarelli B, O'Connor M, Salzman AL. DNA strand breakage, activation of poly(ADP-ribose) synthase, and cellular energy depletion are involved in the cytotoxicity in macrophages and smooth muscle cells exposed to peroxynitrite. *Proc Natl Acad Sci USA* 1996;93:1753–1758.

193. Messmer UK, Ankarcrona M, Nicotera P, Brüne B. p53 Expression in nitric oxide-induced apoptosis. *FEBS Lett* 1994;355:23–26.

194. Salgo MG, Squadrito GL, Pryor WA. Peroxynitrite causes apoptosis in rat thymocytes. *Biochem Biophys Res Commun* 1995;215:1111–1118.

195. Douki T, Cadet J. Peroxynitrite mediated oxidation of purine bases of nucleosides and isolated DNA. *Free Radical Res* 1996;24:369–380.

196. Douki T, Cadet J, Ames BN. An adduct between peroxynitrite and 2′-deoxyguanosine: 4,5-Dihydro-5-hydroxy-4-(nitrosooxy)-2′-deoxyguanosine. *Chem Res Toxicol* 1996;9:3–7.

197. Shigenaga MK, Ames BN. Oxidants and mitogenesis as causes of mutation and cancer: The influence of diet. *Basic Life Sci* 1993;61:419–436.

198. Djuric Z, Heilbrun LK, Reading BA, Boomer A, Valeriote FA, Martino S. Effects of a low-fat diet on levels of oxidative damage to DNA to human peripheral nucleated blood cells. *J Natl Cancer Inst* 1991;83:766–769.

199. Haegele AD, Briggs SP, Thompson HJ. Antioxidant status and dietary lipid unsaturation modulate oxidative DNA damage. *Free Radical Biol Med* 1994;16:111–115.

200. Nair UJ, Obe G, Friesen M, Goldberg MT, Bartsch H. Role of lime in the generation of reactive oxygen species from betel-quid ingredients. *Environ Health Perspect* 1992;98:203–205.

201. Hinrichsen LI, Floyd RA, Sudilovsky O. Is 8-hydroxydeoxyguanosine a mediator of carcinogenesis by a choline-devoid diet in the rat liver? *Carcinogenesis* 1990;11:1879–1881.

202. Nakae D, Yoshiji H, Maruayma H, Kinugasa T, Denda A, Konishi Y. Production of both 8-hydroxydeoxyguanosine in liver DNA and γ-glutamyltransferase-positive hepatocellular lesions in rats given a choline-deficient, L-amino acid-defined diet. *Jpn J Cancer Res* 1990;80:1081–1084.

203. Hirano T, Homma Y, Kasai H. Formation of 8-hydroxyguanine in DNA by aging and oxidative stress. In: Cutler RG, Packer L, Bertram J, Mori A, eds. *Oxidative Stress and Aging.* Basel: Birkhäuser Verlag, 1995;69–76.

204. Nakae D, Mizumoto Y, Yoshiji H. Different roles of 8-hydroxyguanine formation and 2-thiobarbituric acid-reacting substance generation in the early phase of liver carcinogenesis induced by a choline-deficient, L-amino acid-defined diet in rats. *Jpn J Cancer Res* 1994;85:499–505.

205. Simic MG, Bergtold DS. Dietary modulation of DNA damage in human. *Mutat Res* 1991;250:17–24.

206. Djuric Z, Lu MH, Lewis SM, Luongo DA, Chen XW, Heilbrun LK, Reading BA, Duffy PH, Hart RW. Oxidative DNA damage levels in rats fed low-fat, high-fat, or calorie-restricted diets. *Toxicol Appl Pharmacol* 1992;115:156–160.

207. Chung MH, Kasai H, Nishimura S, Yu BP. Protection of DNA damage by dietary restriction. *Free Radical Biol Med* 1992;12:523–525.

208. Sohal RS, Agarwal S, Candas M, Forster MJ, Lal H. Effect of age and caloric restriction on DNA oxidative damage in different tissues of C57BL/6 mice. *Mech Ageing Dev* 1994;76:215–224.

209. Loft S, Velthuis te Wierik EJ, van den Berg H, Poulsen HE. Energy restriction and oxidative DNA damage in humans. *Cancer Epidemiol Biomarkers Prev* 1995;4:515–519.

210. Loft S, Astrup A, Buemann B, Poulsen HE. Oxidative DNA damage correlates with oxygen consumption in humans. *FASEB J* 1994;8:534–537.

211. Inoue T, Mu Z, Sumikawa K, Adachi K, Okochi T. Effect of physical exercise on the content of 8-hydroxydeoxyguanosine in nuclear DNA prepared from human lymphocytes. *Jpn J Cancer Res* 1993;84:720–725.

212. Alessio HM. Exercise-induced oxidative stress. *Med Sci Sports Exerc* 1993;25:218–224.

213. Adachi S, Kawamura K, Takemoto K. Oxidative damage of nuclear DNA in liver of rats exposed to psychological stress. *Cancer Res* 1993;53:4153–4155.

214. Loft S, Vistisen K, Ewertz M, Tjonneland A, Overvad K, Poulsen HE. Oxidative DNA damage estimated by 8-hydroxydeoxyguanine excretion in man: Influence of smoking, gender and body mass index. *Carcinogenesis* 1992;13:2241–2247.
215. Tagesson C, Källberg M, Leanderson P. Determination of urinary 8-hydroxydeoxyguanosine by coupled-column high-performance liquid chromatography with electrochemical detection: A noninvasive assay for in vivo oxidative DNA damage in humans. *Toxicol Meth* 1992;1:242–251.
216. Kiyosawa H, Suko M, Okudaira H, Murata K, Miyamoto T, Chung MH, Kasai H, Nishimura S. Cigarette smoking induces formation of 8-hydroxydeoxyguanosine, one of the oxidative DNA damages in human peripheral leukocytes. *Free Radical Res Commun* 1990;11:23–27.
217. Asami S, Hirano T, Yamaguchi R, Tomioka Y, Itoh H, Kasai H. Increase of a type of oxidative damage, 8-hydroxyguanine, and its repair activity in human leukocytes by cigarette smoking. *Cancer Res* 1996;56:2546–2549.
218. Kiyosawa H, Suko M, Okudaira H, Murata K, Miyamoto T, Chung M-H, Kasai H, Nishimura S. Cigarette smoking induces formation of 8-hydroxydeoxyguanosine, one of the oxidative DNA damages in human peripheral leukocytes. *Free Radical Res Commun* 1990;11:23–27.
219. Leanderson P. Cigarette smoke-induced DNA damage in cultured human lung cells. In: Diana JN, Pryor WA, eds. *Influence of Nutrition on Tobacco Associated Health Risks.* 1993; Ann NY Acad Sci Vol 686 pp. 249–261.
220. Chung FL, Xu Y. Increased 8-oxodeoxyguanosine levels in lung DNA of A/J mice and F344 rats treated with the tobacco-specific nitrosamine 4-(methylnitrosamine)-1-(3-pyridyl)-1-butanone. *Carcinogenesis* 1992;13:1269–1272.
221. Leanderson P, Tagesson C. Cigarette smoke-induced DNA-damage: Role of hydroquinone and catechol in the formation of the oxidative DNA-adduct, 8-hydroxydeoxyguanosine. *Chem Biol Interact* 1990;75:71–81.
222. Leanderson P, Tagesson C. Cigarette smoke-induced DNA damage in cultured human lung cells: Role of hydroxyl radicals and endonuclease activation. *Chem Biol Interact* 1992;81:197–208.
223. Spencer JPE, Jenner A, Chimel K, Aruoma OI, Cross CE, Wu R, Halliwell B. DNA damage in human respiratory tract epithelial cells: Damage by gas phase cigarette smoke apparently involves attack by reactive nitrogen species in addition to oxygen radicals. *FEBS Lett* 1995;375:179–182.
224. Suzuki J, Inoue Y, Suzuki S. Changes in urinary level of 8-hydroxyguanine by exposure to reactive oxygen-generating substances. *Free Radical Biol Med* 1995;18:431–436.
225. Fischer-Nielsen A, Poulsen HE, Loft S. 8-Hydroxydeoxyguanosine in vitro: Effects of glutathione, ascorbate, and 5-aminosalicylic acid. *Free Radical Biol Med* 1992;13:121–126.
226. Muscari C, Guarnieri C, Stefanelli C, Giaccari A, Caldarera CM. Protective effect of spermine on DNA exposed to oxidative stress. *Mol Cell Biochem* 1995;144:125–129.
227. Topinka J, Binkova B, Sram RJ, Erin AN. The influence of α-tocopherol and pyritinol on oxidative DNA damage and lipid peroxidation in human lymphocytes. *Mutat Res* 1989;225:131–136.
228. Samuni A, Godinger D, Aronovitch J, Russo A, Mitchell JB. Nitroxides block DNA scission and protect cells from oxidative damage. *Biochemistry* 1991;30:555–561.
229. Ljungman M, Hanawalt PC. Efficient protection against oxidative DNA damage in chromatin. *Mol Carcinog* 1992;5:264–269.
230. Altman SA, Zastawny TH, Randers-Eichhorn L, Cacciuttolo MA, Dizdaroglu M, Rao G. Formation of DNA-protein cross-links in cultured mammalian cells upon treatment with iron ions. *Free Radical Biol Med* 1992;5:897–902.
231. Fischer-Nielsen A, Loft S, Jensen KG. Effect of ascorbate and 5-aminosalicylic acid on light-induced 8-hydroxydeoxyguanosine formation in V79 Chinese hamster cells. *Carcinogenesis* 1993;14:2431–2433.
232. Fraga CG, Motchnik PA, Shigenaga MK, Helbock HJ, Jacob RA, Ames BN. Ascorbic acid protects against endogenous oxidative DNA damage in human sperm. *Proc Natl Acad Sci USA* 1991;88:11003–11006.
233. Verhagen H, Poulsen HE, Loft S, van Poppel G, Willems MI, van Bladeren PJ. Reduction of oxidative DNA-damage in humans by Brussels sprouts. *Carcinogenesis* 1995;16:969–970.
234. van Poppel G, Poulsen H, Loft S, Verhagen H. No influence of β-carotene on oxidative DNA damage in male smokers. *J Natl Cancer Inst* 1995;87:310–311.

Free Radical Toxicology
Edited by K. B. Wallace
Copyright © 1997 Taylor & Francis

7

Physicochemical Determinants of Free-Radical Cytotoxicity

Enrique Cadenas

Department of Molecular Pharmacology and Toxicology, School of Pharmacy, University of Southern California, Los Angeles, California, USA

INTRODUCTION

The contribution of free-radical species to oxidative cytotoxicity has been amply documented; the occurrence of oxidative radical reactions in a biological setting is usually associated with the formation of byproducts of aerobic metabolism, the metabolism of xenobiotics and other environmental sources, or the response to diverse stimuli by specialized physiological reactions, such as the formation of oxyradicals during the respiratory burst or the release of endothelium-derived releasing factor, identified as nitric oxide or closely related product(s). Recognition of the actual damaging species, its quantitative assessment in terms of its cellular steady-state concentration, and its chemical reactivity toward diverse cellular targets seems essential for evaluating its contribution to oxidative situations and, as a corollary, to implement antioxidant therapies. Although the latter has gained significance because of diverse pathophysiological situations with a proven major oxidative component (1), its implementation is part of a general approach and it awaits deeper understanding of the mechanisms and site of action of free-radical species.

Despite this wealth of information, the actual mechanisms by which free radicals exert toxicity in vivo remais largely hypothetical. A suitable correlation between free-radical chemical reactivity and specific oxidative modifications of cellular targets is still missing. Exceptions are current "fingerprints" of oxidative damage or promising approaches to identify oxidative damage in vivo. Examples of the former are the identification of hydroxy derivatives of nucleic acid bases in urine (2); this evidence is expected to expand with the application of new methodologies to measure oxidative stress in vivo, such as the use of spin traps, antibody-independent visualization of protein carbonyls in situ, and analysis of prostanoid production in blood and urine in humans (3). These approaches furnish information on the actual mechanisms of free-radical damage upon identification of oxidative modifications of specific target molecules.

The steady-state concentration of major byproducts of aerobic metabolism, H_2O_2 and O_2^-, has been estimated as $\sim 1 \times 10^{-8}$ and 2.5×10^{-11} M in liver cytosol, respectively, and $\sim 0.5 \times 10^{-8}$ and 1×10^{-10} M in the liver mitochondrial matrix, respectively (4). The cellular concentration of reactive O_2 species under physiological conditions reflects mainly the contribution of electron-transfer chains and certain enzyme activities inherent in aerobic metabolism. These values were obtained upon identification of two terms of an equation, that is, the measured formation of oxyradicals in aerobic cells and their removal by specific antioxidant enzymic systems. Using a similar steady-state approximation to estimate the cellular concentration of HO· (assuming its formation through a Fenton reaction and an intracellular Fe concentration of 10^{-6} M), a value of $\sim 10^{-18}$ M was obtained (4). An alternative and promising method to calculate steady-state concentrations of oxyradicals is based on the dynamic inactivation—reactivation of aconitase; this offers a specific measure of the steady-state concentration of O_2^- in the mitochondrial matrices of growing mammalian cells (5,6). Steady-state concentrations obtained by this method (5) are similar to those obtained using the rates of O_2^- production and intracellular superoxide dismutase activity in aerobic log phase *Escherichia coli* containing wild-type levels of superoxide dismutase (7).

Overall, it can be stated that about 5% of the O_2 used by cells is reduced to H_2O_2 (8); although the fraction of O_2 consumed by cells channelled to oxidative damage is subject to substantial variations, Floyd (3) estimated that $\sim 1\%$ of the total O_2 consumed by cells appears in the form of oxidized protein and nucleic acids (the latter based on 8-hydroxydeoxyguanosine formation and not taking into account strand breaks).

Careful characterization of free-radical toxicities must of necessity include a correlation between the cellular steady-state concentration of free radicals and the development of particular biochemical changes that are a function of the free-radical physicochemical properties. Hence, knowledge of the critical reactions of free radicals with particular cellular components and their cellular control at multiple levels needs to be recognized as essential for understanding the molecular basis of free-radical toxicity.

This chapter surveys the mechanisms for damage of macromolecules by some type of oxygen-, carbon-, and sulfur-centered radicals as well as the cellular factors known to control these reactions. Some emphasis is given to the addition/substitution reactions involving sulfur nucleophiles and the activated double bond in quinonoid compounds, the oxygen- and sulfur-centered radical production originating from these interactions, and their implication(s) for cytotoxicity.

OXYGEN-CENTERED RADICALS AND OTHER OXIDANTS

The cellular sources of O_2^- and H_2O_2 have been extensively reviewed and their characterization permitted to estimate an intracellular steady-state concentration of these species as well as a ratio for $[H_2O_2]_{ss}/[O_2^-]_{ss}$ of $\sim 10^3$. Although mitochondria are well-established sources of cellular H_2O_2 originating from O_2^- disproportionation (8), an unrecognized function of mitochondrial respiration was recently described consisting of scavenging of cytosolic O_2^- by respiring mitochondria; the latter, via the proton-motive pump, present a polarized, proton-rich surface that enhances nonenzymatic dismutation of extramitochondrial O_2^- (9).

When assessing the reactivity of O_2^- in biological systems, the participation of its conjugated acid ($HO_2^{\cdot}$) should be critically considered, for its pK_a value is only two units below biological pH. The latter could be considerably lower in the proximity of biological membranes, and hence a higher concentration of $HO_2^{\cdot}$ may be expected in this environment. Although the chemical reactivity of O_2^- in protic media is rather restricted, the one-electron reduction of adequate acceptors, such as oxidized transition metals of Fe(III) and Cu(II) (reaction 1a), ferricytochrome c, and quinones with suitable redox potentials, may constitute the basis for some type of cytotoxicity. Likewise, free-radical formation originating from one-electron oxidations by O_2^- of molecules bearing acidic protons, such as ascorbate, and of iron-sulfur clusters (reaction 1b) may have implications for cytotoxicity.

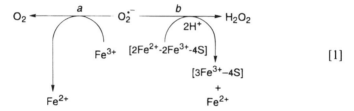

$$[1]$$

Fe(II) released by mechanism a or b in reaction 1 participates in a Fenton reaction (reaction 2), with generation of $HO^{\cdot}$. The concept of an O_2^--driven Fenton-type reaction requires both O_2^- and H_2O_2 as

$$Fe^{2+} + H_2O_2 \rightarrow Fe^{3+} + HO^- + HO^{\cdot} \qquad [2]$$

precursors of $HO^{\cdot}$. It proceeds via an intermediate catalyst, such as a transition metal chelate, which is reduced by O_2^- (reaction 1) and reacts with H_2O_2 (reaction 2). However, reductants other than O_2^- for transition metal chelates abound in a cellular environment; ascorbate and glutathione are such examples. Conversely, Liochev and Fridovich (10) discussed an alternative mechanism leading to $HO^{\cdot}$ formation in vivo and entailing the activity of O_2^- as an oxidant (reaction 1b). The significance of this reaction is twofold; first, O_2^- increases the supply of free iron, and second, O_2^- increases the production of H_2O_2 with a yield at least twice of that from the disproportionation reaction (10).

Catecholamines, dihydroflavins, and tetrahydropterins are susceptible to free-radical chain oxidations initiated by O_2^- (10). By a similar mechanism, O_2^- was proposed as a chain-propagating species in the oxidation of dialuric acid and divicine (11) and several hydroquinones formed during DT-diaphorase catalysis (12). During these processes, the actual steady-state concentration of O_2^- is negligibly small, since it is generated during semiquinone autoxidation (reaction 2) and consumed during hydroquinone oxidation (reaction 4). Expectedly, oxidation of some hydroquinones (at least those formed during DT-diaphorase catalysis) is inhibited by superoxide dismutase upon withdrawal of the propagating species ($O_2^{\cdot-}$) from the chain reaction. Superoxide dismutase may also enhance hydroquinone oxidation in cases where the reduction potential of the $Q/Q^{\cdot-}$ redox couple is less negative than that of the $O_2/O_2^{\cdot-}$ couple (the equilibrium constant K_3 for reaction 3 is below unity: k_{3b} prevails over k_{3f}) (12).

$$Q^{\cdot-} + O_2 \overset{f}{\underset{b}{\rightleftharpoons}} Q + O_2^{\cdot} \qquad\qquad [3]$$

$$QH_2 + O_2^{\cdot-} \rightarrow Q^{\cdot-} + H_2O_2 \qquad\qquad [4]$$

$O_2^{\cdot-}$ can serve as an initiator (via reaction 1a,b) and terminator of lipid peroxidation (via reactions 5,6); according to the latter reactions, it can be expected that scavenging of $O_2^{\cdot-}$ may actually lead to an increase of lipid peroxidation via increased chain length (13). This mechanism explains the dual effect of superoxide dismutase on myocardium reperfusion injury, that is, its protective effect and the exacerbation of injury (13).

$$LO^{\cdot} + O_2^{\cdot-} + H^+ \rightarrow LOH + O_2 \qquad\qquad [5]$$

$$LOO^{\cdot} + O_2^{\cdot-} + H^+ \rightarrow LOOH + O_2 \qquad\qquad [6]$$

Despite its low chemical reactivity, $O_2^{\cdot-}$ can damage some biological targets as illustrated by the $O_2^{\cdot-}$-mediated inactivation of bacterial dehydratases containing iron-sulfur clusters, such as aconitase, dehydroxy acid dehydratase, and 6-phosphogluconate dehydratase (14,15). Also, complex I of the mitochondrial respiratory chain is inactivated by $O_2^{\cdot-}$ probably by a similar mechanism. In addition, the participation of $O_2^{\cdot-}$ in major pathophysiological processes has been described: bactericidal activity [$O_2^{\cdot-}$ generated by NAD(P)H oxidases in leukocytes and macrophages] (16) and reperfusion damage [$O_2^{\cdot-}$ generated by xanthine oxidase (17) and by xanthine oxidase-independent mechanism(s) probably involving the mitochondrial respiratory chain] (18) are some examples. The role of $O_2^{\cdot-}$ in processes as diverse as inflammation, participation in physiological signals through regulation of cell proliferation and apoptosis, and contribution to cell malignancy has been recently reviewed by McCord (19), who bridges these somehow controversial functions of $O_2^{\cdot-}$ in terms of imbalances between cellular production and scavenging of $O_2^{\cdot-}$.

On the other hand, the diversity of effects just outlined does not necessarily mean that $O_2^{\cdot-}$ exhibits different chemical reactivities. The chemistry of $O_2^{\cdot-}$ in protic and aprotic media is well defined, and these diverse effects are rather explained in terms of the physicochemical properties of target(s) that influence the mode of interaction with $O_2^{\cdot-}$ as well as environmental factors that are difficult to identify given the complexity of biological settings.

The cellular steady-state concentration of H_2O_2-originating from $O_2^{\cdot-}$ disproportionation or from reactions of $O_2^{\cdot-}$ as an oxidant or directly upon enzymic reduction of $O_2^{\cdot-}$ is kept at a value of $\sim 10^{-8}$ M in hepatocytes (4). Taking into account the comparable efficiency of catalase and peroxidase in removing H_2O_2 along with their localization in different cellular compartments, the fate of hepatic H_2O_2 will depend on its site of formation. It appears that the metabolism of extraperoxisomal H_2O_2 is the domain of glutathione peroxidase (20).

The moderate chemical reactivity of H_2O_2 is substantially enhanced by two features: on the one hand, its ability to cross freely biological membranes and, on the other hand, its participation in the formation of more potent oxidants, such as $HO^{\cdot}$ (reaction 2) and oxoferryl [Fe(IV) = O] complexes upon its reaction with metal chelates and hemoproteins. The oxoferryl moiety of ferrylmyoglobin (reaction 7) is one of the two electrophilic centers, the other oxidation equivalent being in the form of an aromatic amino acid radical. The specific chemistry attainable by these centers is different, and perhaps the most distinctive feature is their lifetime: Although the oxoferryl complex is a long-lived strong oxidant (with a redox potential of about $+0.99$ V (21), the amino acid radical is short-lived (between 50 and 280 ms) (22).

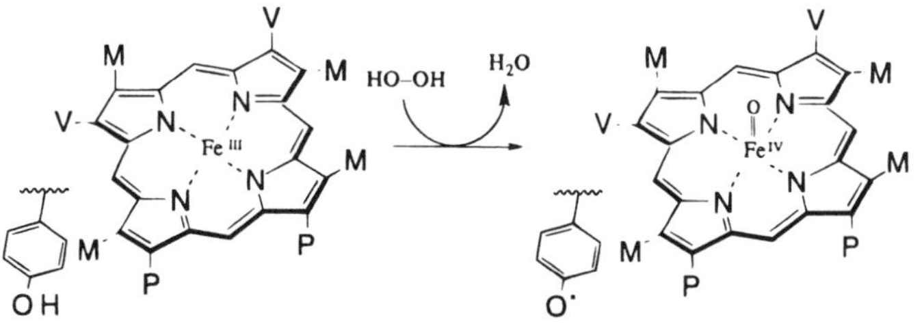

[7]

The oxoferryl complex can easily oxidize phenols, ascorbate, thiols, polyunsaturated fatty acids, and cholesterol (as generalized in reaction 8) and promote sulfoxidation and/or cooxidation of drugs, such as methylcarbazole and chlorpromazine (for a review see 23).

$$HX-Fe(IV)=O + AH^- \rightarrow HX-Fe(III) + A^{\cdot-} \qquad [8]$$

An iron-oxo entity originating from the oxidation of Fe(II)-EDTA by H_2O_2 (reaction 9) might be responsible for the formation of adenine N-1 oxide on DNA exposed to nonlethal levels of H_2O_2 (24) (reaction 10). The oxide is specifically produced by oxidation of DNA with H_2O_2 under nonradical conditions:

$$EDTA-Fe(II) + H_2O_2 \rightarrow EDTA-Fe(IV)=O + H_2O \qquad [9]$$

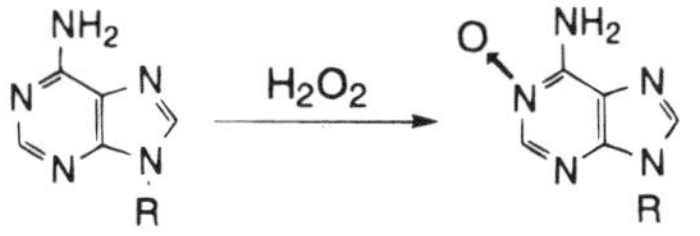

[10]

The formation of $HO^{\cdot}$ in vitro (reactions 1a $\rightarrow$ 2) or as proposed for in vivo conditions (10) (reactions 1b $\rightarrow$ 2) requires H_2O_2 and transition metals. On thermodynamic grounds, semiquinones with a reduction potential between $+460$ and -330

mV can reduce H_2O_2 to $HO^{\cdot}$; experimental evidence for this "organic" Fenton reaction has been provided (25), although counterevidence has also been brought forward (26).

In a biological milieu, the exact chemical nature of an iron pool to catalyze reaction 2 remains unclear (see 27 for a critical discussion). Regardless of the exact nature of the cellular transition metal pool, $HO^{\cdot}$ can be generated in the bulk solution (non-site-specific mechanism of damage), thus accounting for a random attack of target(s). Conversely, $HO^{\cdot}$ may be generated close to a biological target when the metal ion or its complex is bound to the target, which might serve as an effective ligand for, for example, Cu (site-specific mechanism of damage) (28). This distinction is biologically relevant because the production of $HO^{\cdot}$ in the vicinity of DNA may control the type of chemistry observed. Likewise, residues of histidine in proteins are important binding sites for metals, which can localize damage initiated by peroxides on particular functional groups close to the metal-binding amino acid (29,30). Alternatively, protein-bound metals can participate in redox reactions that generate bulk-phase radicals capable of eliciting oxidative damage outside the protein domain (31). The overall process of free-radical-mediated oxidation of proteins is complex, and it depends on the relative localization of radical generation, the occurrence and localization of antioxidants, and the type of target proteins (32).

$HO^{\cdot}$ is endowed with unique properties: Due to a combination of high electrophilicity, high thermochemical reactivity, and a mode of production that can occur in the vicinity of DNA (site-specific mechanism referred to earlier), it can both abstract H atoms from the sugar in the DNA helix and add to DNA bases (33), leading to single-strand nicks and nucleobase oxidation, respectively. Pryor (33) referred to the unusually high ratio for the rate constant of $HO^{\cdot}$ addition to double bonds divided by that for H-abstraction (k_{ad}/k_H) (>10).

The former reaction, H abstraction, is a major route for most aliphatic substrate oxidations by $HO^{\cdot}$ (such as that contemplated in the initiation phase of lipid peroxidation); $HO^{\cdot}$ -mediated oxidation of different electron donors (including antioxidant molecules) has been extensively reported in the pulse radiolysis literature: these reactions usually proceed at diffusion-controlled rates ($>10^9\ M^{-1}s^{-1}$). DNA strand breakage is a multistep process initiated by H abstraction from a sugar or base; DNA-derived radicals are detected by direct electron spin resonance (esr) spectroscopy (34); flow techniques (35), and esr in conjunction with the spin trap *t*-nitrosobutane (36,37). Overall, the detection of radicals at the sugar moiety by esr was aimed at providing some information on the possible routes leading to DNA strand breakage; the C(4') mechanism is centered on the formation of a carbon-centered radical at the position C4' in deoxyribose, with the carbon-bound H-atom abstraction being in itself the rate-determining step (38):

$$[11]$$

The latter reaction, HO˙ addition to bases such as guanine, proceeds at diffusion-controlled rates ($>10^9$ $M^{-1}s^{-1}$). 8-Hydroxydeoxyguanosine, used as a fingerprint of nucleobase oxidative damage, is formed by such an addition reaction (reaction 12). The hydroxyl radical-base adduct is redox ambivalent—that is, it can be both a reducing or oxidizing radical. Oxidation of the C-4 form and loss of a proton leads to imidazole ring re-aromatization and 8-hydroxydeoxyguanosine (39).

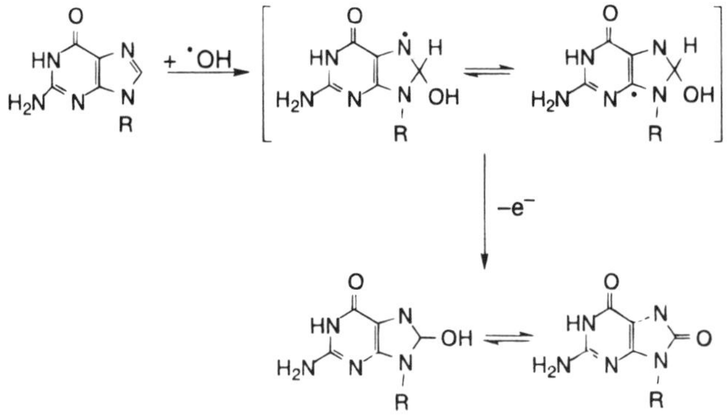

[12]

Not only HO˙ but also singlet oxygen ($^1O_2$) can cause the formation of 8-hydroxy-deoxyguanosine (40). $^1O_2$ reacts with deoxyguanosine with an overall rate constant of 5.2×10^6 $M^{-1}s^{-1}$ (41). An analog of 8-hydroxydeoxyguanosine, 4,8-dihydro-4-hydroxy-8-oxo-guanosine, is formed upon reaction of deoxyguanosine with $^1O_2$ by a Diels—Alder reaction with an endoperoxide intermediate; in reaction 13 the two reducing equivalents required to form the 8-hydroxypurine from the endoperoxide are supplied by a thiol, which was found to enhance significantly $^1O_2$-induced formation of 8-hydroxy derivatives (41).

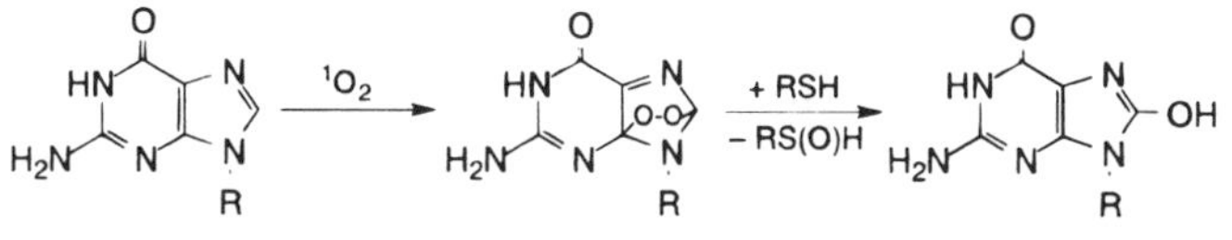

[13]

Although often a fingerprint for oxyradical attack, formation of 8-hydroxydeoxy-guanosine may not be necessarily related to HO˙ addition across the double bond: for example, 8-hydroxyguanine formation during the metabolism of the carcinogen 4-nitroquinoline 1-oxide (4NQO) does not appear to involve HO˙ addition to the base; following bioactivation of 4NQO, the N_4-O-acyl-substituted intermediate is responsible for 8-hydroxydeoxyguanosine formation via a mechanism involving addition of R-NH$^+$ to the 7,8-double bond, H_2O addition, and subsequent elimination of 4-aminoquinoline 1-oxide. The product is a hydroxy-substituted base at the C^8 position (42). This alternative mechanism based on the analogy of the amination of guanosine with dinitrophenoxyamine is shown in reaction 14:

$$[14]$$

Floyd and Schneider (43) proposed a generalized scheme to rationalize 8-hydroxy-deoxyguanosine formation in a $HO^{\cdot}$-independent manner and involving an intermediate C^8 cation radical that following H_2O addition leads to the radical intermediate (within brackets in reaction 12) and, finally, to the 8-hydroxydeoxyguanosine product.

The aforementioned site-specific mechanism for the formation of $HO^{\cdot}$ requires the occurrence of metals bound to suitable targets. Copper ions appear to occur naturally in chromosomes and play a key role in their organization and functions (44). Copper is expected to bind tightly to a mononucleotide by way of both base guanine-cytosine base pair regions (45) and phosphate sites $[K(DNA + Cu^+ \Leftrightarrow DNA\text{-}Cu^+)\ 10^9\ M^{-1}]$ (46). These $DNA-Cu$ complexes were shown to be in dynamic equilibrium and their relative concentration to be modulated by pH and ionic strength, and they might serve as effective ligands supporting a site-specific mechanism of DNA oxidative damage by way of forming $HO^{\cdot}$ in the vicinity of DNA. $HO^{\cdot}$ formation via reaction 15 proceeds slowly ($k_{15} = 1.2$–$1.3\ M^{-1}s^{-1}$) (47), whereas the $O_2^{\cdot-}$-mediated reduction of Cu^{++} bound to DNA (reaction 16) is expected to proceed at higher rates ($k_{16} \sim 10^8\ M^{-1}s^{-1}$) (48).

$$DNA-Cu^+ + H_2O_2 \rightarrow DNA-Cu^{++} + HO^- + HO^{\cdot} \qquad [15]$$

$$DNA-Cu^{++} + O_2^{\cdot-} \rightarrow DNA-Cu^+ + O_2 \qquad [16]$$

Hence, reaction 15 is the rate-limiting step in the sequence of reaction leading to formation of DNA-derived radicals. As discussed earlier, other reductants can replace $O_2^{\cdot-}$ in reaction 16; also, intracomplex electron transfer between Cu^{++} and electronegative regions in DNA (such as guanosine residues) yields Cu^+ attached to an oxidized base, followed by reduction of H_2O_2 by the Cu^+ complex (49).

Mitochondrial DNA (mtDNA) is subjected to more severe oxidative damage than nuclear DNA (50,51). Formation of 8-hydroxydeoxyguanosine in mtDNA could occur as part of a site-specific mechanism of damage, entailing cleavage of the H_2O_2 diffusing into the mitochondrial matrix by metals bound to mitochondrial DNA (52). Although mitochondria generate HO˙, it is difficult to assess the contribution of this species to the oxidative impairment of bases in mitochondrial DNA because the site of HO˙ formation is not specified, although it is dependent on the mitochondrial electron transfer. H_2O_2 is assumed to diffuse outside the mitochondria and into the mitochondrial matrix. In the latter instances, an intramitochondrial steady-state concentration of H_2O_2 of 0.48×10^{-8} M was calculated considering the production and removal of this species by glutathione peroxidase (and catalase in the case of heart mitochondria). The rate of H_2O_2 utilization leading to HO˙ formation was calculated on the basis of a sole target, mtDNA, and the occurrence of active Cu catalytic centers bound to the macromolecule (4). These views suggest that HO˙ formed during mitochondrial electron transfer (52) is not directly responsible for the accumulation of 8-hydroxydeoxyguanosine in mtDNA, which appears to be the result of H_2O_2 difusing into the mitochondrial matrix and reacting via a site-specific mechanism with mtDNA-bound active copper centers. In this regard, a correlation between the rate of H_2O_2 formation during mitochondrial electron transport and accumulation of 8-hydroxydeoxyguanosine was established (52).

Levels of oxidative damage to mtDNA isolated from rat liver or various human brain regions are about 10-fold higher than those of nuclear DNA (50,53), probably due to the lack of protective histones and DNA repair activity along with the location of mtDNA in the vicinity of the site of H_2O_2 generation (51,53). It was established that the level of 8-hydroxydeoxyguanosine in mtDNA increases with age (2), and it is argued that this damage leads to mutations that result in dysfunctional mitochondria. Furthermore, these mutations may lead to protein conformational changes usually associated with an inefficient electron transfer to cytochrome oxidase and, hence, enhanced superoxide/H_2O_2 formation. This cycle is expected to accelerate mitochondrial dysfunction with age (51,53). Other oxidative modifications of rat brain mitochondria challenged with H_2O_2/copper/ascorbate include mtRNA and protein oxidation (54).

Formation of 8-hydroxydeoxyguanosine in DNA in vitro has been observed in association with the metabolism of mutagenic or carcinogenic substances or elicited by ionizing radiation, γ-irradiation, asbestos/H_2O_2 and Cu^+/ascorbate mixtures, and autoxidized unsaturated lipids (see 55). It is likely that in all these instances the formation of 8-hydroxydeoxyguanosine is due to HO˙ addition across the 7,8-double bond of the base as shown in reaction 12.

The detection of 8-hydroxydeoxyguanosine in vivo is obviously important because it relates to mutagenesis/carcinogenesis (56). The oxidized base was detected in vivo in human granulocyte DNA (57) exposed to the tumor promoter 12-*O*-tetradecanoylphorbol 13-acetate (58) or to cigarette smoke (59) as well as in HeLa cells exposed to x-irradiation, Walker carcinoma cells supplemented with Ni(II) compounds under aerobic conditions (60), and human leukemia cell line HL60 (57) incubated with benzene and its phenolic metabolites (61). Likewise, benzene and 1,2,4-benzenetriol increase oxidative DNA damage in the mouse bone marrow in vivo (61). The content of 8-hydroxydeoxyguanosine in the liver of different species was found augmented following γ-irradiation (62) or upon administration of the peroxisomal proliferator ciprofibrate (63), 3-amino-1,2,4-benzotriazine 1,4-oxide (60), Ni(II) compounds (64), iron/Aroclor 1254 (65), diethylstilbestrol (66), the hepatocarcinogen 2-nitropropane (67), or upon modulation of redox enzymes (in the absence or presence of menadione) (68). Overexpression of Cu,Zn-superoxide dismutase and catalase in *Drosophila melanogaster* caused a retardation in the accumulation of 8-hydroxydeoxyguanosine accumulation with aging as well as in the response to the exposure of live flies to x-rays (69).

Smoking, body mass index, and gender are significant predictors of the urinary excretion of 8-hydroxydeoxyguanosine (70), which was found increased in a variety of cancer patients (both before therapy onset and after) compared to healthy individuals (71); also high levels of urinary 8-hydroxydeoxyguanosine were found in patients subjected to whole-body irradiation or receiving chemotherapy (71).

THIOL ADDITION/SUBSTITUTION REACTIONS
AND THIYL RADICALS

The reactions of several xenobiotics with sulfur nucleophiles is of biological significance because of the wide distribution and high intracellular concentration of these compounds in the form of high- and low-molecular-weight thiols. The enzymatic, glutathione-dependent biotransformation of xenobiotics is associated with detoxification of a range of electrophilic substances and it also serves as a bioactivation mechanism for several groups of compounds (for a review see 72). The latter reactions are usually initiated by a glutathione *S*-transferase-catalyzed conjugate formation, and in some instances this is associated with formation of toxic metabolites: electrophilic sulfur mustards, nephrotoxic haloalkenes converted to toxic metabolites in a glutathione multistep mechanism, quinone thioethers, reversible conjugation with isothiocyanates (73). Similar types of reactions take place nonenzymatically in the bioactivation of several electrophiles: 1,4-sulfur reductive addition and *ipso* addition as well as S_N2 attack of thiols occur at considerable rates with a range of quinonoid compounds. In this context, the physicochemical properties of both compound types, electrophilic xenobiotics and sulfur nucleophiles, are important for assessing their participation in critical bimolecular reactions and their implications for cytotoxicity or detoxification. Overall, quinone-mediated cytotoxicity is the expression of several interdependent factors: a particular quinone functional group chemistry, the biochemical pathways involved in the activation of these compounds, and the individual sensitivity of cells to quinone chemical reactivity and the redox properties of the products.

1,4-Sulfur Reductive Addition

The electrophilic arylating reactivity of quinones is partly a function of the cross-conjugated system determined by the alternating single and double bonds including the exocyclic moieties $[(O=C-C=C)_n-C=O]$ and resulting in a polarized double bond (generally $-C_2=C_3-$). This electrophilic center leads to the binding of the quinone moiety to nucleophilic groups in critical molecules. Thiols react chiefly as RS^-; hence, an important property controlling their reactivity is the dissociation constant (pK) of the ionization reaction ($RSH \leftrightarrow RS^- + H^+$). Although this is important for most low-molecular-weight thiols, protein thiols may behave in a manner independent of pK and be susceptible to the environment around the $-SH$ group (74).

The activated or polarized double bond in quinonoid compounds reacts readily with sulfur nucleophiles, such as GSH and cysteine (1,4-reductive addition of the Michael type) (75). The product, a primary thioether or sulfide, customarily named hydroquinone glutathione conjugate, originates from an intermediate transition-state anion stabilized by delocalization of the charge onto an electronegative element:

$$[17]$$

The substituent in the quinone molecule determines both the position in the quinone ring of the glutathionyl adduct and the rate of thiol nucleophilic addition. The preferred site of nucleophilic attack to quinones is the position having the largest, lowest unoccupied molecular orbital coefficient, that is, the lowest electron density. The rate of GSH addition differs between benzo- and naphthoquinones (76–80), and it is influenced by the nature and number of substituents and, in the case of naphthoquinones, whether the substituents are in the quinonoid and/or benzenoid ring.

The glutathionyl substituent exerts little effect on the one-electron reduction potential of quinones, in agreement with the weak electron-withdrawing properties of the thioether substituent; for example, the glutathionyl substituent raises slightly the one-electron reduction potential value relative to that of menadione by about 11 mV (78). Conversely, the half-wave reduction potential values of glutathionyl quinones are more negative than the parent compounds (81), although steric effects of vicinal substituents could alter redox equilibria in a different manner (82).

Sulfur nucleophiles can also add to quinone methides as shown in reaction 18, a mechanism likely to be relevant in connection with the activation of hydroxymethyl-substituted bioalkylating quinones (83,84). Sulfur nucleophilic/substitution reactions also accompany the redox transitions of 2-methyl-1,4-naphthoquinone bioalkylating agents (85).

$$[18]$$

Ipso Addition

The rate-limiting *ipso* sulfur addition across the double bond of the exocyclic imine moiety of *N*-acetyl-*p*-benzoquinoneimine provides an alternative mechanism to the Michael addition depicted in reaction 17, as indicated by the synthesis and characterization of a thiol *ipso* adduct (reaction 19) (86,87). The electrophilic character of this quinoneimine is partly responsible for the observed covalent modification of erythrocyte cytoskeletal proteins and ion transporting systems. A similar mechanism may be operative with halogen-substituted aziridinylbenzoquinones (88) entailing the *ipso* addition of GS$^-$ across the carbonyl double bond followed by attack of GS$^-$ to form a hydroquinone and GSSG (reaction 20):

$$[19]$$

$$[20]$$

Sulfur Nucleophilic Substitution

Halogen-containing aziridinylbenzoquinones are particularly interesting because of the reactivity of halogen atoms at C_3 and C_6 toward sulfur substitution (75). At variance with the reductive addition described in reaction 17, the mono- or dithioether derivative formed is in an oxidized state (reaction 21) (88,89). Although glutathione *S*-transferases can catalyze reactions such as the one shown earlier, various isoenzymes are inhibited irreversibly by a number of arylating quinones.

$$[21]$$

Reactivity of Thioether Derivatives

The subsequent chemical reactivity of the thioether derivative formed in reaction 17 has been extensively discussed (80) and is influenced by the reduction potential of the molecule and its substitution pattern, as well as by environmental factors such as medium polarity, pH, solvent cage, and solvation energy. Following sulfur nucleophile reductive addition (reaction 17), the prevalence of either of these pathways is controlled by various factors and a single mechanism for the oxidation of the glutathionyl-hydroquinone conjugate can be ruled out (80). The transition of the glutathionyl hydroquinone to glutathionyl quinone occurs through the one-electron transfer steps encompassed in cross-oxidation, autoxidation, and disproportionation reactions.

Oxidative elimination and oxidative cyclization are also important decay pathways. The former reactions are limited to those hydroquinones bearing a good leaving group, such as hydroxy, methoxy, chloride, bromide, etc., and are influenced by the electron density of the hydroquinone nucleus, that is, its reduction potential (77,78,90–92).

The latter, oxidative cyclization is an intramolecular 1,4-Michael addition, a process following the primary sulfur nucleophilic addition to some *p*-benzoquinones and 1,4-naphthoquinones and requiring protonation of the quinone and elimination of H$_2$O (acid-catalyzed oxidative cyclization) (reaction 22). 1,4-Benzothiazine is formed during the γ-GT-mediated metabolism of 2-bromo-3-glutathionyl-*p*-benzohydro-quinone by a process involving arrangement *via* oxidative cyclization (93). Although the significance of this product of quinone metabolism *in vivo* remains to be determined, the initial sulfur nucleophilic addition followed by oxidative cyclization removes the electrophilic character of the quinone moiety and, as such, might be considered a detoxication mechanism (93).

[22]

Sulfur nucleophilic addition does not necessarily compete with redox cycling processes, because thioether derivatives are also substrates for one- and two-electron transfer flavoenzymes (e.g., NADPH-cytochrome P450 reductase and DT-diaphorase, respectively) (81,94).

Oxygen- and sulfur-centered radical generation accompany the earlier described thiol/quinone interactions. The latter appears to originate upon electron transfer to O$_2^-$ (reaction 23a) and/or semiquinones (reaction 23b) (85,88,92,95).

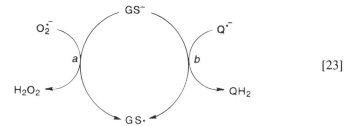

$$[23]$$

Although neither reaction is expected to occur at appreciable rates, there are numerous reports documenting their occurrence in biological settings. The former reaction-analogous to reactions 1b and 4, in which O_2^- acts as an oxidant-proceeds slowly either with cysteine or GSH ($\sim 10^2\ M^{-1}s^{-1}$) (96). The latter is usually thermodynamically unfavorable, but—as exemplified with acetaminophen radical (97)—is controlled by kinetic factors, and its equilibrium is effectively displaced by the rapid conjugation of thiyl radicals with thiolate (98):

$$RS^. + RS^- \rightarrow [RSSR]^{.-} \qquad [24]$$

An alternative route for thiyl radical formation (reaction 25) has been reported for the case of benzoquinone and its methyl-substituted derivatives; a discussion on the competition between reactions 17 and 25 has been provided (99):

$$Q + GHS \leftrightarrow O^{.-} + GS^. + H^+ \qquad [25]$$

Thiyl radical formation is effected differently by superoxide dismutase depending on whether the prevalent pathway involves O_2^- or semiquinone reduction by thiols. During the thiol-mediated reductive decay of the semiquinone (reaction 23b), the focus of superoxide dismutase activity is centered on a reaction down the free-radical chain, that is, displacing the equilibrium of reaction 26:

$$[RSSR]^{.-} + O_2 \rightarrow RSSR + O_2^- \qquad [26]$$

Reactions 23b, 24, and 26 indicate that the radical character is transferred according to the sequence $Q^{.-} \rightarrow GS^. \rightarrow GSSG^{.-} \rightarrow O_2^-$ and, finally, via disproportionation to a nonradical product, H_2O_2. This sequence involves oxidizing and reducing radicals (with positive and negative $E^{o\prime}$ values, respectively). Superoxide dismutase is expected to favor these reactions when $[Q^{.-}]_{ss} >> [O_2^-]_{ss}$. On the other hand, thiyl radical formation during thiol oxidation by O_2^- (reaction 23a) is also suppressed by superoxide dismutase (when $[Q^{.-}]_{ss} < [O_2^-]_{ss}$): in these instances, the effect is accompanied by an inhibition of GSSG accumulation by the enzyme (12). Clearly, the relative steady-state concentrations of O_2^- and semiquinone will influence profoundly the cellular redox state.

Thiyl and disulfide anion radicals may oxidize hydroquinones and reduce quinones, respectively, according to reaction 27. For p-benzoquinone and several methyl-substituted derivatives the rate constants for reaction 27a were $\sim 10^5-10^7$ $M^{-1}\ s^{-1}$ and for reaction 27b, $\sim 10^7-10^9\ M^{-1}s^{-1}$ (99).

$$\text{[27]}$$

The importance of the subsequent redox chemistry of quinone thioethers is illustrated by the formation of DNA strand breaks elicited by oxyradical formation originating from quinone/GSH interactions (88). The 2- and 6-methyl-1,4-naphthoquinone bioalkylating agents react with GSH with rate constants of about 10^2–10^4 $M^{-1}s^{-1}$ (78), and the thioether derivative thereby formed participates in redox transitions yielding oxygen- and sulfur-centered radicals (92).

Thiyl radicals generated nonenzymically as described earlier or enzymically or during the pseudoperoxidatic activity of hemoproteins are strong oxidants ($E^{o'}_{RS'/RSH} = +0.9$ V). The reactions of thiyl radicals have recently been reviewed (98,100). The oxidizing character of thiyl radicals is further substantiated by their ability to react with polyunsaturated fatty acids *via* two reactions: abstraction of a *bis*-allylic hydrogen forming pentadienyl radicals and addition to double bonds (100) (reactions 28 and 29). The rate constants for hydrogen abstraction by RS⁻ from polyunsaturated fatty acids (k_{28}) and those for addition with formation of β-(alkylthio)alkyl radicals (k_{29}) are ~10^7 $M^{-1}s^{-1}$ and 10^8 $M^{-1}s^{-1}$, respectively. The latter reactions are complex and the alkyl radical products may be quenched by molecular O_2 to yield the corresponding peroxyl radicals (100). Protection of membrane lipids against thiyl radical attack may be achieved by vitamin A (retinol), which reacts rapidly with glutathionyl radicals ($k = 1.4 \times 10^9$ $M^{-1}s^{-1}$) (101).

$$\text{[28]}$$

$$\text{[29]}$$

The oxidizing properties of thiyl radicals might have implications for mtDNA oxidative damage. The mitochondrial matrix is endowed with antioxidant activities such as Mn-superoxide dismutase and glutathione peroxidase (and catalase in the case of heart mitochondria). The major importance of mitochondrial GSH and glutathione peroxidase in protection against oxidative damage can be inferred from the fact that mitochondria produce substantial quantities of O_2^- and H_2O_2 and that GSH deficiency-accomplished by prolonged treatment of animals with a transition state inhibitor of γ-glutamylcysteine synthetase-is associated with widespread mitochondrial dysfunction and other types of cell damage (102). Despite the occurrence of the earlier antioxidant enzymes and a large amount of GSH (3 nmol/mg mitochondrial protein equivalent to

3 mM) in the mitochondrial matrix, oxidative damage to mtDNA in the form of 8-hydroxydeoxyguanosine can be observed during mitochondrial electron transfer (52). Although the mechanism for formation of 8-hydroxydeoxyguanosine in mtDNA appears to involve diffusion of H_2O_2 into the matrix space and its subsequent cleavage to HO˙ by DNA-bound Cu (site-specific mechanism), an alternative mechanism for nucleobase oxidative damage or H abstraction from deoxyribose might involve thiyl radicals. Both reactions are likely on thermodynamic grounds and similar to those describing the reactivity of thiyl radicals toward polyunsaturated fatty acids (100) (reactions 27 and 28). These reactions might have further significance for mtDNA considering the lack of protective histones and DNA repair activity along with the location of mtDNA in the vicinity of H_2O_2 (and potentially thiyl radical) generation. It has been reported that GSH enhanced $^1O_2$-induced single strand breaks in plasmid pBR322 DNA (103) (it also enhances the yield of 8-hydroxydeoxyguanosine formation according to reaction 13) (41). Thiyl and derived radicals are likely to participate in this system, although evidence for their occurrence was not available (103).

Conversely, DNA base radicals may be "repaired" by thiols. Although it is not clear which is the actual base radical species, these thiol-dependent repair reactions proceed at high rates (104,105). The H-atom donation from SH compounds to radiation-induced DNA radicals is a process normally blocked by O_2 by the more rapid reaction of O_2 with the DNA radicals. In anaerobic conditions, cysteine, cysteamine, and dithiothreitol repair efficiently DNA lesions, whereas GSH was shown to be significantly less efficient (105). The rate of repair by dithiothreitol of DNA radical precursors to single strand breaks was reported as $2.8 \times 10^6 \, M^{-1}s^{-1}$ (105) and H-atom donation to DNA base radicals by cysteamine and cysteine has a rate of less than 10^6–$10^8 \, M^{-1}s^{-1}$ (106). GSH was reported to catalyze the in vitro formation of 8-hydroxydeoxyguanosine at a low [GSH]/[Cu] ratio; at high [GSH]/[Cu] ratios, GSH behaved as an effective antioxidant (107).

CARBON-CENTERED RADICALS

Carbon-centered radicals are generated during the metabolism of several xenobiotics, such as polycyclic aromatic hydrocarbons, ethanol, carbon tetrachloride, hydrazines, 2-nitropropane, diazoquones, and various peroxides (for a review, see 108). The chemical reactivity of carbon-centered or alkyl radicals is encompassed by hydrogen abstraction and double-bond addition reactions as well as quenching by molecular O_2. The latter occurs at high rates ($>10^9 \, M^{-1}s^{-1}$) and yields peroxyl radicals:

$$R\cdot + O_2 \rightarrow ROO\cdot \qquad [30]$$

DNA base alkylation by alkyl radicals have been reported in several chemical systems. A general mechanism for this type of reaction is exemplified for methyl radicals ($\cdot CH_3$) in reaction 31 (109,110). Despite their low electrophilicity, carbon-centered radicals have a tendency to add to double bonds (33): The ratio of the rate

$$[31]$$

constant for addition to double bonds divided by that for H-abstraction from hydrogen donors (k_{ad}/k_H) is $\sim$ 10 (111).

The formation of 8-hydroxydeoxyguanosine in DNA requires a site-specific mechanism to account for the reactivity of HO· vicinal to the nucleobase. Likewise, the formation of nucleobase-alkyl adducts requires the generation of alkyl radicals in the vicinity of DNA in order to overcome the rapid quenching of carbon-centered radicals by O_2 (reaction 18). Although a "site-specific" type of damage involving addition of alkyl radicals to nucleobases is difficult to envision, support for the biological significance of this reaction has been recently brought forward (108). For the particular case of monoalkyl hydrazine derivatives, it was suggested that DNA—iron complexes could catalyze in situ the oxidation of this compound to methyl radicals (112). Overall, Augusto (108) suggested that redox cycling of metals chelated to DNA might be a relevant mechanism leading to carbon-centered radical-mediated alkylation (113). Alternative mechanisms not involving methyl radicals have been brought forward (114).

Carbon-centered radicals derived from the metabolism of hydrazine derivatives and benzoquinone-imine have been shown to induce DNA strand breakage (115–117) and alkyl-nucleoside adducts (118,119). In some instances, such as the metabolism of hydrazine derivatives, DNA alkylation (formation of C^8-methylguanines) was inhibited in vitro and in vivo by the spin trap α-(4-pyridyl-1-oxide)-*N*-*t*-butylnitrone (120,121); this also provided the first evidence for in vivo DNA alkylation by carbon-centered radicals (120). Both reactions, DNA alkylation and DNA strand breakage—a consequence of carbon-centered radical-mediated double-bond addition and hydrogen abstraction—may be highly significant in chemical carcinogenesis and mutagenesis.

Apparently, several molecular mechanisms underlie the cytotoxicity elicited by *p*-benzoquinoneimine (or *p*-diazoquone or metabolites derived from *p*-aminophenol). On the one hand, *p*-benzoquinoneimine (or its *ortho* analog) is metabolized in a multistep process to a *p*-hydroxyphenyl radical (reaction 32), which both adds readily at the C^8 position of purine nucleosides (reaction 33) with formation of 8-hydroxyphenyldeoxyguanosine (118) and cleaves the phosphodiester bond of lDNA, FX174 RFI DNA, and M13mp8ss DNA (117).

On the other hand, *p*-benzoquinoneimine derived from *p*-aminophenol metabolism is a reactive α,β-unsaturated compound, the toxicity of which appears to be mediated by glutathione-dependent mechanisms, since depletion of GSH by buthioninsulfoximine, which inhibits glutathione synthesis, completely protected rats against *p*-aminophenol nephrotoxicity. The oxidized form of the metabolite 1-amino-3-glutathione-*S*-yl-4-hydroxybenzene is expected to be highly nephrotoxic, probably by a mechanism involving covalent binding to macromolecules (73).

$$[32]$$

$$[33]$$

Hydroxy and alkylderivatives of purines at C^8 have been detected in vivo, suggesting that oxygen- and carbon-centered radicals are likely to play an important role in oxidative DNA damage, although in the latter case these adducts were observed only during the metabolism of 1,2-dimethylhydrazine and not in untreated animals (120). This difference with 8-hydroxydeoxyguanosine, which can be detected under physiological conditions, might reflect a prevalence of oxygen-centered radical formation over carbon-centered radicals under normal metabolic situations. Moreover, this might be an indication of the requirement of a site-specific mechanism of damage, which is difficult to envision in the case of carbon-centered radicals. The involvement of purines with a hydroxy or alkyl substituent at C^8 in mutagenesis (122) and/or carcinogenesis (56) is an important question: Purine substitution at the C^8 position alters base-pairing interactions and, specifically, 8-oxodeoxyguanosine has been shown to be mutagenic by inducing G → T transversions in replication in *E. coli* (55,122) and identical mutations were found in simian kidney cells (123). The occurrence of the hydroxylated purine in template DNA (in actuality 8-hydroxydeoxyguanosine occurs in the C^8 keto form and the *syn* conformation) would cause a miscoded incorporation of nucleotides in the replicated strand (124). In summary, mutagenesis appears to be caused by formation of 8-oxo G—A mispairs. Floyd et al. (133) summarized results of many studies that show a direct correlation between the formation of 8-hydroxydeoxyguanosine and carcinogenesis. Augusto (108) proposed that C^8-alkyl-deoxyguanosine could also be mutagenic via a similar mechanism.

SUMMARY

The reactions described in this chapter emphasize only selected aspects of the biological reactivity of oxygen-, sulfur-, and carbon-centered radicals that may be of physiological and toxicological interest. This narrow focus is especially true for sulfur-centered radicals, the chemistry of which is far more diverse and richer than that of oxygen-centered radicals (98,100,125,126). A large body of evidence for the generation of thiyl radicals in biological systems has been provided by spin-trapping experiments (127,128). Although thiyl radicals are capable of undergoing a large variety of reactions of biological interest, their involvement in particular cellular oxidative stress situationsbased on their chemical reactivity and controlled by environmental factorsremains to be elucidated. Sulfur-centered radicals derived from glutathione have been shown to cause mutagenicity in *Salmonella typhimurium* (129), and those derived from penicillamine may be involved in the oxidation of alcohols (130,131). The biological significance of thiyl radicals may be further substantiated by the occurrence of a thiyl-specific antioxidant enzyme that requires cysteine-47 for its activity (132).

The reaction of HO˙ with guanosine in DNA leads to—among other lesions—the formation of 8-hydroxydeoxyguanosine. It is also likely that formation of 8-hydroxydeoxyguanosine reflects accurately other types of lesions elicited by oxygen radicals in DNA . This adduct appears to have deep biological implications, probably resulting from a combination of several factors: its easy detection in vitro and in vivo made possible by highly sensitive techniques (133), its formation in physiological conditions, its being the most abundant lesion in irradiated chromatine (134), and the occurrence of repair mechanisms (135). The alkyl adducts of purine bases—probably reflecting the occurrence of carbon-centered radicals—appear not to be formed under "physiological" conditions (108) and are detected in vivo during the metabolism of particular carcinogens. The amount of 8-hydroxydeoxyguanosine in DNA is extremely high as compared with DNA adducts formed with alkylating agents and/ or carcinogens; hence, the obvious importance of 8-hydroxydeoxyguanosine in mutagenesis. Evidence for oxidants other than HO˙ in the formation of 8-hydroxydeoxyguanosine is also growing: Peroxynitrite (or an intermediate with the reactivity of HO˙) appears to mediate accumulation of the hydroxy adduct in calf thymus DNA (136), and $^1O_2$ mediates formation of the hydroxy adduct in plasmid DNA, which can be protected by carotenoids (137).

A close look at the chemistry of oxygen-, sulfur-, and carbon-centered radicals (and N-centered radicals with emphasis on nitric oxide) indicates an abundant interaction among these species with formation of secondary oxidants with a chemical reactivity of their own. Obviously, the understanding of the physicochemical parameters for free-radical toxicity is a long-term goal determined by a complex network of oxidants in an already complex biological setting.

ACKNOWLEDGEMENT

Supported by NIH grant HL53467.

REFERENCES

1. Rice-Evans CA, Diplock AT. Current status of antioxidant therapy. *Free Radical Biol Med* 1993;15:77–96.
2. Fraga CG, Shigenaga MK, Park JW, Degan P, Ames BN. Oxidative damage to DNA during aging: 8-Hydroxy-2'-deoxyguanosine in rat organ DNA and urine. *Proc Natl Acad Sci USA* 1990;87:4533–4537.

3. Floyd RA. Measurement of oxidative stress in vivo. In: Davies KJA and Ursini F, eds. *The Oxygen Paradox*. Padova: Cleup University Press, 1995:89–103.

4. Boveris A, Cadenas E. Cellular sources and steady-state levels of reactive oxygen species. In: Massaro DJ, ed. *Oxygen, Gene Expression, and Cellular Function*. New York: Marcel Dekker, 1995.

5. Gardner PR, White CW. Application of the aconitase method to the assay of superoxide in the mitochondrial matrices of cultured cells:effects of oxygen, redox cycling agents, TNF-α, IL-1, LPS and inhibitors of respiration. In: Davies KJA, Ursini F, eds. *The Oxygen Paradox*. Padova: Cleup University Press, 1995:33–50.

6. Gardner PR, Fridovich I. Inactivationreactivation of aconitase in *Escherichia coli*: A sensitive measure of superoxide. *J Biol Chem* 1992; 267:8757–8753.

7. Imlay JA, Fridovich I. Assay of metabolic superoxide production in *Escherichia coli*. *J Biol Chem* 1991;266:6957–6965.

8. Boveris A, Cadenas E. Production of superoxide radicals and hydrogen peroxide in mitochondria. In: Oberley LW ed. *Superoxide Dismutase*, Boca Raton, FL: CRC Press, vol II; 1982:15–30.

9. Guidot DM, Repine JE, Kitlowski AD, Flores SC, Nelson SXK, Wright RM, McCord JM. Mitochondrial respiration scavenges extramitochondrial superoxide anion via a nonenzymatic mechanism. *J Clin Invest* 1995;96:1131–1136.

10. Liochev SI, Fridovich I. The role of superoxide in the production of hydroxyl radical: In vitro and in vivo. *Free Radical Biol Med* 1994;16:29–33.

11. Winterbourn CC. Concerted antioxidant activity of glutathione and superoxide dismutase. In: Packer L, Cadenas E, eds. *Biothiols in Health and Disease*. New York: Marcel Dekker, 1995;117–134.

12. Cadenas E. Antioxidant and prooxidant functions of DT-diaphorase in quinone metabolism. *Biochem Pharmacol* 1995;49:127–140.

13. Nelson SK, Bose SK, McCord JM. The toxicity of high-dose superoxide dismutase suggests that superoxide can both initiate and terminate lipid peroxidation in the reperfused heart. *Free Radical Biol Med* 1994;16:195–200.

14. Gardner PR, Fridovich I. Superoxide dismutase sensitivity of the *Escherichia coli* aconitase. *J Biol Chem* 1991;266:19328–19333.

15. Cuo CF, Mashino T, Fridovich I. α,β-Dihydroxy isovalerate dehydratase: A superoxide-sensitive enzyme. *J Biol Chem* 1987;262:4724–4727.

16. Forman HJ, Thomas MJ. Oxidant production and bactericidal activity of phagocytes. *Annu Rev Physiol* 1986;48:669–680.

17. Omar B, McCord J, Downey J. Ischaemia-reperfusion. In: Sies H ed. *Oxidative Stress: Oxidants and Antioxidants*, London: Academic Press. 1991;493–527.

18. Gonzalez-Flecha B, Cutrin JC, Boveris A. Time course and mechanism of oxidative stress and tissue damage in rat liver subjected to in vivo ischemia reperfusion. *J Clin Invest* 1993;91:454–464.

19. McCord JM. Superoxide radical: Controversies, contradictions, and paradoxes. *Proc Soc Exp Biol Med* 1995;209:112–117.

20. Flohé L. Glutathione peroxidase brought into focus. In: Pryor WA ed. *Free Radicals in Biology*, vol V. New York: Academic Press, 1982:223–275.

21. Koppenol WH, Liebman JF. The oxidizing nature of the hydroxyl radical. A comparison with the ferryl ion (FeO^{2+}). *J Phys Chem* 1984;88:99–101.

22. Miki H, Harada K, Yamazaki I, Tamura M, Watanabe H. Electron spin resonance spectrum of Tyr-151 free radical formed in reactions of sperm whale myoglobin with ethyl hydroperoxide and potassium iridate. *Arch Biochem Biophys* 1989;275:354–362.

23. Cadenas E. Mechanisms of oxygen activation and reactive oxygen species detoxification. In: Ahmad S. ed. *Oxidative Stress and Antioxidant Defenses in Biology*. New York: Chapman & Hall, 1995:1–61.

24. Mouret JF, Odin F, Polverelli M, Cadet J. 32P-postlabeling measurement of adenine N-1 oxide in cellular DNA exposed to hydrogen peroxide. *Chem Res Toxicol* 1990;3:102–110.

25. Kalyanaraman B, Sealy RC, Sinha BK. An electron spin resonance study of the reduction of peroxides by anthracycline semiquinones. *Biochim Biophys Acta* 1984;799:270–275.

26. Sushkov DG, Gritsan NP, Weiner LM. Generation of hydroxyl radical during the enzymic reduction of 9,10-anthraquinone-2-sulfonate. Can semiquinone decompose hydrogen peroxide? *FEBS Lett* 1987;225:139–144.

27. Halliwell B, Gutterdige JMC. Role of free radicals and catalytic metal ions in human disease:an overview. *Methods Enzymol* 1990;186:1–85.

28. Goldstein S, Czapski G. The role and mechanism of metal ions and their complexes in enhancing

damage in biological systems or in protecting these systems from the toxicity of O_2^- *J Free Rad Biol Med* 1986;2:3–11.

29. Stadtman ER. Protein damage and repair. In: Davies KJA ed. *Oxidative Damage and Repair:Chemical, Biological and Medical Aspects.* New York: Pergamon Press, 1991:348–354.

30. Davies KJA. Protein damage and degradation by oxygen radicals. II. Modification of amino acids. *J Biol Chem* 1987;262:9902–9907.

31. Simpson KE, Dean RT. Simulatory and inhibitory actions of proteins and amino acids on copper-catalysed free radical generation in the bulk phase. *Free Radical Res Commun* 1990;10:303–312.

32. Dean RT, Hunt JV, Grant AJ, Yamamoto Y, Niki E. Free radical damage to proteins: The influence of the relative localization of radical generation, antioxidants, and target proteins. *Free Radical Biol Med.* 1991;11:161–168.

33. Pryor WA. Why is the hydroxyl radical the only radical that commonly adds to DNA? Hypothesis:It has a rare combination of high electrophilicity, high thermochemical reactivity, and a mode of production that can occur near DNA. *Free Radical Biol Med* 1988;4:219–223.

34. Fessenden RW, Eiben K. Electron spin resonance studies of transient radicals in aqueous solutions. *J. Phys Chem* 1971;75:1186–1201.

35. Schmidt J, Borg DC. Free radicals from purine nucleosides after hydroxyl radical attack. *Radiat Res* 1976;65:220237.

36. Kuwabara M, Ohshima H, Sato F, Ono A, Matsuda A. Spin-trapping detection of precursors of hydroxyl-radical-induced DNA damage:identification of precursor radicals of DNA strand breaks in oligo(dC)10 and oligo(dT)10. *Biochemistry* 1993;32:10599–10606.

37. Flitter WD, Mason RP. The spin trapping of pyrimidine nucleotide free radicals in a Fenton system. *Biochem J* 1989;261:831–839.

38. Bothe E, Selbach H. Rate and rate-determining step of hydrogen-atom-induced strand breakage in poly(U) in aqueous solution under anoxic conditions. *Z Naturforsch* 1985;40:247–253.

39. Steenken S. Purine bases, nucleosides and nucleotides:aqueous solution redox chemistry and transformation reactions of their radical cations and e- and OH adducts. *Chem Rev* 1989;89:503–520.

40. Floyd RA, West MS, Enff KL, Schneider JE. Methylene blue plus light mediates 8-hydroxyguanine formation in DNA. *Arch Biochem Biophys* 1989;273:106–111.

41. Devasagayam TPA, Steenken S, Obendorf MSW, Schultz WA, Sies H. Formation of 8-hydroxy(deoxy)guanosine and generation of strand breaks at guanine residues in DNA by singlet oxygen. *Biochemistry* 1991;30:6283–6289.

42. Khoda D, Tada M, Kasai H, Nishimura S, Kawazoe Y. Formation of 8-hydroxylguanine residues in cellular DNA exposed to the carcinogen 4-nitroquinoline 1-oxide. *Biochem Biophys Res Commun* 1986;139:626–632.

43. Floyd RA, Schneider JE. Hydroxyl free radical damage to DNA. In: Vigo-Pelfrey C, ed. *Membrane Lipid Oxidation*, Boca Raton, FL: CRC Press, vol. III, 1988;69–85.

44. Bryan SE, Vizard DL, Beary DA, LaBiche RA, Hardy KJ. Partitioning of zinc and copper within subnuclear nucleoprotein particles. *Nucleic Acids Res* 1981;9:5811–5823.

45. Pezzano H, Podo F. Structure of binary complexes of mono- and polynucleotides with metal ions of the first transition group. *Chem Rev* 1980;80:365–401.

46. Stoewe R, Prütz WA. Copper-catalyzed DNA damage by ascorbate and hydrogen peroxide: kinetics and yield. *Free Radical Biol Med* 1987;3:97–105.

47. Prütz WA, Butler J, Land EJ. Interaction of copper(I) with nucleic acids. *Int J Radiat Biol* 1990;58:215–234.

48. Butler J, personal communication, 1995.

49. Sagripanti JL, Kraemer KH. Site-specific oxidative DNA damage at polyguanosines produced by copper plus hydrogen peroxide. *J Biol Chem* 1989;264:1729–1734.

50. Richter C, Park JW, Ames BN. Normal oxidative damage to mitochondrial and nuclear DNA is extensive. *Proc Natl Acad Sci USA* 1988;85:6465–6467.

51. Richter C. Oxidative damage to mitochondrial DNA and its relationship to ageing. *Int J Biochem Cell Biol* 1995;27:647–653.

52. Giulivi C, Boveris A, Cadenas E. Hydroxyl radical generation during mitochondrial electron transfer and the formation of 8-hydroxydesoxyguanosine in mitochondrial DNA. *Arch Biochem Biophys* 1995;316:909–916.

53. Ames BN, Shigenaga MK, Hagen TM. Mitochondrial decay in aging. *Biochim Biophys Acta* 1995;1271:165–170.

54. Richter C, Gogvadze V, Laffranchi R, Schlapbach R, Schweizer M, Suter M, Walter P, Yaffee M. Oxidants in mitochondria:from physiology to diseases. *Biochim Biophys Acta* 1995;1271:67–74.

55. Kasai H; Nishimura S. Formation of 8-hydroxydeoxyguanosine in DNA by oxygen radicals and its biological significance. In: Sies H ed. *Oxidative Stress: Oxidants and Antioxidants*, New York: Academic Press, 1991;99–116.

56. Floyd RA. The role of 8-hydroxyguanine in carcinogenesis. *Carcinogenesis* 1990;11:1447–1450.

57. Takeuchi T, Nakajima M, Ohata Y, Mure K, Takeshita T, Morimoto K. Evaluation of 8-hydroxydeoxyguanosine, a typical oxidative DNA damage, in human leukocytes. *Carcinogenesis* 1994;15:1519–1523.

58. Floyd RA, Watson JJ, Harris J, West M, Wong PK. Formation of 8-hydroxydeoxyguanosine, hydroxyl free radical adduct of DNA in granulocytes exposed to the tumor promoter, tetradeconyl phorbolacetate. *Biochem. Biophys Res Commun* 1986;137:841–846.

59. Kiyosawa H, Suko M, Okudaira H, Murata K, Miyamoto T, Chung MH, Kasai H, Nishimura S.Cigarette smoking induces formation of 8-hydroxydeoxyguanosine, one of the oxidative DNA damages in human peripheral leukocytes. *Free Radical Res Commun* 1990;11:23–27.

60. Cahill A, Jenkins TC, Pickering P, White IN. Genotoxic effects of 3-amino-1,2,4-benzotriazine-1,4-dioxide (SR4233) and nitrogen mustard-N-oxide (nitromin) in Walker carcinoma cells under aerobic and hypoxic conditions. *Chem Biol Interact* 1995;95:97–107.

61. Kolachana P, Subrahmanyam VV, Meyer KB, Zhang L, Smith MT. Benzene and its phenolic metabolites produce oxidative DNA damage in HL60 cells in vitro and in the bone marrow in vivo. *Cancer Res* 1993;53:1023–1026.

62. Kasai H, Crain PF, Kuchino Y, Nishimura S, Ootsuyama A, Tanooka H. Formation of 8-hydroxyguanine moiety in cellular DNA by agents producing oxygen radicals and evidence for its repair. *Carcinogenesis* 1986;7:1849–1851.

63. Kasai H, Okada Y, Nishimura S, Rao MS, Reddy JK. Formation of 8-hydroxydeoxyguanosine in liver DNA of rats following long-term exposure to a peroxisome proliferator. *Cancer Res* 1989;49:2603–2605.

64. Chang J, Watson WP, Randerath E, Randerath K. Bulky DNA-adduct formation induced by Ni(II) in vitro and in vivo as assayed by 32P-postlabeling. *Mutat Res* 1993;291:147–159.

65. Faux SP, Francis JE, Smith AG, Chipman JK. Induction of 8-hydroxydeoxyguanosine in Ah-responsive mouse liver by iron and Aroclor 1254. *Carcinogenesis* 1992;13:247–250.

66. Roy D, Floyd RA, Liehr JG. Elevated 8-hydroxydeoxyguanosine levels in DNA of diethylstilbestrol-treated Syrian hamsters: Covalent DNA damage by free radicals generated by redox cycling of diethylstilbestrol. *Cancer Res* 19911;51:3882–3885.

67. Conaway CC, Nie G, Hussain NS, Fiala ES. Comparison of oxidative damage to rat liver DNA and RNA by primary nitroalkanes, secondary nitroalkanes, cyclopentanone oxime, and related compounds. *Cancer Res* 1991:51:3143–3147.

68. Denda A, Sai KM, Tang Q, Tsujiuchi T, Tsutsumi M, Amanuma T, Murata Y, Nakae D, Maruyama H, Kurokawa Y. Induction of 8-hydroxydeoxyguanosine but not initiation of carcinogenesis by redox enzyme modulations with or without menadione in rat liver. *Carcinogenesis* 1991;12:719–726.

69. Sohal RS, Agarwal A, Agarwal S, Orr WC. Simultaneous overexpression of copper- and zinc-containing superoxide dismutase and catalase retards age-related oxidative damage and increases metabolic potential in *Drosophila melanogaster. J Biol Chem* 1995;270:15671–15674.

70. Loft S, Vistisen K, Ewertz M, Tjnneland A, Overvad K, Poulsen HE. Oxidative DNA damage estimated by 8-hydroxydeoxyguanosine excretion in humans: Influence of smoking, gender, and body mass index. *Carcinogenesis* 1992:13:2241–2247.

71. Tagesson C, Kallberg M, Lintenberg C, Starkhammar H. Determination of urinary 8-hydroxydeoxyguanosine by automated coupled-column high performance liquid chromatography:a powerful technique for assaying in vivo oxidative DNA damage in cancer patients. *Eur J Cancer* 1995;31:934–940.

72. Anders MW, Dekant W, Vamvakas S. Glutathione-dependent bioactivation of xenobiotics. In: Packer L, Cadenas E, eds. *Biothiols in Health and Disease*. New York: Marcel Dekker, 1995;135–163.

73. Koob M, Dekant W. Bioactivation of xenobiotics by formation of toxic glutathione conjugates. *Chem Biol Interact* 1991;77:107–136.

74. Jocelyn EC. *Biochemistry of the SH Group. The Occurrence, Chemical Properties, Metabolism, and Biological Function of Thiols and Disulfides*. London: Academic Press, 1972;47.

75. Finley KT. The addition and substitution chemistry of quinones. In: Patai S, ed. *The Chemistry of Quinonoid Compounds*. London: John Wiley & Sons. 1974;877–1144.

76. Rossi L, Moore GA, Orrenius S, O'Brien PJ. Quinone toxicity in hepatocytes without oxidative stress. *Arch Biochem Biophys* 1986;251:25–35.
77. Brunmark A, Cadenas E. 1,4-Reductive addition of glutathione to quinone epoxides. Mechanistic studies with h.p.l.c. with electrochemical detection under aerobic and anaerobic conditions and evaluation of chemical reactivity in terms of autoxidation reactions. *Free Radical Biol Med* 1989;6:149–165.
78. Wilson I, Wardman P, Tai-Shun L, Sartorelli AC. Reactivity of thiols toward derivatives of 2- and 6-methyl-1,4-naphthoquinone bioreductive alkylating agents. *Chem Biol Interact* 1987;61:229–240.
79. Nickerson WJ, Falcone G, Strauss G. Studies on quinone-thioethers. I. Mechanism of formation and properties of thiodione. *Biochemistry* 1963;2:537–543.
80. Brunmark A, Cadenas E. Biological implications of the nucleophilic addition of glutathione to quinoid compounds. In: Viña J, ed. *Glutathione Metabolism and Physiological Functions.* Boca Raton, FL: CRC Press, 1990;279–294.
81. Buffinton GD, Öllinger K, Brunmark A, Cadenas E. DT-diaphorase-catalyzed reduction of 1,4-naphthoquinone derivatives and glutathionyl-quinone conjugates. Effect of substituents on autoxidation rates. *Biochem J* 1989;257:561–571.
82. Brown ER, Finley KT, Reeves RL. Steric effects of vicinal substituents on redox equilibria in quinonoid compounds. *J Org Chem* 1971;36:2849–2853.
83. Nagakawa Y, Hiraga K, Suga T. On the mechanism of covalent binding of butylated hydroxytoluene to microsomal protein. *Biochem Pharmacol* 1983;32:1417–1421.
84. Peter MG. Chemical modifications of biopolymers by quinones and quinone methides. *Angew Chem* 1989;28:555–570
85. Giulivi C, Cadenas E. One- and two-electron reduction of 2-methyl-1,4-naphthoquinone bioreductive alkylating agents: Kinetic studies, free-radical production, thiol oxidation and DNA strand break formation. *Biochem J* 1994;301:21–30.
86. Novak M, Pelecanou M, Pollack L. Hydrolysis of the model carcinogen *N*-(pivaloyloxy-4-methoxy-acetanilide: Involvement of *N*-acetyl-β-benzoquinone imine. *J Am Chem Soc* 1986;108:112–120.
87. Coles B, Wilson I, Wardman P, Hinson JA, Nelson SD, Ketterer B. The spontaneous and enzymatic reaction of *N*-acetyl-*p*-benzoquinoneimine with glutathione: A stopped-flow kinetic study. *Arch Biochem Biophys* 1988;264:253–260.
88. Goin J, Giulivi C, Butler J, Cadenas E. Enzymic- and thiol-mediated activation of halogen-substituted diaziridinylbenzoquinones: Redox transitions of the semiquinone and semiquinone-thioether species. *Free Radical Biol Med* 1995;18:525–536.
89. Lusthof KJ, de Mol NJ, Jansen LHM, Prins B, Verboom W, Reinhoudt DN. Interactions between potential antitumour 2,5-bis(1-aziridinyl)-1,4-benzoquinone derivatives and glutathione: Reductive activation, conjugation and DNA damage. *Anti-Cancer Drug Design* 1990;5:283–290.
90. Silverman RB. Chemical model studies for the mechanism of vitamin K epoxide reductase. *J Am Chem Soc* 1981;103:5939–5941.
91. Lin J, Cosby LA, Shansky CW and Sartorelli AC. Potential bioreductive alkylating agents. I. Benzoquinone derivatives. *J Med Chem* 1972;15:1247–1248.
92. Goin J, Gibson DD, McCay PB, Cadenas E. Glutathionyl- and hydroxyl radical formation coupled to the redox transitions of 1,4-naphthoquinone bioreductive alkylating agents during glutathione two- electron reductive addition. *Arch Biochem Biophys* 1991;288:386–396.
93. Monks TJ, Highet RJ, Lau SS. Oxidative cyclization, 1,4-benzothiazine formation and dimerization of 2-bromo-3-glutathion-*S*-yl)hydroquinone. *Mol Pharmacol* 1990;38:121–127.
94. Öllinger K, Buffinton G, Ernster L, Cadenas E. Effect of superoxide dismutase on the autoxidation of hydro- and semi-naphthoquinones. *Chem Biol Interact* 1990;73:53–76.
95. Ordoñez ID, Cadenas E. Thiol oxidation coupled to DT-diaphorase-catalysed reduction of diaziquone: Reductive and oxidative pathways of diaziquone semiquinone modulated by glutathione and superoxide dismutase. *Biochem J* 1992;286:481–490.
96. Wardman P. Conjugation and oxidation of glutathione via thiyl free radicals. In: Sies H, Ketterer B, eds. *Glutathione Conjugation. Mechanisms and Biological Significance.* London: Academic Press, 1988;4472.
97. Wilson I, Wardman P, Cohen GM, d'Arcy Doherty M. Reductive role of glutathione in the redox cycling of oxidizable drugs. *Biochem Pharmacol* 1986;35:21–22.
98. Wardman P. Reactions of thiyl radicals. In: Packer L, Cadenas E, eds., *Biothiols in Health and Disease,* New York: Marcel Dekker, 1995;1–19.

99. Butler J, Hoey BM. Reactions of glutathione and glutathione radicals with benzoquinones. *Free Radical Biol Med* 1992;12:337–345.
100. Schöneich C. Thiyl radicals, perthiyl radicals, and oxidative reactions. In: Packer L, Cadenas E, eds., *Biothiols in Health and Disease*, New York: Marcel Dekker, 1995:21–47.
101. D'Aquino M, Dunster C, Willson RL. Vitamin A and glutathione-mediated free radical damage:competing reactions with polyunsaturated fatty acids and vitamin C. *Biochem Biophys Res Commun* 1989;161:1199–1203.
102. Meister A. Mitochondrial changes associated with glutathione deficiency. *Biochim Biophys Acta* 1995;1271:35–42.
103. Devasagayam TPA, DiMascio P, Kaiser S, Sies H. Singlet oxygen induced single-strand breaks in plasmid pBR322 DNA: The enhancing effect of thiols. *Biochim Biophys Acta* 1991;1088:409–412.
104. Willson RL. Free radical repair mechanisms and the interactions of glutathione and vitamins C and E. In: Nygaard OF, Simic MG, eds. *Radioprotectors and Anticarcinogens*. New York: Academic Press, 1993:1–22.
105. Held KD, Harrop HA, Michael BD. Effect of oxygen and sulphydryl-containing compounds on irradiated transforming DNA. II. Glutathione, cysteine and cysteamine. *Int J Radiat Biol* 1984;45:615–626.
106. Greenstock CL, Dunlop I. In: Adams GE, Fielden EM, and Michael BD, eds. *Fast Processes in Radiation Chemistry and Biology*. New York: John Wiley & Sons, 1975:247–258.
107. Spear N, Aust SD. Hydroxylation of deoxyguanosine in DNA by copper and thiols. *Arch Biochem Biophys* 1995;317:142–146.
108. Augusto O. Alkylation and cleavage of DNA by carbon-centered radical metabolites. *Free Radical Biol Med* 1993;15:329–336.
109. Steinmaus H, Rosenthal I, Elad D. Light- and γ-ray-induced reactions of purines and purine nucleosides with alcohols. *J Org Chem* 1971;36:3594–3598.
110. Zady MF, Wong JL. Kinetics and mechanism of carbon-8-methylation of purine bases and nucleosides by methyl radical. *J Am Chem Soc* 1977:5096–6002.
111. Pryor WA, Fuller DL, Stanley JP. Reactivity patterns of the methyl radical. *J Am Chem Soc* 1972;94:1632–1638.
112. Netto LES, Ferreira AMC, Augusto O. Iron(III) binding in DNA solutions: Complex formation and catalytic activity in the oxidation of hydrazine derivatives. *Chem Biol Interact* 1991;79:1–14.
113. Maeda M; Nushi K, Kawazoe Y. Studies on chemical alterations of nucleic acid and their components—VII. C-Alkylation of purine bases through a free radical process catalyzed by ferrous ion. *Tetrahedron* 1974;30:2677–2682.
114. Humphreys WG, Kadlubar FF, Guengerich FP. Mechanism of C^8 alkylation of guanine residues by activated arylamines. Evidence for initial adduct formation at the N7 position. *Proc Natl Acad Sci USA* 1992;89:8278–8282.
115. Augusto O, Faljoni-Alario A, Leite LCC, Nobrega FG. DNA strand scission by the carbon radical derived from 2-phenylhydrazine metabolism. *Carcinogenesis* 1984;5:781–784.
116. Leite LCC, Augusto O. DNA alterations induced by the carbon-centered radical derived from the oxidation of 2-phenylhydrazine. *Arch Biochem Biophys* 1989;270:560–572.
117. Kato T, Kojima K, Hiramoto K, Kikugawa K. DNA strand breakage by hydroxyphenyl radicals generated from mutagenic diazoquinone compounds. *Mutat Res* 1992;268:105–114.
118. Kikugawa K, Kato T, Kojima K. Substitution of *p*- and *o*-hydroxyphenyl radicals at the 8 position of purine nucleosidkes by reaction with mutagenic *p*- and *o*-diazoquinones. *Mutation Res* 1992;268:65–75.
119. Leite LCC, Netto LES, Augusto O. In vitro activation of 1,2-methylhydrazine to methyl radicals and interaction with plasmid DNA. In: Hayaishi O, Niki E, Kondo M, Yoshikawa T, eds. *Medical Biochemical and Chemical Aspects of Free Radicals*. Amsterdam: Elsevier, 1989;1521–1524.
120. Netto LES, Ramakrishna NVS, Kolar C, Cavalieri EL, Rogan EG, Lawson TA, Augusto O. Identification of C^8-methylguanine in the hydrolysates of DNA from rats administered 1,2-dimethylhydrazine. Evidence for in vivo DNA alkylation by methyl radicals. *J Biol Chem* 1992;267:21524–21527.
121. Augusto O, Cavalieri EL, Rogan EG, Ramakrishna NVS, Kolar C. Formation of 8-methylguanine as a result of DNA alkylation by methyl radicals generated during horseradish peroxidase-catalyzed oxidation of methylhydrazine. *J Biol Chem* 1990;265:22093–22096.
122. Wood ML, Dizdaroglu M, Gajewski E, Essigmann JM. Mechanistic studies of ionizing irradiation

and oxidative mutagenesis:genetic effects of a single 8-hydroxyguanine (8-oxoguanine) residue inserted at a unique site in a viral genome. *Biochemistry* 1990;29:7024–7032.

123. Moriya M. Single-stranded shuttle phagemid for mutagenesis studies in mammalian cells: 8-Oxoguanine in DNA induces targeted G-C → T-A transversions in simian kidney cells. *Proc Natl Acad Sci USA* 1993;90:1122–1126.

124. Kuchino Y, Mori F, Kasai H, Inoue H, Iwai S, Miura K, Khtsuka E, Nishimura S. Misreading of DNA templates containing 8-hydroxydeoxyguanosine at the modified base and at adjacent residues. *Nature* 1987;327:77–79.

125. Asmus KD. Sulfur-centered radicals. *Methods Enzymol* 1990;186:168–180.

126. DeGray JA, Mason RP. Biothiyls: Free radical chemistry and biological significance. In: Packer L, Cadenas E, eds. *Biothiols in Health and Disease*. New York: Marcel Dekker, 1995;63–81.

127. Everett SA. Antioxidant drug design: A comparison of thiol and perthiol antiradical and prooxidant reaction mechanisms. In: Packer L, Cadenas E, eds. *Biothiols in Health and Disease*. New York: Marcel Dekker, 1995;49–64.

128. Cadenas E. Thiyl radical formation during thiol oxidation by ferrylmyoglobin. *Methods Enzymol* 1995;251:106–116.

129. Carter MH, Josephy PD. Mutagenicity of thionitrites in the Ames test. The biological activity of thiyl radicals. *Biochem Pharmacol* 1986;35:3847–3851.

130. Schöneich C, Bonifacic M, Asmus KD. Reversible H-atom abstraction from alcohols by thiyl radicals: Determination of absolute rate constants by pulse radiolysis. *Free Radical Res Commun* 1989;6:393–405.

131. Schöneich C, Asmus KD. Determination of absolute rate constants for the reversible hydrogen-atom transfer between thiyl radicals and alcohols or ethers. *J Chem Soc Faraday Trans* 1995;91:1923–1930.

132. Kim K, Kim IH, Lee KY, Rhee SG, Stadtman ER. The isolation and purification of a specific "protector" protein which inhibits enzyme inactivation by a thiol/Fe(III)/O2 mixed-function-oxidation system. *J Biol Chem* 1988;263:4704–4711.

133. Floyd RA, Watson JJ, Wong PK, Altmiller DH, Rickard RC. Hydroxyl free radical adduct of deoxyguanosine:sensitive detection and mechanisms of formation. *Free Radical Res Commun* 1986;1:163–172.

134. Gajewski E, Rao G, Nackerdien Z, Dizdaroglu M. Modification of DNA bases in mammalian chromatin by radiation-generated free radicals. *Biochemistry* 1990;29:7876–7882.

135. Tchou J, Grollman AP. Repair of DNA containing the oxidatively damaged base 8-oxoguanine. *Mutat Res* 1993;299:277–287.

136. Inoue S, Kawanishi S. Oxidative DNA damage induced by simultaneous generation of nitric oxide and superoxide. *FEBS Letts* 1995;371:86–88.

137. Sies H. Damage to plasmid DNA by singlet oxygen and its protection. *Mutat Res* 1993;299:183–191.

Free Radical Toxicology
Edited by K. B. Wallace
Copyright © 1997 Taylor & Francis

8

Free-Radical Defense and Repair Mechanisms

Daniel C. Liebler

Department of Pharmacology and Toxicology, University of Arizona, College of Pharmacy, Tucson, Arizona, USA

Donald J. Reed

Department of Biochemistry and Biophysics, Oregon State University, Corvallis, Oregon, USA

INTRODUCTION

Defense and repair systems are critical modulators of cellular oxidative damage. In this chapter, we discuss the functions and interplay of antioxidants and antioxidant enzymes and emphasize the complementary nature of these systems. To explain the need for such diverse antioxidant defense and repair systems, we describe pertinent aspects of the formation and chemistry of biologically relevant oxidants. We also discuss some aspects of free-radical toxicity that is associated with biotransformation of various chemicals. In doing so, we emphasize those oxidants against which cellular antioxidant defense is directed and perhaps account for Nature's selection of specific antioxidant defenses. Detailed discussions of the formation and chemistry of reactive oxidants are presented elsewhere in this volume.

The continual formation of reactive oxygen species is a physiological necessity and an unavoidable consequence of oxygen metabolism. However, when generated in excess, they can be toxic, particularly in the presence of transition metal ions such as iron or copper (elsewhere in this volume); for a review see Halliwell and Gutteridge (1). Since defense systems are present and functioning under normal conditions, endogenous free radicals do not necessarily place biological tissues and cells at risk. However, these defense systems can be overwhelmed during various pathological conditions caused by xenobiotics, anoxia, radiation, and loss of extracellular calcium. Excess generation of free radicals within tissues can cause damage to vital cellular constituents.

It is estimated that nearly 90% of the total O_2 consumed by mammalian species is delivered to mitochondria, where a four-electron reduction to H_2O by the respiratory chain is coupled to ATP synthesis (2,3). Nearly 4% of mitochondrial O_2 is incompletely reduced by leakage of electrons along the respiratory chain, especially at ubiquinone, forming ROS such as superoxide (O_2^-), hydrogen peroxide (H_2O_2), singlet oxygen, and hydroxyl radical (HO·) (2,3). Richter (4) calculated that during normal metabolism, one rat liver mitochondrion produces 3×10^7 superoxide radicals per day. It is estimated that superoxide and hydrogen peroxide steady state concentrations are in the picomolar and nanomolar range, respectively (5). Jones et al. (6) have estimated the hepatocyte steady state H_2O_2 concentration to be up to 25 μM. These events are thought to contribute over 85% of the free-radical production in mammalian species. Sohal (7) has concluded that there is a variation in the sites of superoxide or hydrogen peroxide generation among mitochondria from different tissues and species. This is a result of the rate of mitochondrial superoxide production is dependent on at least three variables: (1) ambient oxygen concentration; (2) levels of autoxidizable respiratory carriers, especially ubiquinone; and (3) the redox state of the autoxidizable carriers (2,5,7–9).

Toxic chemicals can cause oxidant formation through several mechanisms. In some instances, metabolism drives the formation of oxygen-containing reactive intermediates through a process known as redox cycling. Many other chemicals can also undergo bioactivation to form biological reactive intermediates that bind to macromolecules and indirectly enhance the formation of oxygen radicals. Some chemicals induce inflammatory responses, in which release of reactive oxygen and nitrogen radicals by stimulated phagocytes constitutes an oxidative challenge. Still other chemicals undergo facile photoexcitation reactions that lead to the formation of either singlet oxygen, free radicals, or both. Oxidant generation through any of these scenarios may lead to the oxidation of critical functional groups on macromolecules, to peroxidation of lipids, and to oxidation of other susceptible cellular constituents.

The evolution of bioactivation processes that form biological reactive intermediates, both free radical and ionic, probably necessitated the concomitant evolution of cellular defense and repair systems for cell survival. All tissues and cells contain defense systems for detoxification of biological reactive intermediates and to prevent or limit cellular damage. Toxic processes have reversible and irreversible features that are a consequence of the interplay with cellular defense and repair systems. Reversible toxicity occurs even with chemicals known as "safe" chemicals. Dose determines whether any chemical causes irreversible toxicity. Irreversible toxicity may cause cell death regardless of what antidotal or preventive measures are taken after exposure of cell or tissues to a sufficient dose of the toxic chemical. Death occurs when loss of cellular integrity occurs to such a degree that free exchange between the intracellular constituents and the surrounding milieu prevents cell survival. We review here the mechanisms by which cells are protected by defense and repair systems to prevent or limit cellular damage and death.

THE INITIATION AND PROPAGATION OF OXIDATIVE DAMAGE

In this section we describe general characteristics of the origin of free radicals and related oxidants. Rather than provide a comprehensive documentation of the sources of oxidants, we focus on how the common primordial oxidants superoxide and nitric oxide lead to the formation of a number of more reactive oxidants. We also distinguish between the initiation and propagation of oxidative damage and consider the roles of these processes in oxidative injury. This establishes a framework for describing the interlocking, complementary nature of cellular antioxidant defense.

Superoxide, Nitric Oxide, and Transition Metals as Primordial Oxidant Sources

Major contributors to oxidative injury are (1) xenobiotics or endogenous factors that can cause increased superoxide generation, (2) factors that stimulate the production of nitric oxide, and (3) processes that disrupt heme proteins or other metalloproteins to enhance the contribution of transition metals to oxidant generation. Increased superoxide generation can result from agents that stimulate phagocytic cells including polymorphonuclear leukocytes and macrophages, which generate large quantities of superoxide as a mechanism for destruction of foreign cells. Free-radical generation by neutrophils can be as high as 200 nmol/10^6 cells/h (10,11). It is known that an NADPH oxidase provides the catalysis for the rapid consumption of molecular oxygen (12,13). Even nonphagocytic cells can be stimulated by agents such as phorbol esters to increase superoxide production through the conversion of xanthine dehydrogenase to xanthine oxidase (14). Chemicals also can induce superoxide formation by catalyzing electron transfer from cellular redox proteins to molecular oxygen (redox cycling), as discussed elsewhere in this volume.

Many of the same stimuli that induce macrophages to produce superoxide also stimulate the production of nitric oxide by inducible nitric oxide synthetase (see Morris and Billiar, 15, for a recent review). Nitric oxide produced in relatively high yield by these inducible enzymes may react with oxygen or superoxide to yield more reactive oxidants, as described later. Finally, oxidants, nonoxidizing reactive intermediates, and other mediators of cellular injury may disrupt hemoproteins and other metalloproteins to release transition metal ions, particularly iron and copper, which may amplify damage by catalyzing the formation of highly reactive radicals. Reactions of superoxide, nitric oxide, and metals lead to oxidative injury by forming secondary oxidants that are believed to be responsible for actually causing most biological oxidative damage. These reactions and some of their intermediates are key control points in the initiation and propagation of oxidative damage. These critical reactions and intermediates also are often the targets of antioxidant defense.

Reactions of Superoxide, Nitric Oxide, and Metals: Formation
of Secondary Oxidants

Superoxide is itself a reasonably strong oxidant ($E^{\circ\prime} = 940$ mV at pH 7) (16), but most of its pro-oxidant chemistry is thought to be due to formation of its conjugate acid HOO· (pK_a 4.9), which may initiate lipid peroxidation by hydrogen abstraction from hydroperoxides. Superoxide decomposition gives rise to even more reactive oxidants. Enzyme-catalyzed and nonenzymatic dismutation yield hydrogen peroxide, a nonradical pro-oxidant that may freely diffuse across membranes. Metal-catalyzed cleavage of hydrogen peroxide (the Fenton reaction) forms hydroxyl radical or similarly reactive high-valent metal-oxo complexes, which are the most reactive oxidants known in biological systems (Koppenol, chapter 1, this volume).

Superoxide also may react at diffusion limited rates with nitric oxide to form the highly reactive nonradical peroxynitrite (17). Peroxynitrite is an excellent oxidant for biological thiols, and its conjugate acid peroxynitrous acid forms a reactive oxidant with reactivity similar to hydroxyl radical (18). In addition to its reaction with superoxide, nitric oxide also may autoxidize to nitrogen dioxide, which is a highly reactive initiator of free-radical reactions (19).

Transition metal ions may greatly enhance oxidative damage in two general ways. First, they may reductively cleave hydrogen peroxide and alkyl hydroperoxides to hydroxyl and alkoxyl radicals, respectively (i.e., the Fenton reaction, reviewed by Koppenol, chapter 1, this volume). The extent to which this reaction occurs in vivo depends on the availability of metal ions. However, in all but the most stringently demetalized experimental systems, metal-catalyzed cleavage of lipid hydroperoxides probably is the driving force for most lipid peroxidation studied in vitro (20–22). Metal-catalyzed cleavage of lipid hydroperoxides greatly amplifies lipid peroxidation, and analogous reactions may contribute significantly to the autoxidation of proteins and DNA as well. Metals also may directly oxidize thiols to thiyl radicals, which may add oxygen to form more highly oxidizing intermediates (reviewed in refs. 16 and 23). The reduced forms of the metal ions formed by these reactions may participate in Fenton chemistry as described earlier.

Formation and Reactions of Peroxyl Radicals: Propagation
of Oxidative Damage

The reactive intermediates discussed earlier all contribute to oxidative damage either by direct reaction with oxidizable biomolecules (hydroxyl radical, alkoxyl radical, peroxynitrite, hydroperoxyl radical, nitrogen dioxide) or by serving as immediate precursors to radicals (hydrogen peroxide, organic hydroperoxides, peroxynitrous acid). The radical species react with lipids, proteins, DNA or other biomolecules either by addition, hydrogen abstraction, or electron transfer to form (primarily) biomolecule-derived, carbon-centered radicals. In aerobic environments, these carbon centered radicals reversibly add oxygen to form peroxyl radicals, which then react with adjacent biomolecules:

$$R^. + O_2 \leftrightarrow ROO^. \qquad\qquad [1]$$

$$ROO^. + R'H \leftrightarrow ROOH + R'^. \qquad\qquad [2]$$

This process is termed *propagation* and is normally considered in terms of lipid peroxidation (see Sevanian and McLeod, chapter 4, this volume). However, the same sequence of reactions also can contribute to the spread of oxidative damage in proteins, DNA, and other biomolecules. A free-radical chain initiated by a single hydroxyl radical in a lipid membrane thus may lead to over 20 propagation cycles before the chain is terminated (24). All of the other radicals discussed earlier can initiate radical chains, which then are propagated in the same manner. It is not surprising in this context that peroxyl radical propagation reactions can contribute the bulk of oxidative damage regardless of the specific initiating oxidants involved.

THE ORGANIZATION OF ANTIOXIDANT DEFENSE

Cellular antioxidant defenses are organized into several tiers against oxidant challenges. The juxtaposition of oxidant challenge and antioxidant defense is illustrated in Figure 1. For clarity, we have greatly simplified the highly complex chemistry involved in the initiation and propagation of oxidative damage. Key elements of oxidative challenges are described earlier and depicted in Figure 1. These include (1) the formation of primordial radicals superoxide and nitric oxide, (2) the generation of highly reactive secondary intermediates (e.g., hydroxyl and hydroperoxyl radical, peroxynitrite), which may initiate free-radical chain reactions, and (3) amplification by peroxyl radical dependent chain propagation. Another key element of oxidant challenge is the role of transition metals both in forming highly reactive secondary intermediates (e.g., Fenton chemistry) and in amplifying the propagation of oxidative damage.

Antioxidant defenses are directed against several aspects of the oxidant challenge. A general observation is that the enzyme-mediated antioxidant defenses are directed against the primordial initiator superoxide and the less reactive secondary mediators hydrogen peroxide and organic hydroperoxides. Small-molecule chain-breaking antioxidants are instead directed primarily against peroxyl radicals involved in radical propagation. Cellular antioxidant defenses thus serve complementary functions within the context of a multitiered oxidant challenge. Characteristics of the individual components of cellular antioxidant defense are described later. More extensive discussion of the antioxidant roles of glutathione, vitamin E, and ascorbate is provided in succeeding sections.

Superoxide Dismutases, Catalase and Glutathione Peroxidases

Superoxide dismutases (SOD) catalyze the dismutation of superoxide to oxygen and hydrogen peroxide. A major protective benefit is derived from enzymatic

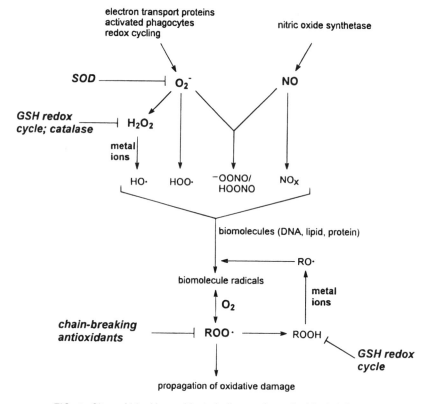

FIG. 1. Sites of blocking oxidant challenges by antioxidant defenses.

catalysis, since the nonenzymatic rate is approximately four orders of magnitude smaller at pH 7.4 (25). Mammalian SOD enzymes include a homodimeric Cu,ZnSOD in the cytosol and a homotetrameric MnSOD in mitochondria (26). Extracellular fluids contain a tetrameric, glycosylated form of the Cu,Zn enzyme (27). The mitochondrial MnSOD is highly inducible by cytokines such as tumor necrosis factor (28) and by mediators of acute oxidative stress, such as superoxide or hydrogen peroxide (29). Catalase is a hemoprotein found in peroxisomes of eukaryotic cells and catalyzes the conversion of hydrogen peroxide to water and oxygen. This enzyme also can be induced in response to cellular hydrogen peroxide exposure (29).

Glutathione peroxidases are selenoproteins found in essentially all tissues. Four isozymes of with glutathione peroxidase activity have been characterized: (a) the classical cellular glutathione peroxidase, GSHPx-1, (b) the phospholipid hydroperoxide glutathione peroxidase, GSHPX, (c) the plasma glutathione peroxidase, GSHPx-P, and (d) GSHPx-GI (30).

The best known of these, glutathione peroxidase, is a homotetramer consisting of 22-kD subunits, each with one selenocysteine residue (31). The enzyme is found in cytosol and mitochondria and reduces hydrogen peroxide and some organic hydroperoxides to water and alcohols, respectively. A similar enzyme found in extracellular fluids and in plasma shares sequence homology with the intracellular enzyme, but is a separate gene product (32). Another enzyme, phospholipid hydroperoxide glutathione peroxidase, is a monomeric protein containing one selenocysteine (33). This enzyme reduces phospholipid hydroperoxides to the corresponding alcohols.

Ursini et al. (33) has purified and characterized an interfacial glutathione peroxidase. This enzyme has been shown to reduce linoleic acid hydroperoxides, cumene hydroperoxide, *tert*-butyl hydroperoxide, and hydrogen peroxide. However, this enzyme, which does not conjugate CDNB with GSH (34), displays glutathione peroxidase activity toward cumene hydroperoxide, hydrogen peroxide, and lipid hydroperoxides and is distinct from the classical glutathione peroxidase (35). Evidence suggests that the enzyme is interfacial in character and can interact directly with liposomes to reduce phospholipid hydroperoxides (33). The addition of this protein to microsomal incubation mixtures inhibited lipid peroxidation (34). Substrate specificities indicate that this enzyme is distinct from the nuclear glutathione transferase (36). In addition to the selenium-dependent glutathione peroxidases, a related extracellular selenoprotein, selenoprotein-P, is found in plasma and in extracellular fluids (37). This monomeric 41 kD glycoprotein contains 10 selenocysteines, and enzyme levels are highly sensitive to changes in dietary selenium status. Although a specific antioxidant activity has not been established for this protein, it is postulated to exert antioxidant effects (37). The soluble intracellular form of Se-glutathione peroxidase is generally regarded as an indispensable defense against hydrogen peroxide (31). Reduction of phospholipid hydroperoxides by phospholipid hydroperoxide glutathione peroxidase, together with peroxyl radical scavenging by vitamin E (discussed later), is thought to constitute a highly efficient defense against membrane lipid peroxidation (38). Weitzel and Wendel (39) have reported findings that phospholipid hydroperoxide-glutathione peroxidase activity regulates the activity of 5-lipoxygenase via regulating the tone of endogenous hydroperoxides. Nevertheless, the relative importance of these different selenoproteins in antioxidant protection remains poorly understood. Awad et al. (40) recently reported that severe dietary selenium deficiency reduced glutathione peroxidase activity to less than 2% of control values without increasing hepatic lipid peroxidation, whereas vitamin E deficiency did increase lipid peroxidation. In another experiment, diquat toxicity in chronically selenium deficient rats was reduced by pretreatment with selenium 12 h prior to diquat exposure. However, the selenium pretreatments did not affect either selenium glutathione peroxidase or phospholipid hydroperoxide glutathione peroxidase, but instead increased plasma levels of selenoprotein-P. A better understanding of the antioxidant role of selenium awaits a clarification of the true function of selenoprotein-P and extracellular selenium glutathione peroxidase and of their interplay with intracellular glutathione peroxidases.

Michiels et al. (41) have reviewed the importance of the defense enzymes Se-glutathione peroxidase, catalase, and Cu,Zn-SOD for cell survival against oxidative stress. From the evidence, they suggest that each enzyme has a specific as well as an irreplaceable function. In part, roles of the enzymes were assessed with the aid of specific enzyme inhibitors including aminotriazole (42) for catalase, diethyldithiocarbamate (43) for Cu,Zn-SOD, mercaptosuccinate (44) for glutathione peroxidase, 1,3-bis(2-chloroethyl)-1-nitrosourea (BCNU) (45) for glutathione reductase, and buthionine sulfoximine (BSO) (46) for GSH synthesis. In transfection studies in which overexpression of a specific enzyme is studied, the physiological responses indicate that the metabolism of reactive oxygen species may have a critical balance. For example, Mn-SOD-transfected mouse cells overexpressing SOD activity were found to be more resistant to hyperoxia (47) and paraquat (47,48). However, Cu,Zn-SOD-enriched bacteria displayed increased sensitivity to hyperoxia (49) and paraquat (50). Warner (51) concurs that SOD has an important role in defense against degenerative disease, but much remains to be understood concerning effects of manipulation of SOD expression as an intervention. Transfection experiments could therefore cause increased or decreased toxicity depending on relative concentrations of hydrogen peroxide and superoxide. In addition, iron (or copper) has the potential for a major influence by being optimized in its redox ratio (Fe^{2+}/Fe^{3+}) and involving various constituents for increasing the reactivity of hydrogen peroxide. Luo et al. (52) have proposed that hydrogen peroxide toxicity is associated with three chemically distinct types of oxidants formed by iron-mediated Fenton reactions in the presence of DNA.

Small-Molecule Antioxidants

Numerous small molecules (<1000 MW) with high reactivity toward oxidants have been described. Three of these, vitamin E, ascorbic acid, and glutathione, play essential antioxidant roles in tissues and in extracellular fluids. The functions of these are discussed in detail next. Numerous other molecules, including carotenoids (53,54), dihydrolipoic acid (55), flavonoids (56), plant polyphenols (57), and ubiquinol (58,59), exert antioxidant effects in vitro and may assume important antioxidant roles in vivo under conditions of increased dietary intake or pharmacological supplementation. Some products of intermediary metabolism, such as bilirubin (60) and uric acid (61), that are toxic at high levels may nevertheless exert antioxidant effects in some tissue microenvironments. Many drugs and other chemicals have been shown to have antioxidant properties in vitro and may also contribute to antioxidant defense under certain circumstances.

In contrast to antioxidant enzymes, which scavenge superoxide and hydrogen peroxide, small molecule antioxidants act for the most part as scavengers of secondary oxidants and inhibitors of radical chain propagation. Such molecules may be classified as *chain-breaking antioxidants*, which are defined as compounds that act by trapping peroxyl radicals. As discussed earlier, peroxyl radicals are the principal chain-propagating species encountered in oxidant challenges and probably the most common ultimate mediators of oxidative damage. Chain breaking antioxidants typically function in a two-step sequence in which the antioxidant traps one peroxyl radical to form an antioxidant-derived radical [Eq. (3)], which then traps a second radical to form nonradical products [Eq. (4)].

$$ROO^{\cdot} + AH \rightarrow ROOH + A^{\cdot} \qquad [3]$$

$$ROO^{\cdot} + A^{\cdot} \rightarrow \text{nonradical products} \qquad [4]$$

Each reaction terminates a radical chain and thus may prevent as many as 20 or more subsequent oxidations. Chain-breaking antioxidants can be effective at relatively low concentrations. For example, membranes typically contain about 1 α-tocopherol per 1000 phospholipids (62,63).

Because small-molecule antioxidants are known to react at high rates with many oxidants (hydroxyl radicals, peroxynitrite, alkoxyl radicals, peroxyl radicals), it perhaps seems surprising that these compounds should act primarily as chain-breaking antioxidants. The apparent specificity of most small-molecule antioxidants for reaction with peroxyl radicals as opposed to other radicals (e.g., hydroxyl radical) is due largely to kinetics. Peroxyl radicals react at relatively slow rates with many biomolecules (e.g., $k \sim 10^2 \, M^{-1} \, s^{-1}$ for linoleic acid (64), but at much higher rates with antioxidants (e.g., $k \sim 10^5\text{-}10^6 \, M^{-1} \, s^{-1}$ for α-tocopherol, depending on the reaction medium (65). Reaction of peroxyl radicals with the antioxidant is kinetically favored, even though the concentration of oxidizable lipid greatly exceeds that of the antioxidant. In contrast, hydroxyl radicals react with most biomolecules and antioxidants at near the diffusion controlled rate [$k \sim 10^9 \, M^{-1} \, s^{-1}$ (66,67)], so there is no kinetic preference for reaction with the antioxidant. Indeed, since other biomolecules outnumber antioxidant molecules, quenching of hydroxyl radicals would occur infrequently. The antioxidant instead would be much more likely to trap peroxyl radicals formed subsequent to initial hydroxyl radical attack. In view of these considerations, the frequently used term "hydroxyl radical scavenger" is probably a misnomer, at least in reference to actions in vivo. Only when relatively high concentrations of scavenger are employed in vitro would effective scavenging of hydroxyl radicals occur.

Small molecule antioxidants react with radicals by a variety of mechanisms [Eqs. (5–10)]. Phenolic antioxidants such as α-tocopherol and thiols such as glutathione usually quench radicals by hydrogen atom transfer (although the reaction also may occur by rapid electron transfer followed by proton transfer) [Eqs. (5) and (6)] (23,68).

$$TH + R^{\cdot} \rightarrow T^{\cdot} + RH \qquad [5]$$

$$GSH + R^{\cdot} \rightarrow GS^{\cdot} + RH \qquad [6]$$

The water soluble antioxidants ascorbate and urate instead react by electron transfer [Eqs. (7) and (8)] (16,61).

$$AH^{\cdot} + R^{\cdot} \rightarrow AH^{\cdot} + R^{\cdot} \qquad [7]$$

$$UH^{\cdot} + R^{\cdot} \rightarrow UH^{\cdot} + R^{\cdot} \qquad [8]$$

Carotenoids react by a combination of electron transfer and radical addition to the carotenoid polyene system [Eqs. (9) and (10)] (69,70).

$$CAR + R^{\cdot} \rightarrow CAR^{+\cdot} + R^{\cdot} \qquad [9]$$

$$CAR + R^{\cdot} \rightarrow R-CAR^{\cdot} \qquad [10]$$

The radical intermediates generated by all these reactions may react with additional radicals in radical-radical termination reactions (e.g., reaction 4) or may undergo disproportionation or reductive "repair" reactions. These reactions of α-tocopherol, glutathione, and ascorbate and their radical intermediates are considered in detail in the following sections.

CELLULAR GLUTATHIONE AND OTHER THIOLS AS DEFENSE AND REPAIR AGENTS

Depending on the cell type, the intracellular concentration of glutathione is maintained in the range of 0.5–10 mM (71). Concentrations in the liver are 4–8 mM. Because of the redox status of glutathione that is maintained by intracellular glutathione reductase and NADPH, nearly all the glutathione is present as reduced glutathione (GSH) with less than 5% of the total is present as glutathione disulfide (GSSG). Constant production of GSSG is a result of continual endogenous production of superoxide from oxygen leading to the formation of hydrogen peroxide and lipid hydroperoxides. The GSH content of various organs and tissues represents at least 90% of the total nonprotein, low-molecular-weight thiols. The GSH content of liver is nearly twice that found in kidney and testes and over threefold greater than in the lung. The importance of hepatic GSH for protection against free radicals has been reviewed extensively (72–75).

The cystathionine pathway is of major importance to pathways of free-radical generation that can cause loss of GSH. Depletion of GSH by rapid conjugation can increase synthesis of GSH to rates as high as 2–3 μmol/h/g wet liver tissue (76). The cysteine pool in the liver, which is about 0.2 μmol/g, has an estimated half-life of 2–3 min at such high rates of synthesis of GSH (72). Although the cystathionine pathway appears to be highly responsive to the need for cysteine biosynthesis in the liver, the organ distribution of the pathway may be limited.

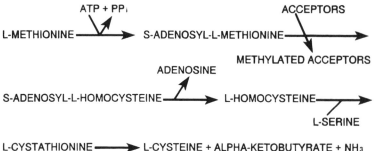

In mammals, such as rats, the liver is the main site of cysteine biosynthesis, which occurs via the cystathionine pathway as shown in the preceding scheme. Maintenance of high concentrations of GSH in the liver, in association with high rates of GSH secretion into plasma and extensive extracellular degradation of GSH and GSSG, supports the concept that liver GSH is a physiological reservoir of cysteine. This idea, which was proposed originally by Tateishi et al. (77) and Higashi et al. (78), was that cells possess two pools of GSH. One has a fast (2-h) and the other a slow (30-h) turnover (78,79). Meredith and Reed (80) observed that in freshly isolated rat hepatocytes the mitochondrial pool of GSH (about 10% of the total cellular pool) had a half-life of 30 h while the half-life of the cytoplasmic pool was 2 h. They concluded that the mitochondrial pool might represent the stable pool of GSH observed in whole animals. Further, cystine has a sparing effect on the requirement of the essential amino acid methionine in the rat (81). This observation is in agreement with the unidirectional process of trans-sulfuration in which methionine sulfur and serine carbon are utilized in cysteine biosynthesis via the cystathionine pathway. For reviews see Reed and Beatty (72) and Reed (75)].

In vivo treatment of rats with an inhibitor of γ-glutamyl transpeptidase (AT-125) prevents degradation of GSH in plasma leading to massive urinary excretion of GSH (82a). This treatment also lowers the hepatic content of GSH because it inhibits recycling of cysteine to the liver (80). A physiologic decrease in interorgan recycling of cysteine to the liver for synthesis of GSH also may account in part for the decrease of hepatic GSH during starvation and for the marked diurnal variation in concentration of GSH in liver. The nadir occurs in the late afternoon, whereas the early morning peak occurs shortly after the animals are fed. The efflux of liver GSH and metabolism of the resulting plasma GSH and GSSG appears to help insure a continuous supply of plasma cysteine. This cysteine pool should in turn minimize the degree of fluctuation of GSH concentrations within the various body organs and cell types that require only cysteine or cystine, or both, rather than methionine for synthesis of GSH.

Glutathione deficiency can be achieved in vivo by the administration of BSO. When newborn rats or guinea pigs are treated with BSO a GSH deficiency develops and the animals develop multiorgan failure and die within a few days. Death can be prevented by the administration of ascorbate (82b).

A controversial approach to assessing the potential for chemicals to cause free-radical damage in vivo is to chemically intoxicate an intact animal and then to measure products of lipid peroxidation in microsomes prepared from the intoxicated animal. In this manner, the depletion of glutathione in vivo with agents that form glutathione conjugates enhances subsequent lipid peroxidation in vitro. Results from such experiments show consistently that an in vivo threshold of 1 μmol GSH/g liver is associated with spontaneous lipid peroxidation in microsomes (83). This critical value of GSH is about 20% of the initial concentration of GSH. Addition of exogenous GSH inhibited the lipid peroxidation in vitro in a concentration-dependent manner; 1 mM GSH yielded 50% inhibition. There also is observed a strong enhancement of spontaneous lipid peroxidation in phenobarbital-induced rats.

The role of GSH as a defense against oxidative stress generated by free radicals has been quantitified by the measurement of lipfuscin. A hypothesis for lipofuscino-genesis that was postulated by Brunk et al. (84) involves the interplay of two processes: (1) the intracellular production of superoxide and hydrogen peroxide and (2) secondary lysosomes that degrade lipids and proteins to a poorly defined sub-stance known as lipofuscin (85). The loss of GSH by BSO treatment of cardiac myocytes resulted in an increase in lipofuscin that appears associated with loss of GSH-dependent defense against increased levels of hydrogen peroxide (85).

GLUTATHIONE REDOX CYCLE DEFENSE AGAINST FREE-RADICAL-INDUCED EVENTS

A major defense system against endogenous reactive oxygen species is the gluta-thione redox cycle (Figure 2) (for a review see Reed, 86). Support for the role of the glutathione redox cycle in defense is that GSH depletion to about 20–30% of normal level of glutathione can impair the cell's defense against the toxic actions of both biological reactive intermediates and reactive oxygen species and may lead to cell injury and death. Endogenous free-radical production, which is a normal physiological process, is a consequence of aerobic metabolism that occurs mostly in the mitochondria of eukaryote cells. Mitochondrially generated H_2O_2, if not decomposed, can lead to the formation of radicals that cause damage to membranes, nucleic acids, and proteins, and alter their functions. A major protective role against exogenous free radicals, which are generated by bioreduction of many xenobiotics followed by redox cycling, is also provided by the ubiquitous glutathione redox cycle (Figure 2). This cycle utilizes NADPH- and, indirectly, NADH-reducing equivalents in the mitochondrial matrix as well as the cytoplasm to provide GSH by the glutathione reductase-catalyzed reduction of GSSG. When the glutathione redox cycle is functioning at maximum capacity to eliminate hydrogen peroxide, a major regulatory effect is imposed on other NADPH-dependent pathways.

Glutathione reductase, which is important in the defense against oxygen-derived free radicals by GSH, is itself regulated by the redox status of the cell. Being similar to other reductases such as nitrate, nitrite, and NADP$^+$ reductase, GSH reductase is inactivated upon reduction by its own electron donor, NADPH. It has been proposed that this autoinactivation of glutathione reductase by NADPH and the protection as well as reactivation by GSSG regulates the enzyme in vivo (87). The activity of glutathione reductase may reflect the physiological needs of the cell especially during oxidative stress. For example, 40-50 μM intracellular NADPH inactivates glutathione reductase in the absence of GSSG and decreases glucose metabolism via the hexose monophosphate pathway. The physiological ratio of GSSG:GSH should provide sufficient GSSG at this level of NADPH to permit retention of significant glutathione reductase activity by preventing inactivation (87).

Cytosolic glutathione peroxidase is a selenium-dependent enzyme that is extremely specific for glutathione and is capable of rapidly detoxifying hydrogen

CELLULAR PROTECTIVE SYSTEMS

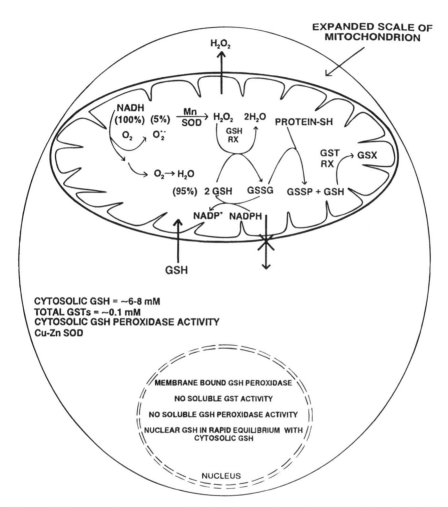

FIG. 2. Cellular protective systems and the glutathione redox cycle. MnSOD in the mitochondria and Cu-ZnSOD in the cytosol provide enzymatic conversion of superoxide to hydrogen peroxidase, which is detoxified by the glutathione redox cycle components glutathione reductase and peroxidase present in the mitochondria matrix (shown) and the cytosol (not shown).

peroxide and certain hydroperoxides as a partner in the glutathione redox cycle with glutathione reductase. As mentioned earlier, selenium-dependent glutathione peroxidase activity is the result of the expression of multiple isozymes.

The antitumor benzanthraquinone, adriamycin, undergoes rapid bioreduction by NADPH-dependent cytochrome P-450 reductase with concomitant consumption of oxygen (88). Adriamycin cytotoxicity may be the result of free radicals formed by bioreduction that overwhelm the cellular antioxidant capacity, including that portion provided by the glutathione redox cycle. Inactivation of glutathione reductase with BCNU has permitted the demonstration of the protective role of the glutathione redox cycle against an adriamycin-mediated challenge (89,90). Depletion of GSH concurrently with inactivation of glutathione reductase can enhance the cellular injury mediated by adriamycin-generated radicals in isolated hepatocytes (90).

The intracellular concentration of GSH in isolated hepatocytes has been examined under conditions that result in enhanced free-radical production. Production of malondialdehyde, which is an index of lipid peroxidation, can be stimulated by addition of a glutathione depletor, diethyl maleate (89). This observation suggests that intracellular concentrations of GSH under these conditions are important for membrane and cellular integrity. That is, GSH protects against free-radical damage to unsaturated fatty acid moieties in biological membranes.

Defense by Glutathione S-Transferases

GSH-dependent protection against lipid peroxidation has been demonstrated in mitochondria (91–93), nuclei (94), microsomes (91,93–98), and cytosol of rat liver (99–101). Lipid peroxidation induced in mitochondria also is inhibited by respiratory substrates such as succinate, which leads indirectly to reduction of ubiquinone to ubiquinol. The latter is a potent antioxidant (102–104). The essential factor in preventing accumulation of lipid peroxides and lysis of membranes in mitochondria, however, is glutathione peroxidase (105). Although the prevention of free-radical attack on membrane lipids may occur by an electron shuttle that utilizes vitamin E and GSH in microsomes, similar activity may not be capable of inhibiting peroxidation in mitochondria (96,106). Instead, mitochondrial GSH S-transferase(s) may prevent lipid peroxidation in mitochondria by a non-selenium glutathione-dependent peroxidase activity. Three GSH S-transferases have been isolated from the mitochondrial matrix (107), and nearly 5% of the mitochondrial outer membrane protein consists of microsomal glutathione S-transferase (108). GSH S-transferase in the outer mitochondrial membrane could provide the GSH-dependent protection of mitochondria by scavenging lipid radicals by a mechanism that requires vitamin E and is abolished by bromosulfophthalein (108).

A limited number of studies have focused on the susceptibility of the cell nucleus to lipid peroxidation. The nuclear membrane regulates the transport of mRNA into the cytoplasm and aids in the process of nuclear division. DNA is also frequently associated with certain regions of the nuclear membrane (109), and it seems likely that nuclear membrane peroxidation may disrupt many of these critical functions. The proximity of the nuclear membrane to DNA could also contribute to the interaction of DNA with reactive compounds generated in lipid peroxidation. Several studies indicate that such lipid peroxidation products can alter the structure and function of DNA (110–113). This fact is of importance since hydroxyl radicals diffuse an average of only 60 Å before reacting with cellular components (114). Assays for

8-hydroxy-2'-deoxyguanosine as a biomarker of oxidative DNA damage include in vivo studies with urine samples (115). Nuclear peroxidation may also increase interactions between more stable peroxidation products and DNA. The cytosolic enzymes aldehyde dehydrogenase (116), glutathione transferase (117), and glutathione peroxidase (91) have all been shown to metabolize various reactive lipid peroxidation products. Such cytosolic enzymes may metabolize peroxidation products generated throughout the cell before they diffuse into the nucleus and interact with DNA.

Glutathione protection of isolated rat liver nuclei against lipid peroxidation is abolished by exposing isolated nuclei to the glutathione transferase inhibitor *S*-octylglutathione (36). *S*-Octylglutathione also inhibited nuclear glutathione transferase activity and glutathione peroxidase activity. A large percentage of the glutathione transferase activity associated with isolated nuclei was solubilized with 0.3% Triton X-100. Since this treatment removes nuclear membranes while preserving the integrity of the remaining nucleus, it appears that the peroxidase activity is associated with the nuclear membrane. This activity in conjunction with GSH may contribute to the inhibition of lipid peroxidation in nuclear membranes and thereby preserve the integrity of this important membrane system. Increasing evidence suggests that this inhibition of peroxidation may in turn protect the structure and function of DNA.

Endogenous α-tocopherol levels in isolated rat liver nuclei have been measured and found to be 0.045 mol E (mol α-tocopherol per mol phospholipid $\times$ 100) (36). This value corresponds to 970 polyunsaturated fatty acid (PUFA) moieties to one molecule of α-tocopherol in the nuclear membrane. These values are higher than values reported for rat liver microsomes (3313) (63) and mitochondria (2100) (118). A threshold level of 0.085 mol% for the prevention of NADPH-induced lipid peroxidation was established for isolated nuclei. That value could be lowered to 0.040 mol% when 1 m*M* GSH was added to assist in the inhibition of lipid peroxidation. The ability of GSH to enhance α-tocopherol-dependent protection against nuclear lipid peroxidation appears to be mainly by a "sparing" effect on the near threshold level of α-tocopherol in the nuclear membrane.

Since lipid hydroperoxides can initiate lipid peroxidation, the reduction of these compounds can contribute to the inhibition of peroxidation (Figure 1). If glutathione peroxidase activity is associated with the phospholipid bilayer of the nuclear membrane, such an association may contribute to the ability of the peroxidase to reduce lipid hydroperoxides. Thus, the association of a glutathione-dependent peroxidase with membranes may encourage the reduction of lipid hydroperoxides located within lipid bilayers.

Glutathione Compartmentation and Defense Against Free-Radical-Induced Injury: Mitochondrial GSH

Several studies have shown that mitochondrial GSH functions as a discrete pool separate from cytosolic GSH. A report by Jocelyn (119) demonstrated that mitochondrial GSH is impermeable to the inner membrane following isolation of mitochondria. However, Kurosawa et al. (120) have reported the transport of glutathione across mitochondrial membranes. Garcia-Ruiz et al. (121) have evidence that the rat hepatic mitochondrial carrier for reduced glutathione (GSH) transport is distinct from the sinusoidal and canalicular transporters. Wahlländer et. al (122) reported the concentration of mitochondrial GSH (10 mM) is higher than cytosolic GSH (7 mM). As previously mentioned, studies by Meredith and Reed (80) demonstrated different rates of GSH turnover in the cytosol and mitochondria confirming the existence of separate intracellular GSH pools. The ratio of GSH:GSSG in mitochondria is approximately 10:1 under normal (untreated) conditions. As reported by Olafsdottir et al. (123), unlike cytosolic GSSG, GSSG is not effluxed from the mitochondrial matrix compartment. This study demonstrated that during oxidative stress induced with t-butyl hydroperoxide, GSSG is accumulated in the mitochondrial matrix and eventually reduced back to GSH. However, as the redox state of the mitochondria increases, an increase in protein mixed disulfides is also observed. This study concluded that mitochondria are more sensitive to redox changes in GSH:GSSG than the cytosol and therefore mitochondria may be more susceptible to the damaging effects of oxidative stress. These findings suggest that under certain experimental conditions, irreversible cell injury due to oxidative challenge may result from irreversible changes in mitochondrial function.

Mitochondria play a critical role in cellular defense free radicals and associated nonradical oxidants. One of the difficulties in experimentally demonstrating the essential role of mitochondrial GSH has been the inability to selectively deplete the mitochondrial pool of GSH. Recently, Shan et al. (124) have utilized the mitochondrial 3-hydroxybutanoate dehydrogenase to generate a GSH-depleting agent, 3-oxo-4-pentenoate, from (R,S)-3-hydroxy-4-pentenoate. By a Michael acceptor reaction of 3-oxo-4-pentenoate with GSH, the mitochondrial GSH pool is selectively depleted. Because mitochondria are a major site for the generation of reactive oxygen species they are susceptible to injury from free radicals. Because of the lack catalase in mitochondria, the entire burden for defense is dependent upon the glutathione redox cycle. Shan et al. (124) observed that the depletion of the mitochondrial, but not the cytosolic, glutathione pool potentiated the cytotoxicity of *tert*-butyl hydroperoxide. As first proposed by Meredith and Reed (80,90), oxidant and electrophile cytotoxicity was correlated with the depletion of GSH in mitochondria but not the cytosol. For reviews see Reed (73–75). In agreement with the mitochondria being a target for free-radical injury, transgenic mice that express high levels of Mn-SOD activity in mitochondria are protected from adriamycin-induced cardiac toxicity (125).

Since mitochondria contain the enzymes and cofactors necessary for the GSH/GSSG redox cycle (126) but do not contain catalase (127), we may assume that a primary function of mitochondrial glutathione (GSH) is the detoxification of endogenously produced H_2O_2. This redox cycle also protects protein sulfhydryls from oxidation (128).

The mitochondrial glutathione redox cycle has a role in regulating mitochondrial oxidations. Various oxidants decrease O_2 uptake by isolated mitochondria and cause a complete turnover of GSH via glutathione peroxidase every 10 min (129). It appears that a continuous flow of reducing equivalents through the glutathione redox cycle is balanced by a continuous formation of mitochondrial NADPH, which is needed for glutathione reductase activity. In addition, metabolism of hydrogen peroxide in mitochondria poses a regulatory function in regard to the oxidation of substrates by lipoamide-dependent ketoacid oxidases (129), which generate NADPH-reducing equivalents. The entire NADPH:NADP$^+$ pool may turn over at least once every minute during a maximum oxidant challenge.

The extent to which bioreduction utilizes mitochondrial reducing equivalents is still uncertain, but evidence is increasing that such effects are very important and relate to both calcium and protein thiol homeostasis of mitochondria. For example, the loss of NADPH, which occurs following addition of menadione to isolated mitochondria, is not related to its consumption via the glutathione redox cycle but more likely is related to bioreductive metabolism by NADH-ubiquinone oxidoreductase (130,131).

Protein Thiols and Toxicity

Thiol groups are well known to be important for normal protein functions, and increasing evidence supports the vital importance of these thiols for cell viability during cytotoxic events. Protein inactivation by oxidation of protein cysteinyl thiols has been shown to occur in more than 240 enzymes (132,133). Membrane-bound enzymes are damaged during lipid peroxidation, and evidence of vitamin E protection strongly supports a free-radical mechanism for protein damage via oxidative stress (134). Oxidative stress can cause loss of protein functions by damaging amino acid residues other than cysteine including methionine, tryptophan, and histidine. An important aspect of such damage is that lipid peroxidative events can amplify free-radical processes that propagate chain reactions. Failure to terminate free-radical processes with a chain-breaking antioxidant, such as vitamin E, can lead to 4 to 10 propagation events occurring per initiation and thus each initiation is amplified (92). Since the reduction of lipid hydroperoxides by GSH utilizes NADPH for the regeneration of GSH from GSSG, the rate of NADPH production can be limiting during oxidative stress (86). Therefore GSSG may be transported from the cell, especially the liver parenchymal cell, when not reduced due to limited levels of NADPH (135). Decreased availability of NADPH and GSH can impair other GSH-dependent detoxication pathways including metabolism of hydrogen peroxide (6), decreased protection of thiols in protein (136,137), and decreased reaction with free radicals (97). Thus, energy-dependent processes involving NADPH, GSH, and thiols in proteins appear to be critically involved in cellular homeostasis during chemical-induced toxicity.

ANTIOXIDANT PROTECTION BY VITAMINS E AND C

Vitamin E is the name given to a family of natural products comprising the tocopherols and tocotrienols. The most potent of these in animal bioassays is α-tocopherol, which has the highest rate constant for reaction with peroxyl radicals (138). Tocopherols are not synthesized de novo in animals, and tissue levels generally reflect dietary intake of grains and plant-derived oils, which are the best natural sources. The liver plays a central role in α-tocopherol distribution by incorporating dietary α-tocopherol into lipoproteins, which then deliver α-tocopherol to tissues. Other tocopherols, principally γ-tocopherol, may be delivered directly to tissues via chylomicrons.

Dietary α-tocopherol deficiency enhances the susceptibility of biological membranes to oxidative damage in vitro and in vivo (for a review, see Chow, 139). Diplock (140), and Rice-Evans and Diplock (141) have reviewed the status of antioxidant nutrients and disease prevention. This section focuses on the interaction of antioxidants for protection against free-radical damage.

α-Tocopherol Threshold and Antioxidant Effect

Although regulation of α-tocopherol distribution at the cellular level is poorly understood, membrane α-tocopherol levels typically range from one to four α-tocopherol molecules per 1000 phospholipids (62,63). This range is thought to correspond to an antioxidant threshold for α-tocopherol (142). Several in vitro studies have demonstrated that α-tocopherol provides effective antioxidant protection only at levels above a threshold concentration (reviewed by Liebler, 143). The α-tocopherol threshold derives from (1) the tendency of α-tocopherol to inhibit peroxyl radical propagation and (2) the tendency of peroxyl radicals to consume α-tocopherol. The threshold essentially represents the α-tocopherol level at which these two opposing tendencies are in balance. Because membrane α-tocopherol levels are apparently kept close to a threshold concentration, relatively modest α-tocopherol depletion could compromise membrane antioxidant defense. Under some circumstances, regeneration of α-tocopherol from its oxidation products may prevent critical depletion of membrane α-tocopherol (discussed later). Moreover, in vitro studies in a liposome model demonstrated that antioxidant synergism between α-tocopherol and ascorbate was most efficient when membrane α-tocopherol levels exceeded the threshold concentration experimentally determined for that system (142). An apparent α-tocopherol threshold for protection against lipid peroxidation in vivo has been deduced from plasma α-tocopherol levels in rats (144,145).

Antioxidant Reactions

TH exerts antioxidant effects primarily by trapping peroxyl radicals [Eqs. (11) and (12)]. α-Tocopherol reacts readily with peroxyl radicals to yield a hydroperoxide and the resonance-stabilized tocopheroxyl radical (T·).

$$\alpha-\text{tocopherol} + \text{ROO}^{\cdot} \rightarrow \alpha-\text{tocopherol}^{\cdot} + \text{ROOH} \qquad [11]$$

$$\alpha-\text{tocopherol}^{\cdot} + \text{ROO}^{\cdot} \rightarrow \text{nonradical products} \qquad [12]$$

The tocoperoxyl radical formed in reaction 11 may be reduced by several biochemical reductants and this is postulated to regenerate α-tocopherol and complete a one-electron redox cycle (discussed later). Direct observation of reactions 11 and 12 in biological systems generally is not feasible, but much has been learned about α-tocopherol antioxidant reactions through analyses of the products formed in reaction 12.

Further reactions of the tocopheroxyl radical yield two groups of nonradical products (146–151). The first consists of 8a-substituted tocopherones, which result either from peroxyl radical addition at C-8a to form 8a-(alkyldioxy)tocopherones (1, Figure 3) (146,148,149,152) or from electron transfer followed by hydrolysis to yield 8a-(hydroxy)tocopherones 2 (151,153,154). Products 1 and 2 hydrolyze and rearrange to form α-tocopherolquinone 3 (155). Formation of 8a-substituted tocopherones 1/2 is analogous to reactions of simple antioxidant phenols (e.g., BHT) with peroxyl radicals and is compatible with the previously reported stoichiometry of two peroxyl radicals trapped for each α-tocopherol oxidized (138,146,156).

The remaining products consist of epoxytocopherones 4/5 and their hydrolysis products 5,6-epoxy-α-tocopherolquinone 6 and 2,3-epoxy-α-tocopherolquinone 7, respectively (149,157). Although the mechanism of α-tocopherol oxidation to epoxides 4/5 is not known, recent studies of product yield and antioxidant stoichiometry indicated that epoxide product yields vary considerably with reaction environment, but the antioxidant stoichiometry remains essentially unchanged at two radicals scavenged per α-tocopherol consumed (158,159).

Peroxyl radical scavenging by α-tocopherol thus forms 8a-substituted tocopherones and epoxytocopherones, which then hydrolyze to more stable α-tocopherolquinone and epoxyquinone products. In recent studies of the peroxyl radical mediated oxidation of α-tocopherol in microsomes in vitro, tocopherone intermediates were found to account for over half of the α-tocopherol consumed (160). Mild acid treatment of microsomal incubation samples effected complete conversion of the tocopherone precursors to α-tocopherolquinone and epoxyquinones (151), which were analyzed by a sensitive stable isotope dilution GC-MS method (160). Analysis of α-tocopherol, together with α-tocopherolquinone, its reduction product α-tocopherolhydroquinone (discussed later), and the epoxyquinones can provide a "snapshot" of the redox distribution of α-tocopherol and its major oxidation products.

Redox Cycles for Vitamin E: One-Electron Redox Cycle

Early observations by Golumbic and Mattill (161) and by Tappel et al. (162) led to the suggestion that α-tocopherol may be regenerated from its oxidation intermediates by other biochemical reductants and that this redox chemistry would maintain through ongoing oxidative stress. The most widely considered redox cycle is the one-electron redox cycle in which α-tocopherol is oxidized by a radical to the tocopheroxyl radical (eq 1), which is then reduced back to α-tocopherol by a reductant such as ascorbate:

$$T^{\cdot} + \text{ascorbate} \rightarrow TH + \text{semidehyroascorbate radical} \qquad [13]$$

Proof of the chemical feasibility of reaction 13 came from pulse radiolysis work by Packer, Slater, and Willson (163). However, evaluation of this one-electron redox cycle in biological systems has been much more difficult. The large body of work on this problem has been reviewed in detail from different perspectives (143,164–166). Several general observations are presented here.

First, in the numerous reported demonstrations of α-tocopherol "sparing" by ascorbate, other low-molecular-weight antioxidants, and redox proteins, the extent to which these co-antioxidants acted by regenerating α-tocopherol or by directly trapping radicals generally was not assessed. This makes it difficult to attribute protection against α-tocopherol depletion to tocopheroxyl radical recycling per se or to independent antioxidant actions of the co-antioxidants. Indeed, it seems likely that both tocopheroxyl radical recycling and direct, co-antioxidant effects of ascorbate may occur to varying degrees in different environments. It is nevertheless noteworthy that in a carefully conducted study of α-tocopherol turnover in several tissues of the guinea pig, dietary ascorbate status did not measurably affect the kinetics of α-tocopherol turnover (167).

Second, reduction of the tocopheroxyl radical by ubiquinol, ascorbate, or other co-antioxidants has been unambiguously demonstrated in human low-density lipoproteins (59). These co-antioxidants reverse the novel pro-oxidant effect of the tocopheroxyl radical in the lipoprotein particle by reducing the tocopheroxyl radical to α-tocopherol and thus "carrying away" the radical from the lipoprotein. In the absence of a coreductant, the tocopheroxyl radical may actually initiate peroxidation of lipoprotein lipid (168).

Third, glutathione and other low-molecular-weight thiols apparently do not reduce the tocopheroxyl radical directly, but instead act to regenerate other antioxidants, such as ascorbate, which then may reduce the tocopheroxyl radical (166,169). Enzymatically mediated synergism between glutathione and α-tocopherol most likely results from parallel antioxidant actions of glutathione peroxidase enzymes (selenium-dependent glutathione peroxidase, selenium-dependent phospholipid hydroperoxide glutathione peroxidase, and some glutathione *S*-transferases) (38).

Redox Cycles for Vitamin E: Two-Electron Cycle

Tocopheroxyl radicals that do not undergo a one-electron reduction to α-tocopherol may instead either disproportionate or react with peroxyl radicals to form a variety of products, as discussed earlier. A large fraction of the products formed are 8a-substituted tocopherones, which may undergo reduction to α-tocopherol to complete a two-electron redox cycle (151,153–155). The possibility that a two-electron redox cycle may contribute to α-tocopherol function has been raised previously and considered in detail recently (143). Although 8a-substituted tocopherones are easily reduced to α-tocopherol in vitro by ascorbate or nordehydroguairetic acid at acidic pH, it is not clear whether an enzyme-catalyzed reduction also can take place in biological systems. Of interest in this regard are the findings of Chan and colleagues, who described the oxidation of α-tocopherol in platelets to a product that was converted back to α-tocopherol by subsequent addition of ascorbate, glutathione, or nordehydroguaretic acid (170). Although the authors proposed that the reducible intermediate was the tocopheroxyl radical, the conditions of the experiment make it more likely that the intermediates were 8a-substituted tocopherones instead, as we have suggested previously (151). This suggests that a two-electron redox cycle involving 8a-substituted tocopherones could contribute to α-tocopherol maintenance during oxidative stress.

α-Tocopherol Esters

Esterified forms of α-tocopherol are resistant to oxidation and display improved stability over α-tocopherol. These forms of vitamin E, particularly α-tocopherol acetate, are frequently used in formulating vitamin supplements and other vitamin E-supplemented products. The esters themselves are inactive as antioxidants. When taken orally, α-tocopherol esters are efficiently hydrolyzed to the active antioxidant α-tocopherol by esterases in the gut, and bioavailability as free α-tocopherol is identical to an equal amount of the unesterified vitamin (171,172). In dosage by other routes, the ester and free α-tocopherol may not be bioequivalent. For example, topical application of free α-tocopherol inhibits photocarcinogenesis induced by repeated exposures to UV-B in a mouse model, whereas topical α-tocopherol acetate is ineffective (173). Polar α-tocopherol esters (e.g., α-tocopherol succinate) have been used in a number of studies in vitro to achieve α-tocopherol supplementation in cell culture systems (136,137,174,175). The water-dispersible hemisuccinate ester confers greater protection against oxidative stress than does either free α-tocopherol or α-tocopherol acetate (176,177). This apparently reflects a greater ability of the water-dispersible ester to release α-tocopherol in proximity to vital locations within cells (178).

Redox Chemistry of α-Tocopherolquinone

α-Tocopherolquinone (8, Figure 3), a stable end-product of α-tocopherol oxidation (discussed earlier) undergoes facile two-electron reduction by ascorbate, sodium borohydride, or other reductants to α-tocopherolhydroquinone at neutral pH (179,180). This hydroquinone would be expected to exert antioxidant effects similar to those of ubiquinols, which have been shown to be effective chain-breaking antioxidants. Hayashi et al. (181) demonstrated that isolated rat hepatocytes contained both α-tocopherolquinone and α-tocopherolhydroquinone in comparable

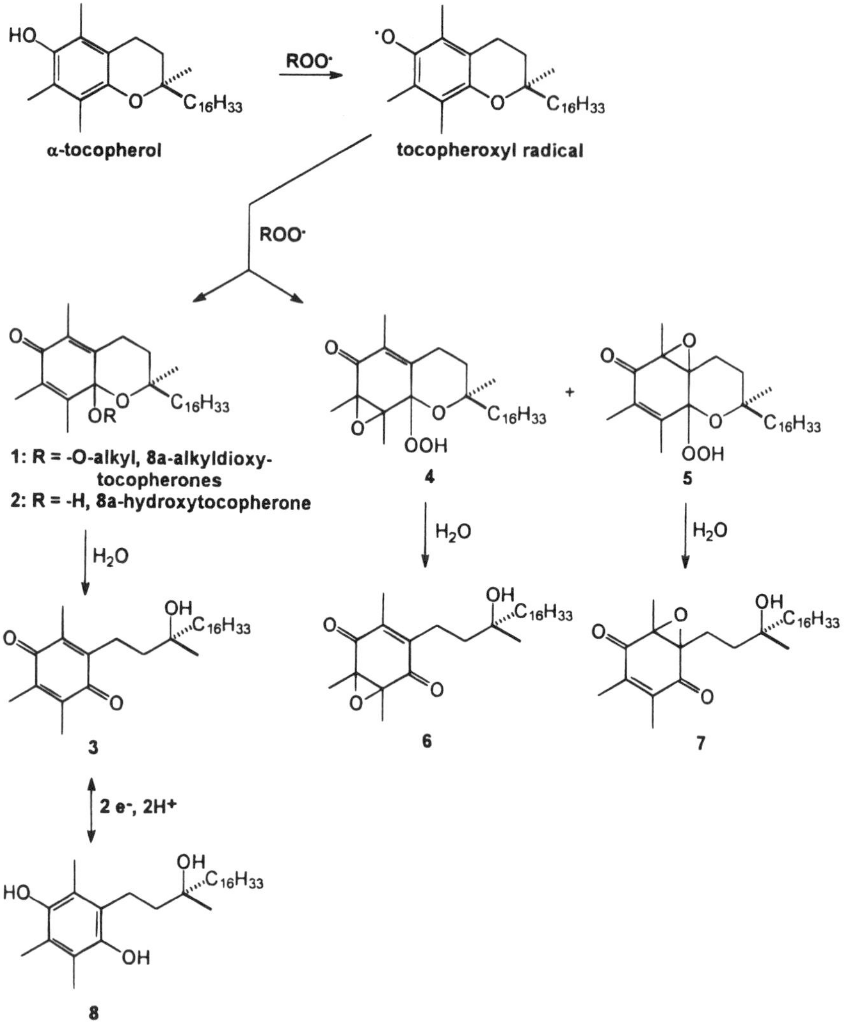

FIG. 3. Reaction products formed during the trapping of peroxyl radicals with α-tocopherol.

amounts and that the cells were capable of rapidly reducing exogenously added α-tocopherolquinone to the hydroquinone. Relatively little is known about the fate and possible role of α-tocopherolquinone formed by oxidative α-tocopherol turnover. Reduction of the quinone to the hydroquinone could provide an important contribution to cellular antioxidant protection, as proposed recently by Kohar et al. (182).

Antioxidant Protection by Vitamin C

In addition to its probable participation in the recycling of α-tocopherol (discussed earlier), ascorbate is thought to exert direct antioxidant effects. This follows from the high reactivity of ascorbate as a one-electron reductant for many biologically relevant oxidants (16). The ability of ascorbate to exert both pro-oxidant and antioxidant effects complicates interpretations of its role as a cellular protectant. Antioxidant effects may be due either to (1) direct reaction with free radicals or nonradical oxidants to produce less reactive products (see Frei, 183, for a recent review), (2) regeneration of phenolic antioxidants such as α-tocopherol (discussed earlier), or (3) shifting the redox balance of transition metal redox couples to disfavor their participation in pro-oxidant reactions (184). As discussed earlier, some combination of the first two mechanisms probably accounts for antioxidant synergy between ascorbate and α-tocopherol. In most experimental systems, it may not be possible to distinguish the relative contributions of these mechanisms. Pro-oxidant effects of ascorbate are often observed in in vitro systems and are thought to be due to (1) reduction of transition metal ions to facilitate participation in Fenton chemistry (see Koppenol, chapter 1, this volume) and (2) formation of reactive oxygen species subsequent to metal catalyzed ascorbate autoxidation. It seems clear that ascorbate can inhibit or enhance metal catalyzed oxidations, depending on the ascorbate concentration (184).

The balance between pro-oxidant and antioxidant effects of ascorbate also may be controlled by the membrane status of α-tocopherol. In studies with a liposome model, in which oxidation was initiated by Fe^{2+} and hydrogen peroxide, ascorbate alone at concentrations of less than 1 mM exerted a marked pro-oxidant effect, apparently by contributing to Fenton chemistry (142). Inclusion of α-tocopherol at a concentration of 0.2 mol%, which is above the α-tocopherol antioxidant threshold for that system, reversed the pro-oxidant effect of ascorbate. This coincided with an ascorbate-dependent prevention of α-tocopherol depletion. In liposomes containing α-tocopherol at lower concentrations, ascorbate was unable either to prevent α-tocopherol depletion or to prevent lipid peroxidation.

Intracellular ascorbate is consumed and recycled by permeant oxidants in activated neutrophiles (185). Since free-radical generation by neutrophils can be as high as 200 nmole/10^6cells/h (10), recycling of ascorbate occurs with rapid reduction of dehydroascorbate by a yet unknown mechanism for reduction. The accumulation of ascorbate and dehydroascorbate occurs by separate mechanisms (11). Winkler et al. (186) recently reviewed the literature on mechanisms for ascorbate reduction in cells. They concluded that there is little convincing evidence for the existence of putative NADH-dependent semidehydroascorbate reductases in mammalian cells, despite the fact that these enzymes are well described in plants. These authors concluded that semidehydroascorbate formed by one-electron oxidations of ascorbate disproportions to dehydroascorbic acid, which then either is reduced nonenzymatically by glutathione or hydrolyzes to nonreducible products. Other mechanisms may maintain reduced ascorbate, including protein disulfide isomerase and glutaredoxin, which have dehydroascorbate-reducing activity (187) that is depdendent on reduced glutathione. Welch et al. (11) have shown that in neutrophils dehydroascorbate reduction is protein mediated and chemical reduction by GSH could not account for the reduction. Also, they have found that dehydroascorbate transport and accumulation is 10-fold greater than for ascorbate. These findings support the concept of extracellular defense against free radicals and other oxidants being an important aspect of the utilization and recycling of ascorbate, with intracellular reducing equivalents being made readily available by a glutathione-dependent reduction process (188).

CONCLUSIONS

Over the past two decades, a large body of work has helped to explain the functions of biological antioxidants and antioxidant enzyme systems. What has more recently emerged is a broader picture of the integration of biological antioxidant defense. Just as biological oxidant challenges encompass a diverse array of primordial oxidants, secondary oxidants, and propagating radicals, so do biological antioxidants comprise a multitiered defense. Specialization in antioxidant function allows specific enzymes and small molecules to scavenge specific oxidants with high efficiency. A diverse antioxidant defense system permits cells to defend against multiple components of oxidant challenges.

In a review of antioxidant therapy, Rice-Evans and Diplock (141) chose to concentrate mainly on coronary heart disease, reperfusion injury, and organ storage for transplantation. They provided ample evidence for free radicals having a major contribution to these conditions and insight on how antioxidant therapy could be beneficial. However, as they point out, "only when the mechanisms and involvement of radicals in the pathogenesis of many disorders described in this review are understood will approaches to antioxidant therapies be designed effectively and targeted successfully." We agree with these comments and we think that they apply equally well to understanding how antioxidant defense affects injury by toxic chemicals. We hope that this review offers perspectives on the functions of cellular antioxidant defense that will prove useful to those investigating chemically induced tissue injury and free-radical-associated diseases.

ACKNOWLEDGMENTS

We wish to thank our many co-workers for their outstanding contributions to the research in our laboratories that has been the basis for our chapter. Our work was supported in part by U.S. Public Health Service grant CA 59585 and Southwest Environmental Health Sciences Center Grant ES 06694 (D. C. Liebler), and U.S. Public Health Service grant ES 01978 and Environmental Health Sciences Center grant ES 00210 (D. J. Reed).

REFERENCES

1. Halliwell B, Gutteridge JMC. Role of free radicals and catalytic metal ions in human disease: An overview. In: Packer L. and Glazer A.N., eds. *Methods in Enzymology.* San Diego: Academic Press, 1990;186(B):1–85.

2. Chance B, Sies H, Boveris A. Hydroperoxide metabolism in mammalian organs. *Physiol Rev* 1979;59:527–605.
3. Cadenas E. Biochemistry of oxygen toxicity. *Annu Rev Biochem* 1989;58:79–110.
4. Richter C. Do mitochondrial DNA fragments promote cancer and aging? *FEBS Lett* 1988;241:1–5.
5. Forman HJ, Boveris A. Superoxide radical and hydrogen peroxide in mitochondria. In: Pryor WA ed., *Free Radicals in Biology.* Vol V, pp. 65–90. New York: Academic Press, 1982.
6. Jones DP, Eklow L, Thor H, Orrenius S. Metabolism of hydrogen peroxide in isolated hepatocytes: Relative contributions of catalase and glutathione peroxidase in decomposition of endogenously generated H_2O_2. *Arch Biochem Biophys* 1981;210:505–516.
7. Sohal RS. Aging, cytochrome oxidase activity, and hydrogen peroxide release by mitochondria. *Free Radical Biol Med* 1993;14:583–588.
8. Turrens JF, McCord JM. Mitochondrial generation of reactive oxygen species. In: Paulet AC, Douste-Blazy L, Paoletti R, eds. *Free Radicals, Lipoproteins, and Membrane Lipids.* New York: Plenum Press, 1990;203–212.
9. Boveris A, Cadenas E. Production of superoxide in mitochondria. In: Oberley, L.W., ed., *Superoxide Dismutase, II.* Boca Raton, FL: CRC Press, 1982;15–30.
10. Mehlhorn RJ. Ascorbate-and dehydroascorbic acid-mediated reduction of free radicals in the human erythrocyte. *J Biol Chem* 1991;266:2724–2731.
11. Welch RW, Wang Y, Crossman Jr A, Park JB, Kirks KL and Levine M. Accumulation of vitamin C (ascorbate) and its oxidized metabolite dehydroascorbic acid occurs by separate mechanisms. *J Biol Chem* 1995;270:12585–12592.
12. Babior BM. Oxidant from phagocytes: Agents of defense and destruction. *Blood* 1984;64:959–966.
13. Babior BM. The respiratory burst oxidase. *Trends Biol Sci* 1987;12:241–242.
14. Frenkel K. Carcinogen-mediated oxidant formation and oxidative DNA damage. *Pharmacol Ther* 1992;53:127–166.
15. Morris SMJr, Billiar TR. New insights into the regulation of inducible nitric oxide synthesis. *Am J Physiol* 1994;266:E829–E839.
16. Beuttner GR. The pecking order of free radicals and antioxidants: Lipid peroxidation, α-tocopherol, and ascorbate. *Arch Biochem Biophys* 1993;300:535–543.
17. Beckman JS, Crow JP. Pathological implications of nitric oxide, superoxide, and peroxynitrite formation. *Biochem Soc Trans* 1993;21:330–334.
18. Koppenol WH, Moreno JJ, Pryor WA, Ischiropoulis H, Beckman JS.. Peroxynitrite, a cloaked oxidant formed by nitric oxide and superoxide. *Chem Res Toxicol* 1992;5:834–842.
19. Pryor WA, Lightsey, JW. Mechanisms of nitrogen dioxide reactions: Initiation of lipid peroxidation and the production of nitrous acid. *Science* 1981;214:435–437.
20. Svingen BA, Beuge JA, O'Neal FO, Aust SD. The mechanism of NADPH-dependent lipid peroxidation. The propagation of lipid peroxidation. *J Biol Chem* 1979;254:5892–5899.
21. Aikens J, Dix TA. Hydrodioxyl (perhydroxyl), peroxyl, and hydroxyl radical-initiated lipid peroxidation of large unilamellar vesicles (liposomes): Comparative and mechanistic studies. *Arch Biochem Biophys* 1993;305:516–525.
22. Wilcox AL, Marnett LJ. Polyunsaturated fatty acid alkoxyl radicals exist as carbon-centered epoxyallylic radicals: A key step in hydroperoxide-amplified lipid peroxidation. *Chem Res Toxicol* 1993;6:413–416.
23. Wardman P. Conjugation and oxidation of glutathione via thiyl free radicals. In: Sies H, Ketterer B, eds. *Glutathione Conjugation: Mechanisms and Biological Significance.* London: Academic Press, 1988;44–72.
24. Pryor WA. Free radicals in autoxidation and aging. In: Armstrong D, Sohal RS, Cutler RG, Slater TF eds., *Free Radicals in Molecular Biology, Aging, and Disease.* New York: Raven Press, 1984;13–41.
25. Fridovich I. Superoxide dismutases. *Adv Enzymol Relat Areas Mol Biol* 1974;41:35–97.
26. Fridovich I. Superoxide dismutase. An adaptation to a paramagnetic gas. *J Biol Chem* 1989;264:7761–7764.
27. Marklund SL. Human copper-containing superoxide dismutase of high molecular weight. *Proc Natl Acad Sci USA* 1982;79:7634–7638.
28. Wong GHW. Protective roles of cytokines against radicaliation: Induction of mitochondrial MnSOD. *Biochim Biophys. Acta* 1995;1271:205–209.
29. Shull S, Heintz NH, Periasamy M, Manohar M, Janssen YMW, Marsh JP, Mossman BT. Differential regulation of antioxidant enzymes in response to oxidants. *J Biol Chem* 1991;266:24398–24403.

30. Chu FF, Doroshow JH, Esworthy RS. Expression, characterization, and tissue distribution of a new cellular selenium-dependent glutathione peroxidase, GSHPx-GI. *J Biol Chem* 1993;268:2571–2576.

31. Wendel A. Glutathione peroxidase. In: Jakoby WB, ed. *Enzymatic Basis of Detoxication.* New York: Academic Press, 1980;333–354.

32. Takahashi K, Akasaka M, Yamamoto Y, Kobayashi C, Mizoguchi J, Koyama J. Primary structure of human plasma glutathione peroxidase deduced from cDNA sequences. *J Biochem* 1990;108:145–148.

33. Ursini F, Maiorino M, Gregolin C. The selenoenzyme phospholipid hydroperoxide glutathione peroxidase. *Biochim Biophys Acta* 1985;839:62–70.

34. Ursini F, Maiorino M, Valente M, Ferri L, Gregolin C. Purification from pig liver of a protein which protects liposomes and biomembranes from peroxidative degradation and exhibits glutathione peroxidase activity on phosphatidylcholine hydroperoxides. *Biochim Biophys Acta* 1982;710:197–211.

35. Nakamura W, Hosoda S, Hayashi K. Purification and properties of rat liver glutathione peroxidase. *Biochim Biophys Acta* 1974;358:251–261.

36. Tirmenstein MA, Reed DJ. Effects of glutathione on the α-tocopherol-dependent inhibition of nuclear lipid peroxidation. *J Lipid Res* 1989;30:959–965.

37. Burk RF, Hill KE. Selenoprotein P. A selenium-rich extracellular glycoprotein. *J Nutr* 1994;124:1891–1897.

38. Maiorino M, Coassin M, Roveri A, Ursini F. Microsomal lipid peroxidation: Effect of vitamin E and its functional interaction with phospholipid hydroperoxide glutathione peroxidase. *Lipids* 1989;24:721–726.

39. Weitzel F, Wendel A. Selenoenzymes regulate the activity of leukocyte 5-lipoxygenase via the peroxide tone. *J Biol Chem* 1992;268:6288–6292.

40. Awad JA, Morrow JD, Hill KE, Roberts LJII, Burk RF. Detection and localization of lipid peroxidation in selenium- and vitamin E-deficient rats using F_2-isoprostanes. *J Nutr* 1994;124:810–816.

41. Michiels C, Raes M, Toussaint O and Remacle J. Importance of Se-glutathione peroxidase, catalase and Cu/Zn-SOD for cell survival against oxidative stress. *Free Radical Biol Med* 1994;17:235–248.

42. Margoliash E, Novogrodsky, A, Schejter, A. Irreversible reaction of 3-amino-1,2,4-triazole and related inhibitors with the protein of catalase. *Biochem J* 1960;74;339–348.

43. Heikkila RE, Cabbat FS, Cohen G. In vivo inhibition of superoxide dismutase in mice by diethyldithiocarbamate. *J Biol Chem* 1976;252:2182–2185.

44. Chaudiere J, Wilhelmsen EC, Tappel AL. Mechanism of selenium-glutathione peroxidase and its inhibition by mercaptocarboxylic acid and other mercaptans. *J Biol Chem* 1984;259:1043–1050.

45. Babson JR, Reed DJ. Inactivation of glutathione reductase by 2-chloroethyl nitrosourea-derived isocyanates. *Biochim Biophys Acta* 1978;83:754–762.

46. Griffith OW. Mechanism of action, metabolism and toxicity of buthionine sulfoximine and its higher analogs, potent inhibitors of glutathione synthesis. *J Biol Chem* 1982;257:3704–3712.

47. Wispe JR, Warner BB, Clark JC, Dey CR, Neuman J, Glasser SW, Crapo JD, Chang L-Y, Whitsett JA. Human Mn-superoxide dismutase in pulmonary epithelial cells of transgenic mice confers protection from oxygen injury. *J Biol Chem* 1992;267:23937–23941.

48. St. Clair DK, Oberley TD, Ho Y-S, Wheeler KT. Overproduction of human MnSOD modulates paraquat-mediated toxicity in mammalian cells. *FEBS Lett* 1991;293:199–203.

49. Scott MD, MEshnick SR, Eaton JW. Superoxide dismutase-rich bacteria. Paradoxical increase in oxidant toxicity. *J Biol Chem* 1987;262;3640–3645.

50. Liochev, SI, Fridovich I. Effects of overproduction of superoxide dismutase on the toxicity of paraquat toward *Escherichia coli. J Biol Chem* 1991;266:8747–8750.

51. Warner HR. Superoxide dismutase, aging, and degenerative disease. *Free Radical Biol Med* 1994;17:249–258.

52. Luo Y, Han Z, Chin SM, Linn S. Three chemically distinct types of oxidants formed by iron-mediated Fenton reactions in the presence of DNA. *Proc Natl Acad Sci USA* 1994;91:12438–42.

53. Krinsky NI. Actions of carotenoids in biological systems. *Annu Rev Nutr* 1993;13:561–587.

54. Liebler DC. Antioxidant reactions of carotenoids. In: Canfield LM, Krinsky NI, Olson JA, eds., *Carotenoids in Human Health. Annals of the New York Academy of Sciences.* New York: New York Academy of Sciences, 1993;20–31.

55. Packer L, Witt EH, Tritschler HJ. Alpha-lipoic acid as a biological antioxidant. *Free Radical Biol Med* 1995;19:227–250.

56. Jovanivic SV, Steenken S, Tosic M, Marjanovic B, Simic, MG. Flavonoids as antioxidants. *J Am Chem Soc* 1994;116:4846–4851.
57. Terao J, Piskula M, Yao Q. Protective effect of epicatechin, epicatechin gallate, and quercetin on lipid peroxidation in phospholipid bilayers. *Arch Biochem Biophys* 1994;308:278–284.
58. Kagan VE, Serbinova EA, Koynova GM, Kitanova SA, Tyurin VA, Stoytchev TS, Quinn PJ, Packer L. Antioxidant action of ubiquinol homologues with different isoprenoid chain length in biomembranes. *Free Radical Biol Med* 1990;9:117–126.
59. Bowry VW, Mohr D, Cleary J, Stocker R. Prevention of tocopherol-mediated peroxidation in ubiquinol-10-free human low density lipoprotein. *J Biol Chem* 1995;270:5756–5763.
60. Stocker R, Yamamoto Y, McDonagh AF, Glazer AN, Ames, BN. Bilirubin is an antioxidant of possible physiological importance. *Science* 1987;235:1043–1046.
61. Simic MG, Jovanovic SV. Antioxidation mechanisms of uric acid. *J Am Chem Soc* 1989; 111:5778–5782.
62. Kornbrust DJ, Mavis RD. Relative susceptibility of microsomes from lung, heart, liver, kidney, brain and testes to lipid peroxidation: correlation with vitamin E content. *Lipids* 1980;15:315–322.
63. evanian A, Hacker A.D, Elsayed N. Influence of vitamin E and nitrogen dioxide on lipid peroxidation in rat lung and liver microsomes. *Lipids* 1982;17:269–277.
64. Howard JA, Ingold KU. Absolute rate constants for hydrocarbon autoxidation. VI. Alkyl aromatic and olefinic hydrocarbons. *Can J Chem* 1967;45:793–802.
65. Iwatsuki M, Tsuchiya J, Komuro E, Yamamoto Y, Niki E. Effects of solvents and media on the antioxidant activity of α-tocopherol. *Biochim Biophys Acta* 1994;1200:19–26.
66. Czapski G. Reaction of OH. *Methods Enzymol* 1984;105:209–215.
67. Simic MG. Antioxidant compounds: An overview. In: Davies KJA, eds. *Oxidative Damage and Repair. Chemical, Biological, and Medical Aspects.* Oxford: Pergamon Press, 1991;47–56.
68. Burton GW, Ingold KU. Vitamin E: Application of the principles of physical organic chemistry to the exploration of its structure and function. *Acc Chem Res* 1986;19:194–201.
69. Hill TJ, Land EJ, McGarveey DJ, Schalch W, Tinkler JH, Truscott TG. Interactions between carotenoids and the CCl_3O_2 radical. *J Am Chem Soc* 1995;117:8322–8326.
70. Liebler DC, McClure TD. Antioxidant reactions of β-carotene: Identification of carotenoid-radical adducts. *Chem Res Toxicol* 1996; 9:8–11.
71. Kosower NS, Kosower EM. Glutathione status of cells. *Int Rev Cytol* 1978;54:109–160.
72. Reed DJ, Beatty PW. Biosynthesis and regulation of glutathione. Toxicological implications. In: Hodgson E, Bend JR, Philpot RM, eds. *Reviews in Biochemical Toxicology.* New York: Elsevier Press, 1980;213–241.
73. Reed DJ. Glutathione: Toxicological implications. *Annu Rev Pharmacol Toxicol* 1990;30:603–631.
74. Reed DJ. Cellular defense mechanisms against reactive metabolites. In: Anders MW, ed. *Bioactivation of Foreign Compounds.* Orlando FL: Academic Press, 1985;71–108.
75. Reed DJ. Toxicity of Oxygen. In: De Matteis F, Smith LL, eds. *Molecular and Cellular Mechanisms of Toxicity.* Boca Raton, FL: CRC Press, 1995;35–68.
76. White INH. Role of liver glutathione in acute toxicity of retrorsine to rats. *Chem Biol Interact* 1976;13:333–342.
77. Tateishi N, Higashi T, Naruse A, et al. Rat-liver glutathione. Possible role as a reservoir of cysteine. *J Nutr* 1977;107:51–60.
78. Higashi T, Tateishi N, Naruse A. et al. Novel physiological role of liver glutathione as a reservoir of L-cysteine. *J Biochem* 1977;82:117–124.
79. Cho ES, Sahyoun N, Stegink LD. Tissue glutathione as a cyst(e)ine reservor during fasting and refeeding of rats. *J Nutr* 1981;111:914–922.
80. Meredith MJ, Reed DJ. Status of the mitochondrial pool of glutathione in the isolated hepatocyte. *J Biol Chem* 1982;257:3747–3753.
81. Womack M, Kremmer KS, Rose WC. The relation of cysteine and methionine to growth. *J Biol Chem* 1937;121:403–410.
82a. Reed DJ, Ellis WW. Influence of γ-glutamyl transpeptidase inactivation on the status of extracellular glutathione and glutathione conjugates, In: Snyder R, Parke CV, Kocsis JJ, et al., eds. *Biological Reactive Intermediates, IIA.* New York: Plenum Press, 1982;75–86.
82b. Meister A. Glutathione-ascorbic acid antioxidant system in animals. *J Biol Chem* 1994; 269:9397–9400.
83. Younes M, Siegers C-P. Mechanistic aspects of enhanced lipid peroxidation following glutathione depletion in vivo. *Chem Biol Interact* 1981;34:257–266.

84. Brunk UT, Jones CB, Sohal RS. A novel hypothesis of lipofuscinogenesis and cellular ageing based on interactions between oxidative stress and autophagocytosis. *Mutat Res* 1992;275:395–403.
85. Gao G, Ollinger K, Brunk UT. Influence of intracellular glutathione concentration of lipofuscin accumulation in cultured neonatal rat cardiac myocytes. *Free Radical Biol Med* 1994;16:187–194.
86. Reed DJ. Regulation of reductive processes by glutathione. *Biochem Pharmacol* 1986;35:7–13.
87. Lopez-Barea J, Lee C-Y. Mouse-liver glutathione reductase. Purification, kinetics, and regulation. *Eur J Biochem* 1979;98:487–499.
88. Bachur NR, Gordon SL, Gee MV. A general mechanism for microsomal activation of quinone anticancer agents to free Radicals. *Cancer Res* 1978;38:1745–1750.
89. Babson JR, Abell NS, Reed DJ. Protective role of the glutathione redox cycle against adriamycin-mediated toxicity in isolated hepatocytes. *Biochem Pharmacol* 1981;30:2299–2304.
90. Meredith MJ, Reed DJ. Depletion *in vitro* of mitochondrial glutathione in rat hepatocytes and enhancement of lipid peroxidation by adriamycin and 1,3-bis(2-chloroethyl)-1-nitrosourea (BCNU). *Biochem Pharmacol* 1983;32:1383–1388.
91. Christophersen BO. Formation of monohydroxy-polyenic fatty acids from lipid peroxides by a glutathione peroxidase. *Biochim Biophys Acta* 1968;164:35–46.
92. McCay PB, Lai EK, Powell SR, et al. Vitamin E functions as an electron shuttle for glutathione-dependent "free radical reductase" activity in biological membrane. *Fed Proc Fed Am Soc Exp Biol* 1976;45:1729.
93. Yonaha M, Tampo Y. Bromosulfophthalein abolishes glutathione-dependent protection against lipid peroxidation in rat liver mitochondria. *Biochem Pharmacol* 1987;36:2831–2837.
94. Tirmenstein MA, Reed DJ. Characterization of glutathione-dependent inhibition of lipid peroxidation of isolated rat liver nuclei. *Arch Biochem Biophys* 1988;261:1–11.
95. McCay PB, Brueggemann G, Lai EK, Powell SR. Evidence that α-tocopherol functions cyclically to quench free Radicals in hepatic microsomes. Requirement for glutathione and a heat-labile factor. *Ann NY Acad Sci* 1989;570:32–45.
96. Reddy CC, Sholz WW, Thomas CB, et al. Vitamin E-dependent reduced glutathione inhibition of rat liver microsomal lipid peroxidation. *Life Sci* 1982;31:571–576.
97. Burk RF. Glutathione-dependent protection by rat liver microsomal protein against lipid peroxidation. *Biochim Biophys Acta* 1983;757:21–28.
98. Burk RF, Trumble KR, Lawrence R A. Rat hepatic cystolic glutathione-dependent enzyme protection against lipid peroxidation in the NADPH-microsomal lipid peroxidation system. *Biochim Biophys Acta* 1980;618:35–41.
99. Haenen GRMM, Bast A. Protection against lipid peroxidation by a microsomal glutathione-dependent labile factor. *FEBS Lett* 1983;159:24–28.
100. Akasaka S. Inactivation of transforming activity of plasmid DNA by lipid peroxidation, *Biochim. Biophys. Acta* 1986;867:201–208.
101. Gibson DD, Hawrylko J, McCay P B. GSH-dependent inhibition of lipid peroxidation: Properties of a potent cytosolic system which protects cell membranes. *Lipids* 1985;20:704–711.
102. Takayanagi R, Takeshige K, Minakami S. NADH- and NADPH-dependent lipid peroxidation in bovine heart submitochondrial particles. Dependence on the rate of electron flow in the respiratory chain and an antioxidant role of ubiquinol. *Biochem J* 1980;192:853–860.
103. Bindoli A, Cavallini L, Jocelyn P. Mitochondrial lipid peroxidation by cumene hydroperoxide and its prevention by succinate. *Biochim Biophys Acta* 1982;681:496–503.
104. Mészaros L, Tihanyi K, Horvath I. Mitochondrial substrate oxidation-dependent protection against lipid peroxidation. *Biochim Biophys Acta* 1982;713:675–677.
105. Flohé L, Zimmermann R. The role of GSH peroxidase in protecting the membrane of rat liver mitochondria. *Biochim Biophys Acta* 1970;223:210–213.
106. McCay P B, Lai EK, Powell SR, et al. Vitamin E functions as an electron shuttle for glutathione-dependent "free radical reductase" activity in biological membranes. *Fed Proc Fed Am Soc Exp Biol* 1986;45:1729.
107. Kraus P. Resolution, purification and some properties of three glutathione transferases from rat liver mitochondria. *Hoppe-Seyler's Z Physiol Chem* 1980;361:9–15.
108. Morgenstern R, Lundqvist G, Andersson G, et al. The distribution of microsomal glutathione transferase among different organelles, different organs, and different organisms. *Biochem Pharmacol* 1984;33:3609–3614.
109. Franke WW. Structure, biochemistry, and functions of the nuclear envelope. *Int Rev Cytol Suppl* 1974;4:71–236.

110. Gibson DD, Hornbrook KR, McCay PB. Glutathione-dependent inhibition of lipid peroxidation by a soluble, heat-labile factor in animal tissues. *Biochim Biophys Acta* 1980;620:572–582.

111. Ueda K, Kobayashi S, Morita J, Komano T. Site-specific DNA damage caused by lipid peroxidation products. *Biochim Biophys Acta* 1984;824:341–348.

112. Brawn K, Fridovich I. DNA strand scission by enzymically generated oxygen radicals. *Arch Biochem Biophys* 1981;206:414–419.

113. Mukai FH, Goldstein BD. Mutagenicity of malonaldehyde, a decomposition product of peroxidized polyunsaturated fatty acids. *Science* 1976;191:868–869.

114. Roots R, Okada S. Estimation of life times and diffusion distances of radicals involved in x-ray-induced DNA strand breaks of killing of mammalian cells. *Radiat Res* 1975;64:306–320.

115. Shigenaga MK, Ames BN. Assays for 8-hydroxy-2'-deoxyguanosine: A biomarker of in vivo oxidative DNA damage. *Free Radical Biol Med* 1991;10:211–216.

116. Hjelle JJ, Petersen DR. Metabolism of malondialdehyde by rat liver aldehyde dehydrogenase. *Toxicol Appl Pharmacol* 1983;70:57–66.

117. Alin P, Danielson UH, Mannervik B. 4-Hydroxyalk-2-enals are substrates for glutathione transferase. *FEBS Lett* 1985;179:267–270.

118. Gruger EH, Tappel AL. Reactions of biological antioxidants: III. Composition of biological membranes. *Lipids* 1971;6:147–148.

119. Jocelyn PC. Some properties of mitochondrial glutathione. *Biochim Biophys Acta* 1975; 396:427–436.

120. Kurosawa K, Hayashi N, Sato N, Kamada T, Tagawa K. Transport of glutathione across mitochondrial membranes. *Biochem Biophys Res Commun* 1990;167:367–372.

121. Garcia-Ruis C, Morales A, Collell A, Rodes J, Yi J, Kaplowitz N, Fernandez-Checa J. Evidence that the rat hepatic mitochondrial carrier is distinct from the sinusoidal and canalicular transporter for reduced glutathione: Expression studies in *Xenopus laevis* oocytes. *J Biol Chem* 1995; 270:15946–15949.

122. Wahlländer A, Sobell S, Sies H, Linke I, Müller M. Hepatic mitochondrial and cytosolic glutathione content and the subcellular distribution of GSH-S-transferases. *FEBS Lett* 1979;97:138–140.

123. Olafsdottir K, Reed DJ. Retention of oxidized glutathione by isolated rat liver mitochondria during hydroperoxide treatment. *Biochim Biophys Acta* 1988;377–382.

124. Shan X, Jones DP, Hashmi M, Anders MW. Selective depletion of mitochondrial glutathione concentrations by (R,S)-3-hydroxy-4-pentenoate potentiates oxidative cell death. *Chem Res Toxicol* 1993;6:75–821.

125. Yen H-C, Oberley TD, Ho Y-S, Vichitbandha S, St. Clair DK. An antioxidant protective mechanism against adriamycin-induced cardiac toxicity. In: *Oxygen'95, 1995; The Annual Meeting of the Oxygen Society,* 1995;58.

126. Flohe L, Schlegel W. Glutathione peroxidase. IV. Intracellular distribution of the glutathione peroxidase system in the rat liver. *Hoppe-Seyler's Z Physiol Chem* 1971;352:1401–1410.

127. Neubert D, Wojtszak AB, Lehninger AL. Purification and enzymatic identity of mitochondrial contraction factors I and II. *Proc Natl Acad Sci USA* 1962;48:1651–1658.

128. Vignais PM, Vignais PV. Fuscin, an inhibitor of mitochondrial SH-dependent transport-linked functions. *Biochim Biophys Acta* 1973;325:357–374.

129. Sies H, Moss KM. A role of mitochondrial glutathione peroxidase in modulating mitochondrial oxidations in liver. *Eur J Biochem* 1978;84:377–383.

130. Moore G A, O'Brien PJ, Orrenius S. Menadione (2-methyl-1,4-naphthoquinone)-induced Ca^{2+} release from rat-liver mitochondria is caused by NAD(P)H oxidation. *Xenobiotica* 1986;16:873–882.

131. Smith PF, Alberts DW, Rush GF. Role of glutathione reductase during menadione-induced NADPH oxidation in isolated rat hepatocytes. *Biochem Pharmacol* 1987;36:3879–3884.

132. Webb JL. Sulfhydryl reagents (Chapter 4), Mercurials (Chapter 7). In: Webb JL, ed. *Enzyme and Metabolic Inhibitors,* Vol. 2. New York: Academic Press, 1965.

133. Webb JL. Iodoacetate and iodoacetamide (Chapter 1), N-Ethylmaleimide (Chapter 3), Arsenicals (Chapter 6), Comparison of SH reagents (Chapter 7), In: Webb JL, ed.: *Enzyme and Metabolic Inhibitors,* Vol. 3. New York: Academic Press, 1966.

134. Dean RT, Cheeseman KH. Vitamin E protects against free radical damage in lipid environments. *Biochem Biophys Res Commun* 1987;148:1277–1282.

135. Akerboom TPM, Bilzer M, Sies H. The relationship of biliary glutathione disulfide efflux and intracellular glutathione disulfide content in perfused rat liver. *J Biol Chem* 1982;257:4248–4252.

136. Pascoe G A, Reed DJ. Relationship between cellular calcium and vitamin E metabolism during protection against cell injury. *Arch Biochem Biophys* 1987;253:287–296.
137. Pascoe GA, Reed, DJ. Vitamin E protection against chemical-indiced injury. II. Evidence for a threshold effect in prevention of adriamycin toxicity. *Arch Biochem Biophys* 1987;256:159–166.
138. Burton GW, Ingold KU. Autoxidation of biological molecules. 1. The antioxidant activity of vitamin E and related chain-breaking phenolic antioxidants in vitro. *J Am Chem Soc* 1981;103:6472–6477.
139. Chow CK. Vitamin E and oxidative stress. *Free Radical Biol Med* 1991;11:215–232.
140. Diplock AT. Antioxidant nutrients and disease prevention: An overview. *Am J Clin Nutr* 1991;53:189S–193S.
141. Rice-Evans CA, Diplock AT. Current status of antioxidant therapy. *Free Radical Biol Med* 1993;15:77–96.
142. Liebler DC, Kling DS, Reed DJ. Antioxidant protection of phospholipid bilayers by α-tocopherol. *J Biol Chem* 1986;261:12114–12119.
143. Liebler DC. The role of metabolism in the antioxidant function of vitamin E. *Crit Rev Toxicol* 1993;23:147–169.
144. Litov RE, Matthews LC, Tappel AL. Vitamin E protection against in vivo lipid peroxidation initiated in rats by methyl ethyl ketone peroxide as monitored by pentane. *Toxicol Appl Pharmacol* 1981;59:96–106.
145. Herschberger LA., Tappel AL. Effect of vitamin E on pentane exhaled by rats treated with methyl ethyl ketone peroxide. *Lipids* 1982;17:686–691.
146. Winterle J, Dulin D, Mill T. Products and stoichiometry of reaction of vitamin E with alkylperoxy radicals. *J Org Chem* 1984;49:491–495.
147. Matsuo M, Matsumoto S, IItaka Y, Niki E. Radical scavenging reactions of vitamin E and its model compound, 2,2,5,7,8-pentamethylchroman-6-ol, in a *tert*-butylperoxyl radical generating system. *J Am Chem Soc* 1989;111:7179–7185.
148. Yamauchi R, Matsui T, Satake Y, Kato K, Ueno Y. Reaction products of alpha-tocopherol with a free radical initiator, 2,2'-azobis(2,4-dimethylvaleronitrile). *Lipids* 1989;24:204–209.
149. Liebler, DC, Baker PF, Kaysen, KL. Oxidation of vitamin E: Evidence for competing autoxidation and peroxyl radical trapping reactions of the tocopheroxyl radical. *J Am Chem Soc* 1990;112:6995–7000.
150. Yamauchi R, Matsui T, Kato K, Ueno Y. Reaction products of alpha-tocopherol with methyl linoleate-peroxyl radicals. *Lipids* 1990;25:152–158.
151. Liebler DC, Burr JA. Oxidation of vitamin E during iron-catalyzed lipid peroxidation: Evidence for elctron-transfer reactions of the tocopheroxyl radical. *Biochemistry* 1992;31:8278–8284.
152. Yamauchi R, Yagi Y, Kato K. Isolation and characterization of addition products of alpha-tocopherol with peroxyl adicals of dilinoleoylphosphatidylcholine in liposomes. *Biochim Biophys Acta* 1994;1212:43–49.
153. Durckheimer W, Cohen LA. The chemistry of 9-hydroxy-alpha-tocopherone, a quinone hemiacetal. *J Am Chem* Soc 1964;86:4388–4393.
154. Marcus MF, Hawley MD. Electrochemical studies of the redox behavior of alpha-tocopherol. *Biochim Biophys Acta* 1970;201:1–8.
155. Liebler DC, Kaysen KL, Kennedy TA. Redox cycles of vitamin E: Hydrolysis and ascorbic acid dependent reduction of 8a-(alkyldioxy)tocopherones. *Biochemistry* 1989;28:9772–9777.
156. Niki E, Tanimura R, Kamiya Y. Oxidation of lipids. II. Rate of inhibition of oxidation by alpha-tocopherol and hindered phenols measured by chemiluminescence. *Bull Chem Soc Jpn* 1982;55:1551–1555.
157. Liebler DC, Kaysen KL, Burr JA. Peroxyl radical trapping and autoxidation reactions of alpha-tocopherol in lipid bilayers. *Chem Res Toxicol* 1991;4:89–93.
158. Liebler DC, Burr JA, Matsumoto S, Matsuo M. Reactions of the vitamin E model compound 2,2,5,7,8-pentamethylchroman-6-ol with peroxyl radicals. *Chem Res Toxicol* 1993;6:351–355.
159. Liebler DC and Burr JA. Antioxidant stoichiometry and the oxidative fate of vitamin E in peroxyl radical scavenging reactions. *Lipids* 1995;30:789–793.
160. Liebler DC, Burr JA, Philips L, Ham AJL. Gas chromatography-mass spectrometry analysis of vitamin E and its oxidation products. *Anal Biochem* 1996;236:27–34.
161. Golumbic C, Mattill HA. Antioxidants and the autoxidation of fats. XIII. The antioxygenic action of ascorbic acid in association with tocopherols, hydroquinones and related compounds. *J Am Chem Soc* 1941;63:1279–1280.

162. Tappel AL, Brown WD, Zalkin H, Maier VP. Unsaturated lipid peroxidation catalyzed by hematin compounds and its inhibition by vitamin E. *J Am Oil Chem Soc* 1961;38:5–9.

163. Packer JE, Slater TF, Willson RL. Direct observation of a free radical interaction between vitamin E and vitamin C. *Nature* 1979;278:737–738.

164. McCay PB. Vitamin E: Interactions with free radicals and ascorbate. *Annu Rev Nutr* 1985;5:323–340.

165. Niki E. Interaction of ascorbate and alpha-tocopherol. *Ann NY Acad Sci* 1987;498:186–199.

166. Packer L, Kagan, VE. Vitamin E: The antioxidant harvesting center of membranes and lipoproteins. In: Fuchs J, Packer L, eds. *Vitamin E in Health and Disease*. New York: Marcel Dekker, 1993;179–192.

167. Burton, GW, Traber MG. Vitamin E: Antioxidant activity, biokinetics, and bioavailability. *Annu Rev Nutr* 1990;10:357–382.

168. Bowry VW, Stocker R. Tocopherol-mediated peroxidation. The pro-oxidant effect of vitamin E on the radical-initiated oxidation of human low-density lipoprotein. *J Am Chem Soc* 1993;115:6029–6044.

169. Barclay LRC. The cooperative antioxidant role of glutathione with a lipid-soluble and a water-soluble antioxidant during peroxidation of liposomes initiated in the aqueous phase and in the lipid phase. *J Biol Chem* 1988;263:16138–16142.

170. Chan AC, Tran K, Raynor T, Ganz PR, Chow CK. Regeneration of vitamin E in human platelets. *J Biol Chem* 1991;266:17290–17295.

171. Burton GW, Ingold KU, Foster DO. Comparison of free alpha-tocopherol and alpha-tocopherol acetate as sources of vitamin E in rats and humans. *Lipids* 1988;23:834–840.

172. Burton GW, Traber MG. Vitamin E antioxidant activity, biokinetics and bioavailability. *Ann. Rev. Nutrition* 1990;10:357–382.

173. Gensler HL, Magdaleno M. Topical vitamin E inhibition of immunosuppression and tumorigenesis induced by ultraviolet irradiation. *Nutr Cancer* 1991;15:97–106.

174. Farris MW, Pascoe GA, Reed DJ. Vitamin E reversal of the effect of extracellular calcium on chemically-induced toxicity in hepatocytes. *Science* 1985;227:751–754.

175. Glascott PA, Gilfor E, Farber, JL. Effects of vitamin E on the killing of cultured hepatocytes by *tert*-butyl hydroperoxide. *Mol Pharmacol* 1992;41:1155–1162.

176. Carini R, Poli G, Dianzani MU, Maddix SP, Slater TF, Cheeseman KH. Comparative evaluation of the antioxidant activity of alpha-tocopherol, alpha-tocopherol polyethylene glycol 1000 succinate and alpha-tocopherol succinate in isolated hepatocytes and liver microsomal suspensions. *Biochem Pharmacol* 1990;39:1597–1601.

177. Fariss MW. Oxygen toxicity: Unique cytoprotective properties of vitamin E succinate in hepatocytes. *Free Radical Biol Med* 1990;9:333–343.

178. Fariss MW, Bryson KF, Gu XY, Smith JD, Walton LP. Superior protection against oxidative injury with hydrophilic tocopherol esters in rat hepatocytes. *Toxicologist* 1995;15:160(abstract).

179. Harrison WH, Gander JE, Blakeley ER, Boyer PD. Interconversions of alpha-tocopherol and its oxidation products. *Biochim Biophys Acta* 1956;21:150–158.

180. Oxman MA, Cohen LA. Reductive cyclization of alpha-tocopherolquinone. *Biochim Biophys Acta* 1966;113:412–413.

181. Hayashi T, Kanetoshi A, Nakamura M, Tamura M, Shirahama H. Reduction of α-tocopherolquinone to a-tocopherolhydroquinone in rat hepatocytes. *Biochem Pharmacol* 1992;44:489–493.

182. Kohar I, Baca M, Suarna C, Stocker R, Southwell-Keely PT. Is α-tocopherol a reservoir for α-tocopherolhydroquinone? *Free Radical Biol Med* 1995;19:197–207.

183. Frei B. Reactive oxygen species and antioxidant vitamins: Mechanisms of action. *Am J Med* 1994;97:5S–13S.

184. Miller DM, Aust SD.. Studies of ascorbate-dependent, iron-catalyzed lipid peroxidation. *Arch Biochem Biophys* 1989;271:113–119.

185. Washko PW, Wang Y, Levine M. Ascorbic acid recycling in human neutrophils. *J Biol Chem* 1993;268:15531–15535.

186. Winkler BS, Orselli SM, Rex TS. The redox couple between glutathione and ascorbic acid: A chemical and physiological perspective. *Free Radical Biol Med* 1994;17:333–349.

187. Wells, WW, Xu, DP, Ynag, Y Rocque, PA. Mammalian thioltransferase (glutatredoxin) and protein disulfide isomerase have dehydroascorbate reductase activity. *J Biol Chem* 1990;265:15361–15364.

188. Reed DJ. Interaction of vitamin E, ascorbic acid, and glutathione in protection against oxidative stress. In: Packer L, ed. *Vitamin E in Health and Disease*. New York: Marcel Dekker, 1992;269–281.

PART III

Selected Examples of Free-Radical-Mediated Tissue Injury

Free Radical Toxicology
Edited by K. B. Wallace
Copyright © 1997 Taylor & Francis

9

Free-Radical-Mediated Liver Injury

Gabriel L. Plaa

*Professor Emeritus Département de pharmacologie, Faculté de médecine,
Université de Montréal, Montréal, Québec, Canada*

It is now commonly held that chemically induced hepatotoxicity, in most instances, is the result of a series of biochemical disruptions due to the appearance of reactive metabolites during the process of biotransformation of the particular chemical involved. The putative chemical species in most cases, however, has not necessarily been identified, but the cascade of events leading to hepatocellular dysfunction is usually reasonably well described based on in vitro and in vivo studies. Nevertheless, what is noticeably lacking, in particular for necrogenic hepatotoxicants, is which of the disruptive intracellular events is ultimately responsible for irreversible cell death in vivo.

Free radicals have been recognized as important biotransformation products known to participate in the pathogenesis of chemically induced liver injury in animals and humans. Perhaps the best studied chemical substance in this regard is the trichloromethyl free radical emanating from carbon tetrachloride. Other free radicals associated with other chemical agents, however, also have been investigated. The purpose of this chapter is not to cover the association of free radicals with chemically induced liver injury in depth. Nor does it deal with reactive metabolites that are not associated with free radicals. Rather, the purpose of this chapter is to illustrate with four different agents—carbon tetrachloride, ethanol, halothane, and acetaminophen—how free radicals have been shown to be involved in the hepatotoxic responses associated with each of these chemical substances.

CARBON TETRACHLORIDE

In a seminal work published in 1961, Butler (1) demonstrated that carbon tetrachloride, administered to dogs, could be reduced in vivo to yield chloroform as a metabolite. He exposed phenobarbital-anesthetized dogs to carbon tetrachloride for a period of 3 h; the expired air was trapped for the subsequent 2 h. A microdistillate of the trapped air was analyzed by gas chromatography and shown to contain fractions that possessed the characteristics of carbon tetrachloride and chloroform.

Additional chemical evidence of identity was obtained by subjecting selected samples of the effluent to the Fujiwara reaction; the development of the crimson color in the fractions and analysis of the absorption spectra confirmed that the material in one of the fractions was chloroform. When carbon tetrachloride was incubated with mouse liver homogenate in vitro, chloroform was formed; the activity diminished, but was not abolished, when the homogenate was heat treated, indicating the presence of enzymatic and nonenzymatic pathways.

Butler postulated that both heterolytic and homolytic fission of the carbon-chlorine bond could be envisioned as possible mechanisms leading to the formation of chloroform from carbon tetrachloride in vivo (1). He favored the position that homolytic fission of the carbon-chlorine bond, leading to the formation of a free radical, occurred in vivo. He further speculated that the high reactivity of the product could be responsible for biochemical derangements that would be injurious to the cell. He suggested that carbon tetrachloride "produced toxic effects on the liver cell not through physical interactions of the unchanged drug molecules with cellular constituents but by virtue of their chemical reactivity." The alkylation of sulfhydryl groups, with the ensuing biochemical consequences, was suggested as a possible reaction responsible for necrotizing effects in the liver.

The homolytic process suggested by Butler (1) was pursued as a hypothetical mechanism of action by Wirtschafter and Cronyn (2), not only for carbon tetrachloride toxicity, but also for other solvents. They studied the hepatotoxic properties of different halogenated hydrocarbons, as had Plaa et al. (3), and suggested that the free-radical reaction could be considered, not as a unimolecular process, but at least as a bimolecular process: a bond-breaking step, coupled with a bond-forming process. They concluded (2) that the relative hepatotoxic potencies of the seven halogenated hydrocarbons previously described (3) corresponded well to the expected reactivity toward a free-radical source.

The theoretical idea of activation of carbon tetrachloride via a free radical was also pursued by Slater (4), who was struck by the fact that a number of diverse chemicals or processes could protect against the necrotic effects of the haloalkane. He speculated that an activation stage consisting of a free-radical form might induce the formation of other free radicals by a chain reaction, which then could result in severe damage near the site of formation. He suggested that the carbon tetrachloride-derived free radical, in the presence of lipid membranes, could eventually lead to peroxidation resulting in necrosis or accumulation of fat. Furthermore, Slater suggested (4) that the endoplasmic reticulum might be more sensitive to damage by free-radical attack because this structure was bounded by a single lipoprotein membrane.

In 1965, before the appearance of Slater's speculative writing, Recknagel and Ghoshal published an abstract (*Fed Proc* 1965;24:abstr 942, cited in ref. 4) describing their discovery that lipid peroxidation occurred in rats after carbon tetrachloride exposure. The work was later published in full (5) and would become the first of a long series of articles emanating from Recknagel's laboratory. In this first work, they demonstrated that diene conjugation, typical of peroxidized polyenoic fatty acids, appeared in microsomal lipids 90 min after rats were exposed to carbon tetrachloride (2.5 ml/kg, po). Furthermore, the haloalkane was shown to act as a pro-oxidant in vitro (followed by malonaldehyde production) when incubated with rat liver microsome-supernatant fractions; the pro-oxidant effect could be counteracted by the addition of α-tocopheryl acetate. The pro-oxidant properties of carbon tetrachloride were not evident in rat brain or rat kidney. These observations, based on the assumption that activation of carbon tetrachloride occurred via the formation of a free radical, supported the hypothesis that homolytic cleavage led to an attack on the methylene bridges of unsaturated fatty acid side chains of microsomal structural lipids, thus initiating peroxidative degeneration.

The lipid peroxidation theory of liver injury is beyond the scope of the present chapter. One can say, however, that the concept has dominated the field of hepatotoxicity for over 25 years, not only for carbon tetrachloride but also for other toxicants. Some investigators thought of the possibility that it might be a more general mechanism of hepatotoxic action. Klaassen and Plaa (6) studied the dose-response relationships of four halogenated hydrocarbons. They confirmed the presence of conjugated dienes in vivo after administration of carbon tetrachloride, and also the depression of glucose 6-phosphatase activity as described by Recknagel's group, but were unable to show the presence of conjugated dienes after chloroform doses sufficiently large to produce steatosis and necrosis; glucose 6-phosphatase was unaffected. They concluded that depression of glucose 6-phosphatase was not a sensitive index of liver injury for all necrogenic substances. Brown et al. (7) reported that rats pretreated with phenobarbital, but not untreated rats, produced conjugated dienes after chloroform exposure; Lavigne and Marchand (8) independently made similar observations. Since chloroform-induced liver injury is more severe in phenobarbital-pretreated rats, the possibility exists that the initial lesion in these animals was only aggravated by the appearance of lipid peroxidation. These findings cast doubt on the general applicability of lipid peroxidation as a mechanism for necrogenic halogenated hydrocarbons. While there is no doubt that lipid peroxidation does occur with some hepatotoxicants, it is evident that with others this component is either absent or of doubtful significance. Lipid peroxidation as a general mechanism of action for hepatotoxicants is less attractive than it was several years ago. The later writings of Recknagel et al. (9) put lipid peroxidation into perspective, even for carbon tetrachloride. They include the possibility that the covalent binding of carbon tetrachloride-derived cleavage products, as well as lipid peroxidation at or near cytochrome P-450, can evoke secondary mechanisms that finally result in end-stage pathological consequences. They state that there are "grounds for caution against undue enthusiasm in favor of generation of toxic lipids or their breakdown products as a dominant mechanism responsible for spread of injury from pin-point sites in the ER to other parts of the cell."

The reactive metabolites of carbon tetrachloride are also known to bind covalently to hepatic macromolecules. Binding to lipids, proteins, and nucleic acids has all been demonstrated (10). Binding to cytochrome P-450, leading to its destruction, occurs very rapidly in vivo. Castro (10) has been a proponent of covalent binding of carbon tetrachloride free radical as an important element of the hepatotoxic mechanism of action of this agent; he recognizes, however, that lipid peroxidation is also of importance.

The trichloromethyl free radical ($\cdot CCl_3$) was successfully identified by spin trapping in rat liver microsomes incubated with carbon tetrachloride and in livers from rats treated with the haloalkane (11, 12). Trichloromethyl free radical reacts extremely rapidly with oxygen to yield a highly reactive trichloromethylperoxy free radical ($\cdot CCl_3O_2$). This species is said to be the initiator of lipid peroxidation (11). In the perfused liver, the carbon dioxide anion radical ($\cdot CO_2^-$) has been described (13,14) following exposure to carbon tetrachloride; the α-phenyl *tert*-butyl nitrone (PBN) adduct of this radical was also identified in the urine of rats treated with the haloalkane. Consequently, the free radical can be formed in vivo. There was a good correlation between the appearance of the radical and hepatotoxicity (14). Nevertheless, the role that the carbon dioxide anion radical may play in carbon tetrachloride-induced cell death is yet to be established; it may only serve as a marker for other radical metabolites of the haloalkane (14).

Regarding some of the reactions subsequent to the formation of trichloromethyl free radical, the source of the hydrogen atom in the chloroform generated anaerobically by the trichloromethyl free radical was studied by Cunningham et al. (15). They demonstrated that the hydrogen atom is produced due to the attack of the free radical on saturated and unsaturated fatty acids; addition of quenchers of free-radical reactions reduced the chloroform production. The mechanism of the reductive inactivation of cytochrome P-450 was investigated by Manno et al. (16). During anaerobic incubation, cytochrome P-450 can be destroyed, even in the absence of lipid peroxidation, and the tetrapyrrolic system of the heme moiety is irreversibly affected by the metabolites of carbon tetrachloride. Although dichlorocarbene ($:CCl_2$) can be formed at the same site, it appears that the trichloromethyl free radical, and not the carbene, is responsible for cytochrome P-450 destruction.

ETHANOL

As with carbon tetrachloride, the interest in an association of free radicals in ethanol-induced liver injury stems, in part, from early observations suggesting that lipid peroxidation might occur in acute ethanol toxicity. DiLuzio and collaborators provided evidence of lipid peroxidation (17,18). Unlike carbon tetrachloride, however, lipid peroxidation as a vector in ethanol hepatotoxicity was not supported by all investigators (19–21). It is not within the scope of this chapter to discuss the various observations pro or con for lipid peroxidation. Suffice it to say that the issue remains less definitive than in the case of carbon tetrachloride, but much of the evidence favors the presence of lipid peroxidation in ethanol hepatotoxicity (21–24).

Albano et al. (25) demonstrated with spin trapping techniques that liver microsomes incubated with ethanol produced the hydroxyethyl free radical, and that its formation was dependent on the presence of cytochrome P-450 activity. Reduced glutathione effectively scavenged the radical. The intensity of the electron spin resonance (ESR) signals of the hydroxyethyl radical adduct was also enhanced in liver microsomes obtained from rats fed 10% ethanol in drinking water for 6 wk. It had been suggested that ethanol might interact with preformed free radicals to yield an ethoxyl radical, but the results obtained by Albano et al. (25) showed that the radical was a carbon-centered hydroxylethyl radical. Knecht et al. (26) were the first to detect the alpha-hydroxylethyl free radical from the bile of alcohol dehydrogenase-deficient deermice given ethanol. Later, the same group isolated the same free radical from the bile of rats consuming ethanol for at least 2 wk (27); the ESR signal intensity correlated with hepatotoxicity. The presence of the radical in the liver of rats after a single ethanol administration by gavage was also reported (28). Cytochrome P-4502E1 is largely responsible for the generation of hydroxyethyl free radical (29). Nevertheless, substrate inhibition studies and experiments performed with P-4502E1-directed antibodies indicated that ESR signals were not decreased by more than 50% compared to normal conditions, suggesting that other P-450 isoforms might also generate the radical. McCay et al. (30) suggested that the biotransformation of ethanol to 1-hydroxyethyl radical also may be mediated in part by hydroxyl radicals produced in a hydrogen peroxide-dependent reaction (hydrogen atom abstraction from ethanol by the hydroxyl radical).

There is also evidence that ethanol intoxication may result in oxidative stress (31–33). Generation of reactive oxygen species (ROS) at cytosolic sites is suggested as accompanying ethanol toxicity. Enhanced superoxide anion production by perfused rat livers was demonstrated after ethanol infusion and likely mediated through arachidonic acid (34). A role for Kupffer cells in these events has been suggested (27,34).

The free radicals generated during ethanol biotransformation are believed to participate in the pathogenesis of ethanol-induced liver injury. As mentioned previously, acute ethanol intoxication can lead to lipid peroxidation (17,18,24), but its role in the pathogenesis of ethanol-induced liver injury is still not well explained. Much more recently, Albano et al. (35) found that chronic ethanol feeding of rats led to increased covalent binding to microsomal protein, but a role in ethanol liver damage is yet to be established. Now that it is known that free radicals are produced from ethanol, one needs to show the toxicological consequences of this event.

HALOTHANE

Lipid peroxidation was observed in hepatic microsomes from phenobarbital-pretreated rats when the pO_2 was below 10 mm Hg (36, 37). This was observed when using malondialdehyde formation or conjugated dienes as indices of lipid peroxidation, accompanied by a 70% loss of microsomal glucose 6-phosphatase activity. When the pO_2 was above 10 mm Hg lipid peroxidation was not observed (36). The effects were attributed to the reductive formation of halothane-derived free radicals ($\cdot CF_3CHCl$) during hypoxia. Lipid peroxidation was also observed in rats in vivo (38, 39); in one study (38) ethane exhalation was the index of lipid peroxidation. Akita et al. (40) showed that treatment of guinea pigs with an inhibitor of cytochrome P-450 (metyrapone) or with a radical trapping agent (BPN) inhibited halothane-induced lipid peroxidation and the incidence or severity of liver injury. Thus it was clear that lipid peroxidation could occur after halothane exposure and that the generation of free radicals was a likely possibility.

Cheeseman et al. (11) described that pulse radiolysis could generate the 1-chloro-2,2,2-trifluoro-1-ethyl radical ($\cdot CF_3CHCl$) from halothane and that this radical reacts rapidly with oxygen to form the $CF_3CHClO_2\cdot$ radical, a radical thought capable of initiating lipid peroxidation if formed in vivo. Janzen et al. (41) used the spin trapping method and detected $\cdot CF_3CHCl$ as well as a carbon-centered radical with a partially assigned structure $\cdot CH_2R$ and an oxygen-centered radical of the $\cdot OR'$ type. Radical adducts arising from the reductive debromination of halothane were detected in bile from hypoxic rats after halothane administration (42).

The relationship of these findings to the hepatotoxic effects of halothane are not clear. The anesthetic produces two different types of hepatotoxic responses in humans. One is a rather mild type of liver injury and is said (43) to occur soon after exposure in about 10–20% of patients exposed to halothane. The second type of injury is much rarer (an incidence of around 1/10,000), later in onset, and a much more severe form, in which an immune mechanism is likely involved (44,45). Although the severe form does depend on the biotransformation of halothane to a reactive acyl chloride (CF_3COCl) that reacts with lysine residues to form trifluoroacetylated (TFA) proteins (45) (the neoantigens cause antibody generation in susceptible humans), the role of free radicals in the process is yet to be investigated. Even with the milder form of liver injury, no studies have been performed to see what role, if any, the free radicals play in the human lesion.

ACETAMINOPHEN

The classic studies of Gillette and collaborators (46–49) set the pattern for investigating the effects of reactive metabolites in acetaminophen hepatotoxicity. Their work showed that drug metabolism was involved (46), that reactive metabolites resulted in covalent binding to macromolecules (47,48), and that glutathione played a key role in the protection of the liver from severe necrogenic injury (49). In isolated hepatocytes, others demonstrated that acetaminophen could promote production of malondialdehyde and conjugated dienes (50). Furthermore, perfusion of mouse livers with the agent resulted in the production of ethane (51). Although some have postulated that lipid peroxidation is part of the hepatotoxic profile of acetaminophen, Kamiyama et al. (52) concluded that it plays a minimal role in rats (1 g/kg, ip), since liver conjugated dienes were unaffected 2 h after treatment; in the same experiments, however, they showed that carbon tetrachloride (1 ml/kg, ip) did result in lipid peroxidation. On the other hand, increased hepatic malondialdehyde was observed by Muriel et al. (53) 4–6 h after acetaminophen intoxication in rats; this effect of acetaminophen was abolished by pretreating the animals with silymarin, an antioxidant. Amimoto et al. (54) found evidence for lipid peroxidation in mice, accompanied by a loss in the reduced form of coenzymes Q_9 and Q_{10}, and reduced glutathione; they concluded that oxidative stress was a component of acetaminophen toxicity in mice. Finally, the presence of oxidative stress was demonstrated (55) in mice within 15 min after treatment with acetaminophen, using liver chemiluminescence and hydrogen peroxide concentrations as endpoints; microsomal superoxide production was enhanced by the presence of acetaminophen.

de Vries is credited (56) with the suggestion (57) that acetaminophen-induced liver injury might be due to a cytochrome P-450-mediated one-electron oxidation to form a semi-iminoquinone radical; the radical might then generate reactive oxygen radicals when proceeding on to *N*-acetyl-*p*-benzoquinone imine (NAPQI). Nelson and collaborators demonstrated (58,59) that a free radical species was detected by ESR spectroscopy; covalent binding to mouse liver proteins was observed, and the NAPQI and hydroquinone were suggested as the reactive species. The semi-iminoquinone radical has been generated and studied by pulse radiolysis (56). The further reaction of NAPQI with oxygen to generate superoxide radical, however, was looked for but not found in the study. A mechanistic scheme was proposed for the metabolic biotransformation to NAPQI (60), consisting of an initial abstraction of a single electron from acetaminophen at the phenolic hydroxyl group to yield an oxygen-centered radical; this scheme is an alternative to others that consist of sequential one-electron transfers. Carbon-centered radicals are proposed for the pathways leading to *p*-benzoquinone and 3-hydroxyacetaminophen, two metabolites of acetaminophen. Discussion of these schemes is beyond the scope of the present brief review, and the interested reader is referred to Hoffmann et al. (60).

There is a general assumption that the hepatotoxic consequences of acetaminophen intoxication are due to NAPQI, the reactive metabolite. Consequently, one could raise the question of whether the intermediate free radicals that occur during the biotransformation of the agent are of toxicological importance; this is apart from the oxidative stress that accompanies the intoxication. The experimental evidence on this point is rather sparse. Harman et al. (61), however, compared the cytotoxic properties of both NAPQI and acetaminophen in parallel studies with cultured hepatic cells. Using the same criteria of oxidative stress for both agents, they concluded that acetaminophen injured cultured hepatocytes by oxidative stress, but that NAPQI did not. The data indicated that acetaminophen and NAPQI are both cytotoxic to cultured hepatocytes but by different mechanisms. These authors speculated that exogenously administered NAPQI might not be a reliable model to pursue the mechanism of action of acetaminophen. Along similar lines, Holme et al. (62) compared the cytotoxic effects of acetaminophen (*N*-acetyl-*p*-aminophenol, APAP), a nonhepatotoxic regioisomer (*N*-acetyl-*m*-aminophenol, AMAP) and their postulated reactive hydroquinone and quinone metabolites in cultured mouse hepatocytes. The found that the relative toxic potencies of the hydroquinone and quinone metabolites of AMAP were comparable to that of NAPQI, yet the cytotoxicity of the parent compounds (AMAP and APAP) differed markedly (10-fold) from each other.

The covalent binding characteristics of acetaminophen have also been studied. As stated previously, Gillette and collaborators were the first to associate acetaminophen hepatotoxicity with covalent binding of acetaminophen-derived material (47,48). Others examined (63–65) the covalent binding of acetaminophen to hepatic proteins and identified two cytosolic protein adducts. Holtzman, however, investigated microsomal protein adducts, which he felt correlated better with acetaminophen toxicity (66). He and his collaborators found that acetaminophen-derived material binds to forms Q-2 and Q-5 of thiol:protein oxidoreductases (TPDO) and to the major hepatic microsomal Ca^{2+}-binding protein, calreticulin; they suggested that the binding of NAPQI to an ϵ-amino lysine group of Q-2 may be a critical event. Furthermore, TPDOs within the lumen of the endoplasmic reticulum might be inhibited and Holtzman sensed (66) that hepatotoxicity is "not due to the immediate inactivation of critical elements, such as the TPDOs, but rather to the failure of the protein synthetic or repair pathways to replace proteins during their natural turnover." Despite these studies, one needs to know which acetaminophen-derived chemical species is binding to the various proteins.

REFERENCES

1. Butler TC. Reduction of carbon tetrachloride in vivo and reduction of carbon tetrachloride and chloroform in vitro by tissues and tissue constituents. *J Pharmacol Exp Ther* 1961;134:311–319.
2. Wirtschafter ZT, Cronyn, MW. A free radical mechanism for solvent toxicity. *Arch Environ Health* 1964;9:186–191.
3. Plaa GL, Evans EA, Hine, CH. Relative hepatotoxicity of seven halogenated hydrocarbons. *J Pharmacol Exp Ther* 1958;123:224–229.
4. Slater TF. Necrogenic action of carbon tetrachloride in the rat: A speculative mechanism based on activation. *Nature* 1966;209:36–40.
5. Recknagel RO, Ghoshal AK. Lipoperoxidation as a vector in carbon tetrachloride hepatotoxicity. *Lab Invest* 1966;15:132–148.
6. Klaassen CD, Plaa GL. Comparison of the biochemical alterations elicited in livers from rats treated with carbon tetrachloride, chloroform, 1,1,2-trichloroethane and 1,1,1-trichloroethane. *Biochem Pharmacol* 1969;18:2019–2027.
7. Brown BR Jr, Sipes IG, Sagalyn AM. Mechanisms of acute hepatic toxicity: Chloroform, halothane, and glutathione. *Anesthesiology* 1974;41:554–561.
8. Lavigne JG, Marchand C. The role of metabolism in chloroform hepatotoxicity. *Toxicol Appl Pharmacol* 1974;29:312–326.
9. Recknagel RO, Glende, EA Jr, Waller RL., Lowrey K. Lipid peroxidation: Biochemistry, measurement, and significance in liver cell injury. In: Plaa GL, Hewitt WR, eds. *Toxicology of the Liver.* New York: Raven Press, 1982;213–241.
10. Castro JA. Mechanistical studies and prevention of free radical cell injury. In: Paton W, Mitchell J, Turner P, eds. *IUPHAR 9th International Congress of Pharmacology, Proceedings.* London: Macmillan Press, 1984;2:243–250.
11. Cheeseman KH, Albano EF, Tomasi A, Slater TF. Biochemical studies on the metabolic activation of halogenated alkanes. *Environ Health Perspect* 1985;64:85–101.
12. Janzen EG, Towner, RA, Krygsman PH, Lai EK, Poyer JL, Brueggemann G, McCay PB. Mass spectroscopy and chromatography of the trichloromethyl radical adduct of phenyl *tert*-butyl nitrone. *Free Radical Res Commun* 1990;9:3–6.
13. Connor HD, Thurman RG, Galizi MD, Mason RP. The formation of a novel free radical metabolite from CCl_4 in the perfused rat liver and in vivo. *J Biol Chem* 1986;261:4542–4548.
14. LaCagnin LB, Connor HD, Mason RP, Thurman RG. The carbon dioxide anion radical adduct in the perfused rat liver: relationship to halocarbon-induced toxicity. *Mol Pharmacol* 1988;33:351–357.
15. Cunningham ML, Chang, SY, Sipes, IG. Covalent adduct formation and chloroform production after

free radical attack on fatty acids by carbon tetrachloride reactive intermediates. *Toxicology* 1985;37;297–305.

16. Manno M, DeMatteis F, King LJ. The mechanism of the suicidal, reductive inactivation of microsomal cytochrome P-450 by carbon tetrachloride. *Biochem Pharmacol* 1988;37:1981–1990.
17. DiLuzio NR, Kalish GH. Enhanced peroxidation of lipid in the pathogenesis of acute ethanol-induced liver injury. *Gastroenterology* 1966;50:392–396.
18. Comporti M, Hartman A, DiLuzio NR. Effect of in vivo and in vitro ethanol administration on liver lipid peroxidation. *Lab Invest* 1967;16:616–624.
19. Hashimoto S, Recknagel RO. No chemical evidence of hepatic peroxidation in acute ethanol toxicity. *Exp Mol Pathol* 1968;8:225–242.
20. Inomata T, Rao GA, Tsukamoto H. Lack of evidence for increased lipid peroxidation in ethanol-induced liver injury. *Liver* 1987;7:233–239.
21. Plaa GL, Witschi HP. Chemicals, drugs, and lipid peroxidation. *Annu Rev Pharmacol Toxicol* 1976;16:125–141.
22. Reinke LA, McCay PB. Free radicals and alcohol liver injury. In: Watson RR, ed. *Drug and Alcohol Abuse Reviews, Vol 2: Liver Pathology and Alcohol.* Clifton, NJ: Humana Press, 1991;133–168.
23. Nordmann R. Alcohol and antioxidant systems. *Alcohol Alcoholism* 1994;29:513–522.
24. Lieber CS. Mechanisms of ethanol-drug-nutrition interactions. *Clin Toxicol* 1994;32:631–681.
25. Albano E, Tomasi A, Goria-Gatti L, Dianzani MU. Spin trapping of free radical species produced during the microsomal metabolism of ethanol. *Chem Biol Interact* 1988;65:223–234.
26. Knecht KT, Bradford BU, Mason RP, Thurman RG. In vivo formation of a free radical metabolite of ethanol. *Mol Pharmacol* 1990;38:26–30.
27. Knecht KT, Adachi Y, Bradford BU, Iimuro Y, Kadiiska M, Qun-Hui X, Thurman RG. Free radical adducts in the bile of rats treated chronically with intragastric alcohol: Inhibition by destruction of Kupffer cells. *Mol Pharmacol* 1995;47:1028–1034.
28. Reinke LA, Kotake Y, McCay PB, Janzen EG. Spin-trapping studies of hepatic free radicals formed following the acute administration of ethanol to rats: in vivo detection of 1-hydroxyethyl radicals with PBN. *Free Radical Biol Med* 1991;11:31–39.
29. Albano E, Tomasi A, Persson, J-O, Terelius Y, Goria-Gatti L, Ingelman-Sundberg M, Dianzani MU. Role of ethanol-inducible cytochrome P450 (P450IIE1) in catalyzing the free radical activation of aliphatic alcohols. *Biochem Pharmacol* 1991;41:1895–1902.
30. McCay PB, Reinke LA, Rau JM. Hydroxyl radicals are generated by hepatic microsomes during NADPH oxidation: Relationship to ethanol metabolism. *Free Radical Res Commun* 1992;15:335–346.
31. Bondy SC. Ethanol toxicity and oxidative stress. *Toxicol Lett* 1992;63:231–241.
32. Younes M, Wagner H, Strubelt O. Enhancement of acute ethanol hepatotoxicity under conditions of low oxygen supply and ischemia/reperfusion—The role of oxygen radicals. *Biochem Pharmacol* 1989;38;3573–3581.
33. Kurase I, Higuchi H, Kato S, Miura S, Ishii H. Ethanol-induced oxidative stress in the liver. *Alcohol Clin Exp Res* 1996;20(suppl S):A77–A85.
34. Bautista AP, Spitzer JJ. Acute ethanol intoxication stimulates superoxide anion production by in situ perfused rat liver. *Hepatology* 1992;15:892–898.
35. Albano E, Parola M, Comoglio A, Dianzani MU. Evidence for the covalent binding of hydroxyethyl radicals to rat liver microsomal proteins. *Alcohol Alcoholism* 1993;28:453–459.
36. de Groot H, Noll T. The crucial role of hypoxia in halothane-induced lipid peroxidation. *Biochem Biophys Res Commun* 1984;119:139–143.
37. de Groot H, Noll T. Halothane-induced lipid peroxidation and glucose-6-phosphatase inactivation in microsomes under hypoxic conditions. *Anesthesiology* 1985;62:44–48.
38. Siegers CP, Heger B, Baretton G, Younes M. Inhibition of halothane-induced lipid peroxidation by misoprostol without hepatoprotection. *Toxicology* 1988;53:213–218.
39. Younes M, Heger B, Wilhelm KP, Siegers CP. Enhanced in vivo-lipid peroxidation associated with halothane hepatotoxicity in rats. *Pharmacol Toxicol* 1988;63:52–56.
40. Akita S, Morio M, Kawahara M, Takeshita T, Fujii K, Yamamoto N. Halothane-induced liver injury as a consequence of enhanced microsomal lipid peroxidation in guinea pigs. *Res Commun Chem Pathol Pharmacol* 1988;61:227–243.
41. Janzen EG, Towner RA, Krygsman PH, Haire DL, Poyer JL. Structure identification of free radicals by ESR and GC/MS of PBN spin adducts from the in vitro and in vivo rat liver metabolism of halothane. *Free Radical Res Commun* 1990;9:343–351.

42. Knecht KT, DeGray JA, Mason RP. Free radical metabolism of halothane in vivo: Radical adducts detected in bile. *Mol Pharmacol* 1992;41:943–949.
43. Frost L, Mahoney J, Field J, Farrell GC. Impaired bile flow and disordered hepatic calcium homeostasis are early features of halothane-induced liver injury in guinea pigs. *Hepatology* 1996;23:80–86.
44. Gut J, Christen U, Huwyler J. Mechanisms of halothane toxicity: Novel insights. *Pharmacol Ther* 1993;58:133–155.
45. Pessayre D. Role of reactive metabolites in drug-induced hepatitis. *J Hepatol* 1995;23(Suppl 1):16–24.
46. Mitchell JR, Jollow DJ, Potter WZ, Davis DC, Gillette JR, Brodie BB. Acetaminophen-induced hepatic necrosis. I. Role of drug metabolism. *J Pharmacol Exp Ther* 1973;187:185–194.
47. Jollow DJ, Mitchell JR, Potter WZ, Davis DC, Gillette JR, Brodie BB. Acetaminophen-induced hepatic necrosis. II. Role of covalent binding in vivo. *J Pharmacol Exp Ther* 1973;187:195–202.
48. Potter WZ, Davis DC, Mitchell JR, Jollow DJ, Gillette JR, Brodie BB. Acetaminophen-induced hepatic necrosis. III. Cytochrome P-450-mediated covalent binding in vitro. *J Pharmacol Exp Ther* 1973;187:203–209.
49. Mitchell JR, Jollow DJ, Potter WZ, Gillette JR, Brodie BB. Acetaminophen-induced hepatic necrosis. IV. Protective role of glutathione. *J Pharmacol Exp Ther* 1973;187:211–217.
50. Albano E, Poli G, Chiarpotte E, Biasi F, Dianzani MU. Paracetamol-stimulated lipid peroxidation in isolated rat and mouse hepatocytes. *Chem Biol Interact* 1983;47:249–263.
51. de Vries J. Hepatotoxic metabolic activation of paracetamol and its derivatives phenacetin and benorilate: Oxygenation or electron capture? *Biochem Pharmacol* 1981;30:399–402.
52. Kamiyama T, Sato C, Liu J, Tajiri K, Miyakawa H, Marumo F. Role of lipid peroxidation in acetaminophen-induced hepatotoxicity: Comparison with carbon tetrachloride. *Toxicol Lett* 1993;66:7–12.
53. Muriel P, Garciapina T, Perez-Alvarez V, Mourelle M. Silymarin protects against paracetamol-induced lipid peroxidation and liver damage. *J Appl Toxicol* 1992;12:439–442.
54. Amimoto T, Matsura T, Koyama, S-Y, Nakanishi T, Yamada K, Kajiyama G. Acetaminophen-induced hepatic injury in mice: The role of lipid peroxidation and effects of pretreatment with coenzyme Q_{10} and α-tocopherol. *Free Radical Biol Med* 1995;19:169–176.
55. Arnaiz SL, Llesuy S, Cutrin JC, Boveris A. Oxidative stress by acute acetaminophen administration in mouse liver. *Free Radical Biol Med* 1995;19:303–310.
56. Bisby RH, Tabassum N. Properties of the radicals formed by one-electron oxidation of acetaminophen-A pulse radiolysis study. *Biochem Pharmacol* 1988;37:2731–2738.
57. de Vries J. Hepatotoxic metabolic activation of paracetamol and its derivatives phenacetin and benorilate: Oxygenation or electron transfer? Biochem Pharmacol 1981;30:399–402.
58. Nelson SD, Dahlin DC, Rauckman EJ, Rosen GM. Peroxidase-mediated formation of reactive metabolites of acetaminophen. *Mol Pharmacol* 1984;20:195–199.
59. Dahlin DC, Miwa GT, Lu AYH, Nelson SD. *N*-Acetyl-*p*-benzoquinone imine: A cytochrome P-450-mediated oxidation product of acetaminophen. *Proc Natl Acad Sci USA* 1984;81:1327–1331.
60. Hoffmann K-J, Axworthy DB, Baillie, TA. Mechanistic studies on the metabolic activation of acetaminophen in vivo. *Chem Res Toxicol* 1990;3:204–211.
61. Harman AW, Kyle ME, Serroni A, Farber JL. The killing of cultured hepatocytes by *N*-acetyl-*p*-benzoquinone imine (NAPQI) as a model of the cytotoxicity of acetaminophen. *Biochem Pharmacol* 1991;41:1111–1117.
62. Holme JA, Hongslo JK, Bjorge C, Nelson SD. Comparative cytotoxic effects of acetaminophen (*N*-acetyl-*p*-aminophenol), a non-hepatotoxic regioisomer acetyl-*m*-aminophenol and their postulated reactive hydroquinone and quinone metabolites in monolayer cultures of mouse hepatocytes. *Biochem Pharmacol* 1991;42:1137–1142.
63. Birge RB, Bulera SJ, Bartolone JB, Ginsberg GL, Cohen SD, Khairallah EA. The arylation of microsomal membrane proteins by acetaminophen is associated with the release of a 44 kDa acetaminophen-binding mouse liver protein complex into the cytosol. *Toxicol Appl Pharmacol* 1991; 109:443–454.
64. Bartolone JB, Birge RB, Bulera SJ, Bruno NK, Nishanian EV, Cohen SD, Khairallah EA. Purification, antibody production, and partial amino acid sequence of the 58-kDa acetaminophen-binding liver proteins. *Toxicol Appl Pharmacol* 1992;113:19–29.
65. Pumford NR, Martin BM, Hinson JA. A metabolite of acetaminophen covalently binds to the 56 kDa selenium binding protein. *Biochem Biophys Res Commun* 1992;182:1348–1355.
66. Holtzman JL. The role of covalent binding to microsomal proteins in the hepatotoxicity of acetaminophen. *Drug Metab Rev* 1995;27:277–297.

Free Radical Toxicology
Edited by K. B. Wallace
Copyright © 1997 Taylor & Francis

10

Free-Radical-Mediated Kidney Injury

J. Fred Nagelkerke and Bob van de Water

*Leiden/Amsterdam Center for Drug Research, Division of Toxicology,
Leiden University, Leiden, The Netherlands*

RENAL MORPHOLOGY AND PHYSIOLOGY IN RELATION TO NEPHROTOXICITY

Major functions of the kidney are related to its role in maintaining the homeostasis of the internal environment. For instance, the kidneys excrete waste products and regulate the electrolyte and acid–base balance. In addition, several regulatory compounds (e.g., renin, erythropoietin, and 1,25-dihydroxy-vitamin D_3) are produced and processed in the kidney (1,2).

The smallest functional unit is the nephron (Figure 1); the kidneys contain 10^4 to 10^6 nephrons (depending on the species). A nephron consist of several distinct parts: the glomerulus, the proximal tubule, the intermediate tubule, the distal tubule, and the collecting duct. It stretches from the outer cortex (glomerulus) deep into the medulla (intermediate tubule), back to the cortex (distal tubule and collecting tubule) (3). Each part of the nephron has its own specialized function.

Some 20% of the incoming renal plasma flow is filtered by the glomeruli to produce an ultrafiltrate. This represents 2–3% of the cardiac output. The ultrafiltrate contains all blood components with a molecular weight below roughly 50 kD, or a size smaller than 75–100 Å when it enters the tubular lumen at the glomerulus. The proximal tubule reabsorbs about 50–60% of the ultrafiltrate. The proximal tubular cells secrete waste products, while nutrients (for instance proteins, peptides, amino acids, and glucose), as well as cations, anions and water, are reabsorbed. In addition these cells possess specific organic ion carriers, which transport compounds from the blood into the tubular lumen. The intermediate tubule is also involved in concentrating the urine: 20–30% of the filtered sodium and potassium, and 15–20% of the filtered water are reabsorbed. In the distal tubule most of the remaining water and sodium is removed, whereas potassium is either secreted or reabsorbed, depending on the need. Finally, the collecting duct also reabsorbs water and sodium, although its contribution is quite small compared to that of the distal tubule.

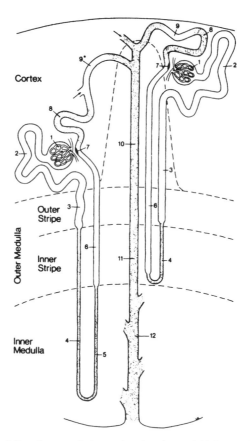

FIG. 1. Scheme depicting the morphology of a short-looped (right) and a long-looped (left) nephron and the location of the different nephron segments within the kidney. Not drawn to scale. Numbers indicate: 1, renal corpuscle including Bowman's capsule and the glomerulus; 2, proximal convoluted tubule consisting of the S_1 and S_2 segment; 3, proximal straight tubule; 4, descending thin limb; 5, ascending thin limb; 6, distal straight tubule; 7, macula densa located within the final portion of the thick ascending limb; 8, distal convoluted tubule; 9, connecting tubule; 10, cortical collecting tubule; 11, outer medullary collecting duct; 12, inner medullary collecting duct. Reprinted from Ref. 3, p. F8, with permission.

Obviously, the transport processes in the kidney cells result in an extensive exposure of the various renal cells to toxicants present in the circulation. For a number of reasons, the cells lining the proximal tubule are especially the target for a wide variety of toxicants. Not only are these the first cells that come into contact with toxicants present in the glomerular filtrate, but also the concentration of a toxicant in the tubulus can increase severalfold due to the reabsorption of water. In addition, carriers present in the proximal tubular cells, such as those for organic ions or amino acids, can carry toxicants into the cells, leading to high intracellular concentrations. Especially in the proximal tubular cells the enzymes that can metabolize compounds to reactive intermediates have a high activity (discussed later). Since reabsorption of all nutrients, ions, and water requires much energy of the proximal tubular cells (PTC), these cells contain many mitochondria, which makes them susceptible to various toxicants, as also discussed later.

NEPHROTOXICITY RELATED TO THE GENERATION OF FREE RADICALS

Ischemia/Reperfusion

Renal ischemia followed by reperfusion (I/R) is often the cause of acute renal failure. The site of cellular damage primarily involves the proximal tubular part of the nephron. Various in vivo and in vitro studies have demonstrated a role for reactive oxygen species (ROS) in I/R-induced renal injury. Thus, treatment of rats with superoxide dismutase (SOD), vitamin E, deferoxamine, or the hydroxyl radical scavengers dimethylthiourea (DMTU) or dimethyl sulfoxide (DMSO) provided partial protection against I/R-induced renal failure (4,5, and refs. therein). In the perfused rat kidney a twofold increase in the generation of hydroxyl radicals during I/R of the kidney was blocked by DMTU (6). In in vitro models of I/R-induced renal injury, SOD and the phenolic antioxidant N,N-diphenyl-p-phenylenediamine (DPPD) prevented the death of renal epithelial cells (7). In primary cultured rat renal proximal tubular cells a two- to threefold increase in the formation of superoxide radicals, hydrogen peroxides, and hydroxyl radicals was observed (8). The increased formation of ROS is, most likely, the cause of lipid peroxidation (LPO); malondialdehyde (MDA) was detected after I/R in various in vitro systems, including human renal tubular cells (9), and in the whole kidney in vivo (10). Yet, in one study no increase in MDA was found in the kidney after 45 min of ischemia followed by 15 min of reflow (11); however, increased formation of MDA occurs primarily immediately after the start of the reperfusion (10).

Chemical-Induced Nephrotoxicity

Haloalkenyl Cysteine Conjugates

Halogenated alkenes are widely used in industry and households. These compounds cause severe tubular necrosis in various mammalian species. They are first metabolized in the liver to corresponding GSH conjugates. Subsequently the conjugates are excreted into blood and/or bile. Depending on the route, they enter the kidney as GSH or cysteine conjugates or as mercapturates (12). The GSH conjugates are metabolized to the cysteine conjugates by γ-glutamyl transpeptidase and cysteinylglycase/aminopeptidase IV. Both cysteine conjugates and mercapturates are specifically taken up by the proximal tubular cell. Inside the cell mercapturates can be deacetylated to regenerate the cysteine conjugates or the cysteine conjugates can be converted into mercapturates; the equilibrium between acetylation/deacetylation depends on the structure of the particular halogenated alkene. The cysteine conjugates are metabolized by renal cysteine conjugate β-lyase (present in both the cytosol and the mitochondria) into pyruvate, ammonia, and a electrophilic reactive metabolite (Figure 2). The reactive metabolites bind covalently to macromolecules thereby initiating the toxic events (12). The haloalkenyl cysteine conjugates, and especially S-(1,2-dichlorovinyl)-L-cysteine (DCVC), have been used by various investigators as a tool to investigate the mechanism of irreversible renal cell injury induced by alkylating chemicals, both in vivo and in vitro (13–27).

In mice, an increased exhalation of ethane and formation of MDA in the renal cortex, indicative for LPO, was found after injection of DCVC (22). Also in renal cortical slices from mice DCVC caused formation of MDA (22). In vitro in LLC-PK1 cells LPO was prevented by various antioxidants, including DPPD, which was associated with protection against cell death (15), indicating a direct relationship between LPO and cell death. Similar observations were made in freshly isolated rabbit proximal tubules and rat proximal tubular cells (16,24). (See the next section for more details on DCVC.)

Acetaminophen

Acetaminophen (N-acetyl-p-aminophenol, APAP, paracetamol) is an antipyretic analgesic. Long-term consumption, especially in combination with other analgesics, can lead to renal dysfunction. Acute overdose leads to very severe liver and renal toxicity depending on the species. In the kidney APAP can undergo three reactions:

1. A two-electron oxidation to the reactive compound N-acetyl-p-benzoquinone imine (NAPQI) through cytochrome P-450-mediated oxidation (28,29).
2. Deacetylation to p-aminophenol (PAP) (30,31).
3. One-electron peroxidation by the prostaglandin H synthase pathway.

This last route is probably only of importance for the long-term toxicity of APAP. Acute toxicity is found in the renal cortex where deacetylase and cytochrome P-450 are present, while long-term abuse affects the renal medulla, where the prostaglandin H synthase complex is located (29).

The two pathways involved in the development of acute toxicity, deacetylation and cytochrome P-450 oxidation, show pronounced species differences. For instance, in CD-1 mice nephrotoxicity of APAP requires oxidation but not deacetylation (32), while in F344 rats inhibition of deacetylase activity prevented development of nephrotoxicity (31–33). In addition susceptibility to APAP nephrotoxicity may differ between males and females: The female Sprague-Dawley rat is more susceptible than the male. The reason for this is unclear; in vitro covalent binding studies did not indicate a difference between male and female in this respect (34). The cytochrome P-450 pathway results in the formation of the reactive metabolite NAPQI. This compound attacks cellular nucleophilic groups, such as those of proteins; glutathione

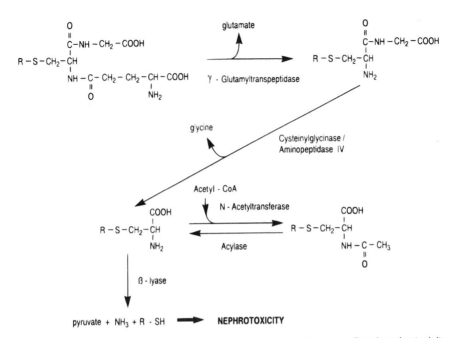

FIG. 2. The mercapturic acid pathway and its involvement in β-lyase mediated nephrotoxicity. GS S-conjugates are subsequently processed by γ-glutamyltranspeptidases and dipeptidases to cysteine S-conjugates. The cysteine S-conjugates are substrate for various enzymes; they may be N-acetylated to mercapturic acids by N-acetyltransferase, oxidized by hydroxy acid oxidase to β-keto acids, or cleaved by β-lyase into reactive intermediates. Reactive thiols may be S-methylated by thiomethyltransferases into thioethers.

protects against this attack, and only after GSH levels have decreased to a critical level, cellular macromolecules are attacked. Recently several proteins were identified that are arylated by NAPQI. A major one is a cytosolic 58-kDa protein, which was identified as a subunit of glutamine synthetase (35–37).

NAPQI is produced by cytochrome P-450 2E1. In C3H/HeJ mice the male is much more susceptible, which correlates with the amount of P-450 2E1 present: males possess 35 times more of this isotype than females (38).

A second mechanism for the toxicity of NAPQI is oxidative stress produced by redox cycling of the quinoneimine. The importance of either one of the mechanisms is still unclear. Some studies indicate that arylation is the main mechanism of toxicity (39,40), while others support oxidative stress (41).

Deacetylation is specific for the kidney. Deacetylase is a cytosolic enzyme that is predominantly located in the proximal tubular cells (30). The resulting p-aminophenol (PAP) is probably, like APAP, oxidized by the cytochrome P-450 system to the reactive p-quinone imine. It was reported by one group that treatment of rats with inducers or inhibitors of cytochrome P-450 had little effect on nephrotoxicity (42), but another group reported protection after inhibition of the enzyme system (43).

The reason for this is not clear. When PAP was given directly to animals it induced toxicity in the proximal tubular cells; also, it decreased glutathione levels and bound covalently in the kidney but not in liver (42,44), suggesting that activation of PAP occurs in the kidney itself. No pathway as described for halogenated alkenes (conjugation with glutathione in the liver, subsequent transport and uptake by the kidney) seems to be involved because neither acivicin nor probenicid, which are inhibitors of these transport systems, could protect against PAP nephrotoxicity in Fischer 344 rats (45). Interestingly, ascorbic acid protected completely against the development of the toxicity and reduced covalent binding (45). After chronic abuse of APAP in combination with other analgesics, necrosis of the renal medulla is found. In this part of the kidney the prostaglandin H synthase (PGS) enzyme complex is located. APAP can act as electron donor for reductions by PGS (46). During this reaction APAP is converted by a one-electron step to a phenoxy radical, which is then further converted to the reactive metabolite NAPQI.

Cisplatin

The antitumor drug cisplatin is effectively and widely used in the treatment of cancer in several tissues, among which head, neck, bladder, ovaries and testes (47). However, nephrotoxicity is dose-limiting and occurs either acutely or after repeated treatments. In rats, cisplatin exerts its effects mainly in the S_3 segment of the proximal tubule, resulting in necrotic lesions (48).

Although a wealth of histopathological data exists about cisplatin induced nephrotoxicity, the biochemical mechanisms are not yet fully understood.

Cisplatin in aqueous solution forms aquated species, which are the reactive forms of the compound. The concentration of chloride ions influences the reactivity of cisplatin, yielding a highly reactive electrophile inside the cells where chloride concentrations are only approximately 3 mM. This electrophile will react with any nucleophile, like sulfydryl groups of glutathione and proteins or nucleophilic groups on nucleic acids (49). Cisplatin transport may be passive as well as active, utilizing both the organic cation and anion transport systems (50). Several antioxidants and radical scavengers alleviated cisplatin-induced nephrotoxicity in vitro (51–56) as well as in vivo (57); however, cisplatin could not induce lipid peroxidation in rat kidney microsomes containing an NADH-generating system (58), while under the same experimental conditions adriamycin was very effective in induction of lipid peroxidation.

At present the experimental evidence suggests that in vivo lipid peroxidation may be involved in the development of nephrotoxicity but that the primary effect of cisplatin is not formation of free radicals but depletion of glutathione and binding to essential proteins.

Aminoglycosides

Aminoglycosides are antibiotics that induce nephrotoxicity in humans (59) mainly in the proximal tubular cells. The cationic compounds bind to the anionic phospholipids from the cell membrane and are internalized by endocytosis (60). In vivo and in vitro this leads to the formation of myeloid bodies: lysosomes filled with phospholipid complexes. These bodies are formed because the aminoglycosides inhibit lysosomal phospholipases (60). The interaction between the cationic aminoglycoside with the anionic phospholipid is essential for the development of toxicity because polyaspartic acid, which prevents binding to the phospholipids, prevents aminoglycoside-induced nephrotoxicity, both in vivo and in vitro (61,62). The formation of the phospholipid-filled lysosomes is probably the first step in the development of cytotoxicity. The lysosomes cannot function properly [which affects degradation of extra- and intracellular components (63)] or the lysosomes burst and release their hydrolytic enzymes. The latter will lead to dysfunction of other cell organelles like the mitochondria.

Formation of lipid peroxides occurs in the kidney of rats injected with gentamicin (64). Also it was observed that the level of unsaturated arachidonic acid decreased by 50% after 2 injections of gentamicin. Furthermore, the level of reduced glutathione was decreased while that of oxidized glutathione was increased (64). However, strategies to prevent lipid peroxidation, such as coadministration of vitamin E or diphenylphenylenediamine with gentamicin, did not prevent nephrotoxicity, although they prevented the decrease in unsaturated lipids (65,66). Others reported contradictory findings; coadministration of the hydroxyl radical scavenger dimethylthiourea (DMTU) or the iron chelator deferoxamine (DFO) with gentamicin prevented development of nephrotoxicity in rats (67). This apparent contrast prompted further experiments by the same researchers that reported lack of protection of vitamin E or DPPD against gentamicin-induced nephrotoxicity (discussed earlier). The experiments with DFO and DMTU were repeated but again no protection could be found (68). The question of the involvement of free radicals as a causative factor in gentamicin-induced nephrotoxicity, therefore, remains presently unanswered. Recent results add to the confusion. Protection in vivo by DMTU (69) was confirmed, but in an in vitro experiment with cultured proximal tubular cells no development of lipid peroxidation after exposure to gentamicin could be detected (70).

Cephalosporins

This class of antibiotics produces nephrotoxicity in humans and in laboratory animals when given in a large dose (71,72). The most potent nephrotoxicants of this group, cephaloridine and cephaloglycin, have been studied in detail (72,73). The severity of nephrotoxicity of these drugs is related to the uptake into the proximal tubular cells. Both are transported into the cell by the organic anion carrier because probenicid, an inhibitor of the carrier, inhibits nephrotoxicity (73). When uptake is stimulated, the toxicity increases (73). Inside the proximal tubular cell the antibiotics accumulate because the release from the cell is relatively slow (73). It has been suggested that inside the cell a reactive intermediate is generated by cytochrome P-450 activity (74). Also, induction of lipid peroxidation through redox cycling (75) is suggested by the following results. The level of conjugated dienes is increased after exposure to cephaloridine, and feeding rats a vitamin E- and/or selenium-deficient diet makes them more susceptible to toxicity of cephaloridine. In addition, antioxidants prevented malondialdehyde formation in renal slices and ameliorated the inhibition of organic ion transport (76). It was postulated that the pyridinium ring of cephaloridine was involved in the production of reactive oxygen species through redox cycling. However, this postulation is weakened by the fact that cephalotin, which is structurally identical to cephaloridin, except for the lack of the pyridinium ring, also induces lipid peroxidation.

It is doubtful whether redox cycling explains the nephrotoxicity of all cephalosporins because administration of cephaloglycin, which is more nephrotoxic than cephaloridine, does not result in any conjugated dienes in the kidney in vivo (77), which indicates at least that oxidative stress is not the major mechanism of induction of nephrotoxicity.

The major mechanisms of induction of nephrotoxicity are probably competition with carnitine, the compound that transports fatty acids into mitochondria (78), and acylation of proteins from the proximal tubular cell, especially those involved in transport of substrates into mitochondria (76,77).

Quinones

Quinones are also conjugated with glutathione (predominantly in the liver). In vivo, the resulting conjugates are transported to the kidney, which ultimately results in toxicity to the proximal tubular cells (79–81). The most studied are bromohydroquinone derived from bromobenzene. When this compound is injected into rats, 2-bromo-diglutathion-S-ylhydroquinone [2-Br-(diGSyl)HQ] and three possible isomers of 2-bromoglutathion-S-ylhydroquinone are formed (79). In vivo, the glutathione conjugates are a few orders of magnitude more nephrotoxic than the parent compound (80). Pretreatment of animals with acivicin, an inhibitor of γ-glutamyl transpeptidase (γ-GT), largely prevented the development of nephrotoxicity indicating that metabolism by γ-GT is required for toxicity (80,81). Similar as with the halogenated alkene conjugates, the balance between acetylation of the cysteine conjugate versus deacetylation of the mercapturate may determine toxicity (82). Thus, more acetylation means less cysteine conjugate available which means less toxicity because either β-elimination or oxidation of this conjugate determines toxicity. The latter reaction is probably the most important; the resulting quinone or semiquinone will arylate cellular macromolecules and/or generate reactive oxygen species (82), respectively. At present, the relative importance of these two pathways is not yet clear; a major factor is the species difference in susceptibility to 2-Br-(diGSyl)HQ-mediated nephrotoxicity (83).

Heavy Metals

Heavy metals are potent nephrotoxicants. In most studies mercury has been used to induce nephrotoxicity. Mercury damages the glomerulus and the proximal tubular cells. The former results from the induction of formation of autoantibodies that are deposited in the glomerulus and affect glomerular filtration (84); in acute toxicity predominantly damage to the proximal tubular cells is found. Mercury binds to nucleophilic groups of glutathione and proteins in the cell, which causes its nephrotoxicity. Major cellular processes that are affected are mitochondrial functioning and intracellular calcium homeostasis. These effects are discussed in the next section.

MECHANISM OF DEVELOPMENT OF RENAL CELL INJURY BY OXIDATIVE STRESS

Studies with Externally Added Peroxides

Because of the possible role of oxidative stress in the pathophysiology of renal tissue injury the direct effect of pro-oxidants on renal cells has been studied by several groups. Both chemicals [H_2O_2, t-butylhydroperoxide (TBHP), cumene hydroperoxide] and enzyme systems (glucose/glucose oxidase and hypoxanthine/xanthine oxidase) have been used to investigate the mechanism of exogenous-induced oxidative stress on renal cells, primarily of proximal tubular origin (24,85–91). H_2O_2, TBHP and cumene hydroperoxide cause LPO in LLC-PK1 cells, and in freshly isolated rat and rabbit renal PTC (24,85,88,90). Moreover, in vivo adminstration of H_2O_2 into the renal artery also produced marked proximal tubular injury, which was associated with a decrease in renal function (91). The LPO is prevented by various (phenolic) antioxidants, including DPPD, n-propyl gallate, butylated hydroxytoluene, lazaroids, and vitamin E, which was associated with complete protection against cell death (24,85,88). Also desferoxamine protected against LPO and cell death (24,86,88), indicating that these are iron-dependent processes.

Site of Formation of Free Radicals During Renal Cell Injury

The mitochondria and the endoplasmatic reticulum (ER) are the predominant intracellular sites implicated in the formation of ROS (Figure 3). It has been estimated that under physiological conditions approximately 2% of the electrons consumed by the mitochondrial respiratory chain during state 4 respiration escape and may react with oxygen to form superoxide anion (92). The respiratory chain is a very likely site for an increased formation of ROS. In renal cortex mitochondria isolated from rats treated with $HgCl_2$ an increased formation of H_2O_2 occurs only if succinate is used as a substrate, suggesting that the formation occurs at a site between complex II and III of the respiratory chain (93). Exposure of isolated renal cortex mitochondria to DCVC results in a decrease of GSH and an increase of GSSG, which is associated with LPO (17). Similar observations were made with $HgCl_2$ and gentamicin (67,93–95). Furthermore, an inhibitor of complex IV of the mitochondrial respiratory chain, potassium cyanide (KCN) (but not the inhibitors of complex I or III, rotenone and antimycin, respectively) protects against LPO and cell death induced by DCVC in

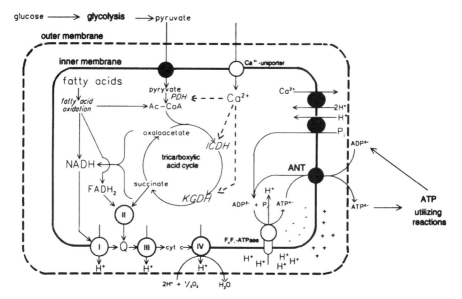

FIG. 3. Mitochondrial enzyme systems which are involved in oxidative phosphorylation and the role of Ca^{2+} in the regulation of various steps. The tricarboxylic acid cycle and the oxidation of fatty acids result in formation of NADH and $FADH_2$, which donate electrons to complex I and II of the mitochondrial respiratory chain (MRC), respectively. The proton gradient due to proton pumping by the complex I, II, and IV of the MRC is used to synthesize ATP. PDH, pyruvate dehydrogenase; ICDH, isocitrate dehydrogenase; KGDH, α-keto-glutarate dehydrogenase; Q, coenzyme Q or ubiquinone; cyt c, cytochrome c; ANT, adenosine nucleotide transporter.

freshly isolated PTC (26). This indicates that mitochondria may be a site of origin of oxidative stress in intact renal cells.

The ER may also play an important role in nephrotoxicant-induced oxidative stress. Thus, exposure of renal cortex microsomes to cyclosporin causes an increase in formation of thiobarbituric-acid-reactive substances (TBARS), indicative for LPO (96). An increase of superoxide anion formation was observed in microsomes isolated from kidneys subjected to I/R, associated with an increase of TBARS (97). ROS formation may occur during redox cycling of cytochrome P-450 moiety, which is predominantly located in the ER. Interestingly, recently a role for cytochrome P-450 disturbance in I/R-mediated renal cell injury was proposed. Thus, an inhibitor of cytochrome P-450, cimetidine, prevented the release of iron, which was associated with a protection against hydroxyl radical production and cell killing caused by hypoxia/reperfusion (98). With regard to the release of iron from cytochrome P-450, an increase of iron was observed in the urine of rats during the reperfusion of ischemic kidneys (5). These observations are consistent with the observed protection of the iron chelator desferroxamine (5). Iron release may also occur from other cellular organelles. Thus, a release of iron was observed in isolated rat renal mitochondria exposed to gentamicin (95). This release seems to be dependent on gentamicin-induced formation of H_2O_2, since catalase (but not heat-inactivated catalase or SOD) prevented the gentamicin-induced iron release.

ROS may also be formed due to increased xanthine oxidase (XO) activity during ischemia and hypoxia in various tissues. XO oxidizes hypoxanthine, formed as a result of the breakdown of AMP during oxygen deprivation, which results in the formation of superoxide anion. XO was proposed as a potential source of ROS during I/R, based on the inhibition of the formation of ROS by an inhibitor of xanthine oxidase, allopurinol. Allopurinol may also scavenge hydroxyl radicals (5). It inhibits I/R-induced renal failure in various species. An increase of XO activity was observed in an in vitro model of hypoxic injury (99,100) and in I/R of the perfused isolated rat kidney (101); however, in an other study no increase in XO activity was found after renal ischemia in vivo, although malondialdehyde formation was increased (10). It is possible that formation of hypoxanthine during the ischemic period in vivo may be sufficient to drive XO-mediated formation of superoxide anion during reperfusion without a dramatic increase of XO activity.

In principle, ROS may also be generated by blood cells in the kidney. Thus, white blood cells, especially neutrophils and macrophages, have been proposed as a source of ROS during tissue injury. Although I/R-induced injury seems independent of circulating cells (5), it is unclear whether influx of these cells in damaged areas is involved in tissue injury caused by nephrotoxicants.

Role of Failure of Antioxidant Enzyme Systems in Progression of ROS-Induced PTC Injury

Depletion of Glutathione in Oxidative Stress

As discussed earlier, almost all nephrotoxicants deplete GSH, which leads to LPO in various cell types. GSH depletion by DCVC or cephaloglycin is not associated with an accumulation of cellular GSSG (14,71, 111), suggesting that the GSH depletion is caused by its reaction with the electrophilic reactive metabolites of DCVC to form conjugates. Prior depletion of renal GSH in vivo in mice by L-buthione-*S,R*-sulfoximine potentiated the DCVC-induced renal injury (13). Similar results were observed in freshly isolated rat renal PTC pretreated with either diamide or (*R,S*)-3-hydroxy-4-pentenoic acid (HPA) (111). The thiol reducing agent dithiothreitol (DTT) protected against LPO and cell death, without inhibiting the covalent binding of reactive metabolites to macromolecules (15, 111). Together, these data strongly suggest that the DCVC-induced cell injury is related to GSH depletion and LPO. A similar role for GSH was found when cells were treated with TBHP or H_2O_2 and menadione (85,89,102). All pro-oxidants cause a rapid depletion of GSH in freshly isolated rat renal PTC. In this case, however, the decrease is associated with a corresponding increase in GSSG levels. Supplementation with GSH prevented the depletion of GSH, while dithiothreitol (DTT) prevented the accumulation of GSSG (89). These latter two conditions provide protection against TBHP-mediated cytotoxicity (85,89,90), while prior depletion of GSH with buthione sulfoximine (BSO) or inhibition of glutathione reductase using bis-(2-chloroethyl)-*N*-nitrosourea (BCNU) aggravated pro-oxidant-induced cytotoxicity (90,102). Together, the data indicate a role for perturbation of the GSH homeostasis in both pro-oxidant- and DCVC-induced cell death.

Role of Inhibition of Antioxidant Enzymes in Oxidative Stress in Renal Cells

PTC possess several enzyme systems that are involved in the detoxification of ROS and LPO products, including GSH peroxidase, GSH reductase, catalase, and superoxide dismutase (SOD). Several nephrotoxicants have been shown to inactivate some of these enzymes. Thus, Cd^{2+}, Zn^{2+}, and different nephrotoxic cysteine conjugates, including DCVC, inhibit GSH peroxidase and GSH reductase activity (103, 111). In the case of DCVC the inactivation of the enzymes of the GSH redox cycle clearly occurred prior to initiation of oxidative stress and cell death. Moreover, pretreatment of PTC with an inhibitor of GSH reductase, BCNU, potentiated oxidative stress and cell death caused by DCVC. A similar observation was made in freshly isolated rat renal PTC treated with menadione and two of its thioether conjugates (102).

Recent findings indicate that the potent endogenous antioxidant vitamin E can be recycled by complex II, which is, in part, dependent on the availability of reduced ubiquinone (ubiquinol) (104). Moreover, studies in isolated mitochondria indicate that only complex II (and not complex I, III, or IV) is involved in the protection by succinate (and several other substrates of the Krebs cycle) against cumene hydroperoxide-induced LPO (105 and refs. therein). Recent observations in PTC exposed to DCVC suggest that also in intact cells complex II is involved in the protection against oxidative stress. Thus, the DCVC-induced LPO and cytotoxicity are preceded by an inhibition of complex II activity (succinate:ubiquinone reductase), whereas complex I is largely unaffected. Pretreatment of cells with an inhibitor of complex II, thenoyltrifluoroacetone (TTFA), potentiated the oxidative stress and cell death (26). Also KCN, an inhibitor of complex IV, protected against oxidative stress and cell death. Interestingly, inhibitors of complex II, either oxaloacetate or TTFA, prevented the KCN-mediated protection, whereas inhibitors of both complex I and III, rotenone and antimycin A, respectively, did not affect KCN protection (26). This indicates that KCN protection is mediated by the activity of complex II. In isolated mitochondria KCN increases the amount of ubiquinol, a potent antioxidant in various in vitro systems (106). In PTC KCN also increases ubiquinol and prevents the depletion of ubiquinol caused by DCVC. However, the observed protection of KCN seems not to be mediated by a simple increase of ubiquinol, because rotenone prevented the KCN-mediated increase of ubiquinol without preventing cytoprotection, whereas oxaloacetate prevented cytoprotection without inhibiting the KCN-mediated increase of ubiquinol (26). Since in isolated mitochondria the activity of complex II is linked to vitamin E recycling, it is likely that interference at complex II will affect the redox state of vitamin E and, thereby, its antioxidant function.

In conclusion, the preceding observations indicate a role for various antioxidant enzymes in the protection against oxidative stress in PTC, while perturbation of the activity of these enzymes will increase the susceptibility to oxidative stress. Further studies are needed to evaluate the effect of other nephrotoxicants on the activity of the discussed enzymes, as well as on catalase, SOD, vitamin E reductase, and DT-diaphorase in relation to oxidative stress and cell death.

Calcium and Oxidative Stress in PTC Injury

The $[Ca^{2+}]_{intra}$ is approximately 10,000 times lower than $[Ca^{2+}]_{extra}$ and varies between 100 and 200 nM under normal circumstances. A sustained perturbation of intracellular Ca^{2+} homeostasis has been implicated in the initiation of cell death of various cell types, including PTC (18,24,25,107). Although the exact role of Ca^{2+} in the induction of renal epithelial cell death is still controversial, several studies suggest a role for Ca^{2+} in the induction of oxidative stress-mediated cell death caused by nephrotoxicants. For instance, in isolated rat renal mitochondria treated with $HgCl_2$ an increase in H_2O_2 formation was observed that was associated with LPO; Ca^{2+} potentiated the LPO while an inhibitor of the mitochondrial Ca^{2+}-uniporter that mediates the uptake of Ca^{2+} into the mitochondrial matrix, ruthenium red (RR), and a calcium chelator, EGTA, prevented the LPO (93). Similar observations were made in intact proximal tubular cells with DCVC. Thus, exposure of freshly isolated rat renal PTC and LLC-PK1 cells to DCVC causes an increase of $[Ca^{2+}]_{intra}$ (18,24,25,107) and an increase of Ca^{2+} in the mitochondrial matrix ($[Ca^{2+}]_{mito}$) (24). Interestingly, chelation of intracellular free calcium with either EDTA/AM, EGTA/AM, or Quin-2/AM prevents LPO and cell death caused by DCVC (18,24). Inhibition of the Ca^{2+}-uniporter with ruthenium red (RR) prevented the DCVC-induced increase of $[Ca^{2+}]_{mito}$ (24), without preventing an increase of the cytosolic free calcium concentration; however, RR protected against LPO and cell death (18,24). Together, these data suggest a role for (especially) mitochondrial Ca^{2+} deregulation in the induction of oxidative stress in PTC. More work is needed to determine whether a similar pathway plays a role in the induction of oxidative stress by I/R or other nephrotoxicants.

MITOCHONDRIAL INJURY

Mitochondria are likely a source of free radicals (see earlier discussion). However, effects on mitochondrial functions, such as generation of ATP and regulation of Ca^{2+} homeostasis (Figure 3), are probably also important factors in the development of nephrotoxicity. Thus, gentamicin, cephaloridin, paracetamol, mercury, DCVC, and cisplatin all bind to mitochondria and/or affect mitochondrial function. Exposure of isolated rat renal cortex mitochondria to an ROS-generating system, HX/XO, causes mitochondrial damage (108,109). This damage is more severe when the mitochondria are exposed to pro-oxidants plus Ca^{2+} (109). The latter results in loss of mitochondrial function, including a loss of the respiratory control, decrease of uncoupled respiration, and a decrease in the activity of NADH-CoQ-reductase, oligomycin-sensitive F_1-ATPase, and adenine nucleotide translocase (109). HX/XO causes the release of Ca^{2+} from the mitochondria, which is associated with an increase of state 4 respiration (108). The released calcium is likely to be taken up again by the mitochondrial uniporter, thereby creating cycling of calcium in and out of the mitochondria. The uniporter can be blocked by ruthenium red, without inhibiting Ca^{2+} release from the matrix. Indeed, ruthenium red prevented the increase in state 4 respiration.

Recently, the preceding observations, which suggest that Ca^{2+} potentiates ROS damage to isolated mitochondria, have been extended to intact freshly isolated rat renal PTC. Thus DCVC causes a decrease of the mitochondrial membrane potential ($\Delta\Psi$) (24), indicative for mitochondrial dysfunction. Both EGTA/AM and RR inhibited the decrease, indicating a role for mitochondrial Ca^{2+} uptake in this process. Moreover, the iron chelator DFO and the phenolic antioxidant DPPD also inhibited the decrease of $\Delta\Psi$, without compromising an increase in $[Ca^{2+}]_{cyto}$ and $[Ca^{2+}]_{mito}$. These observations indicate a relationship between mitochondrial Ca^{2+} deregulation, oxidative stress and mitochondrial damage in intact renal cells. The fact that RR blocked both Ca^{2+}-uptake and oxidative stress suggests a possible role for Ca^{2+}-cycling in the mechanism of the induction oxidative stress (24). In isolated mitochondria Ca^{2+} release is mediated by the mitochondrial permeability transition pore. The release of Ca^{2+} from mitochondria can be prevented by cyclosporin A. Cyclosporin A did not inhibit the DCVC-induced oxidative stress nor the decrease of $\Delta\Psi$ in PTC (Van de Water and Nagelkerke, unpublished observations). Another mechanism of release of Ca^{2+} from the mitochondrial matrix is via the antiport. The release is dependent upon hydrolysis of pyridine nucleotides to ADP-ribose, while the binding of the latter to a specific mitochondrial membrane provokes Ca^{2+} release. This process can be inhibited by mono-iodobenzylguanine, while exposure of intact cells to this compound results in an increase of mitochondrial calcium (110). However, mono-iodobenzylguanine did not inhibit the oxidative stress and cell death caused by DCVC in PTC (Van de Water and Nagelkerke, unpublished observations). These observations suggests that Ca^{2+} cycling is not involved in the initiation of oxidative stress and mitochondrial damage caused by DCVC. Whether a similar interrelationship between Ca^{2+}, oxidative stress, and mitochondrial injury is involved in the mechanism of toxicity for other nephrotoxicants remains to be investigated.

CONCLUSIONS

Clearly, many studies indicate that lipid peroxidation is involved in the development of nephrotoxicity in vivo, although the reports are not all unequivocal. Actually all nephrotoxic compounds, although they differ very much from each other, and I/R affect the amount of glutathione in the cells. As glutathione is an important factor in protection against oxidative stress and lipid peroxidation, which is described elsewhere in this book, it is very tempting to assume that ROS and probably free radicals are generated. However, all evidence is circumstantial and no data are available that clearly demonstrate formation of free radicals, oxygen or otherwise, in cells or tissue. Therefore, at present at best one can say that it is likely that formation of free radicals is involved in the development of nephrotoxicity, but further research is needed to actually prove it.

REFERENCES

1. Brenner BM, Rector FC, eds. *The Kidney* (vols. I and II), 4th ed. Philadelphia: Saunders, 1991.
2. Kinter L B, Short BG. Anatomy and physiology of the Kidney. A brief review. In: Hook JB, Goldstein RS, eds., *Toxicology of the Kidney*, 2nd ed. New York: Raven Press, 1993;1–36.
3. Kriz W, Bankir L. A standard nomenclature for structures in the kidney. *Am J Physiol 254 (Renal Fluid Electrolyte Physiol)* 1988;23:F1–F8.
4. Paller MS, Hoidal JR, Ferris TF. Oxygen free radicals in ischemic acute renal failure in the rat. *J Clin Invest* 1984;74:1156–1164.
5. Greene EL, Paller MS. Oxygen free radicals in acute renal failure. *Miner Electrolyte Metab* 1991;17:124–132.
6. Kadkhodaee M, Endre ZH, Towner RA, Cross M. Hydroxyl radical generation following ischaemia-reperfursion in cell-free perfused rat kidney. *Biochim Biophys Acta* 1995;1243:169–174.
7. Yonehana T, Gemba M. Hypoxia and reoxygenation-induced injury of renal epithelial cells: Effect of free radical scavengers. *Jpn J Pharmacol* 1995;68:231–234.
8. Paller MS, Neumann TV. Reactive oxygen species and rat renal epithelial cells during hypoxia and reoxygenation. *Kidney Int* 1991;40:1041–1049.
9. Grune T, Sommerburg O, Petras T, Siems WG. Postanoxic formation of aldehydic lipid peroxidation products in human renal tubular cells. *Free Radical Biol Med* 1995;18:21–27.
10. Joannidis M, Gstraunthaler G, Pfaller W. Xanthine oxidase: Evidence against a causative role in renal reperfusion injury. *Am J Physiol* 1990;258:F232–F236.
11. Gamelin LM, Zager RA. Evidence against oxidant injury as a critical mediator of postischemic acute renal failure. *Am J Physiol* 1988;255:F450–F460.
12. Lock EA. Mechanism of nephrotoxic action due to organohalogenated compounds. *Toxicol Lett* 1989;46:93–106.
13. Darnerud PO, Brandt I, Feil V, Bakke JE. Dichlorovinyl cysteine (DCVC) in the mouse kidney: tissue-binding and toxicity after glutathione depletion and probenicid treatment. *Arch Toxicol* 1989;63:345–350.
14. Lash LH, Anders MW. Cytotoxicity of S-(1,2-dichlorovinyl)glutathione and S-(1,2-dichlorovinyl)-L-cysteine ion isolated rat kidney cells. *J Biol Chem* 1986;261:13076–13081.
15. Chen Q, Jones TW, Brown PC, Stevens JL. The mechanism of cystein conjugate cytotoxicity in renal epithelial cells. Covalent binding leads to thiol depletion and lipid peroxidation. *J Biol Chem* 1990;265:21603–21611.
16. Groves CE, Lock EA, Schnellmann RG. Role of lipid peroxidation in renal proximal tubule cell death induced by haloalkene cysteine conjugates. *Toxicol Appl Pharmacol* 1991;107:54–62.
17. Lash LH, Anders MW. Mechanism of S-(1.2-dichlorovinyl)-L-cysteine- and S-(1,2-dichlorovinyl)-L-homocysteine-induced renal mitochondrial toxicity. *Mol Pharmacol* 1987;32:549–556.
18. Chen Q, Jons TW, Stevens JL. Early cellular events couple covalent binding of reactive metabolites to cell killing by nephrotoxic cysteine conjugates. *J Appl Physiol* 1994;161:293–302.
19. Yu K, Chen Q, Liu H, Zhan Y, Stevens JL. Signalling the molecular stress response to nephrotoxic and mutagenic cysteine conjugates: Differential roles for protein synthesis and calcium in the induction of *c-fos* and *c-myc* mRNA in LLC-PK1 cells. *J Cell Physiol* 1994;161:303–311.
20. Chen Q, Yu K, Holbrook NJ, Stevens JL. Activation of the growth arrest and DNA-damage-inducible gene *gadd 153* by nephrotoxic cysteine conjugates and dithiothreitol. *J Biol Chem* 1992;267:8207–8212.
21. Chen Q, Yu K, Stevens JL. Regulation of the cellular stress responses by reactive electrophiles. The role of covalent binding and cellular thiols in transcriptional activation of the 70-kilodalton heat shock protein gene by nephrotoxic cysteine conjugates. *J Biol Chem* 1992;267:24322–24327.

22. Beuter W, Cojocel C, Muller W, Donaubauer HH, Mayer D. Peroxidative damage and nephrotoxicity of dichlorovinylcysteine in mice. *J Appl Toxicol* 1989;9:181–186.

23. Davis JW, Blakeman DP, Jolly RA, Packwood WH, Kolaja GJ, Petry TW. *S*-(1,2-dichlorovinyl)-L-cysteine-induced nephrotoxicity in the New Zealand White rabbit: Characterization of proteinuria and examination of the potential role of oxidative stress. *Toxicol Pathol* 1995;23:487–497.

24. Van de Water B, Zoeteweij PJ, De Bont HJGM, Mulder GJ, Nagelkerke JF. Role of mitochondrial Ca^{2+} in the oxidative stress-induced dissipation of the mitochondrial membrane potential. *J Biol Chem* 1994;269:14546–14552.

25. Van de Water B, Zoeteweij JP, De Bont HJGM, Mulder GJ, Nagelkerke JF. The relationship between intracellular Ca^{2+} and the mitochondrial membrane potential in isolated proximal tubular cells from rat kidney exposed to the nephrotoxin 1,2-dichlorovinyl-cysteine. *Biochem Pharmacol* 1993; 45:2259–2267.

26. Van de Water B, Zoeteweij JP, De Bont HJGM, Nagelkerke JF. Inhibition of succinate:ubiquinone reductase and decrease of ubiquinol in nephrotoxic cysteine *S*-conjugate-induced oxidative cell injury. *Mol Pharmacol*, in press.

27. Van de Water B, Jaspers JPTG, Maasdam DH, Mulder GJ, Nagelkerke JF. Detachment of proximal tubular cells and F-actin damage: Implications for renal failure. *Am J Physiol* 1994:267:F888–F899.

28. Zenzer TV, Mattammal MB, David BB. Differential distribution of the mixed-fuction oxidase activities in rabbit kidney. *J Pharmacol Exp Ther* 1978;207:719–725.

29. Mohandas J, Duggin GG, Horvath JS, Tiller DJ. Metabolic oxidation of acetaminophen (paracetamol) mediated by cytochrome P-450 mixed function oxidase and prostaglandin endoperoxidase synthetase in rabbit kidney. *Toxicol Appl Pharmacol* 1981;61:252–259.

30. Carpenter HM, Mudge GH. Acetaminophen nephrotoxicity: Studies on renal acetylation and deacetylation. *J Pharmacol Exp Ther* 1981;218:161–167.

31. Newton JF, Kuo CH, Deshone GM, Hoefle D, Bernstein J, Hook JB. The role of *p*-aminophenol in acetaminophen-induced nephrotoxicity: Effect of bio(*p*-nitro-phenyl) phosphate on acetaminophen and *p*-aminophenol nephrotoxicity and metabolism in Fischer 344 rats. *Toxicol Appl Pharmacol* 1985;81:416–430.

32. Emeigh Hart SG, Beierschmitt WP, Bartolone JB, Wyand DS, Khairallah EA, Cohen SD. Evidence against deacetylation and for cytochrome P450-mediated activation in acetaminophen-induced nephrotoxicity in the CD-1 mouse. *Toxicol Appl Pharmacol* 1991;107:1–15.

33. Newton JF, Baillie MB, Hook JB. Acetaminophen nephrotoxicity in the rat. Renal metabolic activation in vitro. *Toxicol Appl Pharmacol* 1983;70:433–444.

34. Mugford CA, Tarloff JB. Contribution of oxidation and deacetylation to the bioactivation of acetaminophen in vitro in liver and kidney from male and female Sprague-Dawley rats. *Drug Metab Dispos* 1995;23:290–294.

35. Bartolone JB, Beierschmitt WP, Birge RB, Emeigh Hart SG, Wynand DS, Cohen SD, Khairallah EA. Selective acetaminophen metabolite binding to hepatic and extrahepatic proteins: An in vivo and in vitro analysis. *Toxicol Appl Pharmacol* 1989;99:240–249.

36. Bulera SJ, Birge RB, Cohen SD, Khairallah. Identification of the mouse liver 44-kDa acetaminophen-binding protein as a subunit of glutamine synthetase. *Toxicol Appl Pharmacol* 1995;134:313–320

37. Beierschmitt WP, Brady JT, Bartolone JB, Wynand DS, Khairallah EA, Cohen SD. Selective protein arylation and the age dependency of acetaminophen hepatotoxicity in mice. *Toxicol Appl Pharmacol* 1989;98:517–529

38. Hu JJ. Lee M-J, Vapiwala M, Reuhl K, Thomas PE, Yang CS. Sex-related differences in mouse renal metabolism and toxicity of acetaminophen. *Toxicol Appl Pharmacol* 1993;122:16–26.

39. Nicotera P, Rundgren M, Porubek DJ, Cotgreave I, Moldeus P, Orrenius S, Nelson SD. On the role of Ca^{2+} in the toxicity of alkylating and oxidizing quinone imines in isolated hepatocytes. *Chem Res Toxicol* 1989;2:46–50.

40. Gerson RJ, Casini A, Gilfor D, Serrone A, Farber JL. Oxygen-mediated cell injury in the killing of cultured hepatocytes by acetaminophen. *Biochem Biophys Res Commun* 1985;126:1129–1137.

41. Gibson JD, Pumford NR, Hinson JA. Mechanism of acetaminophen hepatotoxicity: covalent binding versus oxidative stress, abstract 807. *Toxicologist* 1995;15:151.

42. Calder IC, Young Ac, Woods RA, Crowe CA, Ham KN, Tange JD. The nephrotoxicity of 4-aminophenol. II. The effect of metabolism inhibitors and inducers. *Chem Biol Interact* 1979; 27:245–254.

43. Newton JF, Kuo C-H, Gemborys MWS, Mudge GH, Hook JB. Nephrotoxicity of 4-aminophenol, a metabolite of acetaminophen in the Fischer 344 rat. *Toxicol Appl Pharmacol* 1982;65:336–344.

44. Crowe CA, Young AC, Calder IC, Ham KN, Tange JD. Nephrotoxicity of 4-aminophenol. I. The effect on microsomal cytochromes, glutathione and covalent binding in kidney and liver. *Chem Biol Interact* 1979;27:235–243.
45. Fowler LM, Foster JR, Lock EA. Effect of ascorbic acid, acivicin and probeecid on the nephrotoxicity of 4-aminophenol in the Fischer 344 rat. *Arch Toxicol* 1993;67:613–621.
46. Moldeus P, Andersson B, Rahimtula A, Berggren M. Prostaglandin synthetase catalyzed activation of paracetamol. *Biochem Pharmacol* 1982;31:1363–1368.
47. Borch RF. The platinum antitumor drugs. In Powis G, Prough RA, eds., *Metabolism & Action of Anticancer Drugs*. London: Taylor & Francis. 1985;163–193.
48. Doyban DC, Levi J, Jacobs C, Kosek J, Weiner MW. Mechanisms of cisplatin-induced nephrotoxicity: II. Morphologic observations. *J Pharmacol Exp Ther* 1980;213:551–556.
49. Chu G. Cellular Responses to cisplatin. The roles of DNA-binding proteins and DNA repair. *J Biol Chem* 1994;269:787–790.
50. McGuinness SJ, Ryan MP. Mechanism of cisplatin nephrotoxicity in rat renal proximal tubule suspensions. *Toxicol In Vitro* 1994;8:1203–1212.
51. Zhang JG, Zhong LF, Zhang M, Xia YX. Protection effects of procaine on oxidative stress and toxicities of renal cortical slices from rats caused by cisplatin in vitro. *Arch Toxicol* 1992;66:354–358.
52. Hannemann J, Baumann K. Nephrotoxicity of cisplatin, carboplatin and transplatin. A comparative in vitro study. *Arch Toxicol* 1990;64:393–400.
53. Hannemann J, Baumann K. Cisplatin-induced lipid peroxidation and decrease of gluconeogenesis in rat kidney cortex: Different effects of antioxidants and radical scavengers. *Toxicology* 1988; 51:119–132.
54. Zhang JG, Zhong LF, Zhang M, Xia YX. Protection effects of procaine on oxidative stress and toxicities of renal cortical slices from rats caused by cisplatin in vitro. *Arch Toxicol* 1992;66:354–358.
55. Sugihara K, Nakano S, Koda M, Tanaka K, Fukuishi N, Gemba M. Stimulatory effect of cisplatin on production of lipid peroxides in renal tissues. *Jpn J Pharmacol* 1987;43:247–252.
56. Kameyama Y, Gemba M. The iron chelator deferoxamine prevents cisplatin-induced lipid peroxidation in rat kidney cortical slices. *Jpn J Pharmacol* 1991;57:259–262.
57. Sugihara K, Nakano S, Gemba M. Effect of cisplatin on in vitro production of lipid peroxides in rat kidney cortex. *Jpn J Pharmacol* 1987;44:71–76.
58. Vermeulen NPE, Baldew G S. The role of lipid peroxidation in the nephrotoxicity of cisplatin. *Biochem Pharmacol* 1992;44:1193–1199.
59. Kahlmeter G, Dahlager J. Aminoglycoside toxicity. A review of clinical studies between 1975–1982. *J Antimicrob Chemother* 1984;13(suppl A):9–22.
60. Kaloyanides GJ. Renal pharmacology of aminoglycoside antibiotics. In: Bianchi C, Bertelli A, Duarte C G, eds. *Contributions to Nephrology 42, Drug-Induced Nephrotoxicity*. Basel: Karger. 1984;148–167.
61. Kishore BK, Kallay Z, Lambricht P, Laurent G, Tulkens PM. Mechanism of protection afforded by polyaspartic acid against gentamicin-induced phospholipidosis. I. Polyaspartic acid binds gentamicin and displaces it from negatively charged phospholipid layers in vitro. *J Pharmacol Exp Ther* 1990;255:867–874.
62. Kishore BK, Lambricht P, Laurent G, Maldague P, Wagner R, Tulkens PM. Mechanism of protection afforded by polyaspartic acid against gentamicin-induced phospholipidosis. II. Comparative in vitro and in vivo studies with poly-L-glutamic acids. *J Pharmacol Exp Ther* 1990;255:875–884.
63. Tulkens GA, van Hoof F, Tulkens PM. Gentamicin-induced lysosomal phospholipidosis in cultured rat fibroblasts. Quantitative ultrastructural and biochemical study. *Lab Invest* 1979;40:481–491.
64. Ramsammy LS, Ling K-Y, Josepovitz C, Levine R, Kaloyanides GJ. Effect of gentamicin on lipid peroxidation in rat renal cortex. *Biochem Pharmacol* 1985;34:3895–3900.
65. Ramsammy LS, Josepovitz C, Ling K-Y, Lane BP, Kaloyanides GJ. Effects of diphenyl-phenylenediamine on gentamicin-induced lipid peroxidation and toxicity in rat renal cortex. *J Pharmacol Exp Ther* 1986;238:83–88.
66. Ramsammy LS, Josepovitz C, Ling K-Y, Lane BP, Kaloyanides GJ. Failure of inhibition of lipid peroxidation by vitamin E to protect against gentamicin nephrotoxicity in the rat. *Biochem Pharmacol* 1987;36:2125–2132.
67. Walker PD, Shah SV. Evidence suggesting a role for hydroxyl radical in gentamicin-induced acute renal failure in rats. *J Clin Invest* 1988;81:334–341.
68. Kaloyanides GJ, Ramsammy LS, Josepovitz C. Assessment of three therapeutic interventions for

modifying gentamicin nephrotoxicity in the rat. In: Bach PH, Cregg NJ, Wilks MF, Delacruz L, eds. *Nephrotoxicity.* New York: Marcel Dekker. 1989;99–104.

69. Nakajima T, Hishida A, Kato A. Mechanisms for protective effects of free radical scavengers on gentamicin-mediated nephropathy in rats. *Am J Physiol (Renal Fluid Electrolyte Physiol.)* 1994; 266:F425–F431.

70. Swann JD, Acosta D. Failure of gentamicin to elevate cellular malondialdehyde content or increase generation of intracellular reactive oxygen species in primary cultures of renal cortical epithelial cells. *Biochem Pharmacol* 1990;40:1523–1526.

71. Silverblatt F, Turck M, Bulger R. Nephrotoxicity due to cephaloridine: A light- and electronmicroscopic study in rabbits. *J Infect Dis* 1970;122:33–44.

72. Tune BM. The nephrotoxicity of beta-lactam antibiotics. In: Hook JB, Goldstein RS, eds. *Toxicology of the Kidney.* New York: Raven Press. 1993; 257–281

73. Tune BM. The nephrotoxicity of cephalosporin antibiotics: Structure-activity relationships. *Commun Toxicol* 1986;1:145–170.

74. McMurtry RJ, Mitchell JR. Renal and hepatic necrosis after metabolic activation of 2-substituted furans and thiophenes, including furosemide and cephaloridine. *Toxicol Appl Pharmacol* 1977;42:285–300.

75. Kuo C-H, Maita K, Slieght SD, Hook JB. Lipid peroxidation: A possible mechanism of cephaloridine-induced nephrotoxicity. *Toxicol Appl Pharmacol* 1983;67:78–88.

76. Browning MC, Tune BM. The reactivity and binding of beta-lactam antibiotics in rabbit renal cortex. *J Pharmacol Exp Ther* 1983;226:640–644.

77. Tune BM, Fravert D, Hsu C-Y. The oxidative and mitochondrial toxic effects of cephalosporin antibiotics in the kidney. A comparative study of cephaloridine and cephaloglycin. *Biochem Pharmacol* 1989;38:795–802

78. Tune BM, Hsu C-Y. Toxicity of cephaloridine to carnitine transport and fatty acid metabolism in rabbit renal cortical mitochondria: Structure-activity relationships. *J Pharmacol Exp Ther* 1994;270:873–880.

79. Monks TJ, Lau SS, Highet RJ, Gilette JR. Gluthatione conjugates of 2-bromohydroquinone are nephrotoxic. *Drug Metab Dispos* 1985;13:553–559

80. Monks TJ, Highet RJ, Lau SS. 2-Bromo-(diglutathin-*S*-yl)hydroquinone nephrotoxicity. Physiological and electrochemical determinants. *Mol Pharmacol* 1988;34:492–500.

81. Lau SS, Hill BA, Highet RJ, Monks TJ. Sequential oxidation and glutathione addition to 1,4-benzoquinone: correlation of toxicity with increased glutathione substitution. *Mol Pharmacol* 1988;34:829–836.

82. Monks TJ, Lo H-H, Lau SS. Oxidation and acetylation as determinants of 2-bromocystein-*S*-ylhydroquinone-mediated nephrotoxicity. *Chem Res Toxicol* 1994;7:495–502.

83. Monks TJ, Lau SS. Nephrotoxicity of quinol/quinone-linked *S*-conjugates. *Toxicology Lett* 1990; 53:59–67.

84. Aten J. Autoantibodies to the laminin P1 fragment in HgCl$_2$-induced membranous glomerulopathy. *Am J Pathol* 1995;146:1467–1480.

85. Chen Q, Stevens JL. Inhibition of iodoacetamide and *t*-butylhydroperoxide toxicity in LLC-PK1 cells by antioxidants: a role for lipid peroxidation in alkylation induced cytotoxicity. *Arch Biochem Biophys* 1991;284:422–430.

86. Walker PD, Shah SV. Hydrogen peroxide cytotoxicity in LLC-PK1 cells: A role for iron. *Kidney Int* 1991;40:891–898.

87. Ueda N, Shah SV. Role of intracellular calcium in hydrogen peroxide-induced renal tubular cell injury. *Am J Physiol* 1992;263:F214–F221.

88. Salahudeen AK. Role of lipid peroxidation in H$_2$O$_2$-induced renal epithelial (LLC-PK1) cell injury. *Am. J Physiol* 1995;268:F30–F38.

89. Lash LH, Tokarz JJ. Oxidative stress in isolated rat renal proximal and distal tubular cells. *Am J Physiol* 1990;259:F338–F347.

90. Messana JM, Cieslinski DA, O Connor RP, Humes HD. Glutathione protects against exogenous oxidant injury to rabbit renal proximal tubules. *Am J Physiol* 1988;255:F874–F884.

91. Salahudeen AK, Clark EC, Nath KA. Hydrogen peroxide-induced renal injury. A protective role for pyruvate in vitro and in vivo. *J Clin Invest* 1991;88:1886–1893.

92. Boveris A, Oshino N, Chance B. The cellular production of hydrogen peroxide. *Biochem J* 1972;128:617–630.

93. Lund BO, Miller DM, Woods JS. Studies on Hg(II)-induced H_2O_2 formation and oxidative stress *in vivo* and *in vitro* in rat kidney mitochondria. *Biochem Pharmacol* 1993;45:2017–2024.
94. Lund BO, Miller DM, Woods JS. Mercury-induced H_2O_2 production and lipid peroxidation in vitro in rat kidney mitochondria. *Biochem Pharmacol* 1991;42:S181–S187.
95. Ueda N, Guidet B, Shah SV. Gentamicin-induced mobilization of iron from renal cortical mitochondria. *Am J Physiol* 1993; 265: F435–439.
96. Walker RJ, Lazzaro VA, Duggin GG, Horvath JS, Tiller DJ. Evidence that alterations in renal metabolism and lipid peroxidation may contribute to cyclosporine nephrotoxicity. *Transplantation* 1990; 50: 487–492.
97. Campos R, Garrido A, Valenzuela A. Increased resistance against oxidative stress is observed during a short period of renal reperfusion after a temporal ischaemia. *Free Radical Res Commun* 1990;10:259–264.
98. Paller MS, Jacob HS. Cytochrome P-450 mediates tissue-damaging hydroxyl radical formation during reoxygenation of the kidney. *Proc Natl Acad Sci USA* 1994;91:7002–7006.
99. Greene EL, Paller MS. Calcium and free radicals in hypoxia/reoxygenation injury of renal epithelial cells. *Am J Physiol* 1994;266:F13−F20.
100. Greene EL, Paller MS. Xanthine oxidase produces O_2^- in posthypoxic injury of renal epithelial cells. *Am J Physiol* 1992;263:F251–F255.
101. Linas SL, Whittenburg D, Repine JE. Role of xanthine oxidase in ischemia/reperfusioon injury. *Am J Physiol* 1990;258:F711–F716.
102. Brown PC, Dulik DM, TW Jones. The toxicity of menadione (2-methyl-1,4-naphtoquinone) and two thioether conjugates studied with isolated renal epithelial cells. *Arch Biochem Biophys* 1991;285:187–196.
103. Splittgerber AG, Tappel AL. Inhibition of glutathione peroxidase by cadmium and other metal ions. *Arch Biochem Biophys* 1979;197:534–542.
104. Maguire JJ, Kagan V, Ackrell BAC, Serbinova E, Packer L. Succinate-ubiquinone reductase linked recycling of α-tocopherol in reconstituted systems and mitochondria: requirement for reduced ubiquinone. *Arch Biochem Biophys* 1992;292:47–53.
105. Bindoli A. Lipid peroxidation in mitochondria. *Free Radical Biol Med* 1988;5:247–261.
106. Beyer RE. The participation of coenzyme Q in free radical production and antioxidation. *Free Radical Biol Med* 1990;8:545–565.
107. Vamvakas S, Sharma VK, Sheu SS, Anders MW. Perturbations of intracellular calcium distribution in kidney cells by nephrotoxic cysteine *S*-conjugates. *Mol Pharmacol* 1990;38:455–461.
108. Vlessis AA, Mela-Riker L. Potential role of mitochondrial calcium metabolism during reperfusion injury. *Am J Physiol* 1989;256:C1196–C1206.
109. Malis CD, Bonventre JV. Mechanism of calcium potentiation of oxygen free radical injury to renal mitochondria. A model for post-ischemic and toxic mitochondrial damage. *J Biol Chem* 1986;261:14201–14208
110. Juedes MJ, Kass GEN, Orrenius S. *m*-Iodobenzylguanidine increases the mitochondrial Ca^{2+} pool in isolated hepatocytes. *FEBS Lett* 1992;313:39–42.
111. Van de Water B, Zoeteweij JP, Nagelkerke JF. Alkylation-induced oxidative cell injury of renal proximal tubular cells: Involvement of glutathione redox-cycle inhibition. *Arch Biochem Biophys* 1996;327:71–80.

Free Radical Toxicology
Edited by K. B. Wallace
Copyright © 1997 Taylor & Francis

11

Free-Radical-Mediated Chemical Cardiomyopathies

Kendall B. Wallace

*Department of Biochemistry and Molecular Biology, University of Minnesota
School of Medicine, Duluth, Minnesota, USA*

The involvement of oxygen-derived free radicals in the progression of assorted cardiovascular diseases is well established and is the topic of numerous recent reviews (1). This chapter avoids this subject and focuses on what is considered to be a neglected but growing area of concern: the implication of free-radical intermediates in xenobiotic-induced cardiac tissue injury. Although less is known regarding the involvement of free-radical intermediates in chemical-induced cardiomyopathies, much of what has been learned from investigating the disease processes can be transposed directly to advance our understanding of chemical-induced cardiac tissue injury.

There are a number of examples wherein the redox status or antioxidant enzyme activities in cardiac tissue are altered following acute or chronic chemical exposure. Other circumstantial evidence that has been interpreted to reflect a free-radical-mediated mechanism of toxicity is the cytoprotective effect of coadministered antioxidants. Oftentimes, these observations are taken as evidence for oxidative, free-radical-mediated toxicity. We must caution, however, that such changes may be no more than a phenomenological consequence to toxic tissue injury. It may have no bearing on whether free radicals are actually generated and are the ultimate mediators of the tissue damage. Ethanol and aromatic amines are two examples of exposures where the evidence for altered redox state of cardiac tissue is irrefutable despite the uncertainty regarding free-radical generation in the chemical mechanism of induction of tissue injury. It is possible that the enhanced rates of free-radical generation by cardiac tissue from chronically treated animals is the result, not the cause, of the tissue damage. In this chapter, we limit the discussion to only those compounds for which there is compelling evidence that the cardiotoxic tissue injury is a direct result of xenobiotic-dependent stimulation of free-radical generation.

The list of chemicals that satisfy these conditions is limited and includes doxorubicin (adriamycin), selected phenyl amines, epinephrine, and some heavy metals.

Before reviewing the evidence for free-radical-mediated mechanisms of toxic tissue damage, we first discuss many of the physiological and biochemical features of the heart that may be important determinants of the target organ toxicity of these compounds.

MORPHOLOGICAL, PHYSIOLOGICAL, AND
BIOCHEMICAL CONSIDERATIONS

The heart is engineered to function optimally in an oxygen-enriched environment. Although it accounts for only 0.4% of the total body mass in adults, the heart receives about 4% of the total cardiac output and extracts an uncharacteristically large portion of oxygen from arterial blood (2). Most tissues extract only 20–25% of the oxygen. The arterial-venous difference across the coronary vasculature, however, is as high as 70%; the pO_2 of coronary venous blood (18–20 mmHg) is lower than that of any other tissue in the nonexercising animal. This exceptionally high rate of oxygen consumption reflects the enormous metabolic demands required to sustain continuous contractile performance and is matched only by strenuously exercising skeletal muscle. Assuming that in humans, total coronary blood flow is 250 ml/min with a cardiac output of 5800 ml/min and the oxygen content of mixed venous blood 4 ml/dl lower than arterial blood, it can be calculated that despite its small size, the heart accounts for 11% of the total body oxygen consumption in the resting individual (2).

It is also estimated that up to 5% of the high-energy phosphates stored as ATP ($\sim$1–3 mM) and creatine phosphate in cardiac tissue is consumed per beat (3). At 90 beats per minute (bpm) in humans and over 300 bpm in rodents, it is obvious that the metabolic demands on the heart are enormous. Recognizing the inefficiency of oxidative metabolism (1–2% of the oxygen consumed by rat liver mitochondria is liberated as H_2O_2) (4), one would expect relatively high rates of oxygen radical liberation, especially under heavy work loads. This may explain the rate-dependent cardiotoxicity observed for many metabolic inhibitors. Interestingly, the rate of H_2O_2 generation by isolated rat liver mitochondria in state 4 (nonphosphorylating respiration) is about one-half of that for cardiac mitochondria (4,5).

This extraordinary energy demand of the heart is met almost exclusively by oxidative phosphorylation (3). Cardiac tissue has a finite capacity for anaerobic glycolysis, providing for no more than 10% of the ATP required to sustain contractile function. This reliance on oxidative phosphorylation is reflected histomorphologically by the fact that mitochondria account for approximately 50% of the cardiomyocyte cell volume. Cardiac glycogen stores are limited and the primary source for reducing equivalents is the oxidation of fatty acids, which yields approximately 70% of the energy requirements of the heart. The remaining 30% is provided mostly through the insulin-dependent accumulation of glucose and aerobic glycolysis. In the diabetic state, virtually all of the energy demands of the heart are met via fatty acid oxidation coupled to the oxidation of acetyl-CoA (acetylcoenzyme A) within the tricarboxylic acid cycle.

Finally, it deserves mentioning that the basal metabolic rate reflects a time-averaged rate. Unlike most tissues, the energy demands of the heart are not constant and metabolic rates vary in synchrony with the contractile cycle. [31]P nuclear magnetic resonance (NMR) spectroscopy reveals that the concentrations of both ATP and creatine phosphate in myocardial tissue are inversely related to aortic pressure (6). Conversely, inorganic phosphate and NAD concentrations peak during systole and reach a minimum during diastole. Accordingly, one would predict that the liberation of free-radical intermediates and any associated tissue damage in heart tissue propagates as wave forms across the contracting myocardium, in synchrony with the contraction cycle and with an intensity that is proportional to the metabolic demands.

CHARACTERISTICS OF FREE-RADICAL GENERATION IN HEART TISSUE

There is compelling evidence indicating that the principal source of free-radical and H_2O_2 generation in cardiomyocytes is the mitochondrion (7,8). The concentration of cytochrome P-450 and the related drug-metabolizing enzyme activities of cardiac microsomes is 20% or less than that of hepatic microsomes (9,10). As would be expected, the activities of cytochrome P-450-dependent drug-metabolizing enzymes and the associated generation of free-radical intermediates in heart tissue is correspondingly lower (9–11). This may explain the number of examples of agents that are known to be substrates for cytochrome P-450-dependent generation of free-radical intermediates but do not elicit substantive cardiotoxicity.

Heart tissue exhibits a comparable scarcity of other subcellular structures that are known to be important sources of free-radical generation in other tissues. Amongst these is xanthine oxidase, which, despite being implicated in experimental models of ischemia-reperfusion damage, is virtually absent from human cardiac tissue (12).

One abundant and potentially important source of free radicals that is unique to skeletal and cardiac muscle is myoglobin. It is well documented that like hemoglobin, the heme iron of myoglobin is subject to sequential univalent oxidations and reductions to liberate a variety of free-radical intermediates of molecular oxygen (13,14). The oxidation of myoglobin by peroxides to the oxoferryl form [Fe(IV) = O], which then liberates highly reactive hydroxyl free radicals, suggests the possibility that myoglobin represents an important physiological source of Fenton iron in vivo. Oxoferrylmyoglobin also catalyzes peroxidase-like reactions, possibly liberating free-radical intermediates of selected xenobiotics. The fact that myoglobin interacts electrochemically with numerous xenobiotics suggests potentially broad toxicological relevance; the reactivity of xenobiotics with myoglobin may be an important factor contributing to the cardioselective toxicity of certain agents (15,16).

Another factor conferring cardioselective toxicity is the mitochondrial-mediated liberation of free-radical intermediates of selected xenobiotic compounds. It is well established that certain xenobiotics, depending on their univalent redox potential, can accept electrons from the mitochondrial electron transport chain, principally from the NADH-ubiquinone oxidoreductase of complex I (17,18). The resulting univalent free-radical intermediate can then either accept a second electron or donate the unpaired electron to a suitable electron acceptor, such as dioxygen, to complete the redox cycle. Anthracycline antibiotics, naphthoquinones, and nitroaromatic compounds are good examples of agents that redox cycle on the mitochondrial inner membrane (19–22). Accordingly, the mitochondrial electron transport chain represents an important subcellular source of excessive free-radical generation in the presence of autoxidizable xenobiotics. In view of the abundance of mitochondria, with cardiac NADH-ubiquinone oxidoreductase activity being 50 times that of liver tissue, the mitochondrion represents an important, if not principal, source of xenobiotic free-radical generation in heart. This is not necessarily the case for tissues such as liver, which have abundant endoplasmic reticulum but sparse mitochondria.

Powis and Appel demonstrated finite ranges of univalent redox potentials for substrates of NADPH-cytochrome P-450 and NADH-cytochrome $b5$ reductases, as well as for mitochondrial NADH-ubiquinone oxidoreductase (23). For each enzyme there exists a range of univalent redox potentials for chemicals that yields the greatest rates of oxygen free-radical generation. Compounds with redox potentials outside this range are poor substrates and elicit minimal free-radical generation. Interestingly, the enzyme systems examined exhibit overlapping but distinct optima. Chemicals with univalent redox potentials between $+25$ mV and -100 mV are good substrates for mitochondrial-mediated free-radical generation. The optimum redox potential is -70 mV. For the microsomal cytochrome P-450 reductase, the range of redox potentials is -70 mV to -300 mV with maximal rates of free-radical generation by chemicals having a redox potential of -200 mV. From these data, it was concluded that an important determinant of the probability for and the subcellular site of generation of free-radical intermediates is the univalent redox potential of the individual agent. For quinone compounds, and possibly others, the mitochondrial electron transport chain is suggested to represent the principal subcellular site of free-radical generation in isolated hepatocytes (20). One might infer from this that, because of the relative abundance of mitochondria, some degree of cardioselectivity may be conferred to those xenobiotics having a univalent redox potential within the optimum range for mitochondrial NADH-ubiquinone oxidoreductase.

A final factor to be considered regarding free-radical-mediated cardioselective toxicity is the demonstration by Nohl et al. (24) of an NADH-oxidoreductase localized on the outer mitochondrial membrane that is unique to heart tissue. This enzyme does not participate in oxidative phosphorylation and is not detectable in any other tissue source. Although there remains some uncertainty as to the physiological purpose of this enzyme, there is growing evidence supporting this rotenone-insensitive exogenous NADH oxidoreductase as a critical factor determining the cardioselective toxicity of selected xenobiotics.

CHARACTERISTICS OF ANTIOXIDANT DEFENSE MECHANISMS IN HEART TISSUE

The relative deficiency of antioxidant defense mechanisms in cardiac tissue (Table 1) has been widely implicated as important not only in myocardial ischemia and perfusion, but also in xenobiotic-induced and malnutritive cardiac tissue injury (25–27). The concentrations of vitamin C (ascorbic acid) and uric acid are lower in heart than most other organs examined in rats 6–15 mo of age (28). Cardiac glutathione concentration (1–2 μmol/g) compares with most other tissues except for liver, which is 5–10 mM GSH in rats and mice (28–31). Antioxidant enzyme activities are also low in heart tissue. Despite the abundance of mitochondria, cardiac SOD activity is one-third that of liver (26,27). Since cardiac myocytes are void of peroxisomes, it is not surprising that catalase activity is barely detectable (26,27). Finally, although the activity of glutathione peroxidase in the soluble fraction of cardiac homogenates (expressed per milligram protein) compares to that of liver (26,27,32,33), cardiac glutathione reductase activity is only about 20% that of liver (27).

These enzymes are vital components of the antioxidant defense systems, which enable tissues to detoxify free-radical intermediates generated during normal physiologic and biochemical activities. Their importance is accentuated in determining the response to external factors that stimulate excessive free-radical generation, whether it be a reperfusion phenomenon or exposure to free-radical-generating xenobiotics. The finite capacity of the antioxidant defense systems determines the capacity of the cells to withstand exaggerated rates of free-radical generation. The limited activities of antioxidant enzymes render the heart highly susceptible to free-radical injury. However, since the antioxidant defense systems are invoked in response to all chemicals capable of stimulating free-radical generation, this alone does not confer cardioselectivity; the critical event in determining cardioselective cell injury must relate to tissue-specific sites of generation, rather than detoxification, of reactive free-radical intermediates.

SELECTED EXAMPLES OF XENOBIOTIC-INDUCED FREE-RADICAL-MEDIATED CARDIOTOXICITY

In this final section, I review the evidence implicating free-radical-mediated tissue injury in the mechanism of action of selected cardiotoxic agents. The review focuses on adriamycin (doxorubicin), which is the most widely studied and best documented example of a free-radical-mediated cardiotoxic agent. Before discussing the individual agents, however, it seems appropriate to briefly describe the reported effects of free-radical generating systems when applied directly to cardiac tissue in vitro.

Application of hydrogen peroxide or the combination of xanthine oxidase plus xanthine suppresses the electrical excitability of cardiomyocytes in culture,

TABLE 1. *Cardiac antioxidant defense mechanisms*

	Heart	Liver
Superoxide dismutase (μg/mg protein)	10	36
Catalase (U/g)	1	173
Glutathione (μmol/g)	1–2	5–10
Glutathione peroxidase (nmol/min/mg protein)	56	64
Glutathione reductase (nmol/min/mg protein)	10	50

Note. Sources of data are referenced in the text.

prolonging the duration of the action potential to the point of decreasing the excitability and rate of contraction (34,35). Perfusion with oxygen free-radical-generating systems ex vivo also depresses the electrical excitability and mechanical contractility of isolated hearts and of cardiac muscle strips (36–39). These responses are suggested to result from the inhibitory effect of free radicals on the Na^+/K^+-ATPase and the Na^+/Ca^{2+}-antiport of the sarcolemma. Free radicals are also known to interfere with calcium accumulation by both the sarcoplasmic reticulum and mitochondria (40,41). Coperfusion of either the muscle strips or cardiomyocyte cell cultures with superoxide dismutase (SOD) or catalase inhibits both the negative inotropic and electrical effects. Therefore, despite the questionable relevance of perfusing cells or tissues with free-radical-generating systems and/or antioxidant enzymes, the evidence does demonstrate the potential for important adverse effects of free radicals liberated in response to xenobiotic exposure on cardiac structure and function.

Catecholamines

Implication of free-radical intermediates in catecholamine toxicity is appropriate only in situations of excessively high catecholamine concentrations. Catecholamines are normally metabolized very efficiently by monoamine oxidase and catechol *O*-methyltransferase. It is only when these enzymes are saturated that catecholamines autoxidize to any appreciable extent. Injection of large boluses of catecholamines cause assorted ultrastructural changes and cardiac arrhythmias that are accentuated in animals deprived of dietary vitamin E (42). The cytotoxicity in isolated cardiomyocytes exposed in vitro to isoproterenol is partially reversed by vitamins A and C or by adding SOD or catalase to the exposure medium (43). Accordingly, cell injury under these conditions likely reflects a free-radical-mediated process, with the radicals being liberated during the metal-catalyzed autoxidation reactions. One might consider that any cardiotoxicity would be secondary to some other neurogenic or endocrine event that elicits a catecholamine storm. Although there are no specific examples of environmental or industrial chemical-induced catecholamine-mediated cardiotoxicity, catecholamine autoxidation and liberation of oxygen free radicals may be vitally important in the pathogenesis of ischemia related cardiac damage. The reader is referred to another monograph in this series for a comprehensive discussion of catecholamine cardiotoxicity (44).

Phenylenediamines

Another class of compounds that undergo extensive autoxidation is the phenylenediamines, which are important in the photographic and dyestuff industries. Like the catecholamines, transition metals catalyze the transfer of electrons from phenylenediamines to molecular oxygen. The products are superoxide anion free radicals and the stable cation radical of the drug (45,46). Additional products of the autoxidation are hydrogen peroxide and hydroxyl free radicals (46). Exposure of isolated erythrocytes to the *N*-methyl-substituted phenylenediamines in vitro results in their autoxidation accompanied by the generation of hydrogen peroxide, the depletion of glutathione (presumably via the H_2O_2-dependent glutathione peroxidase reaction), and the oxidation of hemoglobin (46). This free-radical-mediated oxidative tissue damage is suggested to be responsible for the myocardial and skeletal muscle necrosis that is associated with the administration of phenylenediamines to rats in vivo (47). Structure–activity studies reveal a correlation between the rates of spontaneous autoxidation of *N*-methyl-substituted phenylenediamines and the rates of hydrogen peroxide generation, glutathione depletion, and methemoglobin formation in erythrocytes exposed in vitro (48). More importantly, the extent of histological tissue necrosis and changes in plasma enzymes observed following acute phenylenediamine administration to rats in vivo correlates with the rank order rate of autoxidation in vitro. The tissue necrosis is limited to cardiac and skeletal muscle; there was no evidence for renal or hepatic involvement (48). It should be noted that the phenylenediamines are known to redox cycle on the mitochondrial electron transport chain (49,50), which is consistent with the fact that tissues with high oxidative capacity are most sensitive in vivo. Thus the myotoxicity of these agents may well reflect the inhibition of mitochondrial bioenergetics in tissues that are reliant on oxidative phosphorylation to meet the high metabolic demands. Furthermore, the evidence suggests that the extent of toxicity correlates with the susceptibility of the agents to accept electrons from the respiratory chain to initiate the futile redox cycling of these agents. As suggested by Powis et al. for substituted quinones (20,23), the univalent redox potential may be a useful predictor of the myotoxic potential of the individual substituted phenylenediamine analogs.

Doxorubicin (Adriamycin)

Adriamycin is a potent and broad-spectrum antineoplastic agent effective in treating a number of both solid tumors and leukemias. Unfortunately, the clinical utility is seriously curtailed by the high incidence and severity of a cumulative and irreversible cardiomyopathy that is manifested as a dilated congestive failure. The cardiomyopathy, both in terms of structural and functional deficits, persists far beyond the elimination of residual traces of administered drug. The drug also elicits acute arrhythmogenic effects, but these are transient and responsive to conventional therapies.

It has long been recognized that the mechanism by which adriamycin elicits its toxic effects involves metabolic activation and generation of highly reactive free-radical intermediates (51–53). These mechanisms have been investigated extensively and adriamycin has become a classic, prototypical model for free-radical-mediated cardiotoxicity (54). The following paragraphs present an overview of the mechanistic features of adriamycin toxicity, emphasizing specific factors that may contribute to the cardioselective toxicity caused by the drug.

The metabolic disposition of adriamycin in biological systems is illustrated in Figure 1. The drug is subject to univalent reduction by a number of reducing systems, both chemical and enzymatic, to form a highly reactive and unstable semiquinone

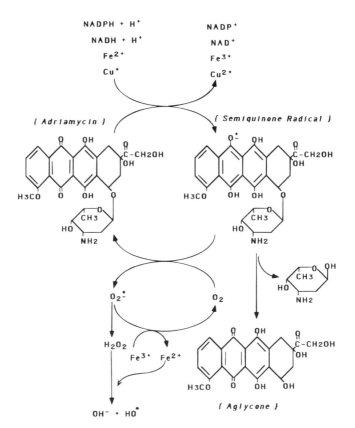

FIG. 1. Schematic representation of the metabolic fate of doxorubicin in biological systems. The anthraquinone is reduced by any one of several enzymatic or metal-catalyzed reactions to the univalently reduced semiquinone free-radical intermediate. In the presence of abundant electron acceptors, such as oxygen, the semiquinone rapidly reoxidizes to the parent quinone at the expense of generating the superoxide anion free radical, which is subject to further reductions to hydrogen peroxide and, in the presence of a Fenton catalyst, the hydroxyl free radical. Under anaerobic conditions, doxorubicin is aglycosylated and subject to extensive protein and nucleic acid binding.

free-radical intermediate. In the presence of a suitable electron acceptor, the unpaired electron transfers from the semiquinone free radical to reduce the electron acceptor to its corresponding free-radical intermediate. With dioxygen as electron acceptor, the product is the superoxide anion free radical. As long as the concentration of electron acceptor is not limiting (e.g., under aerobic conditions), the reaction is characterized by the cyclical univalent reduction and reoxidation of adriamycin at the expense of transferring reducing equivalents to liberate superoxide free radicals with no net metabolism of the drug.

The first metabolic step in initiating the redox cycling of adriamycin is catalyzed by a number of different enzymes, both soluble and membrane bound. Among these, the most prominent in liver is the microsomal NADPH-cytochrome P-450-dependent univalent reduction to the adriamycin semiquinone free radical (51,52). Incubation of isolated liver microsomes or reconstituted enzymes with adriamycin results in the catalytic oxidation of NADPH. In aerobic solutions, this is accompanied by the consumption of dissolved oxygen and liberation of superoxide anion free radicals with no net metabolism of the drug (51–53,55). It is only in oxygen-limited conditions that the adriamycin metabolites are detected (55,56). The limiting step in adriamycin redox cycling is the univalent reduction of the drug, not the transfer of the unpaired electron to molecular oxygen. Thus, the adriamycin semiquinone free radical is highly unstable in aerobic solution and is detectable by electron spin resonance (ESR) spectrometry only when oxygen, along with other alternate electron acceptors, is eliminated from solution (51–53). In biological systems, oxygen appears to be the preferred electron acceptor in that little covalent binding of drug metabolites to cell macromolecules is detected at physiological oxygen partial pressures.

A cytochrome P-450-mediated NADPH-dependent metabolic activation of adriamycin to form the semiquinone free-radical intermediate has also been identified on the nuclear envelope of liver cell fractions (57–59). The nuclear cytochrome P-450-dependent metabolic path is indistinguishable from that characterized for microsomal membranes, except that the rate of metabolism by the nuclear fraction is conspicuously slower (59). Despite this limited metabolic capacity, activation of adriamycin on nuclear membranes may be highly significant in generating the reactive free-radical intermediate(s), which have a finite diffusibility, in the immediate vicinity of the genetic material of the cell (58,59).

Another membrane-associated site of univalent reduction of adriamycin to form the semiquinone free radical is the mitochondrial electron transport chain (18,19). Adriamycin accepts electrons from the NADH:ubiquinone oxidoreductase of complex I to form the semiquinone free radical, which is detectable by ESR spectroscopy in anaerobic solutions (18,19). In the presence of oxygen, the semiquinone free radical rapidly autoxidizes at the expense of generating superoxide anion free radicals. This is a site-specific reduction of adriamycin as revealed by inhibitor isolation experiments in vitro (19). Furthermore, the rate of reduction of adriamycin is proportional to the degree of reduction of complex I of the respiratory chain. Adding either rotenone or antimycin A to NADH-energized mitochondria stimulates adriamycin redox cycling. Succinate-supported redox cycling of adriamycin is enhanced in the presence of antimycin A and attributed to the retrograde transport of electrons to reduce complex I. Adding rotenone to antimycin A-treated mitochondria energized with succinate inhibits the redox cycling of adriamycin, which is evidence that the redox cycling of adriamycin in succinate-energized mitochondria is due to reverse electron transport across complex I.

Besides the membrane-associated reducing systems, there also exist soluble proteins capable of reducing adriamycin to its semiquinone free-radical intermediate, the two most notable examples being xanthine oxidase and ferromyoglobin. In oxygen-limited solutions, adding adriamycin to the combination of xanthine plus xanthine oxidase results in the generation of the adriamycin semiquinone free radical (60). Once formed, the semiquinone free radical of adriamycin is subject to the same metabolic fate as that generated by cytochrome P-450 or the mitochondrial electron transport system. The physiological relevance of this reaction by xanthine oxidase is, however, highly questionable since human heart tissue lacks appreciable amounts of the enzyme activity (12).

It has long been acknowledged that adriamycin associates with free iron or copper to form unstable coordination complexes that spontaneously autoxidize to liberate oxygen free radicals (61–63). This may be of particular significance to heart tissue since adriamycin also interacts with the heme iron of myoglobin to form unstable oxyferro complexes (15,16). Such complexes not only liberate free radicals in solution, but their formation also limits the oxymyoglobin stores available to meet the high oxygen demands of the contracting myocardium. It has been suggested that this heme protein serves as the physiological source of Fenton iron and that its abundance in myocardium may be important in contributing to the cardioselective toxicity of the drug (15,16).

Once formed, the carbon-centered semiquinone or oxygen free-radical intermediates undergo the entire spectrum of reactions discussed in Part I of this volume, including hydrogen atom abstraction, and nucleophilic substitution and addition reactions. Characteristic responses include depletion of glutathione and pyrimidine nucleotide reducing equivalents, stimulation of lipid peroxidation, oxidation of membrane proteins, DNA strand scission, formation of protein and DNA cross links, interference with cell calcium homeostasis, and inhibition of mitochondrial bioenergetics, all of which are believed to be a consequence of the stimulation of free-radical generation by adriamycin (29,30,31,33,54–59). Induction of apoptosis has also been reported (64). The mechanisms by which the adriamycin semiquinone free radical or any of the reactive oxygen radical species catalyze these reactions are not peculiar to either the drug or to heart tissue. Details of the individual reactions are provided in earlier chapters. What merits emphasis in this chapter are the data demonstrating a predilection for the induction and accumulation of oxidative damage in heart tissue. The evidence, although limited, provides some insights into possible determinants of the target organ toxicity.

Adriamycin stimulates the in vitro NADPH-dependent peroxidation of microsomal lipids from various tissue sources, albeit at fairly high drug concentrations (65,66). The degree of stimulation is approximately twofold greater for liver compared to lung and kidney and least with membranes from heart tissue (66). Contrast this with the observation that the covalent binding of adriamycin metabolites to proteins in vitro is sixfold higher with cardiac compared to hepatic microsomal fractions (55). Adriamycin also stimulates the peroxidation of mitochondrial membrane lipids in vitro. In fact, rabbit sarcosomal lipid peroxidation is doubled at an optimum concentration of approximately 100 μM adriamycin, whereas mitochondrial lipid peroxidation is stimulated almost fourfold at 25 μM adriamycin (67). This is consistent with the observation that adriamycin-stimulates a greater rate of oxygen consumption and superoxide anion free-radical generation by cardiac mitochondria compared to the corresponding rates for cardiac sarcosomes (68). These data establish the potential for adriamycin to stimulate the peroxidation of membrane lipids, but they do not reveal important determinants of the cardioselective toxicity of the drug in vivo as evidenced by the preferential accumulation of products of lipid peroxidation in cardiac tissue following acute drug treatment. Four days following a single injection of mice with 15 mg/kg adriamycin (ip) there is a 3-to-30-fold increase in malondialdehyde equivalents in heart tissue, compared to less than a threefold increase in lipid peroxide levels in liver, spleen, or kidney (69,70). Furthermore, the increase in lipid peroxides in heart is sustained over 6 d, whereas that in liver and kidney returns to control pretreatment values by 6 d. There was no increase in lipid peroxide formation in either serum or lung. This preferential stimulation of cardiac lipid peroxidation in vivo varies depending on the species, being most evident in mice and guinea pigs, but not in rats (71).

Finally, it is well established that adriamycin interferes with mitochondrial oxidative phosphorylation and bioenergetics. Interestingly, cardiac mitochondria are far more sensitive than mitochondria from liver or kidney to the in vitro inhibition by adriamycin of succinate-supported oxidative phosphorylation. The IC50 for adriamycin with cardiac mitochondria is approximately 5 μM compared to 500–800 μM for rat liver and kidney mitochondria (72). A similar target organ sensitivity is observed following in vivo drug administration. Mitochondria isolated from heart tissue of rats 1 d following the last of 6 daily injections of 4 mg/kg exhibit a statistically significant decrease in both the coupling and control of oxidative phosphorylation (73). A comparable inhibition of bioenergetics is not manifested for mitochondria isolated from either the liver or kidney of these same animals. The inhibition of mitochondrial glutathione peroxidase activity in vivo also appears to be exclusive to the heart (73).

Collectively, these data reveal that although adriamycin is capable of eliciting free-radical mediated damage to various tissue membranes in vitro, the heart exhibits a preferential sensitivity in vivo, which is most evident in the mitochondrial cell fraction. Accordingly, it may be the abundance and importance of cardiac mitochondria that determines the cardioselective toxicity of the drug. Evidence in support of this hypothesis is the recent demonstration that cardiomyocytes isolated from neonatal rats are protected from adriamycin-induced cell injury by including specific inhibitors of mitochondrial calcium channels in the exposure medium (74). Similarly, cardiomyocytes isolated from adult rats exposed in vivo to subchronic adriamycin express an increased sensitivity to calcium-induced cell injury that is prevented by inhibitors of mitochondrial calcium channels (75,76). Rats treated with the structurally related analog iminodaunorubicin, which does not redox cycle to liberate oxygen free radicals, did not exhibit any change in mitochondrial calcium regulation. We are led to conclude that, although adriamycin indiscriminately stimulates free-radical-mediated tissue damage in vitro, there is ample evidence demonstrating the cardioselective toxicity in vivo. The weight of the experimental evidence implicates the mitochondrion as an important intracellular target conferring the tissue-selective toxicity of this drug.

SUMMARY

This chapter describes a number of features that are important to the manifestation of free-radical-mediated tissue damage to the heart. Some important considerations are the extraordinarily high rate of oxygen consumption by the heart, the presence of myoglobin, the abundance of mitochondria and lack of cytochrome P-450-related drug-metabolizing enzymes, the existence of an NADH-oxidoreductase on the outer mitochondrial membrane that is unique to cardiac tissue, and the deficiency of antioxidant defense mechanisms. Each of these factors, alone or in combination, have been implicated in explaining the cardioselective target organ toxicity observed for selected xenobiotics capable of liberating reactive free-radical intermediates, a few examples of which are described.

REFERENCES

1. Kehrer, JP (1993). Free radicals as mediators of tissue injury and disease. *Crit. Rev. Toxicol.* 23:21–48.
2. Wade, OL, and Bishop, JM (1962). *Cardiac Output and Regional Blood Flow.* Oxford: Blackwell.
3. Morgan, HE, and Neely, JR (1982). Metabolic regulation and myocardial function. In: *The Heart.* New York: McGraw-Hill.
4. Boveris, A, Oshino, N, and Chance, B (1972). The cellular production of hydrogen peroxide. *Biochem. J.* 128:617–630.
5. Cadenas, E, and Boveris, A (1980). Enhancement of hydrogen peroxide formation by protophores and ionophores in antimycin-supplemented mitochondria. *Biochem. J.* 188: 31–37.
6. Fossell, ET, Morgan, HE, and Ingwall, JS (1980). Measurement of changes in high-energy phosphates in the cardiac cycle using gated P-31 nuclear magnetic resonance. *Proc. Natl. Acad. Sci. USA* 77:3654–3658.
7. Turrens, JF, Freeman, BA, and Crapo, JD (1982). Hyperoxia increases H2O2 release by lung mitochondria and microsomes. *Arch. Biochem. Biophys.* 217:411–421.
8. Radi, R, Turrens, JF, Chang, LY, Bush, KM, Crapo, JD, and Freeman, BA (1991). Detection of catalase in rat heart mitochondria. *J. Biol. Chem.* 266:22028–22034.
9. Abraham, NG, Pinto, A, Levere, RD, and Mullane, K (1987). Identification of heme oxygenase and cytochrome P-450 in the rabbit heart. *J. Mol. Cell. Cardiol.* 19:73–81.
10. Namkung, MJ, Yang., HL, and Juchau, MR (1994). Cytochrome P-450-dependent biotransformation of 2-acetylaminofluorene in cell-free preparations of human embryonic hepatic, adrenal, renal, pulmonary, and cardiac tissues. *Drug Metab. Dispos.* 22:331–337.
11. Reinke, LA, Lai, EK, DuBose, CM, and McCay, PB (1987). Reactive free-radical generation in vivo in heart and liver of ethanol-fed rats: Correlation with radical formation in vitro. *Proc. Natl., Acad. Sci. USA* 84:9223–9227.

12. de Jong, JW, van der Meer, P, Nieukoop, AS, Huizer, T, Stroeve, RJ, and Bos, E Xanthine oxidoreductase activity in perfused hearts of various species, including humans. *Circ. Res.* 67:770–773.

13. Galaris, D, Eddy, L, Arduini, A, Cadenas, E, and Hochstein, P (1989). Mechanisms of reoxidation injury in myocardial infarction: Implications of a myoglobin redox cycle. *Biochem. Biophys. Res. Commun.* 160:1163–1168.

14. Davies, MJ (1990). Detection of myoglobin-derived radicals on the reaction of metmyoglobin with hydrogen peroxide and other peroxidic compounds. *Free Radical Res. Commun.* 10:361–370.

15. Trost, LC, and Wallace, KB (1994). Adriamycin-induced oxidation of myoglobin. *Biochem. Biophys. Res. Commun.* 204:30–37.

16. Trost, LC, and Wallace, KB (1994). Stimulation of myoglobin-dependent lipid peroxidation by adriamycin. *Biochem. Biophys. Res. Commun.* 204:23–29.

17. Cadenas, E, Boveris, A, Ragan, CI, and Stoppani, IOM (1977). Production of superoxide radicals and hydrogen peroxide by NADH-ubiquinone reductase and ubiquinol-cytochrome *c* reductase from beef heart mitochondria. *Arch. Biochem. Biophys.* 180:248–257.

18. Doroshow, JH, and Davies, KJA (1986). Redox cycling of anthracyclines by cardiac mitochondria II. Formation of superoxide anion, hydrogen peroxide, and hydroxyl radical. *J. Biol. Chem.* 261:3068–3074.

19. Davies, KJA, and Doroshow, JH (1986). Redox cycling of anthracyclines by cardiac mitochondria I. Anthracycline radical formation by NADH dehydrogenase. *J. Biol. Chem.* 261:3060–3067.

20. Powis, G, Svingen, BA, and Appel, P (1981). Quinone-stimulated superoxide formation by subcellular fractions, isolated hepatocytes, and other cells. *Mol. Pharmacol.* 20:387–394.

21. Henry, TR, and Wallace, KB (1995). Differential mechanisms of induction of the mitochondrial permeability transition by quinones of varying chemical reactivities. *Toxicol. Appl. Pharmacol.* 134:195–203.

22. Bironaite, D, Cenas, NK, and Kulys, JJ (1991). The rotenone-insensitive reduction of quinones and nitrocompounds by mitochondrial NADH:ubiquinone reductase. *Biochim. Biophys. Acta* 1060:203–209.

23. Powis, G, and Appel, P (1980). Relationship of the single electron reduction potential of quinones to their reduction by flavoproteins. *Biochem. Pharmacol.* 29:2567–2572.

24. Nohl, H (1987). A novel superoxide radical generator in heart mitochondria. *FEBS Lett.* 214:269–273.

25. Kaul, N, Siveski-Iliskovic, N, Hill, M, Slezak, J, and Singal, PK (1993). Free radicals in the heart. *J. Pharmacol. Toxicol. Methods* 30:55–67.

26. Doroshow, JH, Locker, GY, and Meyers, CE (1980). Enzymatic defenses of the mouse heart against reactive oxygen metabolites. *J. Clin. Invest.* 65:128–135.

27. Chen, Y, Saari, JT, and Kang, YJ (1994). Weak antioxidant defenses make the heart a target for damage in copper-deficient rats. *Free Radical Biol. Med.* 17:529–536.

28. Rikans, LE, and Moore, DR (1988). Effect of aging on aqueous-phase antioxidants in tissues of male Fischer rats. *Biochim. Biophys. Acta* 966:269–275.

29. Boor, PJ (1979). Cardiac glutathione: Diurnal rhythm and variation in drug-induced cardiomyopathy. *Res. Commun. Chem. Pathol. Pharmacol.* 24:27–36.

30. Doroshow, JH, Locker, GY, Baldinger, J, and Meyers, CE (1979). The effect of doxorubicin on hepatic and cardiac glutathione. *Res. Commun. Chem. Pathol. Pharmacol.* 26:285–295.

31. Olson, RD, MacDonald, JS, VanBoxtel, CJ, Boerth, RC, Harbison, RD, Slonim, AE, Freeman, RW, and Oates, JA (1980). Regulatory role of glutathione and soluble sulfhydryl groups in the toxicity of adriamycin. *J. Pharmacol. Exp. Ther.* 215:450–454.

32. Nohl, H, and Hegner, D (1978). Do mitochondria produce oxygen radicals? *Eur. J. Biochem.* 82:563–567.

33. Yoon, SB, Kajiyama, K, Hino, Y, Sugiyama, Y, and Ogura, R (1983). Effect of adriamycin on lipid peroxide, glutathione peroxidase and respiratory responses of mitochondria from heart, liver and kidney. *Kurume Med. J.* 30:1–4.

34. Barrington, PL, Meier, CF, and Weglicki, B (1988). Abnormal electrical activity induced by free radical generating systems in isolated cardiocytes. *J. Mol. Cell. Cardiol.* 20:1163–1178.

35. Beresewicz, A, and Horackova, M (1991). Alterations in electrical and contractile behavior of isolated cardiomyocytes by hydrogen peroxide: Possible ionic mechanisms. *J. Mol. Cell. Cardiol.* 23:899–918.

36. Blaustein, AS, Schine, L, Brooks, WW, Fanburg, BL, and Bing, OHL (1986). Influence of exogenously generated oxidant species on myocardial function. *Am. J. Physiol.* 250:H595–H599.

FREE RADICAL TOXICOLOGY

37. Gupta, M, and Singal, PK (1989). Time course of structure, function, and metabolic changes due to an exogenous source of oxygen metabolites in rat heart. *Can J. Physiol. Pharmacol.* 67:1549–1559.
38. Kirshenbaum, LA, Thomas, TP, Randhawa, AK, and Singal, PK (1992). Time course of cardiac myocyte injury due to oxidative stress. *Mol. Cell. Biochem.* 111:25–31.
39. Ytrehus, K, Myklebut, R, and Mjos, OD (1986). Influence of oxygen radicals generated by xanthine oxidase in the isolated perfused rat heart. *Cardiovasc. Res.* 20:597–603.
40. Kaneko, M, Singal, PK, and Dhalla, NS (1990). Alterations in heart sarcolemmal Ca^{2+}-ATPase and Ca^{2+} binding activities due to oxygen radicals. *Basic Res. Cardiol.* 85:45–54.
41. Reeves, JP, Bailey, CA, and Hale, CC (1986). Redox modification of sodium-calcium exchange activity in cardiac sarcolemmal vesicles. *J. Biol. Chem.* 201:4948–4955.
42. Singal, PK, Kapur, N, Dhillon, KS, Beamish, RE, and Dhalla, NS (1982). Role of free radicals in catecholamine-induced cardiomyopathy. *Can. J. Physiol. Pharmacol.* 60:1390–1397.
43. Persoon-Rothert, M, van der Valk-Kokshoorn, EJ, Egas-Kenniphaas, JM, Mauve, I, and van der Laarse, A (1989). Isoproterenol-induced cytotoxicity in neonatal rat heart cell cultures is mediated by free radical formation. *J. Mol. Cell. Cardiol.* 21: 285–1291.
44. Dhalla, NS, Yates, JC, Naimark, B, Dhalla, KS, Beamish, RE, and Ostadal, B (1992). Cardiotoxicity of catecholamines and related agents. In: *Cardiovascular Toxicology*, ed. D Acosta, Jr, Target Organ Toxicology series, pp. 239–282. New York: Raven Press.
45. LuValle, JE, Glass, DB, and Weissberger, A (1948). Oxidation processes. XXI. The autoxidation of the *p*-phenylenediamines. *J. Am. Chem. Soc.* 70:2223–2233.
46. Munday, R (1988). Generation of superoxide radical, hydrogen peroxide and hydroxyl radical during the autoxidation of *N,N,N',N'*-tetramethyl *p*-phenylenediamine. *Chem. Biol. Interact.* 65:133–143.
47. Jasmin, G (1961). Action toxique de la paraphenylenediamine chez le rat et quelques autres rongeurs. *Rev. Can. Biol.* 20:37–46.
48. Munday, R, Manns, E, Fowke, EA, and Hoggard, GK (1989). Muscle necrosis by *N*-methylated *p*-phenylenediamines in rats: Structure-activity relationships and correlation with free radical production in vitro. *Toxicology* 57:303–314.
49. Mustafa, MG, and King, TE (1967). Wurster's Blue mediated oxidation of NADH and phosphorylation in miotchondria. *Arch. Biochem. Biophys.* 122:501–508.
50. Mustafa, MG, Cowger, ML, Labbe, RF, and King, TE (1968). General nature of Wurster's Blue shunts in the respiratory chain. *J. Biol. Chem.* 243:1908–1918.
51. Bachur, NR, Gordon, SL, and Gee, MV (1977). Anthracycline antibiotic augmentation of microsomal electron transport and free radical formation. *Mol. Pharmacol.* 13:901–910.
52. Bachur, NR, Gordon, SL, Gee, MV, and Kon, H (1979). NADPH cytochrome P-450 reductase activation of quinone anticancer agents to free radicals. *Proc. Natl. Acad. Sci. USA* 76:954–957.
53. Turner, MJ, Everman, DB, Ellington, SP, and Fields, CE (1990). Detection of free radicals during the cellular metabolism of adriamycin. *Free Radical Biol. Med.* 9:415–421.
54. Singal, PK, Deally, CMR, and Weinberg, LE (1987). Subcellular effects of adriamycin in the heart- A concise review. *J. Mol. Cell. Cardiol.* 19:817–828.
55. Scheulen, ME, Kappus, H, Nienhaus, A, and Schmidt, CG (1982). Covalent protein binding of reactive adriamycin metabolites in rat liver and rat heart microsomes. *J. Cancer Res. Clin. Oncol.* 103:39–48.
56. Wallace, KB, and Johnson, JJ (1986). Oxygen-dependent effect of microsomes on the binding of doxorubicin to rat hepatic nuclear DNA. *Mol. Pharmacol.* 31:307–311.
57. Bachur, NR, Gee, MV, and Friedman, RD (1982). Nuclear catalyzed antibiotic free radical formation. *Cancer Res.* 42:1078–1081.
58. Sinha, BK, Trush, MA, Kennedy, KA, and Mimnaugh, EG (1984). Enzymatic activation and binding of adriamycin to nuclear DNA. *Cancer Res.* 44:2892–2896.
59. Wallace, KB (1986). Aglycosylation and disposition of doxorubicin in isolated rat liver nuclei and microsomes. *Drug Metab. Dispos.* 14:399–404.
60. Pan, S-S, and Bachur, NS (1980). Xanthine oxidase-catalyzed reductive cleavage of anthracycline antibiotics and free radical formation. *Mol. Pharmacol.* 17:95–99.
61. Greenaway, FT, and Dabrowiak, JC (1982). The binding of copper ions to daunomycin and adriamycin. *J. Inorg. Biochem.* 16:91–107.
62. Zweier, JL (1984). Reduction of O_2 by iron-adriamycin. *J. Biol. Chem.* 259:6056–6058.
63. Wallace, KB (1986). Nonenzymatic oxygen activation and stimulation of lipid peroxidation by doxorubicin-copper. *Toxicol. Appl. Pharmacol.* 86:69–79.
64. Thakkar, NS, and Potten, CS (1992). Abrogation of adriamycin cytotoxicity in vivo by cycloheximide. *Biochem. Pharmacol.* 4: 1683–1692.

65. Mimnaugh, EG, Trush, MA, Ginsburg, E, and Gram, TE (1982). Differential effects of anthracycline drugs on rat heart and liver microsomal reduced nicotinamide adenine dinucleotide phosphate-dependent lipid peroxidation. *Cancer Res.* 42:3574–3582.
66. Mimnaugh, EG, Gram. TE, and Trush, MA (1983). Stimulation of mouse heart andliver microsomal lipid peroxidation by anthracycline anticancer drugs: Characterization and effects of reactive oxygen scavengers. *J. Pharmacol. Exp. Ther.* 226:806–816.
67. Kharasch, ED, and Novak, RF (1983). Inhibitory effects of anthracenedione antineoplastic agents on hepatic and cardiac lipid peroxidation. *J. Pharmacol. Exp. Ther.* 226:500–506.
68. Doroshow, JH (1983). Effect of anthracycline antibiotics on oxygen radical formation in rat heart. *Cancer Res.* 43:460–472.
69. Tanizawa, H, Sazuka, Y, and Takino, Y (1983). Change of lipid peroxide levels in mouse organs after adriamycin administration. *Chem. Pharm. Bull.* 31:1714–1718.
70. Lenzhofer, R, Magometschnigg, D, Dudczak, R, Cerni, C, Bolebruch, C, and Moser, K (1983). Indication of reduced doxorubicin-induced cardiac toxicity by additional treatment with antioxidative substances. *Experientia* 39:62–64.
71. Sazuka, Y, Hirose, T, Hashimoto, J, Tanizawa, H, and Takino, Y (1984). Species, strain, sex, and weekly age differences of lipid peroxide levels in animal tissues before and after adriamycin administration. *Chem. Pharm. Bull.* 32:4110–4116.
72. Muhammed, H, Ramasarma, T, and Kurup, CKR (1982). Inhibition of mitochondrial oxidative phosphorylation by adriamycin. *Biochim. Biophys. Acta* 722:43–50.
73. Yoon, SB, Kajiyama, K, Hino, Y, Sugiyama, M, and Ogura, R (1983). Effect of adriamycin on lipid peroxide, glutathione peroxidase and respiratory responses of mitochondria from heart, liver and kidney. *Kurume Med. J.* 30:1–4.
74. Chacon, E, and Acosta, D (1991). Mitochondrial regulation of superoxide by Ca^{2+}: An alternate mechanism for cardiotoxicity of doxorubicin. *Toxicol. Appl. Pharmacol.* 107:117–128.
75. Solem, LE, Henry, TR, and Wallace, KB (1994). Disruption of mitochondrial calcium homeostasis following chronic doxorubicin administration. *Toxicol. Appl. Pharmacol.* 129:214–222.
76. Solem, LE, Heller, LJ, and Wallace, KB (1996). Dose-dependent increase in sensitivity to calcium-induced mitochondrial dysfunction and cardiomyocyte cell injury by doxorubicin. *J. Mol. Cell. Cardiol.* 28:1023–1032.

Free Radical Toxicology
Edited by K. B. Wallace
Copyright © 1997 Taylor & Francis

12

Free-Radical-Mediated Toxic Injury to the Nervous System

Stephen C. Bondy

Department of Community and Environmental Medicine, Center for Occupational and Environmental Medicine, University of California, Irvine, California, USA

INTRODUCTION

The terms *free radicals* and *oxygen radicals* have become commonly used in the past decade as a result of overwhelming data suggesting that short-lived, incompletely reduced oxygen compounds are involved in a variety of disease processes. The works of Freeman and Crapo (1) and Halliwell and Gutteridge (2) especially have addressed the ubiquitous role of free radicals as mediators in a wide range of pathological conditions. Many of the topics broadly considered to date have dealt with the role of free radicals in mechanisms of carcinogenesis, ischemia, and aging. In the field of toxicology, free-radical research has predominantly emphasized the areas of pulmonary, cardiac, and hepatotoxicity.

The liver and the lung have long been known to be organs vulnerable to oxidative stress. However, the brain, with its high lipid content, high rate of oxidative metabolism, and relatively low levels of free-radical eliminating enzymes, may also be a prime target of free-radical-mediated damage. The localization of antioxidant systems is primarily in glial cells rather than neuronal (3,4). While this may provide a first line of defense, neurons may be especially susceptible to toxicants successfully traversing this barrier.

It has been known for many years that mammalian brain contains large amounts of substrates that are susceptible to free-radical attack, such as unsaturated lipids and catecholamines and Halliwell and Gutteridge (5) were the first to discuss the potential role of oxygen radicals in the nervous system. The involvement of these reactive species in hyperoxia, ischemia, trauma, stroke and transition metal-dependent reactions in the brain has recently been a topic of extensive interest (6,7).

The concept that a variety of drug and chemical pathogeneses are associated with free-radical mechanisms has been put forward recently (8). This mediation may significantly contribute to the properties of many neurotoxic agents. Any imbalance of cellular redox status in favor of greater oxidative activity can lead to several kinds of damage to macromolecules, including disruption of genomic function by alterations to DNA, or impairment of membrane properties by attack on proteins or lipids. Lipid peroxidative events are especially hazardous, since lipoperoxy radicals can initiate and propagate oxidative chain reactions (1). Thus, the high lipid content of myelin makes nervous tissue especially susceptible to oxidative stress.

A given neurotoxic compound generally has characteristic and individual properties that result in distinctive morphological and biochemical lesions. However, relatively nonspecific features also constitute part of the overall toxicity of a given agent. Recent attempts to unify the diffuse discipline of neurotoxicology have led to the concept of "final common pathways" that characterize recurring cellular responses to disruption of homeostasis resulting from exposure to xenobiotic agents. The present chapter is built around the idea that oxygen radicals may be mediators of a "final common pathway" in several mechanisms of neurotoxicity.

Free radicals are defined as any species with one or more unpaired electrons. Since the presence of oxygen is found in all aerobic organisms, oxygen-centered free radicals occur commonly and have been implicated in several physiological, toxicological, and pathological phenomena. While superoxide anion and hydroxyl radical qualify as oxygen-centered radicals, hydrogen peroxide is a potent cellular toxicant that lacks unpaired electrons. The terms *reactive oxygen species* (ROS) and *oxygen radicals* have been used to describe all pro-oxidant species whether or not they are oxygen-centered radicals.

The precise nature of oxygen radicals produced in the central nervous system (CNS) is by no means clear. The difficulty of establishing this with certainty is due to the short half-life and rapid interconvertibility of many of the putative key species (9). Relatively stable species such as superoxide and hydrogen peroxide give rise to less clearly defined, highly reactive, transient species that are the primary oxidants. Evaluation of the free-radical-forming potential of neurotoxic agents and determination of whether oxygen radicals are common mediators of neurotoxicity should not be delayed until the precise identity of the terminal very short-lived radicals is unequivocally clarified.

ENDOGENOUS SOURCES OF GENERATION OF REACTIVE OXYGEN SPECIES WITHIN THE CNS

Mitochondrial Oxidative Metabolism

Around 2% of the oxygen consumed by mitochondria is incompletely reduced and appears as oxygen radicals (10). This proportion may be increased when the efficient functioning of mitochondrial electron transport systems is compromised. This could account for the increased lipid peroxidation found in the brains of mice exposed to nonlethal levels of mitochondrial inhibitors such as cyanide (11).

Intracellular pH

Increased cytosolic acidity resulting from excess glycolytic activity may not only accelerate the process of liberating protein-bound iron in organisms but it may also lead to an impairment of oxidative ATP generation, and to the appearance of the pro-oxidant protonated superoxide (12). Chlordecone, a neurotoxic insecticide, elevates pH within synaptosomes, and depresses oxygen radical synthesis (14). However, there is also evidence that the reduction of pH during ATP depletion may be protective and enhance cell survival (13) and the relation between pH and oxidative events is likely to be complex.

Presence of Transition Metal Ions

Liberation of protein-bound iron can occur by enhanced degradation of important iron-binding proteins such as ferritin and transferrin, and small increases in levels of free iron within cells can dramatically accelerate rates of oxygen radical generation (15). A key feature in establishing the rate of production of oxygen radicals by tissue is the cytosolic concentration of free metal ions possessing the capacity to readily change their valence state. Valence ambivalence characterizes transition metals with incomplete inner electron orbits.

Production of Eicosanoids and Neuromodulators

Enhanced phospholipase activity can lead to the release of arachidonic acid. This polyunsaturated fatty acid contains four ethylenic bonds and is readily autooxidizable. In fact, impure preparations of this chemical may explode spontaneously on exposure to air (2). The enzymic conversion of arachidonic acid to many bioactive prostaglandins, leukotrienes, and thromboxanes by cyclooxygenases and lipoxygenases leads to extensive formation of reactive oxygen species (1,16). All major catabolic pathways of arachidonic acid involve the utilization of molecular oxygen and the formation of hydroperoxide or epoxide intermediates. Subsequent metabolism by peroxidases and hydrolases can lead to further formation of free radicals. The physiological relevance of this is illustrated by the finding that antioxidants can protect against arachidonic-acid-induced cerebral edema (17).

Nitric oxide is both an important vasodilator and neuromodulator. Under some circumstances, NO can interact with superoxide anion to form peroxynitrite and subsequently a very short-lived reactive oxygen species, and this is now recognized as a potential source of several types of neurological damage (18).

Increased levels of cytosolic free calcium may result from breakdown of the steep concentration gradient of calcium ions across the plasma membrane, or by liberation of calcium bound intracellularly within mitochondria or endoplasmic reticulum. Elevated calcium levels can activate phospholipases and thus stimulate oxygen radical production. In fact, the activation of phospholipase D has been functionally linked to superoxide anion production (19). A reciprocal relation also exists since free radicals can enhance phospholipase A_2 activity within cerebral capillaries (20). Phospholipase A_2 may in turn selectively inhibit the gamma-aminobutyric acid (GABA) regulated chloride channel, and thus increase cell excitability (21). Such mutually reinforcing changes have the potential to reach a critical level and set in motion an ever-increasing entropic cascade.

Oxidase Activity

Chemical induction of cytochrome P-450-containing mixed function monooxidases can increase the rate of Phase I detoxification reactions. The oxidative metabolism of many lipophilic compounds, while necessary for their conjugation and excretion, often involves the transient formation of highly reactive oxidative intermediates such as epoxides (22).

While mixed-function oxidases predominate in the liver, they are also present in the nervous system, in both neurons and glia (23). At the intracellular level, most of these cerebral oxidases are mitochondrial rather than microsomal, and like the corresponding hepatic enzymes, they are inducible (24).

Xanthine oxidase is a prime generator of superoxide, and it is produced by oxidative or proteolytic degradation of xanthine dehydrogenase (25). It believed to be a significant exacerbating factor in several pathological states.

Phagocytic Activity

Extracellular formation of superoxide anion by phagocytes has long been recognized as an important bactericidal mechanism, and a parallel pro-oxidant activity has been observed in cerebral microglia (2). Astroglial activation is a common event following neural trauma, and reactive astrocytes can act as phagocytes in several ways, such as clearance of cell debris and ultimately in the formation of glial scar tissue. Although the phenomenon of reactive oxygen species generation has not been documented in the injured brain during neuronophagia, the ROS-enhancing potential of such events is worthy of further study.

INTRACELLULAR MECHANISMS FOR REGULATION OF OXIDANT SPECIES OR MITIGATION OF THEIR EFFECTS

Maintenance of oxygen reactive species at an acceptable level is effected by a wide range of cellular mechanisms. Only when such defensive processes are overwhelmed does the potential for significant oxidative damage arise.

Enzymes Removing Oxidative Species

Superoxide dismutase, catalase, and peroxidase are able to destroy the superoxide radical and hydrogen peroxide, respectively. While these oxidant species are not in themselves very active, they are able to interact in the presence of trace amounts of iron, and by the Haber-Weiss reaction give rise to the highly reactive, short-lived hydroxyl radical, which will readily abstract hydrogen from any neighboring molecule. The cerebral content of protective enzymes is rather low (3). Much of the brain's antioxidant capacity lies within cerebral capillaries and glial cells (26), and since the cerebral microvasculature is also a major site of lipid peroxidative activity (27), and mixed-function oxidase activity (28), this arrangement may destroy many pro-oxidants before they are able to diffuse into neurons. Treatment of neurons with nerve growth factor is able to confer resistance to oxidative damage, apparently by induction of antioxidant enzymes (29).

Proteins Capable of Chelating Metals with Pro-Oxidant Potential

Iron- and copper-sequestering proteins such as ferritin, transferrin, and ceruloplasmin are important means of ensuring extremely low levels of free cytosolic transition metals. These metals are key elements in facilitating intracellular generation of reactive oxidant species. Reduced antioxidant activity in the globus pallidus in Parkinson's disease has been related to decreased levels of ferritin (30).

Metallothionein is a protein capable of binding to another class of metals. It can sequester several metals with a high affinity for -SH groups, such as mercury and cadmium. Metallothionein is also induced by these metals. This protein also acts as an antioxidant because of its high sulfhydryl content and also its ability to dismutate superoxide anion. It is only present to a limited extent in nervous tissue.

Soluble Vitamins and Other Cytoplasmic Components

The presence of low-molecular-weight antioxidant vitamins, provitamins, and cofactors provides protection against oxygen radicals. Such molecules may be predominantly lipophilic (β-carotene, α-tocopherol, retinoic acid), or water-soluble (ascorbic acid, coenzyme Q, glutathione). Glutathione is a major source of reducing power and normally exists at high concentrations intracellularly (1–5 mM) (5). Glutathione is maintained largely in the reduced form by glutathione reductase, acting in conjunction with NADPH. Thus, inhibition of NADPH producing events may compromise intracellular levels of glutathione, and overall reducing potential. In contrast, NADPH is also an essential component of many oxidases, including the mixed-function oxidases.

Glutathione reserves can be depleted by excessive oxidative events (31), and such depletion in the brain can cause neurological deficits (32). Glutathione distribution in the CNS is heterogeneous at both the cellular and regional level. Its content is much higher in astroglia than neurons. The brainstem has a low glutathione content and a high mixed-function oxidase content relative to other brain regions. It has been proposed that this may render the region especially vulnerable to oxidative damage, and that this is relevant to damage to the substantia nigra in Parkinson's disease (33,34).

Some serum proteins, notably albumin, can be effective as free-radical scavengers (35). However, the low protein content of cerebrospinal fluid makes both albumin and ferritin largely unavailable to the CNS (36).

PROMOTION OF PRODUCTION OF REACTIVE OXYGEN SPECIES WITHIN THE BRAIN

While several neurotoxic chemicals can stimulate ROS production within the nervous system, this does not imply that such stimulation represents their primary mechanism of toxic action. The pro-oxidant properties of a chemical may: (1) be the primary source of its neurotoxicity, (2) contribute in part to its overall harmfulness, or (3) be an epiphenomenon, not related to the neurotoxiciy of the chemical.

The events underlying the enhancement of ROS induced by toxicants often involve an excess activation of one or more of the ROS-producing processes intrinsic to a cell, or an inhibition of one of the free-radical-regulating systems described earlier.

Neurotoxic Metals

Metal ions can promote the intracellular production of reactive oxygen species by several means. Perhaps the most potent promoters are transition metals, which are able to alter their electronic configurations under biological conditions. Many of these metals are essential cofactors for several enzyme complexes, and this ensures their continuous presence within neural tissue, which can set the stage for deleterious pro-oxidant events following aberrant distribution or metabolic handling. Conversely, relatively stable oxidant species such as superoxide and hydrogen peroxide can be prevented from forming short-lived harmful derivatives by the metal-sequestering abilities of many metalloenzymes concerned with oxidative and reductive processes (37).

The toxicity of any metal is not confined to a single tissue, but while a wide range of tissues may be adversely affected by the abnormal presence of a metal, some organs are clearly more vulnerable to metal-induced oxidative damage. The nervous system and the kidney are, for different reasons, among the most vulnerable to such injury. Both of these organs receive a disproportionate amount of arterial blood and have very high oxidative metabolic rates. In the case of the kidney, the pH changes associated with glomerular filtration and tubular production of urine can lead to concentration and precipitation of metals. The brain is also a susceptible target in part because of its relatively low levels of enzymes protecting against oxidative stress (3), and its high myelin-associated lipid content, and consequent liability to propagation of peroxidative events (38).

Neurotoxicity resulting from the presence of excessive levels of metals, may be associated with several conditions including:

1. Genetic defects involving failure of normal disposition of, and consequent accumulation of a metal.
2. Adverse exposure to metals from environmental or dietary sources.
3. Abnormal presence of iron due to extravasation of hemoglobin into cerebral tissue.
4. Increased excitability of neural tissue with consequent elevation of cytosolic sodium and calcium levels can be a stimulus for generation of excess pro-oxidant events.

The blood-brain barrier is effective in limiting access of many metal cations to the brain, but this protection is incomplete and can be circumvented by several means:

1. Organometals can enter the brain by virtue of their lipophilic properties. Amphiphilic compounds are among the most deleterious forms of metals, perhaps because, possessing both a lipophilic and a water-soluble component, they will concentrate in and align themselves within intracellular membranes.
2. Xenobiotic ions such as thallium can also gain such access to neural cells by entry through ion channels that are not completely specific for normal biologically occurring cations. In the case of thallium, its atomic radius enables it to utilize potassium channels. Several toxic metals bear an atomic resemblance to a biologically essential counterpart.
3. Specific brain regions, notably the hypothalamus, have an incompletely formed blood-brain barrier, probably to allow monitoring of the endocrine composition of circulating blood. This can allow localized entry of ionic species that would otherwise be excluded. The immature brain also has only limited means of excluding charged compounds, and thus the fetus may be particularly vulnerable to penetration by undesirable metal ions.

Damage effected by most neurotoxic metals is unlikely to be solely attributable to generation of excess reactive oxygen species (ROS). However, most toxic metals appear to possess a free-radical inducing component that can contribute to their harmfulness. While the toxicity of each metal is distinctive, and involves a characteristic range of morphological and biochemical abnormalities, the ability to promote ROS formation may be superimposed on this. This can enhance the more specific neurotoxic properties of the agent. Catalyzed generation of ROS may then represent a final common path provoked by disparate metal-containing chemicals. This section describes key features of several neurotoxic metals as far as this may involve their capacity to provoke oxidative stress. Metals have been grouped by classes involving similar mechanisms relating to their pro-oxidant properties.

Metals Where Valence Flux May Underlie Pro-Oxidant Properties
(Fe, Cu, Mn)

Transition metals may induce oxidative stress by cycling between two valence states, thereby alternately donating and receiving electrons. Copper, iron, and manganese are in this class. This property is related to the presence of an unfilled inner electronic shell. The first metal after this series, zinc, has completely filled inner electronic orbitals and thus zinc has no valence ambiguity and no capacity to induce ROS. Other metals such as mercury, tin, thallium, and lead also possess several valence states, but do not readily undergo such valence changes under physiological conditions, and are active in ROS stimulation primarily by other means.

The promotion of redox cycling forms the basis of the neurotoxicity of iron, copper, and manganese. These metals are essential but may owe their effectiveness in their normal biological role, to those very same plurivalence features that when acting in an unregulated manner can promote adverse oxidative events. All three of the transition metals mentioned earlier constitute part of the active sites of many enzymes and transport proteins. These enzymes include those such as superoxide dismutase and catalase, which are important in removal of free radicals or their precursors. In addition, many enzymes involved in bringing about regulated oxidations are metalloenzymes. The need to keep the free concentration of ionic salts of these metals within biological tissues very low is revealed by the existence of distinctive proteins with high affinity for a specific metal, which are able to sequester that metal as an inactive high-molecular-weight complex. Ceruloplasmin is the main copper-chelating plasma protein, while iron is sequestered by several proteins including ferritin. It has been proposed that most biological molecules are not readily autoxidized, and that low-molecular-weight complexes of a transition metal, especially iron, are needed to catalyze all such oxidations, whether beneficial or harmful (39).

While superoxide anion and hydrogen peroxide are not in themselves very active oxidants, they are able to interact in the presence of trace amounts of iron, and, by the Haber-Weiss reaction, give rise to the highly reactive, short-lived hydroxyl radical.

A wide range of enzymic and nonenzymic reactive free-radical-generating processes can thus be activated by Fe^{3+} or Cu^{2+} in the presence of an electron donor. Such activation can lead to lipid peroxidative events and also to the oxidative degradation of proteins, and thence to enzyme inactivation and membrane damage. Metal-ion-catalyzed modification of proteins can be site specific and may occur near an iron-binding lysine residue (40). The oxidation susceptibility of amino acid residues within proteins differs from that of free amino acids. This is because the proximity of amino acid residues to metal binding sites in the peptide chain can influence vulnerability to degradation (41).

The situations under which copper and iron can be neurotoxic do not generally involve excessive ingestion. Iron penetrance into the brain can follow traumatic brain injury or hemorrhagic stroke when low-molecular-weight iron is liberated during degradation of free hemoglobin (42). The consequent elevation of pro-oxidant status may in part account for the delayed appearance of seizure activity, which results in bleeding into brain tissue (43). Excessive levels of unsequestered iron have also been observed in many neurological disorders including various lipofuscinoses such as Batten's disease (44), Alzheimer's disease (45,46), Parkinson's disease (47), seizure disorders (48), stroke (49), ischemia (50), Hallervorden-Spatz disease (51), and edema (52). Evidence exists that ethanol can lead to elevated levels of lipid peroxidation in brain. This has been attributed at least in part, to liberation of protein-bound iron by ethanol (53–56).

Chelation therapy using deferoxamine, a potent iron chelator, is being used experimentally in the treatment of Alzheimer's disease (57) and multiple sclerosis (58). However, deferoxamine, like all chelators, is not completely specific for a single metal. In addition to metal sequestration, its mode of action as an antioxidant may also involve direct scavenging of free radicals (59). Chelation therapy as a means of decorporating toxic metals has many adverse side effects, including the potential for enhancement of ROS formation (60–62). Some of these undesirable side effects are probably due to removal of essential metals (63). Therapeutic intervention for removal of toxic metals with chelators may also allow metals to enter the CNS in the form of sequestered complexes. Thus while acute toxicity is prevented in this way, the possibility of delayed, chronic neurological damage remains. This may constitute a significant hazard, especially since loosely chelated metals can be the most potent inducers of oxidative events.

In interpreting toxicological data, it is important to remember that association does not always imply causation. Thus, while hyperexcitation can elevate intracellular iron levels, iron is not necessarily the cause of the accompanying neuronal damage (48). The molecular state of cytosolic iron is critical. Under normal homeostatic conditions iron is bound to intracellular proteins. However, oxidative events can lead to decompartmentation of this metal and consequent appearance of its pro-oxidant properties. Nitric oxide-induced appearance of low-molecular-weight iron compounds has been proposed to occur in Parkinson's disease (47,64).

Pharmacological treatments may, on occasion, inadvertently stimulate free-radical activity within neural tissues. For example, L-DOPA, used in the therapy of Parkinsonism, is capable of reducing ferric iron, the form in which iron forms a stable complex ferritin. This can lead to the liberation of ferrous iron in the form of a low-molecular-weight species with significant ROS-enhancing potential (65). Since basal iron levels are especially high in the substantia nigra and globus pallidus (66), this may be a significant consideration. Ferritin levels have been reported as being altered (both elevated and depressed) in these regions in Parkinson's disease (30,67).

Copper is present in bodily tissues to a much lesser extent than iron and the only clear appearance of neurotoxicity is due to a genetic defect in copper metabolism, Wilson's disease. This disorder is characterized by the virtual absence of ceruloplasmin leading to greatly elevated levels of low-molecular-weight diffusible copper. The psychiatric and neurological consequences of this disease can be alleviated by chelation of copper with drugs such as penicillamine. Copper is known to enhance catecholamine autoxidation, and such distortion of the normal role of this metal is likely to underlie the neurological features of Wilson's disease (68).

Oxidases are enzymes utilizing molecular oxygen. The scission of the O_2 molecule is an intrinsically hazardous process, and the control of O_2 utilization is regulated at the catalytic center of oxidases that contain a transition metal binding site. However, all oxidases "leak" nonspecific oxidant species to a certain extent. In the mitochondrial respiratory chain, there is very efficient control of this, and the uncoupled leakage rate is less than 2% (10). The presence of both copper as well as iron within cytochrome oxidase may allow this tight regulation, since oxidases containing iron alone, such as the mixed-function oxidases and monoamine oxidases, may be less effective in this respect (69). Inhibition of monoamine oxidase B has proved effective in slowing the rate of progression of Parkinson's disease (70), and antioxidant therapy may also have a beneficial effect (71). Therefore the mechanism of the protective effect of MAO-B blockers may be by way of inhibition of free-radical generation.

Manganese is another member of this group of transition metals. Neurological signs resembling Parkinson's disease are found following excessive exposure to this mineral during the mining, handling, or processing of manganese ore. Manganism presents in several distinct phases, including an initial hyperactive, manic state ("manganese madness"), an intermediate phase involving tremor and incoordination, and a terminal spastic, rigid phase (72). The resemblance of the latter two stages to Parkinson's disease (PD) is pronounced and involves the basal ganglia. There is increasing evidence for the role of oxidative stress in PD, and trials involving antioxidant therapy have met with some success (73). Dopamine and norepinephrine are able to oxidize very readily, and this requires trace amounts of transition metals. Thus, catecholaminergic pathways are especially susceptible to metal-catalyzed oxidative damage. Catalyzed dopamine auto-oxidation may then underlie manganism (74). Manganese can exist in at least four oxidative states (with a valence of 2, 3, 4, or 5), and like iron, has been shown to be capable of enhancing ROS formation in isolated systems. However, the situation is complicated by reports describing significant free-radical scavenging properties of many manganese complexes. Hydrogen peroxide and superoxide may be quenched by such chelates (75). In fact, manganese has been stated to "fulfill the requirements of a physiologically relevant antioxidant" (76). These apparent contradictions can be reconciled by recognition of the essential role of the valence status of metal ions, and the readiness of their interconvertibility, in enabling or retarding oxidative events (15). Vanadium, another transition metal, has also been found to induce lipid peroxidation in the brains of experimental animals (77), although it has not been shown to be neurotoxic in humans.

Metals with a High Affinity for Sulfhydryl Groups and for Selenium (Hg, Tl, Cd, and As)

The capacity of several metals to form covalent linkages to sulfhydryl groups of peptides can lead to the modification of proteins and the inactivation of enzymes.

A key low-molecular-weight tripeptide is glutathione, which is present at millimolar concentrations within the cytosol. Glutathione (GSH) plays three vital roles within the cell; first it is a source of reducing power and thus constitutes an important water-soluble defense against excess ROS. Glutathione is also able to detoxify xenobiotic agents by direct conjugation of xenobiotic agents using glutathione transferase. Finally, glutathione can destroy peroxides in the presence of glutathione peroxidase. Under normal circumstances, the oxidized glutathione formed (GSSG) is reconverted to GSH by glutathione reductase and by this means the reducing power of GSH is sustained. However, excessive ROS levels may overwhelm such GSH regenerative capacity. GSSG usually constitutes a very minor fraction of total intracellular glutathione, but if its level is elevated this nonionic lipophilic molecule can readily become lost to the cell by diffusion across the limiting membrane, rendering it unavailable for GSH formation.

The heavy metals mercury, lead, thallium. and cadmium all have electron-sharing tendencies that, intracellularly, tend to result in the formation of covalent attachments. Metals of this type have an avidity for sulfhydryl groups, and can deplete cellular glutathione levels (78), increase levels of lipid peroxidation (79,80), and accelerate lipofuscinogenesis. This latter effect is exacerbated in the presence of hyperbaric oxygen (81).

α-tocopherol has repeatedly been found to be protective against neurotoxicity induced by this class of metals (82,83). This may reflect the predominantly lipophilic site of the -SH groups reacting with these metals.

Methylmercury can induce generation of ROS within the CNS (84), and this induction can be blocked by deferoxamine. Since deferoxamine does not chelate methylmercury, iron-catalyzed pro-oxidant reactions may play a role in methylmercury neurotoxicity (85).

The degree of the overall toxicity of these metal salts that is expressed as neurotoxicity is related to their ability to cross the bloodbrain barrier. Thus, ionic mercuric chloride is predominantly harmful to nonneural tissues such as the kidney, and inorganic lead has a large range of adverse systemic effects, while the more amphiphilic methyl mercuric halides and triethyllead salts are primarily neurotoxic.

Cadmium salts are also largely nephrotoxic but can enter the CNS by the olfactory route where the bloodbrain barrier is attenuated, and anosmia is characteristic of cadmium intoxication. Interestingly, the complex that cadmium forms with diethyldithiocarbamate increases the access of this metal to the brain but reduces its neurotoxicity (86). However, the extended presence of a relatively inert metal chelate within the CNS may have unforseeable consequences.

The next element of the sulfur-containing family in the periodic table is selenium, and metals binding to sulfur also have an affinity for selenium. These metals can also displace selenium from glutathione peroxidase (87), the only known mammalian enzyme in which selenium is an essential cofactor. This enzyme uses GSH to reduce organic hydroperoxides, and is an important defence against oxidant damage (88), and the consequent inactivation of this enzyme removes a key antioxidant step. This probably accounts for the ability of selenium to protect against the toxicity of methylmercury (89). Selenium has also been shown to attenuate the toxicity of cadmium, arsenic, mercury, thallium, and copper. The protective properties of selenium imply oxidative events as a basis for the toxicity of the already discussed elements.

Cadmium and mercury but not lead, are able to induce metallothionein in several organs (90). This cysteine-rich protein that is capable of sequestering sulfhydryl-binding metals is present only to a minor extent in neural tissues but may be important here since it is present as a CNS-specific variant, metallothionein III.

Complex interactions with both synergistic and antagonistic potential exist between cadmium, mercury and lead (91). Such synergism implies action at different sites, while antagonism of toxicity may be related to competition of a less toxic metal with a more toxic metal, for a common -SH target.

Metals Enhancing Neuronal Excitability: Ca, Pb, Sn (Organic)

Elevation of rates of neuronal firing involves influx of calcium into the presynaptic area, thereby eliciting neurotransmitter release. Under normal circumstances, cytosolic calcium levels are transiently but greatly elevated, before homeostasis is restored by rapid sequestration of excess calcium into endoplasmic reticulum and mitochondria, followed by eventual extrusion of calcium into the extracellular space using ion pumping or exchange processes. There is evidence that chronic excitation may result in failure to maintain low resting levels of calcium. Chronically elevated levels of calcium within the cell can initiate excess ROS generation by several means. These include activation of phospholipases and the arachidonic acid cascade. Calcium can also activate superoxide production by polymorphonuclear lymphocytes, which can be present in postischemic neural tissues (92). By these means, calcium may act as a mediator of oxidative stress in a variety of disease states involving persistent excitation such as ischemia, epilepsy, and chemically induced hyperactivity (93).

Both exogenous antioxidants and calcium chelators can inhibit lipid peroxidation and generation of superoxide anion following postischemic reperfusion (94). The exact degree to which cytosolic calcium elevation and pro-oxidant events occur independently or act in concert is not yet well understood (95).

Several metals can indirectly evoke ROS by way of disruption of normal calcium homeostasis. Although peroxidative events are unlikely to constitute the primary mechanism of lead toxicity, there is evidence that both inorganic and organic lead derivatives can enhance the generation of ROS in nerve tissue. Lead is known to interfere with calcium metabolism, and lead compounds have been reported to enhance rates of lipid peroxidation within the brain (96). Organic lead compounds, which are unlikely to closely mimic calcium, can also induce oxidant conditions in cerebral tissues (97). In this case depolarization-induced excitotoxicity may underlie such elevations in free-radical generation. The mechanism by which lead can generate free radicals may also be indirect since 5-aminolevulinic acid, a heme precursor that accumulates during lead poisoning, is capable of inducing ROS (98).

Both trimethyl- and triethyltin are potent neurotoxic agents. Trimethyl tin is an excitatory agent with a rather high degree of selectivity toward the hippocampus and other limbic structures. This agent can specifically elevate hippocampal ROS in treated rats (86), although it has no ability to induce ROS in isolated preparations. Such very region-specific neurotoxicity is likely to be due to the susceptibility of hippocampal circuitry to excitatory events rather than to any distinctive biochemical features of this area. Elevated calcium levels consequent to energy depletion may be the primary effector of excess production of ROS.

Aluminum

Aluminum does not fit into any of the classes of metals described so far. However, this element may be capable of inducing ROS within neural tissues, and this property may play a role in the etiology of Alzheimer's disease (AD). While such a role is controversial, aluminum has been recognized as a significant factor in dialysis dementia for some time. However, it is uncertain whether an excessive intraneuronal accumulation of aluminum is found in AD, and whether this has a causal relationship to the disease. Recent studies have reported the following:

1. Aluminosilicate complexes are capable of stimulating ROS generation in isolated glial cultures (99).
2. Levels of superoxide dismutase and catalase are elevated in AD brains, implying a response to oxidative stress (100).
3. Chelation therapy with deferoxamine, in order to reduce the body burden of aluminum, may retard the rate of loss of intellectual performance in AD (57). Since iron is also sequestered by this chelator, this report cannot be considered conclusive evidence for a role of aluminum in AD. While aluminum salts in themselves have no ROS-promoting capacity, they have been reported to strongly enhance the pro-oxidant potential of iron salts in an isolated system (101–104).
4. Glutamine synthetase, an enzyme that is very susceptible to oxidative degradation, is depressed in brains from AD patients compared to age-matched controls (105). This depression is confined to the frontal cortex, the location of neuropathologic involvement.
5. The iron binding protein transferrin is depressed in AD (46), and levels of lipid peroxidation are elevated (106).
6. Aluminum and iron have recently been reported to promote the aggregation of β-amyloid peptide (107).

While this evidence is circumstantial, there is a good possibility that pro-oxidant events and derangements of metal ion balance contribute to AD.

The mechanism by which aluminum can promote oxidative stress is unclear. Subtle modification of membrane structures allowing increased availability of peroxidizable fatty acids has been proposed (101,103), and another possibility is that formation of aluminium/iron-containing mineral particulates can promote oxidative injury by stimulation of macrophage-like microglial events (108). The issue of whether ionic or complexed aluminum is the active agent in these events is currently controversial (103,109), and its resolution would clarify our understanding of the role of aluminum in promotion of ROS.

Organic Solvents

The ability of various organic solvents to effect excess ROS synthesis has been described for several tissues (110,111), but the brain has received little attention in this regard. The neurotoxicity of two solvents of environmental significance, ethanol and toluene, has however been reported, and is discussed here. A large range of factors may account for an association between solvent exposure and excess oxidative events. Evidence for varous potential mechanisms of solvent-induced ROS production are listed:

1. Reductions and also increases in glutathione levels have been found in brain following ethanol, toluene or m-dinitrobenzene dosing (112–119). Since compensatory processes can be rapid after induction of excessive ROS, both reductions and increases in cerebral glutathione may be regarded as indices of oxidative stress (120).
2. Elevations in lipid peroxidation following ethanol or toluene treatment are found in brain (115,116). The attenuation of some of these ethanol-induced changes by lipid-soluble antioxidant vitamins A or E and the depletion of antioxidant vitamins in the CNS of ethanol-treated rats (113,121) confirms the presence of induced oxidative stress.
3. Solvent-stimulated lipid mobilization is another phenomenon to be considered as a source of ROS. Ethanol has been shown to activate phospholipases A1 and A2, in an isolated cardiac preparation (122). The effect is blocked in the presence of α-tocopherol. This property has not yet been reported for corresponding cerebral tissue but is likely. Phospholipase activity has been found to be significantly stimulated in synaptosomes isolated from rats exposed to toluene (123), and the consequent liberation of arachidonic acid by phospholipase A2 sets in motion a range of oxidative catabolic processes: the "arachidonic acid cascade." The enzymic conversion of this compound to prostaglandins, leukotrienes, and thromboxanes by cyclooxygenases and lipoxygenases leads to considerable ROS generation (16). Toluene alters synaptosomal phospholipid methyltransferase activity, an event that may be mediated by oxygen radicals (124).

Low-molecular-wieght iron complexes may be essential for the appearance of ethanol-induced ROS, and ethanol may effect the liberation of such complexes within the nervous system, from bound intracellular reserves (55,56), perhaps by way of formation of the superoxide anion, which can release iron from ferritin (125). The protective effects of iron chelators such as deferoxamine on ethanol-related changes in cerebral oxidative events (54,126) also suggest the ethanol-related liberation of low-molecular-weight iron. It has even been proposed that iron-sequestering chemicals can reduce physical dependence on ethanol (127).

Acetaldehyde generated during the metabolism of ethanol may also initiate oxidative stress by reaction with, and depletion of, protective thiols such as cysteine and glutathione. Microsomal mixed-function oxidases may also be a direct target of acetaldehyde. Binding of this ethanol metabolite to these enzymes, forming a stable adduct, can impair their properties (128) and the P-450 2E1 enzyme induced by ethanol is more likely to be malfunctioning (129). The extent to which acetaldehyde found within the brain after ethanol dosing is generated intrinsically rather than systemically transported from the liver is unclear, but its ability to promote cerebral oxidative stress has been reported (118). The reactivity of acetaldehyde with many biological constituents suggests that it is likely to be synthesized close to the site where it is detected. However, following ethanol treatment, acetaldehyde levels of brain interstitial fluid are above those present intacellularly in the CNS (130), suggesting that acetaldehyde can cross the blood-brain barrier. Cysteine and ascorbic acid are protective against the acute behavioral toxicity of acetaldehyde, supporting the concept of the relevance of acetaldehyde-inducible oxidative stress to the brain (131). However, such agents may also have nonantioxidant ameliorative effects by preventing the formation of adducts of acetaldehyde with protein (132).

The catabolic steps involved in the degradation of ethanol, toluene, and other solvents are candidates for the origin of excess ROS. Several major classes of enzyme need to be considered in this context:

1. Since oxidases utilize molecular oxygen directly, their induction has the potential for enhancing ROS production. Ethanol is known to induce a specific microsomal mixed-function oxidase, P-450 2E1, in the liver (133). This enzyme is inducible by ethanol, and can generate oxidizing species in the absence of substrates as long as NADPH is present (134). Under such conditions, P-450 2E1 has been reported to exhibit an unusually high rate of oxidase, and H_2O_2 generating activity (133). More recently, a parallel induction of P-450 2E1 has been found in the CNS where the enzyme is present in much lower concentration (135). The distinct susceptibility of the cerebellum and the hippocampus to ethanol-induced morphological damage may relate to their relatively high content of cytochrome P-450 2E1 monooxygenase. The role of mixed-function oxidases in solvent-stimulated ROS generation within the brain is also indicated by the finding that the capacity of toluene to stimulate cortical ROS production can be blocked by pretreatment of rats with an inhibitor of mixed-function oxidases, namely, metyrapone (136).

2. Increased levels of inducible superoxide dismutase (SOD) are generally taken as indirect evidence of an increased oxidant milieu. However, since this is a sulfhydryl enzyme, depressed levels in a tissue can also reflect oxidative denaturation. Both ethanol-induced increases and decreases in neuronal and glial SOD have been reported (137,138). As with glutathione, biphasic fluxes of SOD levels

are common, and a change in either direction may suggest the presence of excessive levels of ROS.

3. Alcohol dehydrogenase is considered the primary initial step in the catabolism of ethanol. There is evidence that the activity of several dehydrogenases including alcohol dehydrogenase can bring about ROS formation, despite the fact that oxygen is not directly involved (116). The inhibition of ethanol or toluene-effected free-radical production in neural tissue, by an inhibitor of alcohol dehydrogenase, 4-methylpyrazole (139,116), suggests that ROS are generated by this enzyme. However, 4-methylpyrazole is also capable of inhibition of mixed-function oxidases (140), so use of this agent does not allow an unequivocal distinction to be made between the two major routes of ethanol breakdown.

4. Mitochondrial NAD^+-dependent aldehyde dehydrogenase constitutes the major means of oxidation of acetaldehyde by the liver. It is also present in brain (130). Electron spin resonance studies reveal that this dehydrogenase is capable of producing hydroxyl ions (116). Benzaldehyde is a potent agent in enhancing oxygen radical formation in cerebral tissues (116), and this may be the active metabolite responsible for the pro-oxidant properties of toluene.

5. Both xanthine oxidase and aldehyde oxidase are molybdenum and flavin-containing enzymes capable of forming superoxide. The presence of the latter enzyme in the brain is unclear. Xanthine oxidase, derived by the proteolytic modification of xanthine dehydrogenase, can also oxidize acetaldehyde, and is present in all tissues. Ethanol treatment may also bring about the conversion from xanthine dehyrogenase to the oxidase (127), and acetaldehyde appears to be the agent directly responsible for this (141). The further oxidation of ethanol is primarily by way of aldehyde dehydrogenase.

Further suggestion of the ability of ethanol to enhance neural oxidative events comes from results of studies combining ethanol with other toxicants. The toxicity of manganese, 6-hydroxydopamine, and MPP^+, three agents suspected to owe part of their neurotoxicity to oxidative events confined to the dopaminergic system, is enhanced by ethanol or acetaldehyde in a synergistic manner (138,142,143).

A final unresolved issue is the extent to which overall solvent toxicity is related to oxidative stress. The hepatic events consequent to prolonged and high levels of ethanol ingestion such as lipid mobilization are very likely to involve harmful pro-oxidant events. Such dramatic changes are generally not seen in nervous tissue in the absence of thiamine deficiency. However, the brain is an organ with very limited potential for cell replacement and can be vulnerable to gradual, incremental deficits. Such slowly accumulating lesions, although difficult to quantitate, can be irreversible. Many other solvents such as styrene and xylenes also stimulate CNS production of ROS (144), and extended low-level exposures to aromatic and aliphatic solvent mixtures can also effect this in the CNS (145,146). The free-radical inducing property of solvents may not enhance their acute toxicity, but has been proposed to effect more subtle processes such as an acceleration of normal aging processes (110).

Potential Oxidants Selectively Acting on Dopaminergic Neurons

Dopaminergic circuitry is especially vulnerable to neurotoxic damage; this is at least in part due to the readiness with which dopamine is autoxidized in the presence of trace amounts of metals with multivalence potential. In addition, dopamine can be enzymically oxidized by monoamine oxidases to 3,4-dihydroxyphenyl acetaldehyde and H_2O_2.

A role for oxidative stress in the processes underlying 1-methyl-4-phenyl-1,2,3,6-tetrahydropyridine (MPTP) neurotoxicity has been proposed in recent years. This compound, a contaminant of an illicitly manufactured meperidine analogue, has been the subject of much interest since the neurological damage that it can cause closely resembles Parkinson's disease. MPTP is a very specific dopaminergic neurotoxin. There is considerable support for the "mitochondrial theory" of MPTP toxicity, which postulates that 1-methyl-4-phenylpyridinium (MPP^+), the ultimate oxidation product of MPTP, blocks the reoxidation of NADH dehydrogenase by coenzyme Q_{10} and eventually leads to ATP depletion in a rotenone-like fashion (147). However, there are also several studies that suggest oxygen radicals may play a role in the MPTP-induced neuronal damage (148,149). Vitamin E has also been shown to protect against neural oxidative stress induced by MPTP (149). Ganglioside GM1, a membrane-stabilizing agent effective within the CNS, may also mitigate some components of oxidative damage to neural tissue. The conflicting concepts of the primary locus of action of MPP^+, being either by inhibition of a specific mitochondrial enzyme or as an oxidative stressor, may be reconciled by the finding that the metabolic inhibitors rotenone and antimycin can increase the generation rate of oxygen radicals in isolated brain fractions (150,151).

Information relating to mechanisms of MPTP toxicity has led to novel concepts concerning both the etiology and treatment of Parkinson's disease (PD). These include both the possibility of an environmental agent being contributory to the pathogenesis of Parkinsonism (152) and of the potential for antioxidant therapy of this disorder. A contribution of environmentally prevalent agents such as pyridines to the incidence of this disorder has been proposed. PD has been associated with abnormally high levels of superoxide dismutase within the substantia nigra (153), implying an induced response to oxidative stress. The potential utility of several antioxidant therapies in the treatment of PD is currently under investigation (71,73,154). There is evidence that n-hexane may specifically damage dopaminergic neurons and precipitate Parkinsonian symptoms in both humans and experimental animals (155). The environmental relevance of this is underscored by the detection of the neurotoxic metabolite of n-hexane, 2,5-hexanedione, in the urine of persons not known to have had major exposures to organic solvents (156).

The neurotoxicity of methamphetamine, a drug of abuse, may in part be due to oxidative stress relating to dopaminergic and serotonergic circuitry (157), and methamphetamine-induced neuropathologic changes may be attenuated by pretreatment with antioxidants. Neuronal destruction induced by levo-DOPA and 6-hydroxydopamine is also thought to occur via free-radical mechanisms (158), and the administration of hydroxyl radical scavengers, such as phenylthiazolylthiourea, can be protective against such induced damage (159).

There are several reports that neuroleptics may elevate lipid peroxidation in the CNS, and such oxidative stress resulting from the associated increased catecholamine metabolism has been proposed as a cause of tardive dyskinesia (160). α-tocopherol has been reported to attenuate fluphenazine-induced changes in monoamine metabolism (161).

Metabolic Inhibitors

Cerebral lipid peroxidation can be stimulated by cyanide (11,162). This reveals that interruption of the respiratory chain can lead to excess production of free radicals. While acute cyanide exposure is rapidly lethal, more chronic exposures as a result of excess cyanogenic glycosides (e.g., found in cassava) in the diet of some less developed countries can result in ataxic neuropathy (163). This may be related to the high levels of unsaturated fatty acids in myelin that constitute a clear target for ROS-induced lipid peroxidation (59).

Excitatory Compounds

Excitatory events are often associated with neurotoxic exposures. Many agents impair effective mitochondrial oxidation of energy producing substrates. The consequent depletion of ATP due to metabolic insult can lead to dissipation of ionic gradients. Entry of calcium into the cell may increase synaptic firing rates, and lowering of the sodium/potassium gradients will increase axonal excitability. Intracellular calcium overload can also set off a cascade of other events such as phospholipase activation, potentially leading to elevation of free-radical production (164,165). Some neurotoxicants (such as β-N-oxalyl-L-alanine, ODAP) are glutamate agonists while others (such as lindane) act as GABA antagonists. Both types of interaction with neurons can directly depolarize postsynaptic cells, and such depolarization with consequent increased energy demand may intrinsically form the basis of excessive pro-oxidant activity.

Recently, evidence suggesting a role for free radicals in excitotoxic events has been accumulating. Excess neuronal activity is known to have the potential to effect neuronal death, especially in the hippocampus. In addition to the frank neuronal hyperactivity apparent in epilepsy, several other neurological disorders are associated with hyperexcitatory events. Free radicals may play a role in seizure-related brain damage (52,166). Superoxide anion is generated within the brain during seizure activity (167), and attenuation of convulsive activity by phenytoin or corticosteroids also reduces cerebral levels of lipid peroxidation (168). Free-radical generation during transient cerebral ischemia followed by restoration of the vascular oxygen supply may underlie delayed neuronal death (169,170).

Details of the relation between excitatory and oxidant phenomena are gradually emerging. There may be a direct relation between activation of various classes of glutamate receptor and free-radical formation. Glutamic acid as well as several glutamate agonists can directly enhance ROS in isolated cerebral systems (171) and glutamate toxicity in a neuronal cell line has been attributed to inhibition of cysteine transport and consequent oxidative stress (172). Activation of the *N*-methyl-D-aspartate (NMDA) receptor site has been implicated in the post-ischemic elevation of lipid peroxidation in the hippocampus (173), and there is also a report of exacerbation of NMDA toxicity in glutathione-deficient cortical cultures (174).

Calcium stimulation of phospholipase A2, and thence the arachidonic acid cascade, may be a means by which excitatory events promote excess generation of ROS (175). Furthermore, NMDA agonists are able to stimulate nitric oxide synthetase (176), and the resultant nitric oxide free radical can interact with superoxide to form the intensely oxidant nitroperoxyl radical. In this manner, nitric oxide can mediate the neurotoxicity of glutamate (177). Kainate-induced damage to cerebellar neurons may also be mediated, at least in part, by induction of superoxide (178). The shellfish neurotoxin, domoic acid, which predominantly acts as a glutamate agonist at the kainate site (170), is very potent in enhancing synaptosomal ROS (171). When administered to mice, domoic acid has been found to elevate cerebral levels of superoxide dismutase (179), implying the presence of oxidative stress. Excitants that would be worthy of study for their ROS-inducing potential include food additives (monosodium glutamate and aspartame), and β-*N*-oxalyl-L-alanine (ODAP), a glutamergic agonist found in chickling peas and a suspected cause of neurolathyrism.

Transient ischemia elevates cerebral levels of both excitatory amino acids and rates of hydroxyl radical formation (180) but the relation between these two events is not established. Excitatory events may stimulate ROS, and conversely, ROS can lead to release of excitatory amino acids (181). Glutamine synthetase appears to be especially sensitive to ROS-induced damage, and this may increase glutamate concentrations (182). Peroxidative damage can also effect excitation by impairment of GABA-stimulated chloride uptake (21). A bidirectional cooperation between excess neuronal activity and free radicals may thus be relatively common (183).

CONCLUSION

The central nervous system has a very high metabolic rate and also a requirement for this rate to be continuously maintained. This can only be filled by an uninterrupted supply of both glucose and oxygen, and transient deficits in such materials can rapidly compromise brain function. Underlying the brain's unusual energy demand is the need for the maintenance of major ionic gradients across the neuronal plasma membrane. While all cells require such gradients, nerve tissue is distinctive in that the functioning of neural conduction requires that these gradients must transiently be allowed to collapse. The temporary relaxation of the normal sodium gradient is needed for the passage of the axonal action potential, and the very steep calcium gradient must be reduced in order to allow the presynaptic exocytotic release of neurotransmitters into the synaptic cleft. It has been proposed that the initial response to acute insufficiency of energy may primarily involve sodium influx into axons, while more delayed neurodegenerative events may be enabled by the prolonged presence of excess levels of cytosolic calcium (184).

The influx of these cations occurs by opening of ion-selective gates within the external neuronal membrane, and since this increases entropy, these are not energy-requiring events. However, the removal of excess ions from the cytosol by pumping them out into the extracellular space and, in the case of calcium, also by ion-sequestering mechanisms are energy-demanding processes. The ability to maintain an adequate glucose supply to nerve cells is especially critical in view of their limited intraneuronal glycogen reserve and their relative inability to utilize other potential sources of energy such as fatty acids. The supply of oxygen to the brain is equally vital because of its inability to adequately meet its metabolic needs by anaerobic glycolysis.

These CNS features, while they may be considered merely as exaggerations of processes common to many cells, result in the brain possessing a very distinctive set of susceptibilities to impaired energy supply or utilization. Many neurological conditions involve either suboptimal nutrient supply or an excessive energy demand. It is for this reason that, in addition to the specific and definitive characteristics of each neurotoxic chemical, certain recurring pathological features are suspected to be common to a wide range of unrelated neurotoxic agents and neurological disorders.

Several types of metabolic change effected by many agents deleterious to nerve tissue can have the potential for inducing excess oxygen radical production, and the resulting oxidative damage may constitute a varying proportion of the total spectrum of toxicity of a wide range of chemicals. Any chemical disrupting membrane structure or mitochondrial function has the potential for induction of oxygen radicals. This is especially true of the broad range of neurotoxic agents causing the hyperexcitatory state that is generally an intermediate step between neuronal health and death. Figure 1 summarizes the potential routes by which toxicants can influence ROS production in the nervous system and how some of these may be mediated by excitatory states.

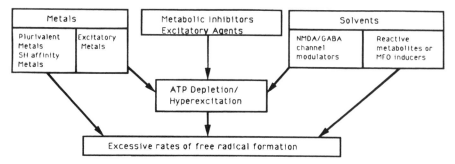

FIG. 1. Potential routes whereby neurotoxicants can induce hazardous levels of reactive oxygen species.

The fact that intrinsic antioxidant defense processes must first be overwhelmed before excess ROS can damage cell functioning increases the likelihood that ROS-related damage may be region specific. Such distinctive regional vulnerability may have either a chemical or an anatomical basis. An example of the first case involves areas rich in catecholamine neurons. These neurotransmitters are prone to oxidation and can give rise to semioxidized products, which can result in continued and potentiated oxidative damage. An example of anatomical susceptibility is the hippocampus, which is especially vulnerable to excitotoxic damage. This is probably by virtue of the distinctive anatomy of the hippocampus, wherein responses to repetitive stimuli are continually augmented rather than undergoing adaptive inhibition, a response characterizing of most other brain regions.

Neurotoxic insult is not an "all-or-none" event, and subtle and insidious gradations of damage can occur. Broad, low-level exposures to hazardous agents are common, so the overall magnitude of harmful neurotoxic exposures across a population is very difficult to estimate. Marginal deficiencies of antioxidant vitamins over extended periods may increase vulnerability to chronic exposure to low levels of free-radical-promoting environmental contaminants. The consequences of this may be expressed as subclinical events that cannot readily be quantitated but that may potentially affect the well-being of an individual. Environmental factors are a suspected contributory element in many neurodegenerative disorders, where chronic low levels of excess pro-oxidant events and excitotoxicity are postulated to be involved (185). This represents an area of great relevance to an aging population with increasing life expectancy, and offers a worthwhile challenge for both mechanistic and therapeutic studies.

ACKNOWLEDGMENTS

This work was supported by grants AA8282 and ES7992 from the National Institutes of Health.

REFERENCES

1. Freeman BA, Crapo JD. Biology of disease: Free radicals and tissue injury. *Lab Invest* 1982; 47:412–426.
2. Halliwell B, Gutteridge JMC. *Free Radicals in Biology and Medicine*. Oxford: Clarendon Press, 1989;266.
3. Savolainen H. Superoxide dismutase and glutathione peroxidase activities in rat brain. *Res Commun Chem Pathol Pharmacol* 1978;21:173–176.
4. Raps SP, Lai JCK, Hertz L, Cooper AJL. Glutathione is present in high concentrations in cultured astrocytes, but not in cultured neurons. *Brain Res* 1989;493:398–401.
5. Halliwell B, Gutteridge JMC. Oxygen radicals and the nervous system. *Trends in Neurosci* 1985;8:22–26.
6. Braughler JM, Hall ED. Central nervous system trauma and stroke. *Free Radical Biol Med* 1989;6:289–301.
7. Floyd RA. Role of oxygen free radicals in carcinogenesis and brain ischemia. *FASEB J* 1990;4:2587–2597.
8. Kehrer JP, Mossman BT, Sevanian A, Trush MA, Smith MT. Free radical mechanisms in chemical pathogenesis. *Toxicol Appl Pharmacol* 1988;95:349–362.

9. LeBel CP, Bondy SC. Persistent protein damage despite reduced oxygen radical formation in the aging rat brain. *Int J Dev Neurosci* 1991;9:139–146.

10. Boveris A, Chance B. The mitochondrial generation of hydrogen peroxide: general properties and the effect of hyperbaric oxygen. *Biochem J* 1973;134:707–716.

11. Johnson JD, Conroy WG, Burris KD, Isom GE. Peroxidation of brain lipids following cyanide intoxication in mice. *Toxicology* 1987;46:21–28.

12. Schisler NJ, Singh SM. Effect of ethanol *in vivo* on enzymes which detoxify oxygen free radicals. *Free Radical Biol Med* 1989;7:117–123.

13. Kehrer JP, Jones DP, Lemasters JJ, Farber JL, Jaeschke H. Mechanisms of hypoxic cell injury. *Toxicol Appl Pharmacol* 1990;106:165–178.

14. Bondy SC, McKee M, LeBel, CP. Changes in synaptosomal pH and rates of oxygen radical formation induced by chlordecone. *Mol Chem Neuropathol* 1990;13:95–106.

15. Minotti G, Aust SD. The role of iron in oxygen radical mediated lipid peroxidation. *Chem Biol Interact* 1989;71:1–19.

16. Saunders R, Horrocks LA. Eicosanoids, plasma membranes, and molecular mechanisms of spinal cord injury. *Neurochem Pathol* 1987;7:1–22.

17. Asano T, Koide T, Gotoh O, Joshita H, Hanamura T, Shigeno T, Takakura K. The role of free radicals and eicosanoids in the pathogenetic mechanism underlying ischemic brain edema. *Mol Chem Neuropathol* 1989;10:101–133.

18. Beckman JS. The double-edged role of nitric oxide in brain function and superoxide-mediated injury. *J Dev Physiol* 1991;15:53–59.

19. Bonser RW, Thompson NT, Randall RW, Garland LG. Phospholipase D activation is functionally linked to superoxide generation in the human neutrophil. *Biochem J* 1989;264:617–620.

20. Au AM, Chan PH, Fishman RA. Stimulation of phospholipase A_2 activity by oxygen-derived free radicals in isolated brain capillaries. *J Cell Biochem* 1985;27:449–453.

21. Schwartz RD, Skolnick P, Paul SM. Regulation of γ-aminobutyric acid/barbiturate receptor-gated chloride ion flux in brain vesicles by phospholipase A_2: Possible role of oxygen radicals. *J Neurochem* 1988;50:565–571.

22. Sevanian A, Nordenbrand K, Kim E, Ernster L, Hochstein P. Microsomal lipid peroxidation: The role of NADPH-cytochrome P-450 reductase and cytochrome P-450. *Free Radical Biol Med* 1990;8:145–152.

23. Warner M, Kohler C, Hansson T, Gustafsson JA. Regional distribution of cytochrome P450 in the brain: Spectral quantitation and contribution of P-450b, e and P450c, d. *J Neurochem* 1988;50:1057–1065.

24. Perrin R, Minn A, Ghersi-Egea JF, Grassiot MC, Siest G. Distribution of cytochrome P450 activities towards alkoxyresorufin derivatives in rat brain regions, subcellular fractions and isolated cerebral microvessels. *Biochem Pharmacol* 1990;40:2145–2151.

25. J. M. McCord. Oxygen-derived radicals: A link between reperfusion injury and inflamation. *Fed Proc* 1987;46:2402–2406.

26. Tayarani I, Chaudiere J, Lefauconnier JM, and Bourre JM. Enzymatic protection against peroxidative damage in isolated brain capillaries. *J Neurochem* 1987;48:1399–1410.

27. Hall ED, Braughler JM. Central nervous system trauma and stroke. II Physiological and pharmacological evidence for involvement of oxygen radicals and lipid peroxidation. *Free Radical Biol Med* 1989;6:303–313.

28. Ghersi-Egea JF, Minn A, Siest G. A new aspect of the protective functions of the blood-brain barrier: Activities of four drug-metabolizing enzymes in isolated rat brain microvessels. *Life Sci* 1988;42:2515–2523.

29. Jackson GR, Apffel L, Werrbach-Perez K, Perez-Polo JR. Role of nerve growth factor in oxidant-antioxidant balance and neuronal injury. I Stimulation of hydrogen peroxide resistance. *J Neurosci Res* 1990;25:360–368.

30. Dexter DT, Carayon A, Vidailhet M, Ruberg M, Agid F, Agid Y, Lees AJ, Wells FR, Jenner P, Marsden CD. Decreased ferritin levels in brain in Parkinson's disease. *J Neurochem* 1990;55:16–20.

31. Maellaro E, Casini AF, Del Bello B, Comporti M. Lipid peroxidation and antioxidant systems in liver injury produced by glutathione depleting agents. *Biochem Pharmacol* 1990;39:1513–1521.

32. Calvin HI, Medvedovsky C, Worgul BV. Near-total glutathione depletion and age-specific cataracts induced by buthionine sulfoximine in mice. *Science* 1986;233:553–555.

33. Perry TL, Godin DV, Hansen S. Parkinson's Disease: a disorder due to nigral glutathione deficiency? *Neurosci Lett* 1982;33:305–310.

34. Ravindranath V, Shivakumar BR, Anandatheerthavarada HK. Low glutathione levels in brain regions of aged rats. *Neurosci Lett* 1989;101:18–190.
35. Halliwell B. Albumin—An important extracellular antioxidant? *Biochem Pharmacol* 1988; 37:569–571.
36. Halliwell B. Oxidants and the central nervous system: Some fundamental questions. Is oxidant damage relevant to Parkinson's disease, Alzheimer's disease, traumatic injury or stroke? *Acta Neurol Scand Suppl* 1989;126:23–33.
37. Czapski G, Goldstein S. When do metal complexes protect the biological system from superoxide toxicity and when do they enhance it? *Free Radical Res Commun* 1986;1:157–161.
38. Bondy SC. Reactive oxygen species relation to aging and neurotoxic damage. *Neurotoxicology* 1992;13:87–100.
39. Aust SD, Miller DM. New horizons in molecular toxicology. *Lilly Research Laboratories Symp* 1991;29–34.
40. Stadtman ER. Metal ion-catalyzed oxidation of proteins:biochemical mechanism and biological consequences. *Free Radical Biol Med* 1990;9:315–325.
41. Stadtman ER. Oxidation of free amino acids and amino acid residues in proteins by radiolysis and by metal-catalyzed reactions. *Annu Rev Biochem* 1993;62:797–821.
42. Sadrzadeh SM, Anderson DK, Panter SS, Hallaway PE, Eaton JW. Hemoglobin potentiates central nervous system damage. *J Clin Invest* 1987;79:662–664.
43. Willmore LJ, Triggs WJ. Iron-induced lipid peroxidation and brain injury responses. *Int J Dev Neurosci* 1991;9:175–180.
44. Gutteridge JM, Westermarck T , Santavuori P. Iron and oxygen radicals in tissue damage: Implications for neuronal ceroid lipofuscinoses. *Acta Neurol Scand* 1983;68:365–370.
45. Grundke-Iqbal I, Fleming J,Tung YC, Lassmann H, Iqbal K, Joshi JG. Ferritin is a component of the neuritic (senile) plaque in Alzheimer dementia. *Acta Neuropathol* 1990;81:105–110.
46. Connor JR, Snyder BS, Beard JL, Fine RE, Mufson EJ. Regional distribution of iron and iron-regulatory proteins in the brain in aging and Alzheimer's disease. *J Neurosci Res* 1992;31:327–335.
47. Youdim MBH, Ben-Shachar D, Reiderer P. Is Parkinson's disease a progressive siderosis of substantia nigra resulting in iron and melanin induced neurodegeneration? *Acta Neurol Scand Suppl* 1989;126:47–54
48. Shoham S, Wertman E, Ebstein RP. Iron accumulation in the rat basal ganglia after excitatory amino acid injections-dissociation from neuronal loss. *Exp Neurol* 1992;118:227–241.
49. Prat AG, Turrens JF. Ascorbate- and hemoglobin-dependent brain chemiluminescence. *Free Radical Biol Med* 1990;8:319–325.
50. Rosenthal RE, Chanderbhan R, Marshall G, Fiskum G. Prevention of post-ischemic brain lipid conjugated diene production and neurological injury by hydroxyethyl starch-conjugated deferoxamine. *Free Radical Biol Med* 1992;12:29–33.
51. Perry TL, Norman MG, Yong VW, Whiting S, Crichton JU, Hansen S, Kish SJ. Hallervorden-Spatz disease: Cysteine accumulation and cysteine dioxygenase deficiency in the globus pallidus. *Ann Neurol* 1985;18:482–489.
52. Ikeda Y, Ikeda K, Long DM. Protective effect of the iron chelator deferoxamine on cold-induced brain edema.*J Neurosurg* 1989;71:233–238.
53. Cederbaum AI. Oxygen radical generation by microsomes: Role of iron and implications for alcohol metabolism and toxicity. *Free Radical Biol Med* 1989;7:559–567.
54. Shaw S. Lipid peroxidation, iron mobilization and radical generation induced by ethanol. *Free Radical Biol Med* 1989;7:541–547.
55. Rouach H, Houze P, Orfanelli MT, Gentil M, Bourdon R, Nordmann R. Effect of acute ethanol administration on the subcellular distribution of iron in rat liver and cerebellum. *Biochem Pharmacol* 1990;39:1095–1100.
56. Bondy SC, Pearson KR. Ethanol-induced oxidative stress and nutritional status. *Alcohol Clin Exp Res* 1993;17:651–654.
57. Crapper-McLachlan DR, Dalton AJ, Kruck TP, Bell MY, Smith WL, Kalow W, Andrews DF. Intramuscular desferrioxamine in patients with Alzheimer's disease. *Lancet* 1991;337:1304–1308.
58. LeVine SM. The role of reactive oxygen species in the pathogenesis of multiple sclerosis. *Med Hypoth* 1992;3:271–274.
59. Halliwell B. Protection against tissue damage in vivo by desferrioxamine: what is its mechanism of action? *Free Radical Biol Med* 1989;7:645–651.

60. Klebanoff SJ, Waltersdorph AM, Michel BR, Rosen H. Oxygen-based free radical generation by ferrous ions and deferoxamine. *J Biol Chem* 1989;264:19765–19771.
61. Wahba ZZ, Murray WJ, Stohs SJ. Desferrioxamine-induced alterations in hepatic iron distribution, DNA damage, and lipid peroxidation in control and 2,3,7,8-tetrachlorodibenzo-*p*-dioxin-treated rats. *J Appl Toxicol* 1990;10:119–124.
62. Kruck TPA, Fisher EA, McLachlan DR. Suppression of deferoxamine mesylate treatment-induced side effects by coadministration of isoniazid in a patient with Alzheimer's disease subject to aluminum removal by ion-specific chelation. *Clin Pharmacol Therap* 1990;48:439–446.
63. Thomas DJ, Chisholm JJ. Lead, zinc and copper decorporation during calcium disodium ethylenediamine tetraacetate treatment of lead-poisoned children. *J Pharmacol Exp Ther* 1986;239:829–835.
64. Reif DW, Simmons RD. Nitric oxide mediates iron release from ferritin. *Arch Biochem Biophys* 1990;283:537–541.
65. Ogawa N, Edamatsu R, Mizukawa K, Asanuma M, Kohno M, Mori A. Degeneration of dopaminergic neurons and free radicals. Possible participation of levodopa. *Adv Neurol* 1993;60:242–250.
66. Wurtman RJ, Wurtman JJ. *Nutrition and the Brain* New York: Raven Press, 1990;59–74.
67. Jellinger KA, Kienzl E, Rumpelmaier G, Paulus W, Reiderer P, Stachelberger H, Youdim MBH, Ben-Shacher D. Iron and ferritin in substantia nigra in Parkinson's disease. *Adv Neurol* 1993;60:267–272.
68. Scheinburg IH. The neurotoxicity of copper. In: Bondy SC, Prasad KN, eds., *Metal Neurotoxicity* Boca Raton, FL: CRC Press, 1988;56–60.
69. Babcock GT and Wikstrom M. Oxygen activation and the conservation of energy in cell respiration. *Nature* 1992;356:301–309.
70. Birkmayer W, Knoll J, Reiderer P, Youdim MBH, Harsand H, Martor J. Increased life expectancy resulting from addition of L-deprenyl to Madopar treatment in Parkinson's disease: A long-term study. *J Neural Transm* 1985;64:113–117.
71. Shoulson I. Deprenyl and tocopherol antioxidative therapy of Parkinsonism (DATATOP) Parkinson Study Group. *Acta Neurol Scand Suppl* 1989;126:171–175.
72. Seth PK, Chandra SV. In: Prasad KN, Bondy SC, eds., *Metal Neurotoxicity.* Boca Raton, FL: CRC Press, 1988;19–33.
73. DATATOP: A multicenter clinical trial in early Parkinson's disease. Parkinson's Study Group. *Arch Neurol* 1989;46:1052–1060.
74. Donaldson J, Labella FS, Gessa D. Enhanced autoxidation of dopamine as a possible basis of manganese neurotoxicity. *Neurotoxicology* 1981;2:53–64.
75. Cheton PLB, Archibald FS. Manganese complexes and the generation and scavenging of hydroxyl free radicals. *Free Radical Biol Med* 1988;5:325–333.
76. Coassin M, Ursini F, Bindoli A. Antioxidant effect of manganese. *Arch Biochem Biophys* 1992;299:330–333.
77. Haider SS, el-Fakhri M. Action of alpha-tocopherol on vanadium-stimulated lipid peroxidation in rat brain. *Neurotoxicology* 1991;12:79–85.
78. Naganuma A, Anderson ME, Meister A. Cellular glutathione as a determinant of sensitivity to mercuric chloride toxicity. Prevention of toxicity by giving glutathione monoester. *Biochem Pharmacol* 1990;40:693–697.
79. Hasan M, Ali SF. Effects of thallium, nickel and cobalt administration on the lipid peroxidation in different regions of the rat brain. *Toxicol Appl Pharmacol* 1981;57:8–13.
80. Yonaha M, Saito M, Sagai M. Stimulation of lipid peroxidation by methylmercury. *Life Sci* 1983;32:1507–1514.
81. Marzabadi MR, Jones CB. Heavy metals and lipofucsinogenesis. A study on myocardial cells cultured under varying oxidative stress. *Mech Ageing Dev* 1992;66:159–171.
82. Chang LW, Gilbert M, Sprecher J. Modification of methylmercury neurotoxicity by vitamin E. *Environ Res* 1978;17:356–366.
83. Shukla GS, Srivastava RS, Chandra SV. Prevention of cadmium-induced effects onregional glutathione status of rat brain by vitamin E. *J Appl Toxicol* 1988;8:355–359.
84. LeBel CP, Ali SF, McKee M, Bondy SC. Organometal-induced increases in oxygen reactive species: The potential of 2',7'-dichlorofluorescin diacetate as an index of neurotoxic damage. *Toxicol Appl Pharmacol* 1990;104:17–24.
85. LeBel CP, Ischiropoulos H, Bondy SC. Evaluation of the probe 2',7'-dichlorofluorescin as an indicator of reactive oxygen species formation and oxidative stress. *Chem Res Toxicol* 1992; 5:227–231.

86. O'Callaghan JP, Miller DB. Diethyldithiocarbamate increases distribution of cadmium to brain but prevents cadmium-induced neurotoxicity. *Brain Res* 1986;370:354–358.
87. Reddy CC, Massaro EJ. Biochemistry of selenium: A brief overview. *Fund Appl Toxicol* 1983; 3:431–436.
88. Hoekstra WG. Biochemical function of selenium and its relation to vitamin E. *Fed Proc* 1975; 34:2083–2089.
89. Chang LW , Suber R. Protective effect of selenium on methylmercury toxicity: A possible mechanism. *Bull Environ Contam Toxicol* 1982;29:285–289.
90. Kojima Y, Kagi JHR. Metallothionein. *Trends Biochem Sci* 1978;3:90–92.
91. Schubert J, Riley EJ, Tyler SA. Combined effects in toxicology—A rapid systematic testing procedure:cadmium, mercury and lead. *J Toxicol Environ Health* 1978;4:763–776.
92. Zimmerman JJ, Zuk SM, Millard JR. In vitro modulation of human neutrophil superoxide anion generation by various calcium channel antagonists used in reperfusion resuscitation. *Biochem Pharmacol* 1989;38:3601–3610.
93. White BC, Aust SD, Arfors KE, Aronson LD. Brain injury by ischemic anoxia hypothesis extensionA tale of two ions? *Ann Emerg Med* 1984;13:862–867.
94. Vanella A, Sorrenti V, Castorina C, Campisi A, Di Giacomo C, Russo A, Perez-Polo JR. Lipid peroxidation in rat cerebral cortex during post-ischemic reperfusion: Effect of exogenous antioxidants and Ca^{2+}-antagonistic drugs. *Int J Dev Neurosci* 1992;10:75–80.
95. Bondy SC, LeBel CP. The relationship between excitotoxicity and oxidative stress in the central nervous system. *Free Radical Biol Med* 1993;14:633–642.
96. Rehman SU. Lead-induced regional lipid peroxidation in brain. *Toxicol Lett* 1984;21:333–337.
97. Ali SF, Bondy SC. Triethyl lead-induced peroxidative damage in various regions of the rat brain. *J Toxicol Environ Health* 1989;26:235–242.
98. Hermes-Lima M, Pereira B, Bechara EJH. Are free radicals involved in lead poisoning? *Xenobiotica* 1991;21:1085–1090.
99. Evans PH, PeterhanS E, Burge T, Klinowski J. Aluminosilicate-induced free radical generation by murine brain glial cells in vitro: potential significance in the aetiopathogenesis of Alzheimer's dementia. *Dementia* 1992;3:1–6.
100. Pappolla MA, Omar RA, Kim KS, Robakis NK. Immunohistochemical evidence of antioxidant stress in Alzheimer's disease. *Am J Pathol* 1992;140:621–628.
101. Gutteridge JMC, Quinlan GJ, Clark I, Halliwell B. Aluminium salts accelerate peroxidation of membrane lipids stimulated by iron salts. *Biochim Biophys Acta* 1985;835:441–447.
102. Fraga CG, Oteiza PI, Golub MS, Gershwin ME, Keen CL. Effects of aluminum on brain lipid peroxidation. *Toxicol Lett* 1990;51:213–219.
103. Oteiza PI, Fraga CG, Keen CL. Aluminum has both oxidant and antioxidant effects in mouse brain membranes. *Arch Biochem Biophys* 1993;300:517–521.
104. Bondy SC, Kirstein S. The promotion of iron-induced generation of reactive oxygen species in nerve tissue by aluminum. *Mol Chem Neuropathol* 1996;27:185–194.
105. Smith CD, Carney JM, TatsumoT, Stadtman ER, Floyd RA, Markesbery WR. Protein oxidation in aging brain. *Ann NY Acad Sci* 1992;663:110–119.
106. SubbaraoKV, Richardson JS, Ang LC. Autopsy samples of Alzheimer's cortex show increased peroxidation in vitro. *J Neurochem* 1990;55:342–355.
107. Mantyh PW, Ghilardi JR, Rogers S, DeMasters E, Allen CJ, Stimson ER, Maggio JE. Aluminum, iron and zinc promote aggregation of physiological concentrations of beta-amyloid peptide. *J Neurochem* 1993;61:1171–1174.
108. Evans PH, Klinowski J, Yano E. Cephaloconiosis: A free radical perspective on the proposed particulate-induced etiopathogenesis of Alzheimer's dementia and related disorders. *Med Hypoth* 1991;34:209–219.
109. Garrel C, Lafond JL, Faure P, Favier A. In vitro study of nitric oxide production by microglial cells stimulated with aluminum salts. *Proc 2nd Int Symp on Reactive Oxygen Species II* 1993;18:xxx.
110. Ahmad FF, Cowan DL, Sun AY. Detection of free radical formation in various tissues after acute carbon tetrachloride administration in the gerbil. *Life Sci* 1987;41:2469–2475.
111. Cojocel C, Beuter W, Muller W, Mayer D. Lipid peroxidation: A possible mechanism of trichloroethylene-induced nephrotoxicity. *Toxicology* 1989;55:131–141.
112. Guerri C, Grisolia S. Changes in glutathione in acute and chronic alcohol intoxication. *Pharmacol Biochem Behav* 1980;13(Suppl 1):53–61.
113. Nordmann R. Oxidative stress from alcohol in the brain. *Alcoholism Alcohol* 1987;(Suppl 1):75–82.

114. Natsuki R. Effect of ethanol on calcium uptake and phospholipid turnover by stimulation of adrenoceptors and muscarinic receptors in mouse brain and heart synaptosomes. *Biochem Pharmacol* 1991;42:39–44.

115. Uysal M, Kutalp G, Odzemirler G, Ayka G. Ethanol-induced changes in lipid peroxidation and glutathione content in rat brain. *Drug Alcohol Depend* 1989;23:227–230.

116. Mattia CJ, Adams JD, Bondy SC. Free radical induction in the brain and liver by products of toluene catabolism. *Biochem Pharmacol* 1993;46:103–110.

117. Ray DE, Abbott NJ, Chan MWK, Romero IA. Increased oxidative metabolism andoxidative stress in *m*-dinitrobenzene neurotoxicity. *Biochem Soc Trans* 1994;22:407S.

118. Bondy SC, Guo SX. Effect of ethanol treatment on indices of cumulative oxidative stress. *Europ J Pharmacol* 1994;270:349–355.

119. Bondy SC, Guo SX. Regional selectivity of ethanol-induced pro-oxidant events within the brain. *Biochem Pharmacol* 1995;49:69–72.

120. Adams JD, Klaidman LK, Odunze IN. Oxidative effects of MPTP in the midbrain. *Res Commun Subst Abuse* 1989;10:169–180.

121. Nadiger HA, Marcus SK, Chavdrakala MV. Lipid peroxidation and ethanol toxicity in at brain: effect of vitamin E deficiency and supplementation. *Med Sci Res* 1988;16:1273–1274.

122. Choy PC, Man RYK, Chan AC. Phosphatidylcholine metabolism in isolated rat heart: Modulation by ethanol and vitamin E. *Biochim Biophys Acta* 1989;1005:225–232.

123. LeBel CP, SchatzRA. Altered synaptosomal phospholipid metabolism after toluene: Possible relationship with membrane fluidity, Na$^+$, K$^+$-adenosine triphosphatase and phospholipid methylation. *J Pharmacol Exp Thep* 1990;253:1189–1197.

124. Kaneko M, Panagia V, Paolillo G, Majumder S, Ou C, Dhalla NS. Inhibition of cardiac phosphatidylethanolamine *N*-methylation by oxygen free radicals. *Biochim Biophys Acta* 1990;1021:33–38.

125. Nordmann R, Ribiere C, Rouach H. Involvement of iron and iron-catalyzed free radical production in ethanol metabolism and toxicity. *Enzyme* 1987;37:57–69.

126. Nordmann R, Ribiere C, Rouach H. *Free Radical Biol Med* 1992;12:219–240.

127. Nordmann R, Ribiere C, Rouach H. Pathophysiological relevance of free radicals to the ethanol-induced disorder in membrane lipids. In: Crastes de Paulet A, Douste-Blazy L, Paoletti R, eds. *Free Radicals, Lipoproteins and Membrane Lipids*. New York: Plenum Press, 1990;309–319.

128. Lucas D, Lamboeuf Y, DeSaint-Blanquat G, Menez JF. Ethanol-inducible cytochrome P-450 activity and increase in acetaldehyde bound to microsomes after chronic administration of acetaldehyde or ethanol. *Alcohol Alcoholism* 1990;25:395–400.

129. Behrens UJ, Hoerner M, Lasker JM, Lieber CS. Formation of acetaldehyde adducts with ethanol inducible P-450IIEI *in vivo*. *Biochem Biophys Res Commun* 1988;154:584–590.

130. Westcott JY, Weiner H, Schultz I, Myers RD. *In vivo* acetaldehyde in the brain of the rat treated with ethanol. *Biochem Pharmacol* 1980;29:411–417.

131. O'Neill PJ, Rahwan RG. Protection against active toxicity of acetaldehyde in mice. *Res Commun Chem Pathol Pharmacol* 1976;13:125–128.

132. Wickramansinghe SN, Hasan R. *In vitro* effects of vitamin C, thioctic acid and dihydrolipoic acid on the cytotoxicity of post-ethanol serum. *Biochem Pharmacol* 1992;43:407–411.

133. Ekstrom G, Ingelman-SundberG M. Rat liver microsomal NADPH-supported oxidase activity and lipid peroxidation dependent on ethanol-inducible cytochrome P-450 (P-450IIE1). *Biochem Pharmacol* 1989;38:1313–1319.

134. Kuthan H, Ullrich V. Oxidase and oxygenase function of the microsomal cytochrome P-450 monoxygenase system. *Eur J Biochem* 1982;126:583–588.

135. Hansson T, Tindberg N, Ingelman-Sundberg M, Kohler C. Regional distribution of ethanol-inducible cytochrome P-450 IIEI in the rat central nervous system. *Neurosci* 1990;34:451–463.

136. Mattia CJ, LeBel CP, Bondy SC. Effects of toluene and its metabolites on cerebral reactive oxygen species generation. *Biochem Pharmacol* 1991;42:879–882.

137. Ledig M, M'Paria JR, Mandel P. Superoxide dismutase activity in rat brain during acute and chronic alcohol intoxication. *Neurochem Res* 1981;6:385–390.

138. Ledig M, Tholey G, Megias-Megias L, Kopp P, Wedler F. Combined effects of ethanol and manganese on cultured neurons and glia. *Neurochem Res* 1991;16:591–596.

139. Gonthier B, Jeunet A, Barret L. Electron spin resonance study of free radicals produced from ethanol and acetaldehyde after exposure to a Fenton system or to brain and liver microsomes. *Alcohol* 1991;8:369–375.

140. Feierman DE, Cederbaum AI. Increased content of cytochrome P-450 and 4-methylpyrazole binding spectrum after 4-methylpyrazole treatment. *Biochem Biophys Res Comm* 1985;126:1076–1081.

141. Sultatos LG. Effects of acute ethanol administration on the hepatic xanthine dehydrogenase oxidase system in the rat. *J Pharmacol Exp Ther* 1988;246:946–949.

142. Zuddas A, Corsini GU, Schinelli S, Barker JL, Kopin IJ, di Porzio U. Acetaldehyde directly enhances MPP$^+$ neurotoxicity and delays its elimination from the striatum. *Brain Res* 1989;501:11–22.

143. Oldfield FF, Cowan DL, Sun AU. The involvement of ethanol in the free radical reaction of 6-hydroxydopamine. *Neurochem Res* 1991;16:83–87.

144. Trenga CA, Kunkel DD, Eaton DL, Costa LG. Effect of styrene oxide on rat brain glutathione. *Neurotoxicol* 1991;12:165–178.

145. Lam HR, Ostergaard G, Guo SX, Ladefoged O, Bondy SC. Three weeks' exposure of rats to dearomatized white spirit modifies indices of oxidative stress in brain, kidney, and liver. *Biochem Pharmacol* 1994;47:651–657.

146. Bondy SC, Lam HR, Ostergard G, Guo SX, Ladefoged O. Changes in markers of oxidative status in brain, liver and kidney of young and aged rats following exposure to aromatic white spirit. *Arch Toxicol* 1995;69:410–414.

147. Heikkila RE, Sieber BA, Manzino L, Sonsalla PK. Some features of the nigrostriatal dopaminergic neurotoxin 1-methyl-4-phenyl-1,2,3,6-tetrahydropyridine (MPTP) in the mouse. *Mol Chem Neuropatholol* 1989;10:171–183.

148. Rios C, Tapia R. Changes in lipid peroxidation induced by 1-methyl-4-phenyl-1,2,3,6-tetrahydropyridine and 1-methyl-4-phenylpyridinium in mouse brain homogenates. *Neurosci Lett* 1987;77:321–326.

149. Odunze IN, Klaidman LK, Adams JD. MPTP toxicity in the mouse brain and vitamin E. *Neurosci Lett* 1990;108:346–349.

150. Cino M, Del Maestro RF. Generation of hydrogen peroxide by brain mitochondria: The effect of reoxygenation following postdecapitative ischemia. *Arch Biochem Biophys* 1989;269:623–638.

151. Ali SF, LeBel CP, Bondy SC. Reactive oxygen species formation as a biomarker of methylmercury and trimethyltin neurotoxicity. *Neurotoxicol* 1992;13:637–648.

152. Tanner CM, Langston JW. Do environmental toxins cause Parkinson's disease? A critical review. *Neurology* 1990;40:17–30(Suppl. 3).

153. Saggu H, Cooksey J, Dexter D, Wells FR, Lees A, Jenner P, Marsden CD. A selective increase in particulate superoxide dismutase activity in parkinsonian substantia nigra. *J Neurochem* 1989;53:692–697.

154. McCrodden JM, Tipton KF, Sullivan JP. The neurotoxicity of MPTP and the relevance to Parkinson's disease. *Pharmacol Toxicol* 1990;67:8–13.

155. Pezzoli G, Ricciardi S, Masotto C, Mariani CB, Cerenzi A. *n*-Hexane induces Parkinsonism in rodents. *Brain Res* 1990;531:355–357.

156. Fedtke N, Bolt HM. Detection of 2,5-hexanedione in the urine of persons not exposed to *n*-hexane. *Int Arch Occup Environ Health* 1986;57:143–148.

157. De Vito MJ, Wagner GC. Methamphetamine-induced neuronal damage: A possible role for free radicals. *Neuropharmacology* 1989;28:1145–1150.

158. Olney JW, Zorumski CF, Stewart GR, Price MT, Wong GJ, Labruyere J. Excitotoxicity of L-DOPA and 6-OH-DOPA: Implications for Parkinson's and Huntington's diseases. *Exp Neurol* 1990;108:269–272.

159. Cohen G. Oxygen radicals and Parkinson's disease. In: Halliwell B, ed., *Oxygen Radicals and Tissue Injury.* Bethesda, MD: FASEB, 1988;130–135.

160. Lohr JB, Kuczenski R, Bracha HS, Moir M, Jeste DV. Increased indices of free radical activity in the cerebrospinal fluid of patients with tardive dyskinesia. *Biol Psychiatry* 1990;28:535–539.

161. Jackson-Lewis V, Przedborski S, Kostic V, Suber F, Fahn S, Cadet JL. Partial attenuation of fluphenazine-induced changes in regional monoamine metabolism by D-alpha tocopherol in rat brain. *Brain Res Bull* 1991;26:251–258.

162. Ardelt BK, Borowitz JL, Isom GE. Brain lipid peroxidation and antioxidant protectant mechanisms following acute cyanide intoxication. *Toxicology* 1989;56:147–154.

163. Montgomery RD. In: Vinken PJ, Bruyn GW, eds., *Handbook of Clinical Neurology, Intoxications of the Nervous System,* Vol. 32, Part I. Amsterdam: North Holland, 1979;515–521.

164. Pazdernik TL, Layton M, Nelson SR, Samson FE. The osmotic/calcium stress theory of brain damage: Are free radicals involved? *Neurochem Res* 1992;17:11–21.

165. Dykens JA. Isolated cerebral and cerebellar mitochondria produce free radicals when exposed to elevated Ca^{2+} and Na^+: Implications for neurodegeneration. *J Neurochem* 1994;63:584–591.
166. Nelson SR, Olson JP. Role of early edema in the development of regional seizure related-brain damage. *Neurochem Res* 1987;12:561–564.
167. Armstead WM, Mirro R, Leffler CW, Busija DW. Cerebral superoxide anion generation during seizures in newborn pigs. *J Cereb Blood Flow Metab* 1989;9:175–179.
168. Willmore LJ, Triggs WJ. Effect of phenytoin and corticosteroids on seizures and lipid peroxidation in experimental post-traumatic epilepsy. *J Neurosurg* 1984;60:467–475.
169. Kitagawa K, Matsumoto M, Oda T, Niinobe M, Hata R, Handa N, Fukunaga R, Isaka Y, Kimura K, Maeda H, Mikoshiba K, Kamado T. Free radical generation during brief period of cerebral ischemia may trigger delayed neuronal death. *Neuroscience* 1990;35:551–558.
170. Sutherland RJ, Hoesing JM, Whishaw IQ. Domoic acid, an environmental toxin, produces hippocampal damage and severe memory impairment. *Neurosci Lett* 1990;120:221–223.
171. Bondy SC, Lee DK. Oxidative stress induced by glutamate receptor agonists. *Brain Res* 1993;610:229–233.
172. Murphy TH, Miyamato M, Sastre A, Schaar RL, Coyle JT. Glutamate toxicity in a neuronal cell line involves inhibition of cystine transport leading to oxidative stress. *Neuron* 1989;2:1547–1558.
173. Haba K, Ogawa N, Mizukawa K, Mori A. Time course of changes in lipid peroxidation, pre- and postsynaptic cholinergic indices, NMDA receptor binding and neuronal death in the gerbil hippocampus following transient ischemia. *Brain Res* 1991;540:116–122.
174. Bridges RJ, Koh JY, Hatalski CG, Cotman CW. Increased excitotoxic vulnerability of cortical cultures with reduced levels of glutathione. *Eur J Pharmacol* 1991;192:199–200.
175. Pellerin L, Wolfe LS. Release of arachidonic acid by NMDA-receptor activation in the rat hippocampus. *Neurochem Res* 1991;16:983–989.
176. Kiedrowski L, Costa E, Wroblewski JT. Glutamate receptor agonists stimulate nitric oxide synthase in primary cultures of cerebellar granule cells. *J Neurochem* 1992;58:335–341.
177. Dawson VL, Dawson TM, London ED, Bredt DS, Snyder SH. Nitric oxide mediates glutamate neurotoxicity in primary cortical culcures. *Proc Natl Acad Sci* 1991;88:6368–6371.
178. Dykens JA, Stern A, Trenkner E. Mechanism of kainate toxicity to cerebellar neurons *in vitro* is analogous to reperfusion tissue injury. *J Neurochem* 1987;49:1222–1228.
179. Bose R, Sutherland GR, Pinsky C. Excitotoxins and free radicals: Accomplices in post-ischemic and other neurodegeneration. *Eur J Pharmacol* 1990;183:1170–1171.
180. Delbarre G, Delbarre B, Calinon F, Ferger A. Accumulation of amino acids and hydroxyl free radicals in brain and retina of gerbil after transient ischemia. *J Ocul Pharmacol* 1991;7:147–155.
181. Pellegrini-Giampietro DE, Cherici G, Alesiani M, Carla V, Moroni F. Excitatory amino acid release and free radical formation may cooperate in the genesis of ischemia-induced neuronal damage. *J Neurosci* 1990;10:1035–1041.
182. N. F. Schor. Inactivation of mammalian brain glutamine synthetase by oxygen radicals. *Brain Res* 1988;456:17–21.
183. Oh SM, Betz AL. Interaction between free radicals and excitatory amino acids in the formation of ischemic brain edema in rats. *Stroke* 1990;22:915–921.
184. Coyle JT, Putfarcken P. Oxidative stress, glutamate and neurodegenerative disorders. *Science* 1993;262:689–695.
185. Hennberry R, Spatz L. The role of environmental factors in neurodegenerative disorders. *Neurobiol Aging* 1990;12:75–79.

Free Radical Toxicology
Edited by K. B. Wallace
Copyright © 1997 Taylor & Francis

13

Free-Radical-Mediated Hematopoietic Toxicity by Drugs, Environmental Pollutants, and Ionizing Radiation

Vangala V. Subrahmanyam

Department of Drug Metabolism, Wyeth Ayerst Research, Monmouth Junction, New Jersey, USA

Martyn T. Smith

Division of Environmental Health Sciences, School of Public Health, University of California, Berkeley, California, USA

OVERVIEW OF HEMATOPOIESIS

Hematopoiesis is the process of formation of blood elements (erythrocytes, leukocytes, and thrombocytes) from pluripotent stem cells. In the human fetus, several organs are sequentially involved in the production of blood cells (1). Initially, the yolk sac produces nucleated red cells, followed by liver, which produces red cells, white cells, and platelets. Subsequently, all the cells are produced in spleen and eventually in bone marrow. In the normal adult, bone marrow is the primary site of hematopoiesis. Bone marrow contains stem cells, which are considered to be the immature precursors of the circulating blood cells, rapidly dividing populations of progenitor cells that give rise to the erythrocytes, thrombocytes, and leukocytes. The bone marrow of a man weighing 70 kg releases more than 200 billion erythrocytes, 400 billion thrombocytes, and 10 billion leukocytes into the circulation every day, indicating a very high degree of proliferative activity in this organ (2). The erythrocytes function in transport of oxygen to tissues, platelets in blood clotting at wound sites, and leukocytes in defense against pathogenic bacteria as well as in immune function by producing antibodies. Thus, any agent that interferes with cell growth, proliferation, and maturation of stem and progenitor cells in bone marrow will result in abnormalities in the production of mature blood cells and therefore in impairment of their functions. One of the interesting features of bone marrow is that the ratio between hematopoietic precursor cells and mature circulating cells is constant throughout life (3), suggesting that the formation of various blood elements from hematopoietic precursor cells is well regulated. Bone marrow also contains a heterogeneous matrix of cells called stroma that provide support for the hematopoietic stem-cell proliferation and differentiation (4–6). The stromal cells include endothelial cells, fibroblasts, adipocytes, and macrophages (6).

The pluripotent stem cells and committed progenitor cells account for about 0.4% and 3% of the total bone marrow cell population, while 95% of the cells in the bone marrow are maturing blood cells (6). The development and maturation of pluripotent (or multipotent) stem cells to early hematopoietic cells (committed stem cells or progenitor cells) is governed by growth factors (cytokines) secreted by stromal cells and mature leukocytes within the bone marrow. Recently, MacEachern and Laskin (6) published an excellent review describing the effects of various cytokines in proliferation and differentiation of hematopoietic stem cells into different lineages. The major cytokines involved in hematopoietic regulation of myeloid elements are colony stimulating factor (CSF-1), granulocyte-CSF (G-CSF), granulocyte-macrophage-CSF (GM-CSF), and interleukin 3 (IL-3). Of all these, IL-3 is believed to contribute to the development of all cell types within the bone marrow, whereas other cytokines are primarily involved in myeloid progenitor cell development. In addition to these several other cytokines have also been identified that play a role in myelopoiesis, including IL-1, IL-6 and IL-8. All these cytokines are responsible for proliferation and differentiation of stem cells as well as progenitor cells. Proliferation and differentiation of stem cells along the lymphocyte lineage is dependent on several interleukins including IL-1 through IL-7.

The cytokines mediate their effects through receptors and protein kinases, which are an integral part of signal transduction (7–10). The loss of these complex interactions and communications between the stromal cells and hematopoietic stem and progenitor cells may contribute to various pathophysiological states of bone marrow including pancytopenia, aplastic anemia, lupus, and leukemias. Free radicals have been thought play a role in the pathophysiology of many hematopoietic toxicants including ionizing radiation (11), environmental pollutants (12,13), and drugs (14,15). Therefore, this review is particularly intended to compile the available evidence to determine the possible mechanisms by which free radicals contribute to hematopoietic toxicities.

FREE RADICALS AND HEMATOPOIETIC TOXICITY

Free radicals have been implicated in various pathophysiological processes including aging (16), Alzheimer's disease (17), atherosclerosis (18), cancer (19,20), cataractogenesis (18), contact dermatitis (18), diabetes (21), glomerulonephritis (18), multiple sclerosis (18), muscular dystrophy (18), pancreatitis (18), Parkinson's disease (22), porphyria (18), rheumatoid arthritis (18), and many more (18). Several agents, such as ionizing radiation and chemicals (environmental pollutants, cigarette smoke, and drugs), are known to generate free radicals intracellularly (11–15,23–27). Evidence indicates free radicals are also involved in various blood dyscrasias such as aplastic anemia, leukemia, lupus, and agranulocytosis. For example, benzene (12), ionizing radiation (11), and cigarette smoke (27) may induce aplastic anemia and leukemia in humans by processes that at least in part involve free-radical generation. Various anticancer drugs that induce secondary leukemias in humans generate free-radical intermediates during their metabolism (28–31). In addition, several drugs that induce lupus, an idiosyncratic reaction, form free radicals during their metabolism (14). Interestingly, people who have aplastic anemia (32) or lupus (33) may eventually develop leukemias, suggesting that early toxicity may be important in increasing risk of leukemia.

Many of the oxygen radical deactivating systems are modulated in leukemic cells. For example, elevated superoxide dismutase (SOD) levels have been found in acute and chronic leukemias (34). Similarly, increased ascorbic acid content was found in the B lymphocytes of patients with chronic lymphocytic leukemia (35). Increased levels of iron were also found in serum of patients with acute nonlymphocytic leukemia (36). Furthermore, oxygen radicals have been shown to be involved in the proliferation (37) and differentiation (38–40) of leukemic cells. Although, these data were obtained from leukemic cells, it is reasonable to postulate that during the neoplastic transformation of normal hematopoietic cells due to free-radical insult, the hematopoietic cells may have attempted to adapt by generating elevated antioxidant systems. The elevated levels of defenses against oxygen radicals in leukemic cells may also have given them growth advantage, by conferring resistance against further free-radical insult.

TYPES OF HEMATOPOIETIC TOXICITY

Pancytopenia and Aplastic Anemia

Pancytopenia is characterized by reduction in the number of all types of cells in circulating blood (3). Aplastic anemia is a condition in which damage to multipotential stem cells causes a reduction in the volume of hematopoietic tissue, a decrease in blood cell production, and pancytopenia (3). The etiology of aplastic anemia may be either due to congenital abnormalities or due to chemical/physical agents, such as radiation and drugs (3,41,42). In idiopathic cases bone marrow aplasia is constitutional and associated with congenital abnormalities (3). Chromosomal abnormalities have been found in such inherited aplastic anemias (3,41,42). Epidemiological studies have also associated aplastic anemia with several drugs including nonsteroidal anti-inflammatory agents, sulfonamides, thyrostatic drugs, certain psychotropics, and specific drugs including penicillamine, allopurinol, and gold (3,41,42). Among these, the antibiotic chloramphenicol is notorious. Mitochondrial injury, which may involve oxygen radical production, related to inhibition of protein synthesis has been implicated as the major causative factor of chloramphenicol-induced aplastic anemia (3). However, chromosomal damage is also likely to play a role (43,44).

Among environmental pollutants, benzene is a bone-marrow poison that causes aplastic anemia in humans at high levels of exposure (45,46). Exposure to ionizing radiation also results in aplastic anemia in humans (41). In addition, benzene (12,47–50), chloramphenicol (44), and ionizing radiation (51) all induce chromosomal aberrations in hematopoietic cells in vivo. Both benzene (12,52), and ionizing radiation (11,53) produce oxygen radicals, which may contribute to producing chromosomal aberrations and aplastic anemia induced by these agents.

Leukemia

Cigarette smoke, drugs, environmental pollutants, ionizing radiation and viruses have long been considered as possible etiological factors in the induction of leukemias in humans (11–15,23–27,54). Many of these agents are mainly implicated in the production of leukemias of the myeloid series, but in some cases also of the lymphoid series. Free radicals have been implicated as potential culprits in virtually all of the etiologic factors involved in the pathogenesis of leukemia including viruses (11–15,23–27,54,55). DNA is believed to be the primary target for free-radical-mediated cellular damage, but other intracellular targets that may also be involved include topoisomerase II, histones, tubulin, DNA-polymerases, DNA-ligase, and poly(ADP-ribose) polymerase. These effects of free radicals may result in specific chromosomal abnormalities resulting in the induction of several different types of leukemias, depending upon the type of agent involved.

Acute Myeloid Leukemias

Acute myeloid leukemia (AML) refers to malignancies of adults and children affecting myeloid or nonlymphoid progenitor cells and involves an immature blast cell (56). Between 45 and 55% of cases of de novo AML have a detectable chromosomally abnormal clone present in bone marrow, of which 85% are nonrandom changes (56). Some chromosomal abnormalities are restricted to de novo AML and are rarely seen outside this class. Other chromosomal abnormalities, including rearrangements of 3(q21q26), del(5q), t(6;9), del(7q), monosomy 7, trisomy 8, del(9q), trisomy 11, i(17q), and del(20q), are seen in AML, but are also seen with other myeloid disorders, such as myelodysplastic syndrome (MDS) and myeloproliferative disorders (MPD). Both MDS and MPD may evolve to AML eventually and are considered to be preleukemic states. For example, children with Down's syndrome, an MPD, have trisomy 21 as the major chromosomal abnormality, and show increased incidence of acute megakaryoblastic leukemia and acute lymphoblastic leukemia (ALL) (56). Some patients having chromosome instability syndromes such as Bloom's syndrome and Fanconi's anemia, also develop acute myeloid leukemias (56).

Acute myeloid leukemias are believed to arise due to a defect either at the committed or multipotent stem cell level (57). In cases with t(15;17), inv(16), and t(8; 21) the leukemic clone may be derived from a committed stem cell (57). On the other hand, the presence of monosomy 5, del (5q), monosomy 7, del(7q), trisomy 8, t(6;9), or inv(3) is probably associated with leukemia arising in a multipotent stem cell (57). It is interesting that people who have developed AML due to cigarette smoking have been reported to have the chromosomal abnormalities monosomy 7, del(7q), -Y, or trisomy 13 (58). Workers exposed to high levels of benzene show aneuploidy of chromosomes 7, 8, and 9, when analyzed in their lymphocytes (59). Chromosome 7 appears to be more sensitive than chromosome 8 and 9 to the aneuploidogenic effects of benzene. The common effect of both cigarette smoke and benzene on chromosome 7 suggests that multipotent stem cells are the probable targets of these agents, but this remains to be determined.

Therapy-Related Acute Myeloid Leukemias

The therapy-related secondary acute myeloid leukemias (t-AML), however, show chromosomal abnormalities related to MDS but not of de novo AML (56). Characteristic chromosomal abnormalities seen in t-AML include −7, +7, der(7), t(1;7)(p11;11), monosomy 5, del(5q), del(7q), and abnormalities of 3q, 11q23, 12p, and 17. Many of these chromosomal changes may also be seen in some cases of de novo AML, which may indicate a role for environmental factors, similar in nature to the therapeutic agents. This group also induces chromosomal abnormalities associated with chromosome 11, mainly t(9;11) but also t(11;19), t(11;17), t(11;21), t(X;11), inv(11), and 11q−. Further, the common chromosomal abnormalities seen in MDS include del(5)(q(11q33), del(7)(q22q36), trisomy 8, del (11)(q14) or (q23), del (13) del(20)(q11), and monosomy Y (56).

Interestingly, there are some differences in chromosomal aberrations found in t-AML induced by different classes of anticancer drugs (60,61). While the t-AML induced by alkylating agents (melphalan, mechloroethamine, chlorambucil, cyclophosphamide, carmustine, lomustine, semustine, procarbazine, dacarbazine, mitolactol, etc.) is characterized by aneuploidy of chromosomes 5 and 7, the t-AML induced by topoisomerase II inhibitors (etoposide, teniposide, actinomycin D, doxorubicin, 4-epi-doxorubicin, mitoxantrone, etc.) is characterized by 11q23 and 21q22 translocations.

The observations of deletions and monosomies of chromosomes of 5 and 7 and of 11q23 breakpoints may indicate previous exposure to mutagenic agents (56). In cases with the same abnormalities in people who have not been exposed to anticancer drugs or radiotherapy, exposure to other mutagenic agents may be involved. Therefore, analysis of chromosomal abnormalities may provide indications to the nature of the etiologic agent involved in the induction of specific types of leukemias.

Chronic Myeloid Leukemias

Chronic myeloid leukemia (CML), which is classified among the MPD, was seen in surviving children exposed to ionizing radiation due to atomic bombs at Hiroshima and Nagasaki (62). CML is characterized by an abnormality popularly known as the Philadelphia (Ph') chromosome, which is actually a translocation, t(9;22), and is present in 90% of cases (51). It is well established that in chronic granulocytic leukemia, a type of CML, the Ph' chromosome is present in all myeloid lineages: the erythroid series, megakaryocytes, granulocytes (neutrophils, eosinophil,s and basophils), monocytes, macrophages, and B-lineage lymphoblasts, indicating that the initial leukemogenic event must have occurred in a pluripotent stem cell, although the differentiation during the chronic phase is into myeloid cells (57).

Acute Lymphoblastic Leukemias

The lymphocytes are the main cellular elements of the body's immune system. B-lineage lymphocytes are responsible for immunoglobulin (Ig) mediated immunity and the T-lineage lymphocytes play a role in cellular immunity. They also regulate B cells modulating the Ig-mediated immune response via helper and suppressor T cells. The genes for Ig are located on chromosomes 14q32 (Ig heavy chain gene), 2p12 (κ light chain gene), and 22q11 (λ light chain gene) (63,64). In B-cell maturation, somatic recombination of the Ig gene loci precedes Ig production. In T-cell differentiation three gene loci—14q11.2 α-chain locus, 7q35 β-chain locus, and 7p15 γ-chain locus—are essential for the production of T-cell receptor molecules.

Based on immunological characteristics ALL can be classified into at least seven types (63): (1) early B-precursor ALL; (2) common ALL; (3) pre-B ALL; (4) B-cell-ALL; (5) early thymocyte ALL; (6) common thymocyte ALL; (7) mature thymocyte ALL.

Therapy-Related Acute Lymphoblastic Leukemias

While the t-AML having aberrations in chromosomes 5 and 7 is exclusively found in myeloid lineage, the aberrations involving t11q23 are not restricted to t-AML (61). Many cases of therapy-related ALL were found with t11q23 aberrations in patients treated with doxorubicin and teniposide for neuroblastoma and breast cancer. This is not surprising, however, given the involvement of 11q23 in both de novo AML and ALL. Indeed, the clinical presentation, morphology, and immunophenotype of therapy-related leukemias with 11q23 translocations are indistinguishable from de novo cases. Most cases of infant leukemias have abnormalities involving chromosomal rearrangements of 11q23. As pointed out by Greaves (65), in utero exposure is the most likely cause of these leukemias.

Lymphomas and Chronic Lymphoproliferative Disorders

Lymphomas and chronic lymphoproliferative disorders both arise as a result of neoplastic proliferation of lymphatic cells, particularly of lymph nodes, bone marrow, and peripheral blood (64). Lymphomas may also arise in spleen, liver, intestinal tract, and skin and are broadly classified into Hodgkin's disease and non-Hodgkin's lymphomas (NHL).

Chronic lymphoproliferative disorders are a diverse group of diseases representing the mature cell of the lymphocyte lineage, which accumulate in bone marrow and peripheral blood. Chronic lymphocytic leukemia is the most common of the lymphoproliferative disorders and is associated with trisomy 12, 14q+ , 13q− chromosomal abnormalities.

Lupus

Systemic lupus erythematosus (SLE) is a chronic autoimmune disease, characterized by the formation of autoantibodies against nuclear histone components (66). The basic defect in SLE in humans is a deficiency in suppressor T-cell function, which leads to proliferation and hyperactivity of B lymphocytes. Many drug-induced lupus (DIL) cases are clinically indistinguishable from idiopathic SLE. DIL is classified as an idiosyncratic adverse reaction that occurs after prolonged exposure to a drug. The drugs implicated in DIL include antibiotics (isoniazid, griseofulvin, streptomycin, tetracycline, minocycline, sulfonamides, nitrofurantoin); anti-inflammatory agents (D-penicillamine, gold salts); psychotropic drugs (chlorpromazine, lithium); antiarrhythymics (procainamide, quinidine, acebutolol, practolol); and antihypertensive agents (hydralazine, alpha-methyldopa, and some beta-blockers).

Drug-induced lupus is clearly a systemic disease with no apparent liver involvement. It has been suggested that bioactivation locally in the immune compartment is responsible for DIL. In support of this, many of the lupus-inducing drugs (procainamide, propylthiouracil, isoniazid, hydralazine, quinidine and chlorpromazine) have been shown to undergo myeloperoxidase (MPO) mediated metabolism by stimulated neutrophils to reactive free-radical intermediates (66).

Patients with SLE are reported to have an increased risk of cancer, especially lymphomas (33). Similarly, patients with rheumatoid arthritis have an increased risk of developing neoplasia of both lymphatic and hematopoietic systems (67). Boumpos et al. (67) found increased expression of many proto-oncogenes (c-*myc*, c-*myb*, and c-*raf*), in T and B lymphocytes of SLE patients, suggesting damage to these cells. For example, increased c-*myc* expression is associated with translocation of c-*myc* from chromosome 8 to chromosomes 14, 2, or 22, next to the genes of immunoglobulin α-heavy chain, κ-, and λ-light chain, respectively (63, 64).

Agranulocytosis

In addition to lupus, several drugs including aminopyrine (68), acetaminophen (69), benzene (70), clozapine (71), carbamazapine (72), vesnarinone (73), and omeprazole (74) are known to induce another idiosyncratic adverse reaction known as agranulocytosis. Agranulocytosis is actually severe granulocytopenia (15) in which blood granulocyte count falls below 500/mm³. Agranulocytosis is also believed to be an autoimmune disease, similar to lupus, in which autoantibodies are produced specifically against neutrophil contents, for example, MPO (15,75,76). However, other mechanisms such as bone-marrow cell damage or neutrophil-cell killing by activated killer T cells are also implicated (16, 75–77). Nevertheless, MPO-mediated metabolism in neutrophils and bone-marrow progenitor cells, which generates reactive free-radical metabolites, has been implicated as a possible mechanism of drug-induced agranulocytosis (78–81).

AGENTS THAT CAUSE HEMATOPOIETIC TOXICITY

Ionizing Radiation

Exposure of humans to ionizing radiation induces bone-marrow depression and leukemias (82,83). Patients undergoing radiation therapy, with doses in the low- to midlethal range, will have depression of bone-marrow function with cessation of blood-cell production leading to pancytopenia (82). Changes in peripheral blood profile usually occur within 24 h postirradiation. Lymphocytes are depressed most rapidly, followed by leukocytes, thrombocytes, and erythrocytes.

Long-term effects of radiation either after a single exposure or multiple low doses results in the induction of leukemias (83). The leukemias most often associated are ALL, AML, CML, and MDS. Other conditions occasionally showing association include myeloma, some high-grade non-Hodgkin's lymphoma, and polycythemia rubra vera.

A single exposure of high-dose gamma irradiation from the atomic bombings in Japan clearly demonstrated an excess of various types of leukemia, but mainly AML and ALL (62). Many studies have shown that radiation induces reactive oxygen species production in hematopoietic cells. A seven- to eightfold increase in SOD activity was found in the bone marrow of rats following 3 d of irradiation of these animals (84). Further, SOD activity in mouse bone marrow increased by 40% 1 h after a lethal dose of radiation (85). Glutathione peroxidase and catalase were also increased. Increases in glucose-6-phosphate dehydrogenase activity in normal (86) and tumor tissues (87) on exposure to ionizing radiation have also been noted, presumably to enhance the endogenous capacity to eliminate the radiation-induced peroxide via the hexose monophosphate shunt pathway. In humans, following exposure to ionizing radiation for 5 h, erythrocyte SOD content decreased about 75–89%, suggesting damage to SOD (88). In another study Petkau (89) reported higher levels of SOD in atomic radiation workers when compared to controls. These data suggest that SOD activity is modulated, presumably due to increased oxygen radical production in humans and animals.

There are two modes of DNA damage by ionizing radiation; one is the so-called ionization and excitation of DNA directly by ionizing radiation (53). This process can lead to breakage of chemical bonds in DNA, and reactive short-lived free radicals are formed. These short-lived free radicals can further damage DNA. The second mode of DNA damage, which is believed to be the major intracellular radiation damage, is due to radiolysis of water leading to the formation of three short-lived reactive species, the hydrated electron (e-aq), the H· atom, and the hydroxyl radical, all of which can damage DNA. The hydroxyl radical appears to be the most physiologically relevant oxidant that induces DNA damage. The chemistry of DNA damage by the hydroxyl radical is very complex and generates multiple products. Early radiation–chemical studies with aqueous DNA solutions showed that the radiation-produced hydroxyl radicals reacted with both the base and sugar components but predominantly with the former in the ratio 3 to 1 (121). The extents of destruction of the pyrimidines were somewhat higher than those of the purines, and in solutions containing oxygen, peroxidation of the pyrimidines occurred. On the other hand, hydroxyl radical attack on sugar moiety was found to lead to strand breakage and also to the release of free bases. Formation of 8-hydroxydeoxyguanosine (8-OHdG) and 5-hydroxymethyluracil (from thymine) moieties has been detected in DNA following its γ-irradiation in aqueous solution (91,92). Severalfold increases in 8-OHdG production were observed in DNA of irradiated cells in vitro or in vivo in mice and humans exposed to ionizing radiation (23,24,93). These studies thus demonstrated that massive oxidative DNA damage by oxygen free radicals can be induced following exposure to ionizing radiation.

Radiation has been shown in vitro to induce cell transformation of many cell types including hematopoietic stem cells (94). Most of the research in vitro, relating free radicals in cell transformation by radiation, however, has been done in nonhematopoietc cell lines. For example, ascorbic acid, a free-radical scavenger, suppresses neoplastic transformation of C3H10T1/2 cells and Balb/c 3T3 cells by radiation (94). Overexpression of mitochondrial SOD has been shown to suppress the radiation-induced neoplastic transformation (94). Furthermore, addition of SOD was found to protect phospholipid membranes and macrophage progenitor cells of mouse bone marrow from radiation damage (94). These results suggest that oxygen radicals play an important role in cellular damage and neoplastic transformation induced by ionizing radiation.

Administration of antioxidant enzymes or antioxidant mimics to animals or humans has been shown to offer protection against radiation induced lethality or damage, suggesting that oxygen radicals play a role in cellular damage in intact animals (95). Intravenous administration of SOD protected mice against radiation-induced lethality (95). Marginal protection was reported when polyethylene glycol-catalase was given to female B6C3F1 mice before irradiation (95). Selenium (Se) administration to mice increased the catalase activity 24 h after the administration and presumably is involved in detoxification of radiation-induced formation of hydrogen peroxide (95).

Hydroxyl radicals have 10- to 60-fold higher reaction rates with many thiols than with DNA, and therefore thiols can afford protection against DNA damage (121).

For example, WR-2721, a phosphorothionate derivative of cysteamine, provides protection against radiation lethality in mice (96). The use of this drug in humans was limited by its side effects such as nausea and vomiting. Administration of Se 6 h prior to WR-2721 administration increased the radioprotection by WR-2721 and reduced its acute toxicity. Selenium GSHPx in bone marrow increased 30–40% 24 h after the administration of Se. It was found that this drug in combination with 2-mercaptopropionylglycine (MPG), another thiol drug, was able to reduce chromosomal aberrations induced by radiation in mouse bone marrow (96). The consequences of oxidative DNA damage by ionizing radiation include, among many others, chromosomal aberrations, oncogene activation and/or tumor suppressor gene deactivation, programmed cell death (apoptosis), and alteration of cytokine production, all of which have been proposed to contribute to hematopoietic toxicity and neoplasia. These effects and their relative contributions in different types of hematopoietic toxicity and neoplasia are dealt with in detail later in this review.

Chemicals

A wide spectrum of chemicals including environmental pollutants (benzene, benzo[a]pyrene) and drugs (phenylhydrazine, chloramphenicol, phenylbutazone, procarbazine, aspirin, indomethacin, tolmetin, fenoprofen, gold salts, chloroquine, clozapine, procainamide, and some alkylating anticancer drugs) are known to produce agranulocytosis, aplastic anemia, and leukemia in humans. Most of these chemicals require metabolism to become hemotoxic and are known to generate free radicals during this metabolism. A wide variety of structurally diverse chemicals are excellent substrates for MPO in circulating neutrophils and bone marrow and are metabolized to free radicals contributing to cellular damage. Here, we briefly review the role of neutrophils, bone-marrow cells, and purified MPO in the catalysis of several environmental pollutants and drugs that cause myelotoxicity.

FREE-RADICAL FORMATION DURING METABOLISM OF DRUGS BY NEUTROPHILS, BONE-MARROW CELLS, AND MYELOPEROXIDASE

The neutrophil-catalyzed metabolism of drugs was first demonstrated by Klebanoff (97), who showed that estradiol is activated to a protein-reactive intermediate following oxidative burst of human leukocytes. We and others have demonstrated that many other chemicals including polynuclear aromatic hydrocarbons, arylamines, diethylstilbestrol, bleomycin A and several lupus-inducing drugs are all metabolized by stimulated human and guinea pig neutrophils to protein and DNA-reactive intermediates (98). This metabolism was mediated by MPO in the neutrophils, which utilized the hydrogen peroxide generated during the oxidative burst.

MPO is a heme-containing enzyme that oxidizes its substrates by one-electron oxidation, resulting in the formation of free radicals (12). The mechanism involves an initial complex formation by hydrogen peroxide with heme iron, followed by loss of water, resulting in iron-oxo formation. Two subsequent one-electron abstractions of substrate result in the formation of corresponding substrate derived free radicals, with the regeneration of the native enzyme. These free radicals have been shown to react with cellular thiols, lipids, or molecular oxygen, thus inducing oxidative stress (12). All these free radicals further react with cellular protein and DNA, resulting in oxidative damage. In some cases, free radicals dismutate to the corresponding electrophilic species, which covalently interact with cellular proteins and DNA.

Benzene

Extensive literature testifies to the role of benzene (BZ) metabolism in exerting its hematopoietic toxicities (99,100). Initial metabolism occurs in the liver by cytochrome P-4502E1 (CYP2E1) to several phenolic metabolites including phenol (PH), hydroquinone (HQ), catechol (CAT), and 1,2,4-benzenetriol (BT), and to a ring-opened product, *trans,trans* -muconaldehyde (*t,t*-MA). Recently, Medinsky and colleagues (101), using genetically engineered mice lacking the gene for CYP2E1, showed marked reduction in benzene metabolism and toxicity, indicating the importance of initial hepatic metabolism of benzene. The phenolic metabolites have been detected in bone marrow following benzene administration, indicating that they travel from liver to bone marrow (102). In bone marrow, the phenolic metabolites are further activated to reactive free radicals and quinones by MPO (12). However, *t,t*-MA is highly reactive and is unlikely to travel to bone marrow from liver. In addition, bone marrow contains little or no CYP2E1 (103), and therefore *t,t*-MA is unlikely to be produced in bone marrow.

We have extensively studied the mechanisms of MPO-catalyzed metabolism of benzene's phenolic metabolites in neutrophils, bone-marrow cells, and by purified human MPO. We have previously reviewed the mechanisms of free-radical formation by benzene metabolites in bone marrow, in detail (12). The peroxidatic metabolism of benzene's phenolic metabolites in bone marrow by MPO results in the formation of phenoxyl radicals from PH and corresponding semiquinone radicals from HQ, CAT, and BT (12). These radicals then undergo reactions with molecular oxygen directly or indirectly in the presence of reducing agents such as glutathione. Reactions with glutathione produce thiyl radicals, which subsequently undergo reaction with molecular oxygen. The phenoxyl radicals may also initiate lipid peroxidation by reacting with cellular membranes. Reactions with oxygen generate oxygen radicals. Phenoxyl radicals dimerize to 2,2'-biphenol and 4,4'-biphenol. 2,2'-Biphenol seems to polymerize rapidly, whereas 4,4'-biphenol is further metabolized peroxidatively to 4,4'-diphenoquinone. The semiquinone radicals derived from HQ and CAT undergo dismutation to the corresponding 1,4- and 1,2-BQ, respectively.

The most likely key molecular targets of quinones and oxygen radicals generated from benzene are DNA, tubulin, topoisomerase-II, DNA and RNA polymerases, histone proteins, and other DNA-associated proteins. Damage to these proteins would potentially cause DNA strand breakage, mitotic recombination, chromosome translocations, and malsegregation of chromosomes at anaphase to produce aneuploidy. If these effects take place in stem or early progenitor cells, a leukemic clone with selective advantage to grow may arise, as a result of proto-oncogene activation, gene fusion, and suppressor gene activation. Therefore, the identification of critical target cell populations and intracellular targets for individual metabolites of benzene is crucial for understanding the molecular mechanisms of benzene toxicity.

Binding with DNA

Due to an association between neoplastic development and the ability of many chemical carcinogens to bind to DNA, considerable research has focused on the interaction of BZ and its metabolites with DNA (104). A number of early studies demonstrated that BZ (or metabolites) was capable of binding to bone marrow DNA following in vivo administration (105–107). Subsequently, several in vitro studies have indicated that 1,4-BQ, HQ, PH, BT, MA, and CAT are all capable of forming adducts with deoxynucleotides and DNA (108–113). Bodell et al. (114) found DNA adducts in bone marrow of B6C3F1 mice dosed with benzene, using ^{32}P-postlabeled technique, corresponding to the adducts formed with HQ and BT. Nevertheless, Reddy and co-workers (115,116), using the same technique, were unable to detect any DNA adducts in the liver, kidney, bone marrow, and mammary gland of rats treated with benzene or PH and HQ, suggesting at most a limited level of covalent binding to DNA by benzene metabolites. However, Subrahmanyam and O'Brien (117) have shown that polymeric PH oxidation products are able to noncovalently, but very strongly, associate with DNA, following peroxidative metabolism of PH. Therefore, the DNA binding observed in early studies following benzene administration could be due to noncovalent association of polymeric PH oxidation products with DNA. Nevertheless, such noncovalent binding of phenolic polymers to DNA may occur at very high doses of benzene, and the exact physiologic relevance of such interactions in bone marrow toxicity of benzene remains to be determined.

Oxidative DNA Damage

The peroxidative metabolism of PH, HQ, and BT can result in the formation of reactive free radicals (12). These free radicals may then interact with molecular oxygen either directly or in the presence of reducing agents such as glutathione (12). These oxygen radicals may also damage DNA, producing oxidative DNA damage. Recently, we demonstrated the formation of 8-OHdG, a marker of oxidative DNA damage, in bone marrow DNA of mice administered benzene, BT, or combinations of phenolic metabolites (52). The 8-OHdG formation in DNA occurred within 1 h following administration and returned to background levels rapidly. These results provided direct evidence for oxygen radical formation by benzene and its phenolic metabolites in vivo. This oxidative DNA damage also occurred in HL-60 cells, which contain MPO, when incubated with phenolic metabolites of benzene (12,52). These results support the hypothesis that free radicals at least in part contribute to cellular damage induced by benzene. Cigarette smoke, which also induces acute myelogenous leukemia in humans, similar to benzene, contains many products including HQ and CAT, and has also been shown to produce free radicals and subsequent oxidative DNA damage in vitro and in vivo in human peripheral lymphocytes (118). The presence of 8-OHdG in DNA has been shown to cause DNA-polymerase to miscode nucleotide incorporation in the replicated strand and to result in mutagenesis (119,120).

Oxygen radicals not only damage DNA but also cellular protein, contributing to oxidative protein damage. However, the contribution to oxidative protein damage by oxygen radicals produced during benzene exposure is not known.

Microtubule Disruption

Benzene exposure to humans and animals has been shown to result in various structural and numerical chromosomal abnormalities and sister chromatid exchanges in lymphocytes and bone-marrow cells (121–125). There are numerous mechanisms by which benzene metabolites can induce aneuploidy in cells. These include damage to microtubules in the mitotic spindle, kinetochore detachment, and centriole damage. More than 15 years ago, Irons and co-workers (126) showed that 1,4-BQ would selectively target tubulin and disrupt microtubules in vitro. Further, they showed that 1,4-BQ was one of the most potent disrupters known and proposed tubulin as a key target in benzene toxicity. Recently, we demonstrated that HQ and BT would disrupt the microtubular structure of intact human cells using fluorescent immunocytochemistry with an anti-tubulin antibody (127). A generic mechanism for aneuploidy production by benzene may therefore be microtubule disruption.

It is difficult to imagine, however, how disruption of microtubules would lead to selective aneuploidy as has been indicated by our recent results (59). Indeed, it may not. Benzene's quinonoid metabolites may produce general aneuploidy of all chromosomes, but some alterations may be lethal or cause premature apoptosis. Only cells with nonlethal chromosome abnormalities would then survive to be detectable. It seems almost certain, however, that chromosome-specific aneuploidy plays a key role in the development and progression of leukemia, and does so for many other cancers (128).

Inhibition of Topoisomerase II

Another attractive hypothesis for explaining benzene's clastogenic effects is by topoisomerase-II inhibition. Recent studies by Chen and Eastmond (129) have shown that PH, 2,2'-biphenol, and 4,4'-biphenol are the most effective inhibitors of topoisomerase II, following peroxidative metabolism of these compounds. At least 50

μM concentrations of PH and 2,2'-biphenol were required for inhibition of topoisomerase II, whereas concentrations as low as 10 μM of 4,4'-biphenol exerted significant inhibitory effects. Both 2,2'-biphenol and 4,4'-biphenol are formed during the peroxidative metabolism of PH and therefore could have contributed to PH-mediated topoisomerase II inhibition. The nature of the reactive species involved in inhibition of topoisomerase II is not clear but may be 4,4'-diphenoquinone, since peroxidative metabolism of 4,4'-biphenol produces stoichiometric quantities of 4,4-dipheniquinone and is known to bind albumin by interacting with its sulfhydryl groups. In support of this, glutathione, a sulfhydryl-containing agent, protected topoisomerase II from inhibition by 4,4'-biphenol metabolites. On the other hand, HQ, 1,4'-BQ, and BT inhibited topoisomeraseII only at higher concentrations, requiring at least 250 μM, indicating that these metabolites are unlikely to play a role in the inhibition of topoisomerase-II in vivo following benzene exposure. In addition, the lack of effect of BT, which is autoxidized rapidly and produces oxygen radicals (130), suggests that oxygen radicals may not play a major role in the inhibition of topoisomerase II. However, the role, if any, of inhibition of topoisomerase II in benzene-induced myelotoxic and leukemogenic effects requires further investigation.

Inhibition of DNA Polymerases

Benzene metabolites have also been shown to inhibit the activities of DNA polymerases α and γ (131–133) and DNA synthesis, in vivo in bone marrow following benzene administration to mice, in cultured bone-marrow cells and in L5178YS cells. The in vitro inhibition of DNA synthesis has been shown to occur with CAT, HQ, BT, and 1,4-BQ. Pellack-Walker et al. (133) have shown that HQ, BT, CAT, and PH are cytotoxic to L51785S cells, inhibit DNA synthesis, and induce DNA strand breaks in these cells. The inhibition of DNA synthesis by these BZ metabolites correlated inversely with their respective one-electron redox potentials: HQ is most potent, followed by BT, CAT, and PH. These authors suggested that oxygen radicals play a major role in the cytotoxicity and DNA strand breaks induced by these BZ metabolites in these cells.

Apoptosis

As indicated earlier, benzene produces aplastic anemia in humans by decreasing the production of all types of blood cells. This may occur by direct action of benzene metabolites on bone-marrow progenitor cells, resulting in cell death due to cellular necrosis or apoptosis. Ross and colleagues (134) have recently shown that bone-marrow progenitor (CD34) cells are prone to undergo apoptotic cell death following exposure to benzene metabolites. Similarly, lymphocytes irradiated with low doses of ionizing radiation are known to undergo apoptotic cell death. Alternatively, apoptotic cell death may also occur due to imbalance of production of cytokines involved in growth and differentiation of bone-marrow cells (135). Nevertheless, many biochemical studies have related apoptotic cell death to the formation of free radicals (136). Therefore, MPO-dependent metabolism of benzene's phenolic metabolites to free radicals may result in apoptotic cell death. In support of this, Hockenbery et al. (137), have shown that the antioxidants N-acetylcysteine and GSHPx protected cells from undergoing apoptotic death, indicating free-radical involvement in cell death. We have shown that oxygen free radicals are produced in bone marrow of benzene-treated mice (52). Therefore, MPO-dependent metabolism of benzene's phenolic metabolites to free radicals may result in apoptotic cell death. This may explain initial bone marrow suppression produced by benzene. However, it is not clear how it is related to the fixing of genetic damage, long-term anemia, or eventual progression to the leukemic state.

Chromosomal Translocations

The most likely consequence of aberrant recombination caused by benzene metabolites is the production of stable chromosome translocations (138,139). The Philadelphia chromosome, which results from a reciprocal translocation between chromosomes 9 and 22, is involved in CML, AML, and ALL. The most common translocation found in acute myelogenous leukemia is a reciprocal translocation between chromosomes 8 and 21, t(8;21) (139,140). This results in fusion of the AML-1 and ETO genes and produces a highly active transcription factor that promotes excessive growth and differentiation paralysis in myeloid progenitor cells (139–141). The t(8;21) translocation and translocations at 11q23 are commonly found in myeloid leukemias resulting from treatment with epidophyllotoxins (60). Since benzene metabolites appear to act in a similar fashion to epidophyllotoxins, inhibiting topoisomerase II and causing DNA strand breaks and structural aberrations, we hypothesized that benzene may also cause the t(8;21) translocation.

We are currently testing this hypothesis using chromosome painting to detect translocations between chromosomes 8 and 21 in the peripheral blood cells of workers exposed to high levels of benzene. Preliminary results suggest that benzene increases the rate of translocations between 8 and 21 in highly exposed workers (142). The t(8;21) has also been observed in conventional cytogenetic analyses of leukemia associated with benzene or other chemical exposures (143,144). The production of t(8;21) translocations is therefore likely to be involved in at least one pathway of benzene-induced leukemogenesis.

The Role of Aneuploidy

Another common genetic abnormality found in leukemias is aneuploidy, the loss and gain of whole chromosomes. Numerical changes in C-group chromosomes 6–12 and X have been detected in the blood and bone marrow of patients with benzene-induced myelogenous leukemia, myelodysplastic syndrome, and pancytopenia. One of these patients showed a clonal expansion of cells with trisomy 9, and a nonclone

was found in another. We have reported that benzene metabolite BT induces aneuploidy of chromosome 9 in HL-60 cells (127). Eastmond and co-workers reported
similar findings following exposure of human lymphocytes to HQ (145). We also
found that benzene induces aneuploidy of chromosome 9 in the lymphocytes of
exposed workers in a dose-dependent manner (146). Benzene and its metabolites
are therefore able to produce chromosome-specific aneuploidy, which most likely
plays a role in leukemogenesis.

Role of Bone-Marrow Stromal Cells in Benzene Metabolism and Toxicity

Many studies have suggested that alterations of stromal cell functions are responsible for hematopoietic dyscrasias observed following benzene exposure. Evidence
for this comes from studies by Garnett et al. (147), who showed that bone-marrow
stromal cells from mice exposed to benzene were unable to sustain hematopoiesis
in vitro. Further in vitro studies by Wierda and colleagues (148) revealed that stromal
cells exposed in vitro to benzene metabolites such as HQ, 1,4-BQ, CAT, and BT
have reduced capacity to support progenitor-cell development and differentiation.
These studies suggested that damage to bone-marrow stroma is a significant factor
in benzene-induced myelotoxicity. Bone-marrow stroma contains many cell types,
of which macrophages play an important role in hematopoiesis (6). Studies from
Wierda's laboratory have shown that macrophages are more sensitive than fibroblastoid stromal cells to the toxic effects of HQ (149). Interestingly, bone-marrow
macrophages contain appreciable peroxidase activity, while fibroblastoid cells do
not (150). Hydrogen peroxide-dependent bioactivation of HQ occurred readily in
bone-marrow macrophages, but not in fibroblastoid stromal cells, indicating macrophages contain an active peroxidase.

The selective toxicity of HQ to bone-marrow macrophages rather than fibroblastoid stromal cells could be a result of both increased peroxidative activation of
HQ to 1,4-BQ in the macrophage and an increased deactivation of 1,4-BQ in the
fibroblast by the obligate two-electron reductase, DT-diaphorase (151). Inhibition
of DT-diaphorase by dicumarol in the stromal fibroblast, but not in the stromal
macrophage, has been shown to lead to increased covalent binding of HQ to protein
(152,153). These data suggest that activation and deactivation mechanisms such as
peroxidase and DT-diaphorase, respectively, in individual cell types are an important
determinant of the cell-specific toxicity of phenolic metabolites of benzene.

Although, several in vitro and ex vivo studies show that stromal cells are damaged
following exposure to benzene and other hematopoietic toxins, it is not known with
certainty how critical this damage is in altering hematopoietic progenitor cell growth
and differentiation. For example, many patients with aplastic anemias and leukemias
transplanted with bone-marrow progenitor cells survive by producing all the elements
of blood, and stromal cell function and growth factor production are normal in almost
all patients with aplastic anemia (154,155,156). This has led these investigators to
argue that stromal-cell damage may not be critical in hematopoietic toxicity. In

addition, some of the cytokines are produced not only by bone-marrow stromal cells, but also by other tissues such as liver, lung, skin, and circulating blood cells (157), which may substitute for cytokine production in cases of stromal-cell damage. Therefore, the actual contribution of stromal cells in bone-marrow progenitor cell growth and differentiation is not clear. If the defect lies in the bone-marrow progenitor cells, it is not known with certainty at what stage of development this defect is produced.

Polynuclear Aromatic Hydrocarbons

Polynuclear aromatic hydrocarbons (PAHs) are also known to induce leukemias in animal models, albeit less frequently than benzene. Benzo[a]pyrene (BaP), a well-studied PAH, induces myelotoxicity and leukemias in mice (158). The myelotoxicity includes marked reduction in myeloid precursors and promegakaryocytes. In addition, BaP induces chromosomal damage in vivo in mouse bone marrow (159), and in vitro in cellular systems (160). The antioxidant, vitamin E, reduced the BaP-induced chromosomal aberrations in vitro in Chinese hamster lung (Don) and Chinese hamster ovary (CHO) cells, suggesting a role for free radicals in chromosomal damage. In addition, BaP administration in mice, following phenobarbital (PB) induction, resulted in increased chemiluminescence in plasma, liver, lungs and kidneys (161). This increased chemiluminescence was suppressed by free-radical scavengers, TIRON, and butylated hydroxytoluene, indicating the formation of free radicals during BaP metabolism (161).

The widely accepted mechanism of BaP carcinogenesis involves a two-electron oxidation by cytochrome P-450, to an epoxide, which undergoes hydration to BaP-7,8-dihydrodiol (BaP-diol) followed by further epoxidation to generate ultimate carcinogenic metabolite, BaP-diol epoxide (162). However, evidence exists that BaP is also metabolized by peroxidases to a cation-radical intermediate, which covalently binds to macromolecules including DNA (163). In addition, BaP is also metabolized by murine bone-marrow homogenates to redox-active quinones and BaP-diol (158–164). Twerdok and Trush (13) have shown that BaP-diol is activated to a covalent binding intermediate by neutrophil oxidants requiring MPO. These results suggest that both BaP and BaP-diol are metabolized locally in bone marrow to reactive free-radical intermediates and presumably result in oxidative cellular damage that may contribute to the chromosomal damage that occurs following administration with BaP.

Drugs Producing Agranulocytosis and Lupus

As indicated earlier, several drugs are known to induce idiosyncratic adverse reactions, such as agranulocytosis and lupus. While lupus is clearly an autoimmune disease, there is no unequivocal evidence to support the autoimmune nature of agranulocytosis. Nevertheless, it appears that all these drugs must be metabolized locally in the immune compartment either by circulating neutrophils or by bone-marrow cells that contain MPO. The peroxidatic reaction of MPO catalyzes the conversion of these drugs to reactive free radicals that result in covalent binding to cellular macromolecules either in neutrophils or of other cells in the surrounding immune compartment. The covalently bound drug may act as hapten and produce antibodies against the cellular components. Rubin (66) has developed a bioassay in which they show that MPO-mediated metabolism in neutrophils of several lupus-inducing drugs results in cytotoxicity to externally added EL4 cells (a mouse lymphoma cell line). We and others have shown that several drugs and carcinogens when activated in neutrophils result in covalent binding to neutrophil proteins. The covalent binding and the cytotoxicity were inhibited by azide and cyanide, showing that MPO is involved in the bioactivation of these chemicals. Rubin (66) has also correlated MPO-mediated metabolism with cytotoxicity of lupus-inducing drugs with corresponding analogs of non-lupus-inducing drugs. For example, procainamide, propylthiouracil, isoniazid, hydralazine, quinidine, and chlorpromazine induce rapid cytotoxicity in EL4 cells when activated by stimulated neutrophils. Little or no cytotoxicity was observed in the absence of stimulated neutrophils. The corresponding non-lupus-inducing analogs, N-acetylprocainamide, propyluracil, isonicotinamide, phthalazine, quinoline, and promazine, are less cytotoxic to EL4 cells, supporting the theory that neutrophil-mediated metabolism is necessary for DIL. Apparently, the functional groups such as $-NH_2$, $-NHNH_2$, $-SH$, $-Cl$, or $-OCH_3$ required for MPO-mediated metabolism are blocked in these non-lupus-inducing analogs.

Although the majority of these chemicals are catalyzed by classical peroxidase compound I and compound II-mediated one-electron abstractions resulting in the formation of free radicals, some of them are metabolized by other pathways requiring chloride ion. For example, neutrophil-catalyzed vesnarinone oxidation is proposed to involve initial oxidation by hypochlorous acid generated from stimulated neutrophils, followed by release of HCl generating iminium ion. Further one-electron oxidation of iminium ion releases a cation radical. Fischer et al. (81) reported that clozapine is metabolized by MPO and horseradish peroxidase in a classical pathway generating a free radical. They identified this free radical by ESR spectroscopy following its reaction with glutathione and ascorbate, which produces thiyl and ascorbate radicals. Similarly, a peroxidatic oxidation of acetaminophen and other arylamines in the presence of thiols or NADPH generates free radicals (165). Oxidation of isoniazid by peroxidases also generates free radicals (166). The phenolic metabolites of benzene (PH, HQ, CAT and BT) all are capable of producing free radicals and covalent binding intermediates during MPO-catalyzed metabolism in neutrophils. Therefore free radicals generated during the metabolism of many of these drugs and carcinogens may contribute to DIL and agranulocytosis.

Anticancer Drugs

Cancer chemotherapy is often complicated by the induction of secondary cancers, particularly of the hematopoietic system. A highly increased risk of t-MDS and t-AML has been demonstrated following therapy with alkylating agents (e.g.., mechloreth-amine, cyclophosphamide, melphalan, chlorambucil, prednimustine, busulfan, dihy-droxybusulfan, carmustine, lomustine, procarbazine, dacarbazine, mitolactol, etc.). The therapy with these compounds primarily results in loss of whole chromosomes 5 and/or 7 or various parts of the long arms of these chromosomes. However, following therapy with epidophyllotoxins (e.g.. etoposide, teniposide, actinomycin D, doxorubi-cin, 4-epi-doxorubicin, mitoxantrone, etc.), *t*-AML arise without preceding *t*-MDS and often show balanced chromosomal aberrations of bands 11q23 and 21q22.

The mechanism of epidophyllotoxins inducing *t*-AML has been attributed to their action on topoisomerase II. The major function of topoisomerases is to modulate the topological state of DNA by breaking and resealing DNA strands (167,168). These enzymes also participate in DNA replication (169), transcription (169), chromosome segregation (170), DNA repair (171–173) and genomic stability (174). The inhibition of topoisomerase II has been linked to chromosomal abnormalities including sister chromatid exchanges (175), deletions (176), micronucleus formation (177), poly-ploidy (178,179), nonhomologous recombination (180), and gene amplification (181).

Many compounds that inhibit topoisomerase II are either quinones or quinone-form-ing compounds (31,167,182,183). In vitro studies show that these agents stabilize a ternary complex where topoisomerase II is covalently linked to DNA (28). This ternary complex represents an intermediate in the topoisomerase II-catalyzed DNA supercoil relaxation reaction. The stabilization induces large DNA rearrangements and dele-tions, possibly due to topoisomerase-subunit exchange at drug-stabilized ternary com-plexes or from attempts by the cell to bypass the replication block caused by stabilized ternary complexes. However, studies in bacterial mutation assays show that topoisom-erase-interactive agents may also induce mutations, through simple DNA intercalation or via generation of oxygen radicals (28). It also has been suggested that the stabilized ternary complexes of topoisomerase inhibitors may likely induce apoptosis, which is characterized by DNA fragmentation (29). It is interesting that many of the topoisomer-ase II inhibitors are also peroxidase substrates. For example, mitoxantrone is metabo-lized by human MPO to reactive intermediates that covalently and noncovalently bind to DNA (30). The major peroxidative metabolite, hexahydronaphtho[2,3-f]quinoxa-line-7,12-dione, was also found in urine of patients treated with mitoxantrone, impli-cating MPO in this metabolism (30). Similarly, etoposide is also known to be metabolized by peroxidases to reactive metabolites that covalently bind to cellular macromolecules (31). These data suggest that peroxidative metabolism is common in the induction of leukemias by chemicals. Further, many leukemogens act by a mecha-nism involving, but not limited to, topoisomerase II inhibition.

ROLE OF CYTOKINES IN HEMATOPOIETIC TOXICITY AND THERAPY

The complex network of cytokines provides important safeguards for normal hemopoiesis (4). Production of specific cell types has to be induced when new cells are required and has to stop when sufficient cells are produced, thus maintaining a constant ratio between hematopoietic precursor cells and mature circulating cells throughout life. It is interesting that many of the genes for cytokines are located on chromosomes that are common sites for chromosomal aberrations. For example, genes for GM-CSF, M-CSF, CSF, IL-3, IL-4, and IL-5 are located on chromosome 5 and genes for G-CSF, erythropoietin, and IL-6 are located on chromosome 7 (4). Interestingly, the chromosomal aberrations that are most commonly involved in myeloid leukemias are chromosomes 5 and 7. Therefore, it is reasonable to argue that the chromosomal aberrations may result in altered production in cytokines that affect differentiation and development of bone-marrow progenitor cells.

Alternatively, it has been postulated that the damaged cell itself may continuously produce the cytokine due to the activation of signal transduction pathways—which is known as autocrine growth (8). It is now known that many oncogenes code for protein kinases involved in signal-transduction pathways, which are located near chromosomal break points and can be activated. The kinases coded by the activated oncogenes phosphorylate their targets in a constitutive manner, namely, continuously and independently of the presence or lack of cytokine, indicating that mechanisms that control proliferation are short-circuited. Hence it is due not to a continuous signal evoked by the cytokine, but to the presence of a broken receptor in the cell membrane that is blocked in its active form. Thus, the phosphorylation of tyrosine kinase due to activated oncogene expression can produce the signal that is necessary for cellular proliferation, which eventually becomes indefinitely out of control.

Some in vitro and in vivo studies have also shown that exogenous addition or injection of cytokines induces leukemic cells to differentiate to mature cells (4). This effect of cytokines has been exploited in the therapy of aplastic anemias and leukemias. However, these differentiated cells still contain the same chromosomal abnormalities that the undifferentiated leukemic cell had (4). The differentiated cells, however, subsequently die via apoptosis (4). Furthermore, differentiation is induced only in early leukemic cells but not in the cells belonging to late-stage leukemia. In addition, treatment of aplastic anemias with G-CSF, a cytokine, resulted in increased rate of incidence of MDS, and acute myeloblastic leukemia in humans (184). In contrast, therapy with G-CSF in combination with erythropoietin had favorable results in patients with moderate aplastic anemia but not in patients with severe aplastic anemia (185). These data suggest that cytokine therapy is not always beneficial in treating hematopoietic disorders. The data also suggest that alteration of cytokine production is secondary to chromosomal damage in the production of aplastic anemias and leukemias.

ROLE OF ONCOGENE ACTIVATION AND TUMOR SUPPRESSOR GENE SUPPRESSION IN HEMATOPOIETIC TOXICITY

A growing number of studies have implicated proto-oncogene activation in the induction of leukemias. Irons and Stillman (186) recently reviewed this literature and concluded that there is no consistent pattern of proto-oncogene and tumor suppressor gene involvement associated with AML development. The reason for this is that activation of *N-RAS*, a proto-oncogene, has been reported to occur in about 25% cases of de novo AML. In addition, *ras* mutations are present only in subclone of the leukemic cells. Similarly inactivation of p53, a tumor suppressor gene, is encountered in the 20–30% cases of CML, but is encountered only in a few cases of MDS/AML. They presented similar arguments for *c-fms* and retinoblastoma genes, which are proto-oncogene and tumor-suppressor genes, respectively. They argued that mutations in many of these genes are important only in the late stages of development of AML.

In contrast, however, *c-myc* activation in some NHLs, particularly in Burkitt's lymphoma, has been associated with early as well as late events of lymphomagenesis (187). The c-*myc* gene is located on the long arm of chromosome 8, which encodes for a nuclear protein with DNA-binding properties. In general, high c-*myc* expression is associated with cell proliferation and low c-*myc* expression with cell differentiation. Therefore, oncogene activation may indeed play an important role in the initial and late stages of leukemogenesis. Nevertheless, it appears that chromosomal aberrations precede the oncogene activation and tumor suppressor gene deactivation, whether they belong to initial or late stages of disease evolution.

Since free radicals play an important role in hematopoietic dyscrasias, it is not surprising that free-radical damage is involved in oncogene activation or deactivation of tumor suppressor genes. For example, reactions of pEC plasmids containing c-*Ha-ras-1* proto-oncogene with Cu^{2+} and hydrogen peroxide, a oxygen-radical-generating system, resulted in G $\rightarrow$ T mutations and A $\rightarrow$ T transversions in the DNA (188,189). This mutated DNA when transfected into NIH/3T3 cells resulted in the formation of 11 transformed foci. These transformed foci when characterized were found to contain G $\rightarrow$ T mutations at the second codon 12 in 2 foci, A $\rightarrow$ T transversions at the second base of codon 61 in 5 foci, and G $\rightarrow$ T mutations at the third position of codon 61 in 4 foci. The mutations at the second and third base of codon 61(CAG) are present in significant proportions in human skin carcinomas (190–193), suggesting that oxygen radicals play an important role in the carcinogenic progression of these tumors. In addition to these mutations, oxygen radicals are also known to induce tandem double CC $\rightarrow$ TT substitutions (194–197) and these mutations are found in p53 gene of skin squamous-cell carcinomas (198). Thus free radicals may contribute to proto-oncogene activation or tumor suppressor gene deactivation at different stages of neoplastic processes of different organs including hematopoietic system. In the hematopoietic system, since many oncogenes code for cytokine receptors and protein kinases, alteration in the production of these factors may contribute to autonomous proliferation of cells and other events that contribute to neoplastic transformation.

CONCLUSIONS

An understanding of the molecular mechanisms of hematopoietic toxicity and carcinogenesis is developing at a rapid pace. Several targets involved in these processes have been identified and characterized. Free radicals seems to play a role in most forms of hematopoietic dyscrasias. Other mechanisms such as topoisomerase II inhibition may also contribute to the induction of leukemias. The differences in the types of leukemias and chromosomal aberrations produced by different classes of chemicals suggest that each class contains a distinct target at both cellular and intracellular levels. With the advent of genetic manipulation and powerful molecular biological techniques combined with recent advances in cytogenetic analysis, the coming years promise to be exciting, as these targets are identified and the molecular pathways of hematopoietic dyscrasias are determined.

ACKNOWLEDGMENTS

This publication was made possible by grant numbers P42 ES04705, ROI ES06721, and P30 ES01896 from the National Institute of Environmental Health Sciences. Its contents are solely the responsibility of the authors and do not necessarily represent the official views of NIEHS. Martyn T. Smith also thanks the National Foundation for Cancer Research for the continued support of his research.

REFERENCES

1. Smith, RP (1991). Toxic responses of the blood, In: *Casarett and Doull's Toxicology: Basic Science of Poisons*, ed. MO Amdur et al., pp. 257–281. New York: McGraw-Hill.
2. Seitz, JF (1970). The bone marrow: In: *Biochemistry of Blood and Bone*. American Lecture Series 759, pp. 213–239
3. Freikhofen, N, Liu, JM, and Young NS (1990). Etiologic mechanisms of hematopoietic failure. *Am. J. Pediatr. Hematol. Oncol.*, 12:385–390.
4. Dexter, TM, Coutinho, LH, Spooncer, E, Heyworth, CM, Daniel, CP, Schiro, R, Chang, J, and Allen, TD (1990). Stromal cells in haemopoiesis. In: *Molecular Control of Haemopoiesis*, Ciba Foundation Symposium 148, eds. G Bock and J Marsh, pp. 76–95. New York: John Wiley & Sons.
5. Zipori, D (1989). Stromal cells from the bone marrow: Evidence for a restrictive role in regulation of hemopoiesis. *Eur. J. Haematol.* 42:225–232.
6. MacEachern, L, and Laskin, DL (1994): Bone marrow phagocytes, inflammatory mediators, and benzene toxicity. In: *Xenobiotics and Inflammation*, eds. LB Schook and DL Laskin, pp. 149–171. New York: Academic Press.
7. Pierce, JH (1989). Oncogenes, growth factors and hematopoietic cell transformation. *Biochim. Biophys. Acta* 989:179–208.
8. Dunn, AR (1987). The role of growth factors in normal and neoplastic haemopoiesis, *Ann. N.Y. Acad. Sci.* 511:1–9.
9. Comoglio, PM, Renzo, DFM, and Gaudino, G (1987). Protein tyrosine kinases associated with human malignancies, *Ann. N.Y. Acad. Sci.* 511:256–261.
10. Sachs, L (1993). The molecular control of hemopoiesis and leukemia. *C.R. Acad. Sci. Paris* 316:882–891.
11. Greenstock, CL (1984). Free-radical processes in radiation and chemical carcinogenesis. *Adv. Radical Biol.* 11:269–293.
12. Subrahmanyam, VV, Ross, D, Eastmond, DA, and Smith, MT (1991). Potential role of free radicals in benzene induced myelotoxicity and leukemia. *Free Radical Biol. Med.* 11:495–515.
13. Twerdok, LE, and Trush, MA (1988). Neutrophil-derived oxidants as mediators of chemical activation in bone marrow. *Chem. Biol. Interact.* 65:261–273.
14. Jiang, X, Khursigara, G, and Rubin, RL (1994). Transformation of lupus-inducing drugs to cytotoxic products by activated neutrophils. *Science* 266:810–813.

15. Mason, RP and Fischer, V (1992). Possible role of free radical formation in drug-induced agranulocytosis. *Drug Safety* 7(suppl. 1):45–50.
16. Harman, D (1988). Free radical theory of aging: Current status. In: *Lipofuscin—1987: State of the Art*, ed. Z Nagy, pp. 3–21. Amsterdam: Elsevier.
17. Volicer, L and Crino, P (1990). Involvement of free radicals in dementia of the Alzheimer type: a hypothesis. *Neurobiol. Aging* 11:567–571.
18. Halliwell, B and Gutteridge, JM (1990). Role of free radicals and catalytic metal ions in human disease: an overview. *Methods Enzymol.* 186:1–85.
19. Goldstein, BD and Witz, G (1990). Free radicals and carcinogenesis. *Free Radical Res. Commun.* 11:3–10.
20. O'Brien, PJ (1982). Peroxide-mediated metabolic activation of carcinogens. In *Lipid Peroxides in Biology and Medicine*, ed. K Yagi, pp. 317–338. New York: Academic Press.
21. Oberley, LW (1988). Free radicals and diabetes. *Free Radical Biol. Med.* 5:113–124.
22. Adams, JD, and Odunze, IN (1991). Oxygen free radicals and Parkinson's disease. *Free Radical Biol. Med.* 10:161–169.
23. Wilson, VL, Taffe, BG, Shields, PG, Povey, AC, and Harris, CC (1991). Detection and quantitation of 8-hydroxydeoxyguanosine adducts in peripheral blood of people exposed to ionizing radiation. In: *Biomonitoring and Susceptibility Markers in Human Cancer: Applications in Molecular Epidemiology and Risk Assessment*. Kailua-Kona, Hawaii. Abstr. P44.
24. Taffe, BG, Sheilds, PG, Kasai, H, Povey, AC, Yeager, H, Trivers, G, Nishimura, S, Harris, CC, and Wilson, VL (1991). Analysis of 8-hydroxydeoxyguanosine DNA adducts in humans following exposure to oxidants: An interlaboratory study. *Proc. Amer. Assoc. Cancer Res.* 32:Abstr. 1339.
25. Tsuruta, Y, Subrahmanyam, VV, Marshall, W and O'Brien, PJ (1985). Peroxidase-mediated irreversible binding of arylamine carcinogens to DNA in intact polymorphonuclear leukocytes activated by a tumor promoter. *Chem. Biol. Interact.* 53:25–35.
26. Eastmond, DA and Smith, MT (1990). Xenobiotic activation by stimulated human polymorphonuclear leukocytes and myeloperoxidase. *Methods Enzymol.* 186:579–585.
27. Kiyosawa, H, Suko, M, Okudaira, H, Murata, K, Miyamoto, T, Chung, M-H, Kasai, H and Nishimura, S. (1990). Cigarette smoking induces formation of 8-hydroxydeoxyguanosine, one of the oxidative DNA damages in human peripheral leukocytes. *Free Radical Res. Commun.* 11:23–27.
28. Anderson, RD and Berger, NA (1994). International commission for protection against environmental mutagens and carcinogens. Mutagenicity and carcinogenicity of topoisomerase-interactive agents. *Mutat. Res.* 309:109–142.
29. Charcosset, JY, Soues, S and Laval, F (1993). Poisons of DNA topoisomerases I and II. *Bull. Cancer* 80:923–954.
30. Panousis, C, Kettle, AJ, and Phillips, DR (1994). Oxidative metabolism of mitoxantrone by the human neutrophil enzyme myeloperoxidase. *Biochem. Pharmacol.* 48:2223–2230.
31. Haim, N, Nemee, J, Roman, J, and Sinha, B (1987). Peroxidase- catalyzed metabolism of etoposide (VP-16-123) and covalent binding of reactive intermediates to cellular macromolecules. *Cancer Res.* 47:5835–5840.
32. De Planque, MM, Kluin Nelemans, HC, van Kricken, HJM, Kluin, PM, Brand, A, Berrestock, GC, Willemze, R, and Van Rood, JJ (1988). Evolution of acquired severe aplastic anaemia to myelodisplasia and subsequent leukaemias in adults. *Br. J. Haematol.* 70:55–62.
33. Petterson, T, Pukkala, E, Teppo, L, and Friman, C (1992). Increased risk of cancer in patients with systemic lupus erythematosus. *Ann. Rheumat. Dis.* 51:437–439.
34. Kokoglu, E, Aktuglu, G, and Belce, A (1989). Leukocyte superoxide dismutase levels in acute and chronic leukemias. *Leuk. Res.* 13:457–458.
35. Liebes, L, Krigel, R Kuo, S Nevrla, D, Pelle, E, and Silber, R (1981). Increased ascorbic acid content in chronic lymphocytic leukemia B lymphocytes. *Proc. Natl. Acad. Sci. USA.* 78:6481–6484.
36. Gordeuk, VR, and Brittenham, GM (1992). Bleomycin-reactive iron in patients with acute non-lymphocytic leukemia. *FEBS Lett.* 308:4–6.
37. Alcain, FJ, Buroin, MI, Rodriguez-Aguilera, JC, Villalba, JM, and Navas, P (1990). Ascorbate free radical stimulates the growth of a human promyelocytic leukemia cell line. *Cancer Res.* 50:5887–5891.
38. Nishihira, J, Ishibashi, T, Takeichi, N, Sakamoto, W, and Nakamura, M (1994). A role for oxygen radicals in in rat monocytic leukemia cell differentiation under stimulation with platelet activating factor. *Biochim. Biophys. Acta.* 1220:286–290.
39. Kobayashi, M, Nishihira, J, Fujii, Y, Maeda, H, Hosokawa, M, and Takeichi, N (1994): Involvement

of oxygen radicals in the differentiation of rat myelomonocytic leukemia cells *in vitro* and in vivo. *Leuk. Res.* 18:199–203.

40. Nagy, K, Pasti-G, Bene-L, and Zs-Nagy, I (1993). Induction of granulocytic maturation in HL-60 human leukemia cells by free radicals: A hypothesis of cell differentiation involving hydroxyl radicals. *Free Radical Res. Commun.* 19:1–15.

41. Young, NS (1995). Aplastic anaemia. *Lancet* 346:228–232.

42. Kaufman, DW, Kelly, JP, Levy, M, and Shapiro, S (1991). *The Drug Etiology of Agranulocytosis and Aplastic Anemia*. New York: Oxford.

43. Catalan-J, Moreno, C, and Aruga, MV (1993). Sister chromatid exchanges induced by chloramphenicol on bovine lymphocytes. *Mutat. Res.* 319:11–18.

44. Sbrana, I, Caretto, S, Rainaldi, G, and Loprieno, N (1991). Induction of chromosomal aberrations and SCE by chloramphenicol. *Mutat. Res.* 248:145–153.

45. Toxicological profile for benzene (1989). In: *Agency for Toxic Substances and Disease Registry,* U.S. Public Health.

46. Aksoy, M (1989). Hematotoxicity and carcinogenicity of benzene. *Environ. Health Perspect.* 82:193–197.

47. Aksoy, M (1988). Benzene carcinogenicity. In: *Benzene Carcinogenicity*, ed. M Aksoy, pp. 113–148. Boca Raton, FL: CRC Press.

48. Tice, RR, Costa, DL, and Drew, RT (1980) Cytogenetic effects of inhaled benzene in murine bone marrow: induction of sister chromatid exchanges, chromosomal aberrations, and cellular proliferation inhibition in DBA/2 mice. *Proc. Natl. Acad. Sci. USA* 77:2148–2152.

49. Chen, W, Rupa, DS, Tomar, R, and Eastmond, DA (1994). Chromosomal loss and breakage in mouse bone marrow and spleen cells exposed to benzene in vivo. *Cancer Res.* 54:3533–3539.

50. Chen, H, and Eastmond, DA (1995). Synergistic increase in chromosomal breakage within the euchromatin induced by an interaction of the benzene metabolites phenol and hydroquinone in mice. *Carcinogenesis* 16:1963–1969.

51. Holmberg, M (1992). Is the primary event in radiation-induced chronic myelogenous leukemia the induction of the t(9;22) translocation? *Leuk. Res.* 16:333–336.

52. Kolachana, P, Subrahmanyam, VV, Meyer, KB, Zhang, L, and Smith, MT (1993). Benzene and its phenolic metabolites produce oxidative DNA damage in HL-60 cells *in vitro* and in the bone marrow *in vivo*. *Cancer Res.* 53:1023–1026.

53. Scholes, G (1983). Radiation effects on DNA. *Br. J. Radiol.* 56:221–231.

54. Sandler, DP, Shore, DL, Anderson, JR, Davey, FR, Arthur, D, Mayer, RJ, Silver, RT, Weiss, RB, Moore, JO, and Schiffer, CA (1993). Cigarette smoking and risk of acute leukemia: associations with morphology and cytogenetic abnormalities in bone marrow. *J. Natl. Cancer Inst.* 85:1994–2003.

55. Peterhans, E, Grob, M Burge, TH, and Zanoni, R (1987). Virus-induced formation of reactive oxygen intermediates in phagocytic cells. *Free Radical Res. Commun.* 3:39–46.

56. Potter, AM and Watmore, A (1992). Cytogenetics in myeloid leukaemia. In: *Human cytogenetics. A practical approach*, Vol. II: *Malignancy and Acquired Abnormalities*, eds. DE Rooney and BH Czepulkowski, 2nd ed., pp. 27–66. New York: Oxford University Press.

57. Bain, BJ (1992). The role of cytogenetics in the assessment of haematological disorders. In: *Human Cytogenetics. A practical approach*, Vol. II: *Malignancy and acquired abnormalities*, eds. DE Rooney and BH Czepulkowski, 2nd ed., pp. 121–153. New York: Oxford University Press.

58. Sandler, DP, Shore, DL, Anderson, JR, Davey, FR, Arthur, D, Mayer, RJ, Silver, RT, Weiss, RB, Moore, JO, and Schiffer, CA, (1993). Cigarette smoking and risk of acute leukemia: Associations with morphology and cytogenetic abnormalities in bone marrow. *J. Natl. Cancer Inst.* 85:1994–2003.

59. Smith, MT, Zhang, L, Rothman, N Wang, Y, Hayes, RB, Li, GL, and Yin, SN, (1995). Interphase cytogenetics of workers exposed to benzene. *Toxicologist* 15: 87, Abstr. 463.

60. Pedersen-Bjergaard, J, and Rowley, JD (1994). The balanced and unbalanced chromosome aberrations of acute myeloid leukemia may develop in different ways and may contribute differently to malignant transformation. *Blood* 83:2780–2786.

61. Thirman, MJ, and Larson, RA (1996). Therapy-related myeloid leukemia. *Hematol./Oncol. Clin. North Am.* 10:293–319.

62. United Nations Scientific Committee on the Effects of Atomic Radiation (UNSCEAR). (1988). *Sources, Effects and Risks of Ionizing Radiation*. New York: United Nations.

63. Gibbons, B, and Czepulkowski, BH (1992). Cytogenetics in acute lymphoblastic leukaemia. In: *Human Cytogenetics. A Practical Approach*, Vol. II: *Malignancy and acquired abnormalities*, eds. DE Rooney and BH Czepulkowski, 2nd ed., pp. 67–95. New York: Oxford University Press.

64. Harrison, CJ (1992). The lymphomas and chronic lymphoproliferative disorders. In: *Human cytogenetics. A Practical Approach*, Vol. II: *Malignancy and Acquired Abnormalities*, eds. DE Rooney and BH Czepulkowski, 2nd ed., pp. 97–120. New York: Oxford University Press.
65. Greaves, M (1993). A natural history of for pediatric acute leukemia. *Blood* 82:1043–1051.
66. Rubin, RL (1992). Autoantibody specificity in drug-induced lupus and neutrophil-mediated metabolism of lupus-inducing drugs. *Clin. Biochem.* 25:223–234.
67. Boumpos, DT, Tsokos, GC, Mann, DL, Eleftheriades, EG, Harris, CC, and Mark, GE (1986). Increased proto-oncogene expression in peripheral blood lymphocytes from patients with systemic lupus erythematosus and other autoimmune diseases. *Arthritis Rheum.* 29:755–760.
68. Barrett, JA, Weller, E, Rozengurt, N, Longhurst, P, and Humble, JG (1976). Aminopyrine agranulocytosis: drug inhibition of granulocyte colonies in the presence of patient's serum. *Br. Med. J.* 2:850–851.
69. Lacotte, J, Perrinc, C, Mosquet, B, Moulin, M, and Bazin, C (1990). Agranulocytosis caused by paracetamol. A case report (letter). *Therapie* 45:438–439.
70. Gill, DP, Jenkins, VK, Kwmpen, RR, and Ellis, S (1980). The importance of pluripotential stem cells in benzene toxicity. *Toxicology* 16:163–171.
71. Pisciotta, AV, Konings, SA, Ciesemier, LL, Cronkite, CE, and Lieberman, JA (1992). On the possible mechanisms and predictability of clozapine-induced agranulocytosis. *Drug Safety* 7:33–44.
72. Pisciotta, V (1978). Drug-induced agranulocytosis. *Drugs* 15:132–143.
73. Uetrecht, JP, Zahid, N, and Whitfield, D (1994). Metabolism of vesnarinone by activated neutrophils: implications for vesnarinone-induced agranulocytosis. *J. Pharmacol. Exp. Ther.*, 270:865–872.
74. Ottenvager, JP, Stricker, BHC, Kappelle, JW, and Claas, FHJ (1995). Omeprazole-associated agranulocytosis. *Eur. J. Haematol.* 54:279–280.
75. Uetrecht, JP (1989). Mechanism of hypersensitivity reactions: proposed involvement of reactive metabolites generated by activated leukocytes. *Trends Pharmacol. Sci.* 10:463–467.
76. Uetrecht, JP (1989). Idiosyncratic drug reactions: possible role of reactive metabolites generated by leukocytes. *Pharm. Res.* 6:265–273.
77. Gerson, SL, and Meltzer, H (1992). Mechanisms of clozapine-induced agranulocytosis. *Drug Safety* 7(Suppl. 1):17–25.
78. Uetrecht, JP (1992). Metabolism of clozapine by neutrophils: Possible implications for clozapine-indured agranulocytosis. *Drug Safety* 7(Suppl. 1):51–56.
79. Furst, SM, and Uetrecht, JP (1993). Carbamazepine metabolism to a reactive intermediate by the myeloperoxidase system of activated neutrophils. *Biochem. Pharmacol.* 45:1267–1275.
80. Uetrecht, JP Zahid, N, and Whitfield, D (1994). Metabolism of vesnarinone by activated neutrophils: Implications for vesnarinone-induced agranulocytosis. *J. Pharmacol. Exp. Ther.* 270:865–872.
81. Fischer, V, Haar, JA, Greiner, L, Lloyd, RV, and Mason, RP (1991). Possible role of free radical formation in clozapine (clozaril)—induced agranulocytosis. *Mol. Pharmacol.* 40:846–853.
82. Walker, RI (1988). Acute radiation injuries. *Pharm. Ther.* 39:9–12.
83. Cartwright, RA (1992). Leukemia epidemiology and radiation risks. *Blood Rev.* 6:10–14.
84. Krizala, J, Stoklasova, A, Kovarova, W, and Ledvina, M (1982). The effect of gamma-irradiation and cystamine on superoxide dismutase activity in the bone marrow and erythrocytes of rats. *Radiat. Res.* 91:507–515.
85. Kumar, KS, Vaishnav, YN, and Weiss, JF (1988). Radiation protection by antioxidant enzymes and enzyme mimetics. *Pharm. Ther.* 39:301–309.
86. Savitskii, IV, Musiko, VA, and Erigova, SG (1985). Changes in fructose diphosphate aldolase and glucose-6-phosphate dehydrogenase activity after irradiation of animals with an absolutely lethal dose of gamma rays. *Radiobiologiia* 25:245–249.
87. Szeinfeld, D, and Bleekenhorst, G (1987). Effect of X-irradiation on adenosine triphosphate and glucose-6-phosphate dehydrogenase in the CaNT mouse tumor. *Radiat. Res.* 110:305–309.
88. Schweitzer, K, Benko, Gy and Bohos, P (1985). Investigation into the superoxide dismutase (SOD) activity of human erythrocytes at work places exposed to radiation hazard. *Radiobiol. Radiother.* 26:629–632.
89. Petkau, A (1987). Role of superoxide dismutase in modification of radiation injury. *Br. J. Cancer* 5 (Suppl. VIII):87–95.
90. Fahey, RC (1988). Protection of DNA by thiols. *Pharm. Ther.* 39:101–108.
91. Dizdaroglu, M (1985). Formation of an 8-hydroxyguanine moiety in deoxyribonucleic acid on gamma-irradiation in aqueous solution. *Biochemistry* 24:4476–4481.

92. Tofigh, S, and Frenkel, K (1989). Effect of metals on nucleoside hydroperoxide, a product of ionizing radiation in DNA. *Free Radical Biol. Med.* 7:131–143.

93. Kasai, H, Crain, PF, Kuchino, Y Nishimura, S Ootsuyama, A, and Tanooka, H (1986): Formation of 8-hydroxyguanine moiety in cellular DNA by agents producing oxygen radicals and evidence for its repair. *Carcinogenesis* 7:1849–1851.

94. Borek, C (1985). Oncogenes and cellular controls in radiogenic transformation of rodent and human cells. *Carcinogenesis* 10:303–316.

95. Biaglow, JE, Varnes, ME, Epp. ER, and Clark, EP (1988). Antioxidant and redox enzymes in radioprotection. *Pharm. Ther.* 39:275–286.

96. Devi, PU and Thomas, B (1988). Bone marrow cell protection And modification of drug toxicity by combination of protectors. *Pharm. Ther.* 39:213–214.

97. Klebanoff, SJ (1979). Effect of estrogens on the myeloperoxidase-mediated antimicrobial system. *Infect. Immun.* 25:153–156.

98. Eastmond, DA, French, RC, Ross, D and Smith, MT (1987). Metabolic activation of diethylstilbestrol by stimulated human leukocytes. *Cancer Lett.* 35:79–86.

99. Cooper, KR and Snyder, R (1988): Benzene metabolism (toxicokinetics and molecular aspects of benzene toxicity). In: *Benzene Carcinogenicity*, ed. M Aksoy, pp. 33–58. Boca Raton, FL: CRC Press.

100. Rothman, N, Li, G-L, Dosemeci, M, Bechtold, WE, Marti, GE, Wang, Y-Z, Linet, M, Xi, L-Q, Lu, W, Smith, MT, Titenko-Holland, N, Zhang, L-P, Blot, W, Yin, S-N, and Hayes, RB (1996). Hematotoxicity among Chinese workers heavily exposed to benzene. *Am. J. Ind. Med.* 29:236–246.

101. Valentine, JL, Seaton, MJ, Asgharian, B, Lee, S S-T, Gonjalez, FJ, and Medinsky, MJ (1996). Benzene metabolism and toxicity in transgenic CYP2E1 knockout mice. *Toxicologist* 30(1):Abstr. 377.

102. Rickert, DE, Baker, TS, Bus, JS, Barrow, CS, and Irons, RD (1979). Benzene disposition in the rat after exposure by inhalation. *Toxicol. Appl. Pharmacol.* 49:417–423.

103. Ross, D, Siegel, D, Schattenberg, DG, and Moran, JL (1996). Cell specific metabolism in benzene toxicity. A metabolic basis for benzene-induced toxicity at the level of the progenitor cell in human bone marrow. *Toxicologist* 30(1):Abstr. 1740.

104. Lutz, WK (1979). In vivo covalent binding of organic chemicals to DNA as a quantitative indicator in the process of chemical carcinogenesis. *Mutat. Res.* 65:289–356.

105. Lutz, WK, and Schlatter, CH (1977): Mechanism of the carcinogenic action of benzene: Irreversible binding to rat liver DNA. *Chem. Biol. Interact.* 18:241–245.

106. Gill, DP, and Ahmed, AE (1981). Covalent binding of [^{14}C] benzene to cellular nucleic acids. *Biochem. Pharmacol.*, 30:1127–1131.

107. Arfellini, G, Grill, S, Colacci, A, Mazzullo, M, and Prodi, G (1985) In vivo and vitro binding of benzene to nucleic acids and proteins of various rat and mouse organs. *Cancer Lett.* 28: 159–168.

108. Rushmore, T, Snyder, R, and Kalf, G (1984). Covalent binding of benzene and its metabolites to DNA in rabbit bone marrow mitochondria *in vitro*. *Chem. Biol. Interact.* 49:133–154.

109. Snyder, R, Jowa, L, Witz, G, Kalf, G, and Rushmore, T (1987). Formation of reactive metabolites from benzene. *Arch. Toxicol.* 60:61–64.

110. Latriano, L, Witz, G, Goldstein, BD, and Jeffrey, AM (1989). Chromatographic and spectrophotometric characterization of adducts formed during the reaction of trans, trans-muconaldehyde with ^{14}C-deoxyguanosine 5'-phosphate. *Environ. Health Perspect.* 82:249–252.

111. Jowa, L, Winkle, S, Kalf, G, Witz, G, and Snyder, R (1986). Deoxyguanosine adducts formed from benzoquinone and hydroquinone. In: *Biological Reactive Intermediates*, Vol. III, pp. 825–832. New York: Plenum Press.

112. Pongraca, K; Kaur, S, Burlingame, AL, and Bodell, WJ (1990). Detection of (3'-hydroxy)-3N^4-benzetheno-2'-deoxycytidine-3'-phosphate by ^{32}P-postlabelling of DNA reacted with p-benzoquinone. *Carcinogenesis* 11:1469–1472.

113. Bauer, H, and Snyder, R (1989). Studies on the formation of adducts formed during the oxidation of the benzene metabolites, 1,2- or 1,4-benzenediiol and purine or pyrimidine-3'-monophosphates. *Proc. Am. Assoc. Cancer Res.* 30:Abstr. 11.

114. Pathak, DN, Levay, G and Bodell, WJ (1995). DNA adduct formation in the bone marrow of B6C3F1 mice treated with benzene. *Carcinogenesis* 16:1803–1808.

115. Reddy, MV, Bleicher, WT, Blackburn, GR, and Mackerer, CR (1990). DNA adduction by phenol, hydroquinone or benzoquinone *in vitro* but not *in vivo*: nuclease P$_1$-enhanced ^{32}P-postlabelling of adducts as labelled nucleoside bisphosphates, dinucleotides and nucleoside monophosphates. *Carcinogenesis* 11:1349–1357.

116. Reddy, MV, Blackburn, GR, Schreiner, CA, Mehlman, MA, and Mackerer, CR (1989). ^{32}P-analysis of DNA adducts in tissues of benzene-treated rats. *Environ. Hlth. Perspect.* 82:253–257.
117. Subrahmanyam, VV, and O'Brien, PJ (1985). Phenol oxidation product(s) formed by a peroxidase reaction, that bind to DNA. *Xenobiotica* 15:873–885.
118. Ong, CN, Lee, BL, Shi, CY, Ong, HY and Lee, HP (1994). Elevated levels of benzene-related compounds in the urine of cigarette smokers. *Int. J. Cancer.* 59:177–180.
119. Kuchino, Y, Mori, F, Kasai, H, Inoue, H, Iwai, S, Miura, K, Ohtsuka, E, and Nishimura, S (1987). Misreading of DNA templates containing 8-hydroxydeoxyguanosine at the modified base and at adjacent residues. *Nature* 237:77–79.
120. Floyd, RA (1990). The role of 8-hydroxyguanine in carcinogenesis. *Carcinogenesis* 11:1447–1450.
121. Dean, BJ (1985). Recent findings on the genetic toxicology of benzene, toluene, xylenes and phenols. *Mutat. Res.* 154:153–181.
122. Forni, A, Cappellini, A, Facifico, E, and Vigliani, EC (1971). Chromosomal changes and their evolution in subjects with past exposure to benzene. *Arch. Environ. Health* 23:385–391.
123. Morimoto, K, and Wolff, S (1980). Increase of sister chromatid exchanges and perturbations of cell division kinetics in human lymphocytes by benzene metabolites. *Cancer Res.* 40:1189–1193.
124. Yardley-Jones, A, Anderson, D, Lovell, DP, and Jenkinson, PC (1990). Analysis of chromosomal aberrations in workers exposed to low levels of benzene. *Brit. J. Ind. Med.* 47:48–51.
125. Tice, R, Costa, D, and Drew, R (1980): Cytogenetic effects of inhaled benzene on murine bone marrow: Induction of sister chromatid exchanges, chromosomal aberrations and cellular proliferation inhibition in DBA/2 mice. *Proc. Natl. Acad. Sci. USA* 77:2148–2155.
126. Irons, RD, and Neptune, DA (1980). Effects of the principal hydroxy- metabolites of bensene on microtubule polymerization. *Arch. Toxicol.* 45:297–305.
127. Zhang, L, Venkatesh, P, Creek, MLR, and Smith, MT (1994). Detection of 1,2,4-benzenetriol induced aneuploidy and microtubule disruption by fluorescence *in situ* hybridization and immunocytochemistry. *Mutat. Res.* 320:315–327.
128. Fearon, ER, and Vogelstein, B (1990). A genetic model for colorectal tumorigenesis. *Cell* 61: 759–767.
129. Chen, H, and Eastmond, DA (1995). Topoisomerase inhibition by phenolic metabolites: A potential mechanism for benzene's clastogenic effects. *Carcinogenesis* 16:2301–2307.
130. Zhang, L, Smith, MT, Bandy, B, Tamaki, SJ, and Davison, AJ (1994). Role of quinones, active oxygen species and metals in the genotoxicity of 1,2,4-benzenetriol, a metabolite of benzene. In: *Free Radicals in the Environment, Medicine and Toxicology*, Vol. 8, eds. H Nohl, H Esterbauer, and C Rice-Evans, pp. 521–562. London: Richelieu.
131. Lee, EW, Johnson, JT, and Garner, CD (1989). Inhibitory effect of benzene metabolites on nuclear DNA synthesis in bone marrow cells. *J. Toxicol. Environ. Health.* 26:277–291.
132. Kalf, GF (1987). Recent advances in the metabolism and toxicity of benzene. *CRC Crit. Rev. Toxicol.* 18:141–159.
133. Pellack-Walker, P, Walker, JK, Evans, HH, and Blumer, JL (1985). Relationship between the oxidation potential of benzene metabolites and their inhibitory effect on DNA synthesis in L5178YS cells. *Mol. Pharmacol.* 28:560–566.
134. Moran, JL, Siegel, D, Sun, X-M, and Ross, D (1996). Induction of apoptosis by benzene metabolites in HL60 and CD34+ human bone marrow progenitor cells. *Mol. Pharmacol.* 50:610–615.
135. Allen, PD, Bustin, SA, and Newland, AC (1993). The role of apoptosis (programmed cell death) in haemopoiesis and the immune system. *Blood Rev.* 7:63–73.
136. Wood, KA and Youle, RJ (1994). Apoptosis and free radicals. *Ann. N.Y. Acad. Sci.* 738:400–407.
137. Hockenbery, DM, Oltval, ZN, Yin, X-M, Milliman, CL, and Korsmeyer, SJ (1993). Bcl-2 functions in an antioxidant pathway to prevent apoptosis. *Cell* 75:241–251.
138. Rabbits, TH (1995). Chromosomal translocations in human cancer. *Nature* 372:143–149.
139. Nucifera, G, and Rowley, JD (1995). AML1 and the 8;21 and 3;21 translocations in acute and chronic myeloid leukemia. *Blood* 86:1–14.
140. Downing, JR, Head, DR, Curcio-Brint, AM, Hulshof, MG, Motroni, TA, Raimondi, SC, Carroll, AJ, Drabkin, HA, William, C, Theil, KS, et al. (1993). An AML1/ETO fusion transcript is consistently detected by RNA-based polymerase chain reaction in acute myelogenous leukemia containing the (8;21)(q22;q22) translocation. *Blood* 81:2860–2865.
141. Erickson, PF, Robinson, M, Owens, G, and Drabkin, HA (1994). The ETO portion of acute myeloid leukemia t(8;21) fusion transcript encodes a highly evolutionarily conserved, putative transcription factor. *Cancer Res.* 54:1782–1786.

142. Smith, MT, Rothman, N, Zhang, L, Wang, Y, Hayes, R, and Yin, S-N (1996). Molecular cytogenetics of humans exposed to benzene. *Toxicologist* 30(1):Abstr. 911.
143. Mitelman, F, Nilsson, PG, Brandt, L, Alimena, G, Gastaldi, R, and Dallapiccola, B (1981). Chromosome pattern, occupation, and clinical features in patients with acute nonlymphocytic leukemia. *Cancer Genet. Cytogenet.* 4:197–214.
144. Li, Y-S, Zhao, Y-L, Jiang, Q-P, and Yang, C-L (1989). Specific chromosome changes and non occupational exposure to potentially carcinogenic agents in acute leukemia in China. *Leuk. Res.* 13:367–376.
145. Eastmond, DA, Rupa, DS, and Hasegawa, LS (1994). Detection of hyperdiploidy and chromosome breakage in interphase human lymphocytes following exposure to the benzene metabolite hydroquinone using multicolor fluorescence *in situ* hybridization with DNA probes. *Mutat. Res.* 322:9–20.
146. Zhang, LP, Rothman, N, Wang, Y, Hayes, RB, Bechtold, W, Venkatesh, P, Yin, S-N, Wang, Y-Z, Dosemeci, M, Li, G-L, Lu, W, Smith, MT (1996). Interphase cytogenetics of workers exposed to benzene. *Environ. Health Perspect.* 104(Suppl. 6):1325–1329.
147. Garnett, HM, Cronkite, EP, and Drew, RT (1983). Effect of *in vivo* exposure to benzene on the characteristics of bone marrow adherent cells. *Leuk. Res.* 7:803–810.
148. Gaido, K, and Wierda, D (1984). In vitro effects of benzene metabolites on mouse bone marrow stromal cells. *Toxicol. Appl. Pharmacol.* 76:45–55.
149. Thomas, DJ, Reasor, MJ, and Wierda, D (1989). Macrophage regulation of myelopoiesis is altered by exposure to the benzene metabolite hydroquinone. *Toxicol. Appl. Pharmacol.* 97:440–443.
150. Thomas, DJ, Sadler, A, Subrahmanyam, VV, Siegel, D, Reasor, MJ, Wierda, D, and Ross, D (1990). Bone marrow stromal cell bioactivation and detoxification of the benzene metabolite hydroquinone: Comparison of macrophages and fibroblastoid cells. *Mol. Pharmacol.* 37:255–262.
151. Smart, RC, and Zannoni, V (1984). DT-diaphorase and peroxiase influence the covalent binding of metabolites of phenol, the major metabolite of benzene. *Mol. Pharmacol.* 26:105–111.
152. Rothman, N, Traver, RD, Smith, MT, Hayes, RB, Li, G-L, Campleman, S, Dosemeci, M, Zhang, L, Linet, M, Wacholder, S, Yin, S-N, and Ross, D (1996). Lack of NAD(P)H:quinone oxidoreductase activity (NQO1) is associated with increased risk of benzene hematotoxicity. *Proc. Amer. Assoc. Cancer Res.* 37:258(Abstr. 1761).
153. Traver, RD, Rothman, N, Smith, MT, Yin, SY, Hayes, RB, Li, GL, Franklin, WF, and Ross, D (1996). Incidence of a polymorphism in NAD(P)H:quinone oxidoreductase (NQO1). *Proc. Am. Assoc. Res.* 37: 278(Abstr. 1894).
154. Young, NS, and Barrett, AJ (1995). The treatment of severe acquired aplastic anemia. *Blood.* 85:3367–3377.
155. Marsh, JCW, Chang, J, Testa, NG, Hows, JM, and Dexter, TM (1991). In vitro assessment of marrow "stem cell" and stromal cell function in aplastic anemia. *Br. J. Hematol.* 78:258–267.
156. Holmberg, LA, Seidel, K, Leisenring, W, and Torok-Storb, B (1994). Aplastic anemia: Analysis of stromal cell function in long-term marrow cultures. *Blood* 84:3685–3690.
157. Brandes, ME, and Wahl, SM (1994). Inflammatory cytokines. In: *Xenobiotics and Inflammation*, eds. LB Shook and DB Laskin, pp. 33–70. New York: Academic Press.
158. Nebert, DW, and Jensen, NM (1979). Benzo(a)pyrene-initiated leukemia in mice, association with allelic differences at the Ah locus. *Biochem. Pharmacol.* 27:149–151.
159. Kleisch, U, Roupova, I and Adler, ID (1982). Induction of chromosome damage in mouse bone marrow by benzo(a)pyrene. *Mutat. Res.* 102:265–273.
160. Smalls, E, and Patterson, RM (1982): Reduction of benzo(a)pyrene induced chromosomal aberrations by DL-alpha-tocopherol. *Eur. J. Cell Biol.* 28:92–97.
161. Yoshida, LS, Miyazawa, T, Fujimoto, K, and Kaneda, T (1989). Spontaneous and luminol-dependent chemiluminescences from tissue preparations of benzo(a)pyrene-injected mice. *J. Nutr. Sci. and Vitaminol.* 35:569–578.
162. Conney, AH (1982). Induction of microsomal enzymes by foreign chemicals and carcinogenesis by polycyclic aromatic hydrocarbons. *Cancer Res.* 42:4875–4917.
163. Cavalieri, EL, Devanesan, PD, and Rogan, EG (1988). Radical cations in the horseradish peroxidase and prostaglandin H synthase mediated metabolism and binding of benzo(a)pyrene to deoxyribonucleic acid. *Biochem. Pharmacol.* 37:2183–2187.
164. Nebert, DW, Levitt, RC, Orlando, MM, and Felton, JS (1977). Effects of environmental chemicals on the genetic regulation of microsomal enzyme systems. *Clin. Pharmacol. Ther.* 22:640–658.
165. Subrahmanyam, VV, and O'Brien, PJ (1985). Peroxidase-catalyzed oxygen activation by arylamine carcinogens and phenol. *Chem. Biol. Interact.* 56:185–196.

166. Hofstra, AH Li-Muller, SMA, and Uetrecht, JP (1992). Metabolism of isoniazid by activated leukocytes: Possible role in drug-induced lupus. *Drug Metab. Dispos.* 20:205–210.
167. D'Arpa, P, and Liu, LF (1989). Topoisomerase-targeting antitumor drugs. *Biochem. Biophys. Acta.* 989:163–177.
168. Pommier, Y, and Bertrand, R (1993). The mechanisms of formation of chromosomal aberrations: role of eukaryotic DNA topoisomerases. In *The Causes and Consequences of Chromosomal Aberrations*, ed. IR Kirsch, pp. 277–309. Boca Raton: FL: CRC Press.
169. Anderson, HJ, and Roberge, M (1992). DNA topoisomerase II: A review of its involvement in chromosome structure, DNA replication, transcription and mitosis. *Cell Biol. Int. Rep.* 16:717–724.
170. Downes, CS, Mullinger, AM, and Johnson, RT (1991). Inhibitors of DNA topoisomerase II prevent chromatid separation in mammalian cells but do not prevent exit from mitosis. *Proc. Natl. Acad. Sci. USA* 88:8895–8899.
171. Downes, CS, and Johnson, RT (1988). DNA topoisomerase and DNA repair. *Bioessays* 8:179–184.
172. Stevnsner, T, and Bohr, VA (1993). Studies on the role of topoisomerases in general, gene- and strand-specific DNA repair. *Carcinogenesis* 14:1841–1850.
173. Theilmann, HW, Popanda, O, Gersbach, H, and Gilberg, F (1993). Various inhibitors of topoisomerases diminish repair-specific DNA incision in UV-irradiated human fibroblasts. *Carcinogenesis* 14:2341–2351.
174. Wang, JC, Caron, PR, and Kim, RA (1990). The role of DNA topoisomerases in recombination and genomic stability: A double-edged sword? *Cell* 63:403–406.
175. Mukherjee, A, Sen, S, and Agarwal, K (1993). Ciprofloxacin: Mammalian DNA topoisomerase II poison *in vivo. Mutat. Res.* 301:87–92.
176. Shibuya, ML, Ueno, AM, Vannais, DB, Craven, PA, and Waldren, CA (1994). Megabase pair deletions in mutant mammalian cells following exposure to amsacrine, an inhibitor of DNA topoisomerase II. *Cancer Res.* 54:1092–1097.
177. Holmstrom, L, and Winters, V (1992). Micronucleus induction by camptothecin and amsacrine in bone marrow of male and female CD-1 mice. *Mutagenesis* 7:189–193.
178. Zucker, RM, Adams, DJ, Bair, KW, and Elstein, KH (1991). Polyploidy induction as a consequence of topoisomerase inhibition. A flow cytometric assessment. *Biochem. Pharmacol.* 42:2199–2208.
179. Zucker, RM, and Elstein, KH (1991): A new action of topoisomerase inhibitors. *Chem. Biol. Interact.* 79:31–40.
180. Bae, YS, Kawasaki, I, Ikeda, H, and Liu, LF (1988). Illegitimate recombination mediated by calf thymus DNA topoisomerase II *in vitro. Proc. Natl. Acad. Sci. USA* 85:2076–2080.
181. Ikeda, H (1990). DNA topoisomerase mediated illegitimate recombination. In: *DNA Topology and Its Biological Effects*, eds. NR Cozzarelli and JC Wang, pp. 341–370. Cold Spring Harbor, NY: Cold Spring Harbor Laboratory Press.
182. Li, CJ, Averboukh, L, and Pardee, AB (1993). B-Lacaphone, a novel topoisomerase I inhibitor with a mode of action different from camptothecin. *J. Biol. Chem.* 268:22463–22468.
183. Stoyanovski, D, Yalowich, J, Gantchev, T, and Kagan, V (1993). Tyrosine-induced phenoxyl radicals of etoposide (VP-16): Interaction with reductants in model systems, K 562 leukemic cell and nuclear homogenates. *Free Radical Res. Commun.* 19:371–386.
184. Imashuku, S, Hibi, S, Kataoka-Morimoto, Y, Yoshihara, T, and Ikushima, S (1995). Myelodysplasia and acute myeloid leukemia in cases of aplastic anemia and congenital neutropenia following G-CSF administration. *Br. J. Haematol.* 89:188–190.
185. Imamura, M, Kobayashi, M, Kobayashi, S, Yoshida, K, Mikuni, C, Ishikawa, Y, Matsumoto, S, Sakamaki, S, Niitsu, Y, Hinoda, Y, Yachi, A, Kudoh, T, Chiba, S, Kasai, M, Oka, T, Okuno, A, Maekawa, I, Sakurada, K, and Miyazaki, T (1995). Combination therapy with recombinant human granulocyte colony-stimulating factor and erythropoietin in aplastic anemia. *Am. J. Hematol.* 48:29–33.
186. Irons, RD, and Stillman, WS (1996). The process of leukemogenesis. *Environ. Health Perspect.* 104(Suppl. 6):1239–1246.
187. Van Krieken, JHJM, and Kluin, PM (1992). The association of *c-myc* rearrangements with specific types of human non-Hodgkin's lymphomas. *Leukemia Lymphoma* 7:371–376.
188. Kamiya, H, Miura, H, Suzuki, M, Murata, N, Ishikawa, H, Shimizu, M, Komatsu, Y, Murata, T, Sasaki, T, Inoue H, et al. (1992). Mutations induced by DNA lesions in hot spots of the c-Ha-ras gene. *Nucleic Acids Symp Ser.* 27:179–180.
189. Du, M-Q, Carmichael, PL, and Phillips, DH (1994). Induction of activating mutations in the human c-Ha-ras-1 proto-oncogene by oxygen free radicals. *Mol. Carcinogen.* 11:170–175.

190. Scotto, J, and Fears, TR (1978). Skin cancer epidemiology: Research need. *Natl. Cancer Inst. Monogr.* 50:169–177.
191. White, SI, and Balmain, A (1988). G to T mutation in codon 12 of the human Harvey ras oncogene derived from a basal cell carcinoma. *J. Invest. Dermatol.* 91:407.
192. van der Schoeff G, Even LM, Boot, AJM, and Bos, JL (1990). Ras oncogene mutations in basal cell carcinomas and squaous cell carcinomas of human skin. *J. Invest. Dermatol.* 94:423–425.
193. Ananthaswamy, HN, and Pierceall, WE (1992). Molecular alterations in human skin tumors. *Progress Clin. Biol. Res.* 376:61–84.
194. McBride, TJ, Preston, BD, and Loeb, LA (1991) Mutagenic spectrum resulting from DNA damage by oxygen radicals. *Biochemistry* 30:207–213.
195. Tkeshelashvili, LK, McBride, T, Spence, K and Loeb, LA (1992). Mutation spectrum of copper-induced DNA damage. *J. Biol. Chem.* 267:13778.
196. Reid, TM, and Loeb, LA (1992). Mutagenic specificity of oxygen radicals produced by leukemic cells. *Cancer Res.* 52:1082–1086.
197. Reid, TM and Loeb, LA (1993). Tandem double CC → TT mutations are produced by reactive oxygen species. *Proc. Natl. Acad. Sci. USA* 88:10124–10128.
198. Brash, DE, Rudolph, JA, Simon, JA, Lin, A, McKenna, GJ, Baden, HP, Halperin, AJ, and Ponten, J (1991). A role for sunlight in skin cancer: UV-induced p53 mutations in squamous cell carcinoma. *Proc. Natl. Acad. Sci. USA.* 88:10124–10128.

Free Radical Toxicology
Edited by K. B. Wallace
Copyright © 1997 Taylor & Francis

14

Selected Examples of Free-Radical-Mediated Lung Injury

Hanspeter Witschi

Institute of Toxicology and Environmental Health and Department of Molecular Biosciences, School of Veterinary Medicine, University of California, Davis, Davis, California, USA

INTRODUCTION

Free radicals play an important role in the pathogenesis of some forms of acute and chronic lung injury. Our environment puts daily an oxidative burden upon the tissues of the respiratory tract where free radicals may be generated by the action of air pollutants such as ozone or NO_2, tobacco smoke, or even by lung defense cells themselves. When formed, reactive and unstable free radicals, with subsequent chain reactions leading to uncontrolled destructive oxidation, then become initiating or propagating mechanisms in lung disease. The pivotal roles of superoxide, nitric oxide, peroxynitrate, and hydroxyl radicals, and perhaps of singlet oxygen, in mediating tissue damage are well recognized (1). The potential role of free radicals in lung damage is further illustrated by responses such as the increased activity of free radical-scavenging enzymes in lungs of animals exposed to oxygen, O_3, NO_2, or other toxicants (2).

Within cells, the partial reduction of O_2 to reactive species occurs normally as a by-product of cellular metabolism during cytosolic, microsomal, and mitochondrial electron transfer reactions. When cellular injury of any type occurs, the release of otherwise contained cellular constituents, such as iron, into the extracellular space may lead to extracellular generation of deleterious reactive O_2 species. Among pulmonary defense cells, neutrophils, monocytes, and macrophages seem particularly adept at converting molecular O_2 to reactive O_2 metabolites, probably related to both their phagocytosis and antimicrobial activities. As a by-product of this capability, toxic O_2 species are released. Oxidative damage may represent a significant component of all types of pneumotoxic lung injury accompanied by a phagocyte-mediated inflammatory component.

One of the most dramatic examples of lung injury caused by reactive oxygen metabolites is the condition commonly known as adult respiratory distress syndrome (ARDS). It is frequently precipitated by sepsis, trauma, shock, aspiration of gastric contents, or inhalation of toxic agents and is a condition characterized by diffuse alveolar damage and pulmonary edema; the disease still carries about 50–90% mortality (3). Reactive oxygen species generated from neutrophils accumulating in the damaged lung appear to play a key role in producing tissue lesions (4). In lungs challenged with less dramatic and less acute insults, such as in people exposed chronically to oxidant air pollutants, inflammation is often a characteristic event (5). While the degree of inflammatory changes and therefore the eventual tissue lesions may vary with the nature and dose of the pollutant, the species examined, and the predominant localization of the injury, it is conceivable that many of the subsequent events are triggered by reactive oxygen species. In general, free radicals represent an important component in the pathogenesis of lung disease. In the following, a few examples of lung diseases involving free radicals are provided.

PULMONARY OXYGEN TOXICITY

Oxygen is necessary for life. The cells that line the conducting airways and the alveolar surface are continuously in contact with oxygen and do not seem to suffer. However, should the partial pressure of oxygen rise above normal, this otherwise vital gas becomes toxic. By now a large body of experimental evidence has firmly established that pulmonary oxygen toxicity is mediated through partially reduced oxygen products, such as the superoxide anion, perhydroxy and hydroxyl radicals, and possibly singlet molecular oxygen (6–10).

Hypoxemia is often seen in humans when some form of respiratory dysfunction prevents the diffusion of adequate amounts of oxygen from air to blood. An increase in the partial oxygen pressure in the inspired air may help to ameliorate the problem, although often at the risk of pulmonary oxygen toxicity. This toxicity is characterized by extensive initial damage to the capillary endothelial cells, followed by damage to the alveolar type II cell population. There follows proliferation of type II cells and eventual repair, partially or fully, of the damaged epithelium (11,12).

All cells of the lung appear to be susceptible to oxygen toxicity, although sensitivity between the different cell types may vary. Often it is difficult to differentiate oxygen toxicity per se from the changes produced by the disease process that required oxygen therapy in the first place. There is good evidence to suggest that administration of oxygen can aggravate preexisting lung injury (13). This may lead to a vicious circle in which increasing lung injury with inflammatory and edematous changes may call for increased administration of oxygen. Potentiation of acute lung injury by oxygen has been demonstrated in several animal models, and the consequences may be long-lasting and essentially irreversible fibrotic changes (14,15). In neonate children, mostly premature infants that require supplemental oxygen therapy after birth, a syndrome known as bronchopulmonary dysplasia often develops (16). Lung pathology of this disorder is characterized by a necrotizing bronchiolitis, fibroblast proliferation, squamous metaplasia of bronchial lining cells, and destruction of alveolar ducts. Long-term sequelae of pulmonary oxygen toxicity may be mild to moderate pulmonary fibrosis. In baboons exposed for up to 14 to 60% hyperoxia, a chronic proliferation of the type II cell population was found. When animals were allowed to recover in air following exposure to oxygen, progressive changes in the interstitium involving both cellular and extracellular elements were observed (17).

The morphologic changes produced by continuous exposure to hyperoxia have been studied extensively in the respiratory tract of experimental animals. In rodents exposed to an atmosphere containing 95–100% oxygen, diffuse and eventually fatal pulmonary damage develops usually within 3–4 d. In rat lungs, the earliest signs of oxygen toxicity are significant injury of the capillary endothelial cells. The number of endothelial cells and the capillary surface area decrease. It remains unclear why capillary endothelial cells and not the cells in immediate contact with oxygen, that is, the alveolar epithelial cells, are the first ones to become damaged. Capillary lesions are followed by leakage of proteinaceous fluid and of formed blood elements into the alveolar space. Hyaline membranes, formed by cellular debris and protein-aceous exudate, are a characteristic morphologic sign of pulmonary oxygen toxicity. Formation of hyaline membranes greatly diminishes oxygen diffusion. Changes in the epithelial cell population appear to be more limited, and at death the epithelial cell population shows comparatively little structural injury (18). A somewhat different picture is seen in baboon lungs, where endothelial cell swelling and aggregation of neutrophils are the earliest signs of oxygen toxicity, but the number of endothelial cells does not appear to be diminished. With progressing time (between 66 and 80 h of exposure to hyperoxia) there is a marked increase in cellularity within the alveolar interstitium. Epithelial cells display enhanced permeability to solutes. Eventually, there is widespread damage to the type I alveolar epithelial cells and large areas of the alveolar septum become denuded of cellular lining (19). It thus appears that in rats the major targets for oxygen are capillary endothelial cells, whereas in primates, including humans, epithelial damage is a prominent feature.

When animals exposed to hyperoxia are removed into air before they die and are allowed to recover, the alveolar lesions are eventually repaired. The pattern of recovery was first analyzed in detail in mice (20,21). Beginning 2–3 d after hyperoxia, the overall number of dividing cells in the alveolar parenchyma increases dramatically. Identification of the labeled cells showed that an initial burst of proliferative activity occurred in the alveolar type II epithelial cell population, followed some 24 h later by a proliferative burst of the capillary endothelial cells. Such a pattern might not be common to all species. To examine this possibility, four species—rats, mice, hamsters, and marmosets—were exposed to 100% oxygen for 48 h. The animals were then removed into air and allowed to recover. Analysis of the pattern of cell replication showed significant differences between rats on one side and mice, hamsters, and marmosets on the other hand (22,23). In rats, the predominant population regenerating after oxygen injury was the capillary endothelial cells. This agrees with the observation that endothelial cell damage is a prominent feature in rat pulmonary oxygen toxicity (18). As judged by the overall extent of the lesions, rats were also more sensitive to oxygen than were the other species. In mice, hamsters, and marmosets, the largest number of cells that divided during the recovery period were type II epithelial cells (22,23). These observations suggested that repair to injury might be species specific. Other evidence suggests that oxygen toxicity may be not only species specific, but even strain specific (24).

Species differences also appear to exist in the development of oxygen tolerance. It was first observed by Crapo and Tierney (25) that rats become tolerant to 100% oxygen following pretreatment with 85% oxygen. On the other hand, mice and hamsters do not develop oxygen tolerance if preexposed to low levels of oxygen. A second agent capable to provide oxygen tolerance in rats is bacterial endotoxin (26). Induction of antioxidant defense mechanisms, most notably the superoxide dismutases, is thought to play a substantial role in the development of tolerance. This was most dramatically illustrated in transgenic mice that express human manganese superoxide dismutase (Mn-SOD) in their pulmonary epithelial cells. Such animals survived almost twice as long in an atmosphere of 95% oxygen than did normal control animals (27). However, overexpression or induction of SOD does not seem to be the only mechanism in the development of tolerance. For example, interleukin 1 appears to be involved in protecting rats (28). Tolerance can also be produced following extensive diffuse lung injury. Initially, mice with extensive alveolar damage are more sensitive to hyperoxia than are controls. About 1 wk after the lung injury, when epithelial repair has mostly been accomplished, the animals become resistant to 100% [survival time 9.6 d, similar to the survival time seen in transgenic mice expressing SOD (27) vs. 4.5 d in controls]. After 3 wk, the animals have lost tolerance again (29). No evidence for increased activity in antioxidant enzymes was found in the lungs of the resistant mice. Tolerance to oxygen independent of antioxidant activity has also been described in rabbits, where the effect was thought to be dependent upon increased surfactant synthesis (30). Inducers of cytochrome P-450 enzymes also can convey oxygen tolerance (31,32).

PULMONARY OZONE TOXICITY

Ozone air pollution is a major problem in many parts of the world. An extensive database exists on both potential adverse effects of ozone in humans and on studies with experimental animals (33). Ozone in the troposphere is the product of a photochemical reaction between oxides of nitrogen or of hydrocarbons and sunlight; contributors to ozone air pollution are mostly exhaust gases from internal combustion engines, but also hydrocarbons emanating from trees and plants.

The predominant lesions produced by ozone are inflammatory changes in the airways. In humans such changes have been observed already a few hours after a 2-h exposure to 0.4 ppm ozone (34). The acute and chronic toxicity of ozone has been extensively studied in experimental animals, including in primates. The pulmonary lesions produced by ozone are not as uniformly distributed throughout the lung as are lung lesions in oxygen toxicity. Rather, at least at lower concentrations of ozone (below 0.8 ppm), the lesions are mostly confined to a well-defined anatomical region, the centriacinar region of the lung (35). Ozone-induced lesions are usually seen at the bronchiolo-alveolar duct junction and involve damage to the terminal bronchioli and to the tip of the alveolar septum. The few histopathological findings available on potential ozone effects on human lung suggest that the centriacinar region is also the target in humans (36).

In experimental animals, it has been found that the extent of alveolar epithelial cell injury at the bronchiolo-alveolar junction provides an excellent internal dosimeter for cumulative ozone exposure (37). The importance of this region as a prime target for ozone-induced lung injury is underlined by observations made in long-term studies. Chronic exposure to ozone concentrations, as may be encountered on occasion in heavily polluted urban areas, produces permanent damage to the bronchiolar epithelium and interstitial fibrosis in rats (38). Quantitative studies on ozone toxicity in several animal models have suggested that different species display different sensitivities towards ozone. Particularly, monkeys appear to be considerably more sensitive to ozone than are rats (39). This is an important observation because if monkeys are indeed more sensitive to ozone than are rats, caution must be exercised when extrapolating quantitative observations from rats to humans.

Ozone, while not a free radical, is a highly reactive molecule. As such, it apparently penetrates only for a very short distance across the air/tissue boundary layer in the lung; it is unlikely that ozone per se can penetrate a lipid bilayer thicker than 0.1 μm (40). Ozone can react with every type of hydrocarbon, particularly rapidly with hydrocarbons containing double carbon–carbon bonds. With unsaturated compounds such as polyunsaturated fatty acids, ozone reacts in a process called Crieege ozonation. There is only a limited number of reactive groups in biological molecules whose rate constants are high enough ($>10^5$ M^{-1} s^{-1}) to be candidates as primary reactants with ozone. These include carbon-to-carbon double bonds in unsaturated fatty acids, as reactive amino acid side chains such as the SH groups in cysteine; in the phenolic hydroxyl group in tyrosine and the ring nitrogen atoms in histidine and tryptophan; as well as in naturally occurring reducing agents such as ascorbic acid, vitamin E, and uric acid. The possibility also needs to be considered that multiple reaction mechanisms yield secondary products. Lipid hydroperoxides may be formed in lipid layers, and in aqueous solutions ozone can react with carbon-to-carbon double bonds to give Crieege ozonides, which ultimately give rise to various reactive aldehydes as secondary toxicants. Formation of these molecules may lead to activation of phospholipases and triggering of the arachidonic acids cascade with ensuing tissue damage, including damage to cellular DNA (41).

The initial interaction of ozone with molecules present in the pulmonary fluid lining layer is followed by a cascade of events in the lung such as release of ozonolysis products, which then may become involved in acute toxicity (42). Cell damage may manifest itself in alterations in glucose, lipid, and protein metabolism. Antioxidants present in the lung lining layer or within cells such as antioxidant defense enzymes, glutathione, vitamin E, or uric acid may protect against ozone toxicity. In experimental studies with vitamin E-depleted rats that are more sensitive to ozone, it has been possible to provide protection by restoring vitamin E levels in the feed. However, overfeeding with vitamin E does not convey protection above that seen in normal animals. To what extent supplementation of the diet with vitamin E might protect humans against ozone toxicity remains, for the time being, unclear (43).

Prolonged exposure to ozone produces morphological and biochemical changes within the tissues of the respiratory tract that eventually convey some protection against further ozone injury. In short-term experiments, adaptation to ozone can be seen usually within a few days; the cells lining the airways and alveoli following initial ozone injury appear to be less vulnerable to the pollutant. In rats exposed for 20 mo to the comparatively high concentration of 1 ppm of ozone for 6 h/d, 5 d/wk, extensive remodeling of the centriacinar region of the lung was observed. The remodeling process apparently allowed the animals to survive continuous exposure without any progression and deterioration of the lesions (44).

Of some interest is the observation that the effects of ozone can be greatly enhanced by concomitant exposure to NO_2 (45,46). It is likely that ozone and NO_2 react to form a more toxic species, most likely N_2O_5. However, there may exist a large number of minor reactions of NO_2 and nitrate radical; furthermore, it is unclear to what extent these reactions, which are favored to occur in the dark, might also occur in strong sunlight. Nevertheless, the observations show that exposure to air pollutants is not only exposure to single compounds, but that the biological response may be driven by interactions between different pollutants, many of them possibly free radicals. Prolonged exposure to a combination of ozone and NO_2 produces pulmonary changes similar to the ones seen in human idiopathic pulmonary fibrosis (47).

CIGARETTE SMOKE

Inhaled tobacco smoke, a complex chemical mixture containing more than 5000 compounds, imposes a considerable oxidative burden onto the lung. Active smoking is the single most serious risk factor for the development of cancer in the lung and in other sites such as mouth, larynx, esophagus, stomach, pancreas, kidney, and urinary bladder. Chronic obstructive lung disease and cardiovascular disease are also considered to be closely associated with inhalation of tobacco smoke. It has been estimated that the death toll from active smoking in the United States, entirely preventable, may run as high as 400,000 deaths annually (48). More recently, concern has focused on the adverse health effects that may possibly be induced by involuntary exposure to tobacco smoke, by "passive smoking." The available data have been reviewed in several official documents. Practically all conclusions are based on an analysis of available human epidemiological data. Exposure to environmental tobacco smoke has been causally linked to an increased risk of developing lung cancer, cardiovascular disease, respiratory disease in children, reduced birthweight, sudden infant death syndrome (SIDS), and increased childhood cancers. Environmental tobacco smoke has been classified by the U.S. Environmental Protection

Agency (EPA) as a known human carcinogen (49). Deaths from passive smoking have been estimated in the United States to be as high as 53,000 annually (50). Of particular concern appears to be the observation that nonsmokers may be at risk because they are not "adapted" to some of the active ingredients present in cigarette smoke (51). This analysis of the epidemiological evidence and the numerical projections of disease and death have not gone unchallenged (52,53).

So far, animal experimentation has not shown that cigarette sidestream smoke (SS) produces an increased incidence of lung tumors in experimental animals (54). There is some evidence that SS enhances the development of sclerotic lesions in the arteries of cockerels (55) and of rabbits (56), and intensifies the development of myocardial infarct size (57). SS also adversely affects the growing fetus. Exposure of rats to SS reduces birthweights (58) and adversely affects lung development (59). A combined in utero–postnatal exposure of rats to SS increases airway reactivity and reduces pulmonary compliance. Proliferation of pulmonary neuroendocrine cells may be a possible underlying mechanism for these anomalies in pulmonary function (60). On the other hand, several studies have suggested that inhalation of SS at considerably higher concentrations than can be found in the day-to-day environment actually produces no or only transient changes in the lungs of experimental animals (61,62).

It is conceivable that many of the acute effects of tobacco smoke are free-radical mediated, although the complexity of smoke makes it impossible to attribute any specific event to a given smoke constituent. Tobacco smoke is usually fractionated into two phases: the gas phase and the tar phase, that is, the material that can be collected by drawing smoke through a glass-filter type Cambridge filter. At the high temperatures at which tobacco is burned, free gas-phase radicals are formed at the tip of the burning cigarette. They appear to have a very short half-life, but as cigarette smokes ages the concentration of free radicals increases, reaching a maximum after 1–2 min. The free radical nitric oxide, present in very high concentrations in fresh cigarette smoke, is slowly oxidized to the more reactive NO_2 radical. The tar phase of cigarette smoke is a rich source of comparatively more stable free radicals, mostly associated with a mixture of quinone, semiquinone radical, and hydroquinone moieties. Certain tar components are able to associate with DNA and to produce the highly damaging hydroxyl radical (63).

While active smoking undoubtedly places a high oxidative burden onto the lung, it is much less certain to what extent second-hand smoke has the same effect. Sidestream smoke differs from mainstream smoke in two important aspects: It is generated at much lower burning temperatures than mainstream smoke, and it rapidly ages. Presumably because of differences in burning temperature, the concentrations of several carcinogens, among them polycyclic aromatic hydrocarbons, cadmium, nickel, polonium-210, and NNK (4-[methylnitrosamino-1-(3-pyridyl)-1-butanone], a potent animal lung carcinogen) are higher in sidestream smoke than in mainstream smoke (49). As it ages, the smoke mixture rapidly undergoes multiple physical and chemical changes. In the general environment, sidestream smoke usually is considerably diluted, and it has been maintained that "passive smokers" are exposed to only fractions of what active smokers daily inhale (64). On the other hand, the concentration of sidestream smoke in air decreases with the square of the distance from the source. This would expose children of smoking mothers to higher concentrations of smoke than are usually measured in homes and would explain why this particular population is mostly at risk from environmental tobacco smoke (49). In adults, an association has been found between passive smoke exposure at the workplace and chronic respiratory symptoms such as wheezing and cough; the severity of the signs was dependent upon hours per day of smoke exposure (65).

PARAQUAT

Paraquat has found widespread use as an efficient herbicide. In chemistry, the bipyridylium compound has been used for a long time as a redox indicator under the name of methyl viologen. As a widely used herbicide, it is safe if handled properly. However, if it enters the body, most often by voluntary or involuntary oral ingestion, it is highly toxic. During the last few decades, the compound has gotten some notoriety because it caused several accidental and quite a few suicidal deaths. If ingested in toxic amounts, acute paraquat toxicity in humans is a multiorgan toxicity with acute kidney and liver damage, adrenal and cerebral hemorrhages, and acute diffuse lung lesions. The cause of death is often difficult to establish at this stage. If patients survive the first few days of acute paraquat poisoning, they eventually develop diffuse and, more importantly, irreversible and therapy-resistant pulmonary fibrosis. Death is due to respiratory failure. Studies in experimental animals have shown that the initial lung injury is widespread necrosis of both the type I and type II alveolar epithelium. This is followed by an extensive proliferation of fibroblasts, both within the alveolar interstitium and within collapsed alveoli (66).

Diquat is a related compound that also can undergo redox cycling. It has a lower redox potential than paraquat. When ingested, diquat causes predominantly diffuse kidney lesions. Although paraquat and diquat probably share similar mechanisms of toxicity, the differences in target organs between diquat and paraquat are a consequence of their different toxicokinetics. The main reason for the characteristic pulmonary toxicity of paraquat seems to be active uptake by and accumulation of the herbicide in the lung. Both lung slices in vitro (67) and the lungs of animals exposed to paraquat in vivo accumulate the compound (68). A series of investigations has shown that certain endogenous compounds such as the polyamines putrescine, spermine, and spermidine effectively compete with paraquat for pulmonary uptake. The apparent K_m for paraquat is approximately 10 times higher than it is for putrescine. Type I and type II alveolar epithelial cells and bronchiolar Clara cells are rich in this uptake system, and this may explain why these cells are predominantly damaged by the herbicide. Curiously, capillary endothelial cells, through which paraquat must pass from the blood before entering the epithelial cells, do not seem to become damaged, nor do these cells apparently take up the compound actively (69).

The deleterious cellular lesions produced by paraquat are a result of continuous redox cycling of the compound. In the absence of oxygen, paraquat undergoes a single electron reduction and forms a stable blue radical. In the presence of oxygen, paraquat will accept an electron from NADPH and is rapidly reoxidized with the concomitant formation of superoxide anion. This may lead to the formation of additional free radicals, to cellular lipid peroxidation, and to NADPH depletion in the affected cells. Evidence that lipid peroxidation is a critical event in paraquat toxicity has mostly been obtained from studying in vitro systems (70,71). The experimental evidence to show that lipid peroxidation is a major factor in the pathogenesis of lung lesions in vivo is more indirect and less complete. A reduction in the NADPH:NADP ratio has been demonstrated directly in vivo in the lungs treated with paraquat (72). There was also some loss of total NADPH observed. Diquat, although used in doses not known to be associated with acute lung injury, caused a similar drop in the ratio of NADPH:NADP. However, this was not accompanied by depletion of NADPH, suggesting NADPH depletion is a potentially crucial event. Additional evidence for such a mechanism was obtained in other in vivo studies where paraquat was found to produce intracellular NADPH depletion coupled with a stimulation of the pentose shunt pathway and a concomitant decrease of fatty acid synthesis. All these events occur very early after exposure of rats to paraquat and may thus be instrumental in producing lung lesions (73).

Evidence for a critical role of redox cycling in paraquat toxicity is suggested by the observation that pulmonary toxicity is greatly enhanced in rats treated with paraquat and exposed to hyperoxia (74). Following intravenous injection of a comparatively high dose of paraquat, 80 mg/kg, animals kept in 100% oxygen die from acute pulmonary edema and diffuse pulmonary hemorrhage within 4 h. Hyperoxia also can produce lung toxicity in animals injected with diquat, although the compound does not accumulate in the lung. Given 80 mg/kg of diquat intravenously and placed into 100% oxygen, rats will die even more quickly, within 2 h, than do animals treated with 80 mg/kg of paraquat (75). The lower redox potential of diquat probably accounts for this phenomenon.

BLEOMYCIN

Bleomycin, actually a mixture of several structurally similar compounds, is a widely used cancer chemotherapeutic agent. While it produces little damage to the bone marrow, the drug can precipitate, as its most serious side effect, interstitial pulmonary fibrosis. Mortality as high as 1–2% has been reported. The sequence of lung injury includes necrosis of capillary endothelial cells, type I and type II alveolar cells, edema formation, and hemorrhage. One to 2 wk following the acute injury, a delayed proliferation of type II epithelial cells may restore some of the damaged alveolar septum. However, there often is extensive accumulation of fibrous tissue in the lung interstitium, with the result being diffuse interstitial pulmonary fibrosis (76).

In many tissues, the cytosolic enzyme bleomycin hydrolase inactivates bleomycin. In lung and skin, two target organs for bleomycin toxicity, the activity of this enzyme is low compared to other organs (77). Bleomycin stimulates, in the lung, the production of collagen. Prior to increased collagen biosynthesis, steady-state levels of mRNA coding for fibronectin and procollagens are increased, presumably subsequent to a bleomycin-mediated release of cytokines such as transforming growth factor beta and tumor necrosis factor (78).

The damaging action of bleomycin is due to a simultaneous binding of the drug with Fe(II) and with DNA. "Activated bleomycin," an oxygen-ligated ferric–bleomycin complex, is thought to be the DNA attacking species. In the presence of molecular oxygen, this may lead to the release of hydroxyl radicals, and single and double DNA strand breaks are produced via a free-radical reaction (76,78). The role of oxygen in bleomycin toxicity is most dramatically illustrated by the fact that exposure to hyperoxia greatly potentiates bleomycin pulmonary toxicity (15).

Since the development of pulmonary injury caused by bleomycin depends heavily on both iron and the presence of oxygen, it might be anticipated that antioxidants and iron-chelating agents would be effective preventive treatments. Unfortunately, there has been very little success with the use of antioxidants, reducing agents such as *N*-acetylcysteine, radioprotective agents, or iron chelators (76). What seems to be a most efficient treatment in order to prevent collagen accumulation in bleomycin-exposed hamster lung is administration of a diet containing niacin and taurine (79). Supplementation of the diet with these two agents not only reduces overall collagen accumulation, but prevents the increase in collagen cross-links (80). It is thought that protection is afforded by the capability of niacin to maintain intracellular levels of NAD and ATP and by taurine to scavenge HOCl or by stabilizing membranes and preventing the influx of Ca^{2+} (81,82); in combination, the two agents may practically abolish all biochemical and morphological signs of bleomycin-induced pulmonary fibrosis (82). On the other hand, there is some experimental evidence that bleomycin-induced pulmonary fibrosis also can be mitigated by cyclosporin A. This suggests that T lymphocytes may play a role in the development of the fibrotic lesion (83).

PERSPECTIVES

There is no doubt that free-radical toxicity plays a role in lung injury. To some extent, recognition of the role of free radicals has revolutionized our understanding of the molecular basis of the biology of lung disease. A closer inspection of the provided examples, however, shows that we are far from being able to explain, in terms of free-radical biology, most aspects of the disease processes that were discussed.

Pulmonary oxygen toxicity and paraquat lung injury are probably the most obvious examples where we can directly link lung injury with the generation of free radicals, followed by deleterious secondary events. The most convincing evidence for a radical-mediated mechanism is the observation that diquat, which also cycles from a reduced to an oxidized form, produces as much if not more lung injury in the presence of a sufficiently high oxygen partial pressure as does paraquat (75). At normal oxygen pressure, the selective pulmonary toxicity of paraquat is readily explained by its preferential uptake into the lung. What remains largely unknown, however, is the precise physiological role of the polyamine uptake system that allows paraquat to get into the lung in the first place. The study of paraquat toxicity has given us a comparatively satisfactory explanation for the role a free radical can play in causing death from pulmonary damage, but it has also opened some as yet unanswered questions about a normal physiological process.

As is the case with paraquat, bleomycin toxicity can also satisfactorily explained by a free-radical mechanism. Bleomycin pulmonary toxicity, mediated by Fe and oxygen radicals, is greatly enhanced in the presence of hyperoxia (15). Understanding bleomycin's mechanism of toxicity in terms of free-radical toxicology immediately suggests that there might be rational treatments—administration of iron chelators, antioxidant agents, and free radical scavengers. Unfortunately, none of these rational approaches has been able to ameliorate bleomycin toxicity (76). What appears to be an efficient curative treatment is protocols that focus on the second stage of pulmonary bleomycin toxicity, proliferation of fibroblast and deposition of abnormal amounts of collagen. There is a rational biochemical basis for this strategy with several plausible mechanistic explanations, most of them not necessarily explained by the toxicity of free radicals alone (82). What is obvious from this example is that to focus exclusively on formation of free radicals and subsequent initiation of lesions should not be the only strategy to be pursued if eventually we want to prevent and perhaps even cure free-radical-precipitated lung disease.

The two oxidant inhalants, oxygen and ozone, raise a different issue: Can pulmonary resistance to the deleterious effects of either agent, initiated by free radicals, be explained solely in terms of antioxidant defense mechanisms? In ozone toxicity, cells appear to become resistant within a few days (84). Biochemical studies with whole-lung homogenates suggested early on that antioxidant defense mechanisms play an important role in the development of ozone adaptation (85). The exact cellular events that produce adaptation within a few days and then are able to maintain the altered state for up to many months remain mostly unresolved. The question must be asked, how can the lung mount effective countermeasures against the continuing onslaught of free-radical-mediated toxicity and eventually reach a status quo without any apparent progression of lesions with time? In the development of oxygen tolerance, there are even some more puzzling questions, such as sensitivity of different species—what makes rats unique in that they appear to be the only species that can be made resistant to hyperoxia by preexposure to lower amounts of oxygen, whereas a similar treatment in other species has no such effect. It is also interesting to note that two entirely different experimental approaches produce essentially the same result: Transgenic mice overexpressing human SOD live exactly as long in 100% oxygen (27) as do mice 1 wk following acute lung injury and repair (29). The question also remains open of why "tolerant" mouse lungs lose their adaptation after 3 wk, the time it takes for newborn, oxygen-resistant mice to become oxygen sensitive (86).

Cigarette smoke, with its abundance of free radicals, has the undoubted potential to cause acute lung injury. Active smokers receive, with each inhalation, large amounts of free radicals delivered to the epithelia lining airways and alveoli. A plausible mechanism has been suggested: Leukocytes or cigarette smoke releases active oxygen species, and active oxygen species diffuse into to the cell nucleus and together with Fe produce hydroxyl radicals. Hydroxyl radicals then cause DNA strand breaks, leading to oncogene activation and tumor suppressor gene inactivation, the end result eventually being cancer (87). Such a sequence of events is well supported by numerous studies, mostly involving in vitro systems. But these apparent mechanisms must be reconciled with the fact that most tobacco-smoke-associated lung cancers take years to develop, that lung cancers originating at multiple sites are extremely rare in humans (although inhaled smoke certainly becomes distributed throughout the lung), and that the majority of smokers do not develop lung cancer (they may die from tobacco-smoke-related diseases before cancer can be expressed). In this case, free-radical-mediated toxicity, although possibly crucial in initiating events, might represent only a comparatively trivial part in the development of a long disease process. This should be kept in mind when developing strategies for prevention and therapeutic intervention.

REFERENCES

1. Halliwell B, and Cross CE. Oxygen-derived species: their relation to human disease and environmental stress. *Environ Health Perspect* 1994;102(Suppl 10):5–12.
2. Heffner JE, and Repine JE. Pulmonary strategies of antioxidant defense. *Am Rev Respir Dis* 1989;140:531–554.
3. Macnaughton PD, and Evans TW. Management of adult respiratory distress syndrome. *Lancet* 1992;339:469–472.
4. Repine JE. Scientific perspectives on adult respiratory distress syndrome. *Lancet* 1992;339:466–469.
5. Crapo J, Miller FJ, Mossman B, Pryor WA, and Kiley JP. NHLBI workshop summary. Environmental lung diseases. Relationship between acute inflammatory responses to air pollutants and chronic lung disease. *Am Rev Respir Dis* 1992;145:1506–1512.
6. Fisher AB. Pulmonary oxygen toxicity. In: *Pulmonary Diseases and Disorders*, ed. AP Fishman. New York: McGraw-Hill, 1988, pp. 2331–2338.
7. Fracica PJ, Piantadosi CA, and Crapo JD. Oxygen toxicity. In: *The Lung, Scientific Foundations*, eds. RG Crystal and JB West. New York: Raven Press, 1991, pp. 2155–2161.
8. Jamieson D. Oxygen toxicity and reactive oxygen metabolites in mammals. *Free Radical Biol Med* 1989;7:87–108.
9. Doelman CJ, and Bast A. Oxygen radicals in lung pathology. *Free Radical Biol Med* 1990;9:381–400.
10. Tsan MF. Superoxide dismutase and pulmonary oxygen toxicity [published erratum appears in *Proc Soc Exp Biol Med* 1993;203(4):512]. *Proc Soc Exp Biol Med* 1993;203:286–290.
11. Bachofen A, and Weibel ER. Alterations of the gas exchange apparatus in adult respiratory insufficiency associated with septicemia. *Am Rev Respir Dis* 1977;116:589–615.
12. Gould VE, Tosco R, Wheelis RF, Gould NS, and Kapanci Y. Oxygen pneumonitis in man. Ultrastructural observations on the development of alveolar lesions. *Lab Invest* 1972;26:499–508.
13. Pratt PC, Vollmer RT, Shelburne JD, and Crapo JD. Pulmonary morphology in a multihospital collaborative extracorporeal membrane oxygenation project. I. Light microscopy. *Am J Pathol* 1979;95:191–214.
14. Witschi HP, Haschek WM, Klein-Szanto AJP, and Hakkinen PJ. Potentiation of diffuse lung damage by oxygen; Determining variables. *Am Rev Respir Dis* 1981;123:98–103.
15. Tryka AF, Skornik WA, Godleski JJ, and Brain JD. Potentiation of bleomycin-induced lung injury by exposure to 70% oxygen. Morphologic assessment. *Am Rev Respir Dis* 1982;126:1074–1079.

16. Frank L. Developmental aspects of experimental pulmonary oxygen toxicity. *Free Radical Biol Med* 1991;11:463–494.
17. Crapo JD, Hayatdavoudi G, Knapp MJ, Fracica PJ, Wolfe WG, and Piantadosi CA. Progressive alveolar septal injury in primates exposed to 60% oxygen for 14 days. *Am J Physiol* 1994; 267:L797–L806.
18. Crapo JD, Barry BE, Foscue HA, and Shelburne J. Structural and biochemical changes in rat lungs occurring during exposures to lethal and adaptive doses of oxygen. *Am Rev Respir Dis* 1980; 122:123–143.
19. Fracica PJ, Knapp MJ, and Crapo JD, Patterns of progression and markers of lung injury in rodents and subhuman primates exposed to hyperoxia. *Exp Lung Res* 1988;14(Suppl):869–885.
20. Adamson IY, and Bowden DH. The type 2 cell as progenitor of alveolar epithelial regeneration. A cytodynamic study in mice after exposure to oxygen. *Lab Invest* 1974;30:35–42.
21. Bowden DH, and Adamson IY. Endothelial regeneration as a marker of the differential vascular responses in oxygen-induced pulmonary edema. *Lab Invest* 1974;30:350–357.
22. Tryka AF, Witschi H, Gosslee DG, McArthur AH, and Clapp NK. Patterns of cell proliferation during recovery from oxygen injury. Species differences. *Am Rev Respir Dis* 1986;133:1055–1059.
23. Tryka AF, and Witschi H. Modulation of cellular repair response patterns. *Chest* 1991;99:28S–30S.
24. He LS, Chang SW, Ortiz de Montellano P., Burke TJ, and Voelkel NF. Lung injury in Fischer but not Sprague-Dawley rats after short-term hyperoxia. *Am J Physiol* 1990;259:L451–L458.
25. Crapo JD, and Tierney DF. Superoxide dismutase and pulmonary oxygen toxicity. *Am J Physiol* 1974;226:1401–1407.
26. Frank L, and Roberts RJ. Oxygen toxicity: protection of the lung by bacterial lipopolysaccharide (endotoxin). *Toxicol Appl Pharmacol* 1979;50:371–380.
27. Wispe JR, Warner BB, Clark JC, Dey CR, Neuman J, Glasser SW, Crapo JD, Chang LY, and Whitsett JA. Human Mn-superoxide dismutase in pulmonary epithelial cells of transgenic mice confers protection from oxygen injury. *J Biol Chem* 1992;267:23937–23941.
28. Tsan MF, Lee CY, and White JE. Interleukin 1 protects rats against oxygen toxicity. *J Appl Physiol* 1991;71:688–697.
29. Margaretten N, Tryka AF, and Witschi H. Oxygen tolerance in mice following exposure to butylated hydroxytoluene. *Toxicol Appl Pharmacol* 1988;96:147–158.
30. Baker RR, Holm BA, Panus PC, and Matalon S. Development of O_2 tolerance in rabbits with no increase in antioxidant enzymes. *J Appl Physiol* 1989;66:1679–1684.
31. Gonder JC, Proctor RA, and Will JA. Genetic differences in oxygen toxicity are correlated with cytochrome P-450 inducibility. *Proc Natl Acad Sci USA* 1985;82:6315–6319.
32. Mansour H, Brun-Pascaud M, Marquetty C, Gougerot-Pocidalo MA, Hakim J, and Pocidalo JJ. Protection of rat from oxygen toxicity by inducers of cytochrome P-450 system. *Am Rev Respir Dis* 1988;137:688–694.
33. Lippmann M. Ozone. In: *Environmental Toxicants, Human Exposures and Their Health Effects*, ed. M. Lippmann. New York: Van Nostrand Reinhold, 1992, pp. 465–519.
34. Koren HS, Devlin RB, Graham DE, Mann R, McGee MP, Horstman DH, Kozumbo WJ, Becker S, House DE, McDonnell WF, and Bromberg PA. Ozone-induced inflammation in the lower airways of human subjects. *Am Rev Respir Dis* 1989;139:407–415.
35. Pinkerton KE, Mercer RH, Plopper CG, and Crapo JD. Distribution of injury and microdosimetry of ozone in the ventilatory unit of the rat. *J Appl Physiol* 1992;73:817–824.
36. Sherwin RP, and Richters V. Centriacinar (CAR) disease in the lungs of young adults: A preliminary report. In: *Tropospheric Ozone and the Environment*, eds. RL Berlund, DR Lawson, and DJ McKee. Pittsburgh, PA: Air and Waste Management Association, 1991, pp. 178–196.
37. Chang L, Miller FJ, Ultman J, Huang Y, Stockstill BL, Grose E, Graham JA, Ospital JJ, and Crapo JD. Alveolar epithelial cell injuries by subchronic exposure to low concentrations of ozone correlate with cumulative exposure. *Toxicol Appl Pharmacol* 1991;109:219–234.
38. Chang LY, Huang Y, Stockstill BL, Graham JA, Grose EC, Menache MG, Miller FJ, Costa DL, and Crapo JD. Epithelial injury and interstitial fibrosis in the proximal alveolar regions of rats chronically exposed to a simulated pattern of urban ambient ozone. *Toxicol Appl Pharmacol* 1992;115:241–252.
39. Plopper CG, Harkema JR, Last JA, et al. The respiratory system of non-human primates responds more to ambient concentrations of ozone than does that of rats. In: *Tropospheric Ozone and the Environment*, eds. RL Berglund, DR Lawson, and DJ McKee, pp. 137–150. Pittsburgh, PA: Air & Waste Management Association, 1991.

40. Pryor WA. How far does ozone penetrate into the pulmonary air/tissue boundary before it reacts? *Free Radical Biol Med* 1992;12:83–88.
41. Uppu RM, and Pryor WA. The reactions of ozone with proteins and unsaturated fatty acids in reverse micelles. *Chem Res Toxicol* 1994;7:47–55.
42. Leikauf GD, Zhao Q, Zhou S, and Santrock J. Ozonolysis products of membrane fatty acids activate eicosanoid metabolism in human airway epithelial cells. *Am J Respir Cell Mol Biol* 1993;9:594–602.
43. Pryor WA. Can vitamin E protect humans against the pathological effects of ozone in smog? *Am J Clin Nutr* 1991;53:702–722.
44. Pinkerton KE, Dodge DE, Cederdahl-Demmler J, Wong VJ, Peake J, Haselton CJ, Mellick PW, Singh G, and Plopper CG. Differentiated bronchiolar epithelium in alveolar ducts of rats exposed to ozone for 20 months. *Am J Pathol* 1993;142:947–956.
45. Gelzleichter TR, Witschi H, and Last JA. Concentration-response relationships of rat lungs to exposure to oxidant air pollutants: A critical test of Haber's Law for ozone and nitrogen dioxide. *Toxicol Appl Pharmacol* 1992;112:73–80.
46. Gelzleichter TR, Witschi H, and Last JA. Synergistic interaction of nitrogen dioxide and ozone on rat lungs: acute responses. *Toxicol Appl Pharmacol* 1992;116:1–9.
47. Last JA, Gelzleichter TR, Pinkerton KE, Walker RM, and Witschi H. A new model of progressive pulmonary fibrosis in rats. *Am Rev Respir Dis* 1993;148:487–494.
48. Peto R, Lopez AD, Boreham J, Thun M, and Heath CJ. Mortality from tobacco in developed countries: Indirect estimation from national vital statistics [see comments]. *Lancet* 1992; 339:1268–1278.
49. U.S. Environmental Protection Agency (EPA/600/6-90/006F). *Respiratory Health Effects of Passive Smoking: Lung Cancer and Other Disorders*. Washington, DC: Office of Health and Environmental Assessment, U.S. EPA, 1992.
50. Glantz SA, and Parmley WW. Passive smoking and heart disease. Epidemiology, physiology, and biochemistry. *Circulation* 1991;83:1–12.
51. Glantz SA, and Parmley WW. Passive smoking and heart disease. Mechanisms and risk. *J Am Med Assoc* 1995;273:1047–1053.
52. Gori GB. Science, policy, and ethics: The case of environmental tobacco smoke. *J Clin Epidemiol* 1994;47:325–334.
53. Huber GL, Brockie RE, and Mahajan VK. Smoke and mirrors. The EPA's flawed study of environmental tobacco smoke and lung cancer. *Regulation* 1993;3:44–54.
54. Witschi HP, Oreffo VIC, and Pinkerton KE. Six month exposure of strain A/J mice to cigarette sidestream smoke: Cell kinetics and lung tumor data. *Fundam Appl Toxicol* 1995;26:32–40.
55. Penn A, Chen LC, and Snyder CA. Inhalation of steady-state sidestream smoke from one cigarette promotes arteriosclerotic plaque development. *Circulation* 1994;90:1363–1367.
56. Zhu BQ, Sun YP, Sievers RE, Isenberg WM, Glantz SA, and Parmley WW. Passive smoking increases experimental atherosclerosis in cholesterol-fed rabbits. *J Am Coll Cardiol* 1993;21:225–232.
57. Zhu BQ, Sun YP, Sievers RE, Glantz SA, Parmley WW, and Wolfe CL. Exposure to environmental tobacco smoke increases myocardial infarct size in rats. *Circulation* 1994;89:1282–1290.
58. Rajini P, Last JA, Pinkerton KE, Hendrickx AG, and Witschi H. Decreased fetal weights in rats exposed to sidestream cigarette smoke. *Fundam Appl Toxicol* 1994;22:400–404.
59. Ji CM, Plopper CG, Witschi HP, and Pinkerton KE. Exposure to sidestream cigarette smoke alters bronchiolar epithelial cell differentiation in the postnatal rat lung. *Am J Respir Cell Mol Biol* 1994;11:312–320.
60. Joad JP, Ji C, Kott KS, Bric JM, and Pinkerton KE. In utero and postnatal effects of sidestream cigarette smoke exposure on lung function, hyperresponsiveness, and neuroendocrine cells in rats. *Toxicol Appl Pharmacol* 1995;132:63–71.
61. Lee CK, Brown BG, Reed EA, Coggins CR, Doolittle DJ, and Hayes AW. Ninety-day inhalation study in rats, using aged and diluted sidestream smoke from a reference cigarette: DNA adducts and alveolar macrophage cytogenetics. *Fundam Appl Toxicol* 1993;20:393–401.
62. von Meyerinck L, Scherer G, Adlkofer F, Wenzel-Hartung R, Brune H, and Thomas C. Exposure of rats and hamsters to sidestream smoke from cigarettes in a subchronic inhalation study. *Exp Pathol* 1989;37:186–189.
63. Church DW, and Pryor WA. The oxidative stress placed on the lung by cigarette smoke. In: *The Lung, Scientific Foundations*, eds. RG Crystal and JB West. New York: Raven Press, 1991, pp. 1975–1979.

64. Gori GB, and Mantel N. Mainstream and environmental tobacco smoke. *Regul Toxicol Pharmacol* 1991;14:88–105.
65. Leuenberger P, Schwartz J, Ackermann-Liebrich U, Blaser K, Bolognini G, Bongard JP, Brandli O, Braun P, Bron C, and Brutsche M. Passive smoking exposure in adults and chronic respiratory symptoms (SAPALDIA Study). *Am J Respir Crit Care Med* 1994;150:1221–1228.
66. Smith P, and Heath D. Paraquat. *CRC Crit Rev Toxicol* 1976;4:411–445.
67. Rose MS, Smith LL, and Wyatt I. Evidence for energy-dependent accumulation of paraquat into rat lung. *Nature* 1974;252:314–315.
68. Rose MS, Lock EA, Smith LL, and Wyatt I. Paraquat accumulation: tissue and species specificity. *Biochem Pharmacol* 1976;25:419–423.
69. Smith LL, Lewis C, Wyatt I, and Cohen GM. The importance of epithelial uptake systems in lung toxicity. In: *Basic Science in Toxicology*, eds. GN Volans, J Sims, FM Sullivan, and P Turner. London: Taylor & Francis, 1990, pp. 233–241.
70. Trush MA, Mimnaugh EG, Ginsburg E, and Gram TE. In vitro stimulation by paraquat of reactive oxygen-mediated lipid peroxidation in rat lung microsomes. *Toxicol Appl Pharmacol* 1981; 60:279–286.
71. Aldrich TK, Fisher AB, Cadenas E, and Chance B. Evidence for lipid peroxidation by paraquat in the perfused rat lung. *J Lab Clin Med* 1983;101:66–73.
72. Witschi H, Kacew S, Hirai KI, and Côté MG. In vivo oxidation of reduced nicotinamide-adenine dinucleotide phosphate by paraquat and diquat in rat lung. *Chem Biol Interact* 1977;19:143–160.
73. Keeling PL, Smith LL, and Aldridge WN. The formation of mixed disulphides in rat lung following paraquat administration. Correlation with changes in intermediary metabolism. *Biochim. Biophys Acta* 1982;716:249–257.
74. Fisher HK, Clements JA, and Wright RR. Enhancement of oxygen toxicity by the herbicide paraquat. *Am Rev Respir Dis* 1973;107:246–252.
75. Kehrer JP, Haschek WM, and Witschi H. The influence of hyperoxia on the acute toxicity of paraquat and diquat. *Drug Chem Toxicol* 1979;2:397–408.
76. Hay J, Shahzeidi S, and Laurent G. Mechanisms of bleomycin-induced lung damage. *Arch Toxicol* 1991;65:81–94.
77. Lazo JS, and Humphreys CJ. Lack of metabolism as the biochemical basis of bleomycin-induced pulmonary toxicity. *Proc Natl Acad Sci USA* 1983;80:3064–3068.
78. Lazo JS, Hoyt DG, Sebti SM, and Pitt BR. The use of bleomycin in model systems to study the pathogenesis of interstitial pulmonary fibrosis. In: *Metabolic Activation and Toxicity of Chemical Agents to Lung Tissue and Cells*, ed. TE Gram. New York: Pergamon Press, 1993, pp. 267–283.
79. Wang QJ, Giri SN, Hyde DM, and Li C. Amelioration of bleomycin-induced pulmonary fibrosis in hamsters by combined treatment with taurine and niacin. *Biochem Pharmacol* 1991;42:1115–1122.
80. Blaisdell RJ, Schiedt MJ, and Giri SN. Dietary supplementation with taurine and niacin prevents the increase in lung collagen cross-links in the multidose bleomycin hamster model of pulmonary fibrosis. *J Biochem Toxicol* 1994;9:79–86.
81. O'Neill CA, and Giri SN. Biochemical mechanisms for the attenuation of bleomycin-induced lung fibrosis by treatment with niacin in hamsters: The role of NAD and ATP. *Exp Lung Res* 1994;20:41–56.
82. Giri SN, Blaisdell R, Rucker RB, Wang Q, and Hyde DM. Amelioration of bleomycin-induced lung fibrosis in hamsters by dietary supplementation with taurine and niacin: biochemical mechanisms. *Environ Health Perspect* 1994;102(Suppl 10):137–147.
83. Sendelbach LE, Lindenschmidt RC, and Witschi HP. The effect of cyclosporin A on pulmonary fibrosis induced by butylated hydroxytoluene, bleomycin and beryllium sulfate. *Toxicol Lett* 1985;26:169–173.
84. Rajini P, and Witschi HP. Cumulative labeling indices in epithelial cell populations of the respiratory tract after exposure to ozone at low concentrations. *Toxicol Appl Pharmacol* 1995;130:32–40.
85. Mustafa MG. Biochemical basis of ozone toxicity. *Free Radical Biol Med* 1990;9:245–265.
86. Frank L, Bucher JR, and Roberts RJ. Oxygen toxicity in neonatal and adult animals of various species. *J Appl Physiol* 1978;45:699–704.
87. Jackson JH. Potential molecular mechanisms of oxidant-induced carcinogenesis. *Environ Health Perspect* 1994;102(Suppl 10):155–157.

Free Radical Toxicology
Edited by K. B. Wallace
Copyright © 1997 Taylor & Francis

15

Activation of the Inflammatory Response by Asbestos and Silicate Mineral Dusts

James Varani and Peter A. Ward

Department of Pathology, University of Michigan Medical School, Ann Arbor, Michigan, USA

INTRODUCTION

The entire aerodigestive tract is in contact with the external environment and is continually exposed to noxious soluble and particulate stimuli. The terminal air spaces of the lungs, in particular, are constantly exposed to potentially injurious stimuli. These delicate structures, separated from the lung microvasculature by only a single epithelial cell layer and single basement membrane, would be irreversibly damaged early in life if not protected by a variety of defense mechanisms. One of the most important of these is the inflammatory system, consisting of tissue macrophages (found in the interstitum of the lung and in the alveolar spaces) and circulating neutrophils.

While the inflammatory system is well designed for its function of protecting the tissues against outside invaders, it is a double-edged sword. Under certain conditions, the same inflammatory effector mechanisms that are used to rid the body of foreign invaders can also produce tremendous damage to the tissues. Inflammatory injury can be seen in any tissue, but it is the terminal air space of the lung that frequently suffers severe inflammatory injury. Inflammatory injury in the lungs can take several forms. On the one hand, it can be rapid and fulminant. The acute form of of the disease, referred to as acute respiratory distress syndrome (ARDS), can be precipitated in a number of ways. It may follow acute lung infection with bacterial or viral pathogens, or occur as a result of systemic infection (sepsis) or widespread burn/trauma injury. The acute form of the disease can be rapidly life-threatening.

Acute inflammatory tissue injury is followed by the body's attempt to repair the damage. The repair process that follows inflammation is similar to wound healing after other types of tissue injury. Resident macrophages, epithelial cells, fibroblasts, and vascular endothelial cells all become activated in an attempt to regenerate the normal tissue architecture. This may occur almost completely, leaving little trace of the initial damage. Alternatively, the repair process may not be able to completely return the tissue to its preinjury architecture. If the damage has been too extensive, a collagenous scar may be left in conjunction with a decrease in function. Whether this is clinically important or not depends on the extent of injury, the degree of scarring in the repair process, and the tissue site.

Chronic lung inflammation (such as seen in asbestosis and silicosis) differs from the acute form of the disease in a number of important ways. While the initial injury may be less severe, chronic diseases are characterized by continual or repetitive stimulation of the tissue-injuring inflammatory response. Tissue injury and tissue repair occur simultaneously. Under such conditions restorative recovery of the lung is never possible. Rather than regenerating the normal architecture, the result of this abnormal healing process is a loss of functional alveoli and extensive deposition of fibrous connective tissue in their place. To fully appreciate the clinical picture seen in chronic diseases such as asbestosis and silicosis, one needs to examine both injury and repair processes. To do so, however, is beyond the scope of a single review. In this review, we focus on injury. There are two major themes: (1) production and metabolism of reactive oxygen species in inflammation, and (2) tissue injury by oxidants in inflammation. With both, information on acute inflammation is presented first since there is a much larger literature. This information will be used to set the stage for discussions related to oxygen radical generation and oxygen radical-induced tissue injury in chronic diseases such as asbestosis and silicosis. In focusing primarily on inflammation (rather then on repair), we must keep in mind that this is only a part of the picture. For information on normal and abnormal repair in chronic lung inflammation, recent reviews are available (1).

PRODUCTION AND METABOLISM OF REACTIVE OXYGEN SPECIES IN ACUTE INFLAMMATION

Effector Mechanisms of Macrophages and Neutrophils

Neutrophils and macrophages are both well equipped with a variety of effector responses. Both cells can generate extracellular oxidants through a similar pathway (e.g., the surface NADPH oxidase) (2–4). Both cells can also release proteolytic enzymes, other potent hydrolases, and a variety of other effector molecules (5). A major difference is that in the neutrophil, preformed effector molecules are stored in granules and rapidly released to the surface upon cell activation. In contrast, effector molecules are synthesized by macrophages in response to cell stimulation. Another major difference between macrophages and netutrophils is that the former also synthesize and release large amounts of numerous growth factors and cytokines, while the cytokine profile of the neutrophil is much more limited (6). Macrophage cytokines/growth factors attract neutrophils to sites of inflammation and influence virtually every aspect of their behavior once they arrive there. Macrophage products also influence the activities of other cells present at the inflammatory site. Because of this, the macrophage may be considered to be the major orchestrator of the inflammatory cascade as well as for the wound-healing response that follows. Table 1 lists effector molecules found in neutrophil granules and Table 2 lists many of the growth factors and cytokines synthesized by activated macrophages. As discussed later in this review, the potent hydrolytic enzymes produced by macrophages and neutrophils contribute to the tissue injury that occurs in inflammation. In some cases, these enzymes can function alone to produce tissue damage. As will be seen, however, in many cases, they act in concert with oxidants to bring about their effect.

Oxidant Generation and Metabolism

The initial oxidant generated by activated neutrophils and macrophages is superoxide anion (O_2^-). This is accomplished during cell activation by increased glucose metabolism through the hexose monophosphate shunt (leading to increased NADPH

TABLE 1. *Neutrophil granule contents*

Primary (azurophilic) granules
Acid hydrolases
  Cathepsin B
  Cathepsin D
  N-Acetyl glucosaminidase
  α-Mannosidase
  β-Glucuronidase
Neutrophil hydrolases
  Cathepsin G
  Elastase
  Myeloperoxidase
Cationic proteins
  Defensins
  Bactericidal/permeability increasing protein
  Lysozyme

Secondary (specific) granules
Lysozyme
Collagenase
Lactoferrin
Vitamin B_{12} binding protein
C5a-cleaving enzyme
Plasminogen activator
Cytochrome b_{558}
Membrane receptors
  FMLP receptor
  C3bi receptor
  Laminin receptor
Alkaline phosphatase

Tertiary granules
Gelatinase
Membrane receptors
  C3bi receptor
  Laminin receptor

TABLE 2. *Macrophage growth factors*

Fibroblast growth factor
Granulocyte/macrophage colony-stimulating factor
Granulocyte colony-stimulating factor
Insulin-like growth factor-1
Interleukin-1α
Interleukin-1β
Interleukin-6
Interleukin-8
Interferon-α
Interferon-γ
Macrophage inflammatory protein-1α
Macrophage inflammatory protein-1β
Neutrophil-activating factor
Platelet-derived growth factor
Tumor necrosis factor-α
Transforming growth factor-α
Transforming growth factor-β

generation) associated with increased oxygen consumption (the respiratory burst) and concomitant organization of the components of the surface NADPH oxidase enzyme complex into a functional enzyme on the cell surface (4). The end result of this is production of a large amount of extracellular O_2^-. At physiological pH or at acidic pH, O_2^- accepts a single electron and spontaneously dismutates to hydrogen peroxide (H_2O_2). The enzyme superoxide dismutase (SOD) catalzyzes this reaction. The formation of O_2^- and H_2O_2 is shown schematically as part of Figure 1 (reactions A and B).

Studies by Fridovich (2), subsequently expanded on by numerous investigators, showed that most oxidant damage in biological systems is not directly due to O_2^- or H_2O_2 as both are too slowly reactive under physiological conditions. A more reactive species produced from these two reactants was therefore considered likely. The hydroxyl radical ($\cdot OH$) was thought to be the reactive species. The formation of $\cdot OH$ from O_2^- and H_2O_2 was originally postulated by Haber and Weiss (7). However, since the rate constant for $\cdot OH$ formation is lower than the rate constant for dissociation, the reactant would not be expected to form in significant quantites by itself under in vivo conditions. A modification of the Haber-Weiss reaction, referred to as the Fenton reaction, overcomes this limitation. The Fenton reaction uses molecular iron in the presence of O_2^- and H_2O_2 to form $\cdot OH$ (8). A key to this reaction is the ability of iron to exist in two main valency states-as Fe^{2+} and as Fe^{3+}-and the capacity of O_2^- to reduce Fe^{3+} to Fe^{2+}. Reduction of H_2O_2 to $\cdot OH$ then

$\longrightarrow$

FIG. 1. Pathways for the generation and metabolism of oxidants in acute inflammation. Pathways A and B represent the major mechanism leading to H_2O_2 formation by inflammatory cells. Pathways C, D, and E represent potential routes of detoxification. Pathways F and G are routes to the generation of toxic metabolites.

OXIDANT GENERATION AND METABOLISM IN INFLAMMATION

A. $O_2 \xrightarrow[\text{NADPH oxidase}]{\overset{\text{NADPH} \quad \text{NADP}}{+1e^-}} O_2^-$

B. $O_2^- + 2H^+ \xrightarrow[\substack{\text{Spontaneous} \\ \text{or} \\ \text{Superoxide dismutase}}]{+1e^-} H_2O_2$

C. $2H_2O_2 \xrightarrow{\text{Catalase}} 2H_2O + O_2$

D. $2H_2O_2 \xrightarrow[\substack{\text{Glutathione} \\ \text{peroxidase}}]{\overset{\text{2GSH} \quad \text{GSSG}}{}} 2H_2O + O_2$

E. $AA\text{-}Mn^{2+} + H_2O_2 \longrightarrow \overbrace{AA\text{-}Mn^{3+}\cdots\cdot OH\cdots OH^-}^{\text{Coordinate complex}}$

$\alpha\text{-keto acid} + NH_3 + Mn^{2+} \longleftarrow \cdot AA\text{-}Mn^{3+} + H_2O$

F. $H_2O_2 \xrightarrow[\text{MPO}]{Cl^-} HOCl \xrightarrow{\text{Amino acid}} \text{Chloramine}$

G. $O_2^- + Fe^{3+} \longrightarrow O_2 + Fe^{2+}$

$O_2^- + 2H^+ \longrightarrow H_2O_2$

$\longrightarrow Fe^{3+} + \cdot OH + OH^-$

proceeds with Fe^{2+} as the catalyst and regenerates Fe^{3+} in the process. The two-reaction summary is shown as part of Figure 1 (reaction G). $\cdot OH$ is so reactive that it is believed to react within 1–5 molecular diameters of its site of formation.

Because reactive oxygen species have the potential to be so damaging, various defense mechanisms exist to control these reactants. Copper-zinc superoxide dismutase (SOD) in the cytoplasm and manganese SOD in mitochondria keep intracellular levels of O_2^- to approximately 10^{-11} M. Intracellular H_2O_2 generated by these enzymes is detoxified by reaction with either the heme enzyme, catalase, or the selenium-containing enzyme, glutathione peroxidase. There are no specific enzyme inhibitors of $\cdot OH$. However, levels of this reactant can be controlled in a variety of ways. Rapid removal of its precursors (O_2^- and H_2O_2) is one way. Sequestration of iron is another mechanism for preventing $\cdot OH$ generation. Intracellular iron (Fe^{3+}) is stored bound to macromolecular ferritin. The presence of "nonessential" molecules within the cell to serve as scavengers also prevents the build up of $\cdot OH$.

Another possible mechanism for preventing the buildup of $\cdot OH$ involves a manganese (II) and bicarbonate-catalyzed disproportionation of H_2O_2 (9). In the presence of physiological concentrations of bicarbonate, manganese(II) forms a coordinate complex with amino acids and catalyzes the direct transfer of electrons from H_2O_2 to one of the bound amino acids. The manganese(II)-catalzyed reaction is analogous to the reduction of H_2O_2 by Fe^{2+} but instead of forming a "free" radical, the transfer of electrons occurs within the complex. The end result is destruction of a molecule of amino acid with the concomitant sparing of more important cellular targets. That this novel pathway of H_2O_2 detoxification may have biological relevance is suggested by experimental studies showing that addition of manganese(II) to cultured cells or experimental animals in the presence of amino acids and bicarbonate buffer affords strong protection against H_2O_2-induced injury (10). Oxidant detoxification pathways are included as part of Figure 1 (reactions C, D, and E).

OXIDANT GENERATION IN MINERAL DUST EXPOSURE

Silicosis and asbestosis are chronic lung diseases that occur as a consequence of years of occupational exposure to silicon-containing mineral dusts. Silica (SiO_2) occurs mainly in one of three cystalline forms: quartz, tridymite, and cristobalite. The most common form, quartz, has a crystalline tetrahedron structure with a centrallylocated silicon atom. The silicon atom shares oxygen atoms with neighboring atoms of silicon. Asbestos is the collective term for a group of naturally occurring fibrous silicate minerals including chrysotile, crocidolite, anthophyllite, tremolite, and actinolite. All of the minerals of asbestos consist of sheets of silica tetrahedra in which oxygen is covalently bound either to two silicon atoms or to one silicon atom and carries a net negative charge. Both silicate quartz and asbestos fibers are capable of producing a debilitating lung disease characterized by chronic inflammation, leading to interstitial fibrosis with concomitant obliteration of alveoli, alveolar ducts, and respiratory bronchioles. Silicosis and asbestosis are members of a family of lung diseases that include those caused by dusts of other metals, coal mine dust, and tannins (cotton mill dusts).

In extrapolating from acute inflammatory lung injury to progressive pulmonary diseases resulting from silica and asbestos exposure, there are many factors to consider. One is the nature of the activation stimuli. While acute inflammatory responses are triggered by soluble factors and phagocytosable/digestible microbial particles, silica crystals and asbestos fibers are, for the most part, insoluble and indigestible. There are additional features of these mineral dusts that make them potentially unique; specifically, the chemical composition of these mineral dusts is such that there is always a high concentration of iron present. The availability of iron as part of the surface chemistry of asbestos fibers raises the possibility that oxygen radicals might be generated in a phagocyte-independent mechanism or that oxidants generated by activated phagocytes (O_2^- and H_2O_2) might be efficiently converted in the presence of mineral dusts to more toxic forms.

Leukocyte Activation by Mineral Dusts: Comparison with Soluble Stimuli and Phagocytic Particles

Both neutrophils and macrophages produce reactive oxygen metabolites (as well as several other potentially injurious agents) when activated. The question is: Do all stimuli lead to an idential response or is there specificity of response based on the stimuli? If there are not qualitative differences in response to different stimuli, there are, at least, quantitative differences. Specifically, different soluble agonists induce a chemotactic response in neutrophils and monocytes, and a number of these also induce both a weak oxidant burst and exocytosis. *N*-Formyl peptides, the complement peptide C5a, platelet-activating factor (PAF), the cytokine interleukin-8 (IL-8), and leukotriene B4 are such agonists. Particulate stimuli, including aggregated immunoglobin G (IgG), immune complexes containing IgG/anti-IgG, and opsonized microbial cells or cell walls elicit a more extensive oxidant burst. In an earlier study (11) we compared a number of soluble and particulate leukocyte agonists for ability to induce an oxidant burst and enzyme release on the one hand, and for ability to kill endothelial cells on the other. To summarize the data from this study, soluble stimuli were more effective in stimulating a chemotactic response; soluble and particulate stimuli were equally effective at inducing release of stored enzymes from granules; and particulate stimuli induced more extensive oxidant production. Production of oxidants, in particular H_2O_2, correlated with a cytotoxic outcome (for the endothelial cells). It would appear that soluble stimuli are designed to optimally recruit cells to inflammatory sites, while particulate stimuli promote functions that allow the recruited cells to remove the inducers of the inflammation.

In regard to asbestos, Perkins, Scheule, and Holian (12,13) have examined the in vitro response of normal alveolar macrophages to positively charged chrysotile and negatively charged crocidolite asbestos fibers. Findings from this work include the following: (1) Both types of fibers induce O_2^- production by alveolar macrophages in vitro, but the response is greater with the positively-charged fibers than with the negatively-charged species; (2) both types of fibers are capable of binding proteins and lipids present in bronchoalveolar secretions; IgG, a major constituent of the lavage fluid, binds to both types of particles and greatly increases O_2^- synthesis; and (3) the relative effectiveness of subclasses of IgG for enhancing O_2^- production in response to the fibers varies directly with capacity to bind to Fc receptors on macrophages. Taken together, these findings support the notion that asbestos fibers stimulate oxidant generation as the cells try to engulf them. Interaction of the particles with cells through Fc receptors enhances binding and concomitantly O_2^- production. The fact that the positively-charged chrysotile fibers are more stimulatory than the negatively charged crocidolite fibers in the absence of protein binding is of interest because cationic particles, in general, are highly stimulatory for leukocytes (14–18). Of additional interest is the observation that silicate, which like asbestos is fibrogenic, does not stimulate an O_2^- response by alveolar macrophages by itself but does so when bound to IgG (12,13). However, in contrast to what is observed with the asbestos fibers, other lung lavage constituents compete with IgG binding to silicate and, when present in high concentration, reduce O_2^- generation. Difference such as this may account for the different patterns of fibrosis that characterize silicate-induced disease and that induced by asbestos fibers.

In addition to direct stimulation of O_2^- production, asbestos fibers and silica particles can act as priming agents (priming agents being factors that do not by themselves activate inflammatory cells but that render inflammatory cells increasingly sensitive to factors that do). This has been shown following in vivo exposure in sheep (19). Animals repeatedly exposed to chrysotile fibers or to a single dose of quartz were lavaged at various times after exposure. The lavaged cells, which consisted of mixtures of alveolar macrophages and neutrophils, did not spontaneously produce O_2^- in vitro at a rate different from control cells. However, the amount of oxidants generated in response to stimulation with phorbol esters was higher with the cells from the asbestos/silica-exposed animals than with cells from control sheep. The priming effect was seen throughout the entire period of the study (18 mo). Priming may have been a direct consequence of mineral dust exposure, but could also reflect the presence of multiple cytokines in the lavage fluid of the chronically injured lungs. Cytokines such as TNF-α are known to be potent priming agents (20,21).

In addition to simply acting as a stimulus for phagocytosis, there are other potential mechanisms by which the mineral dusts can influence inflammatory cell oxidant generation and action. For example, the iron associated with the mineral fibers can enhance generation of toxic oxidants through concentration of iron in the target cells. Small silicate particles can be endocytosed by lung cells and carry iron into these cells. As discussed in a later section, cell injury by leukocytes in acute inflammation involves O_2^- generation by the stimulated phagocytic cell and its eventual conversion to $\cdot OH$ within the target cell. Iron contributed by the target cell serves as catalyst. By concentrating iron within the target cell, the mineral dusts may act to enhance target cell sensitivity. Finally, iron on the mineral surface may allow ·OH to be generated without the contribution of iron by the target cell. That this might have clinical significance is suggested by studies showing the increased iron content in the lungs of workers chronically exposed to mineral dusts (22).

Cell-Free Generation of Oxidants in the Presence of Asbestos and Silica

As indicated earlier, a unique feature of asbestos fibers and silicate crystals (in regard to oxidant generation) is their high iron content. For example, in amphibole asbestos fibers such as crocidolite and amosite, iron may account for up to 27% of the total weight (23–26). Though much lower (2–6%), iron content in serpentine (chrysotile) asbestos fibers is still significant (23–27). Although the actual content of surface iron may be important, total iron content may ultimately be less important than the form in which it exists. In aqueous buffers, mineral oxides are covered with surface hydroxyl groups. Silanol groups (-Si-OH) bind ferric iron to produce a silicon-oxygen-iron coordination complex (28). The coordination chemistry of these complexes has been wellstudied, though it is still incompletely understood. It is thought that when one of the iron coordination sites is unoccupied or loosely occupied (as with water), the complex can efficiently catalyze electron transfer reactions. Thus, the possibility exists that asbestos fibers and silicate minerals can directly catalzye oxygen radical formation independent of inflammatory cells. Several studies have provided strong evidence that iron-containing minerals can, in fact, reduce H_2O_2 to ·OH under completely cell-free conditions (29–33). Mineral-catalyzed ·OH generation, as indicated by electron spin trapping with DMPO, has been shown to occur in direct relation to the amount of iron in association with the fibers. In these studies pretreatment of the minerals with deferoxamine to chelate the iron dramatically reduced ·OH production, as did treatment with ·OH scavengers. Pretreatment with inorganic iron to increase iron content increased ·OH production.

The ability of asbestos fibers to serve as Fenton catalysts in ·OH generation is of interest in that it might augment the rate-limiting reaction in free-radical formation. Potentially of equal interest are the observations of Zalma et al. (32,33) and Pezerate et al. (34), which showed that certain iron-mineral dust coordination complexes were able to directly catalyze the transfer of an electron to molecular oxygen to produce O_2^-. Following spontaneous dismutation to H_2O_2, adjacent surface iron could further reduce the peroxide to ·OH (as described earlier). According to this scheme (Figure 2), oxygen radicals including the presumably highly toxic ·OH could be generated in a purely cell-free system using the mineral dust surface as catalyst. While the level of radical production from these cell-free systems might be expected to be low as compared to what fully activated leukocytes are capable of generating, it could provide either enough radical to sustain a low level of injury (as one sees in chronic injury) or might be sufficient to initiate the injury process and lead to leukocyte recruitment/activation. These possibilities are discussed more fully in the section on cell and tissue damage in inflammation. It should be noted also that injury due to exposure to a single noxious particle is not often found in

POSSIBLE MECHANISM FOR GENERATION OF
O_2^- AND •OH AT THE SURFACE OF ASBESTOS FIBERS

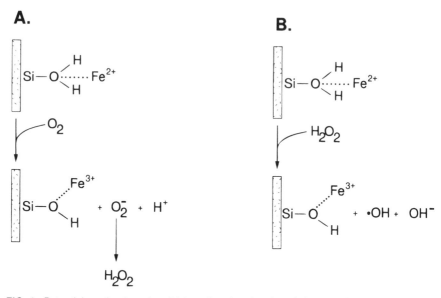

FIG. 2. Potential mechanisms by which surface iron in mineral dusts such as asbestos might catalyze the formation of oxidants under cell-free conditions. See references 22 and 32–34 for details.

the environmental setting. In practice, the lungs are often bombarded with mineral dusts in conjunction with other agents that are by themselves injurious or, if not injurious, capable of synergizing with mineral dusts to exacerbate the effects of the dusts. Cigarette smoke has been the environmental pollutant most wellstudied in this regard (35–40), and indeed, the level of radicals generated in the presence of cigarette smoke and mineral dusts is greater than those generated by the mineral dusts alone. Other pollutants, though less well studied, may be equally effective.

OXIDANT-INDUCED CELL INJURY IN ACUTE INFLAMMATION

In preceding sections of this review the focus was on generation of reactive oxygen species. Oxidant generation and metabolism in acute inflammation served as a basis for the subsequent discussion of the more limited information dealing specifically with asbestos and mineral dusts. In the following two sections, the focus is on oxidant-induced cell and tissue injury. Injury in acute inflammationis discussed first. This is used as a basis for understanding the process of cell injury in chronic conditions.

Evidence from Animal Models That Acute Lung Injury Is Oxidant Mediated

A large number of studies have shown that oxidants play a major role in inflama-
tory cell and tissue injury. Convincing evidence comes from studies in experimental
animals. Lung injury in rats induced either through systemic complement activation
or through formation of immune complexes in the alveolar wall can be suppressed
with catalase, as well as with iron chelators and scavengers of ·OH (41–45). Neutrophil depletion procedures (41–44) and interference with neutrophil adhesion to the
pulmonary vasculature (46) also ameliorate injury, arguing strongly that in these
experimental models, tissue injury is dependent on leukocyte accumulation and
oxygen radical production. Studies from other tissue sites and from other experimental animals support the critical role for leukocyte oxidants in acute inflammatory
cell injury (47–49).

An important role for oxidants in most forms of acute inflammatory tissue injury
is reasonably certain. This does not imply, however, that oxidants are the only
mediators of tissue injury or that they function in isolation. Quite the contrary, the
inflammatory nidus is a milieu of oxidants, proteinases, other hydrolytic enzymes,
phospholipids, phospholipid breakdown products, cationic peptides, polyamines,
growth factors, and cytokines. Tissue injury in acute inflammation, no doubt, reflects
the actions of all of these agents. Studies from our own laboratory (50) have shown
that blocking either serine proteinases with secreted leukoproteinase inhibitor (SLPI)
or matrix metalloproteinases with tissue inhibitor of metalloproteinase-2 (TIMP-2)
will partially reduce lung injury in a model that is known to be primarily oxidant
mediated (42,44).

In experimental models of acute lung inflammation, just as in cases of acute lung
injury in humans (i.e., ARDS), histological examination often reveals widespread
damage of the lung parenchyma. Typical findings include denudation of alveoli,
influx of plasma, leukocytes, and erythrocytes into the interstitum and alveolar
space, and extensive deposition of fibrin. Mononuclear and polymorphonuclear
leukocytes are abundant. While damage to all of the structures of the lung is often
seen, it appears that the lung microvascular endothelium is the initial target. Structural
abnormalities can be seen in the vasculature early in the disease process. These
include endothelial cell detachment from the underlying basement membrane, endothelial blebbing, and necrosis. A loss of endothelial cell biochemical function accompanies these structural changes. Figures 3 and 4 demonstrates typical histological
and ultrastructural features that one sees in acute lung injury, and Figure 5 shows
ultrastructural evidence of early damage to the vasculature. Because endothelial
cells appear to be a critical early target of the acute inflammatory response in the
lung, extensive efforts have been made to elucidate the cellular and biochemical
events that result in their destruction.

Endothelial Cell Injury in Acute Inflammation—Oxidant Pathway

Endothelial cell injury in culture has been extensively investigated over the past
20 years. Studies from a number of laboratories have shown that unstimulated

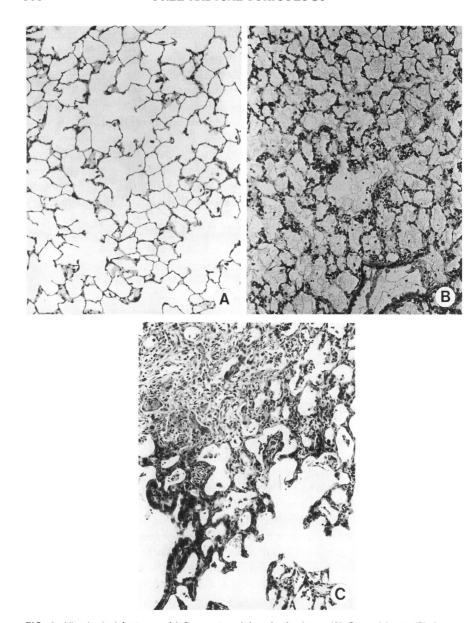

FIG. 3. Histological features of inflammatory injury in the lung. (A) Control lung. (B) Acute inflammation in the lung. Characteristic features include hemorrhage and fibrin deposition in the interstitium and alveolar space as well as an influx of inflammatory cells (mostly neutrophils). (C) Chronic inflammation in the lung. Collapse of alveolar spaces with consolidation and collagen deposition in the interstitium are characteristic features.

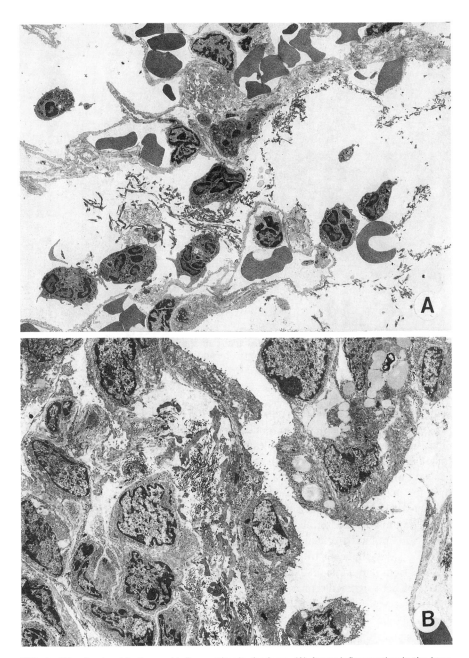

FIG. 4. Ultrastructural features of inflammation in the lung. (A) Acute inflammation in the lung. (B) Chronic inflammation in the lung.

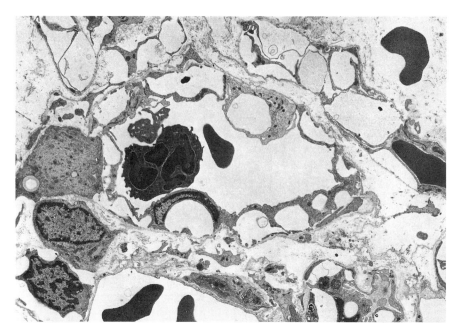

FIG. 5. Ultrastructural features of early vascular damage in acute inflammatory lung injury. Characteristic features include bleb formation in the endothelium, endothelial cell necrosis, and separation of the endothelial cells from the underlying basement membrane.

neutrophils are not cytotoxic to cultured endothelial cells at virtually any effector:target cell ratio. On the other hand, neutrophils stimulated with a variety of soluble or particulate agonists produce widespread injury to endothelial cell monolayers. Endothelial cell separation from the underlying matrix is routinely seen. This can occur in the absence of cell lysis, but lethal injury normally accompanies release from the underlying matrix. Based primarily on inhibitor studies and studies with oxidant-deficient cells, it can be stated that endothelial cell detachment from the underlying matrix is a serine proteinase-mediated event (51,52), while endothelial cell lysis is primarily oxidant driven (11,53–55).

Using endothelial cells from several species (human, bovine, porcine, mouse, and rat) and from both large and small vessels, an overall picture of the injury process caused by activated neutrophils has emerged. These studies have, for the most part, shown that neutrophil-derived H_2O_2 is a central intermediate in the injury process but that a more reactive species (such as $\cdot OH$) seems to be directly responsible for the damage. As discussed earlier, $\cdot OH$ can be generated wherever iron in its transition state comes into contact with hydrogen peroxide. For the most part, however, it appears that the $\cdot OH$ radical is generated within the target cell (via the Fenton reaction) and that the target cell provides both the iron and a source of O_2^-. Iron chelators and $\cdot OH$ scavengers that readily cross cell membranes are highly protective, while chelators and scavengers that do not cross the plasma membrane are ineffective

(11,56). While the overall mechanism of injury appears to be of a general nature, there are cell-specific features. For example, the source of the intracellularly generated oxidant may differ from cell to cell. Rat and bovine cells contain substantial amounts of xanthine oxidase and agents that are effective inhibitors of this enzyme are protective (57,58). Human endothelial cells also contain this enzyme, although it appears to be present in very low levels in resting endothelial cells and upregulated in hypoxia (59). Thus, it may not be the primary source of O_2^- in support of neutrophil-mediated killing of these targets. Other possibilities include cyclooxygenase and lipoxygenase enzymes, mitochondrial enzymes, and mixed-function oxidases.

Our laboratory has utilized endothelial cells from several different sources as targets for injury by activated neutrophils. Figure 6 provides an overview of the findings that have been made in these studies. As depicted in part A of this figure, activated neutrophils adhere tightly to the target endothelium. It is known from a variety of studies that the same agonists that activate the neutrophil for cytotoxicity also cause upregulation and activation of β2 integrins and that the tight adhesion to the target cell is a reflection of this (60–63). These same stimuli activate the respiratory burst, leading to O_2^- and H_2O_2 production (11).

H_2O_2 crosses the plasma membrane of the target cell (Figure 6, part B), where it serves two functions. First, it is the substrate that is ultimately reduced to ·OH. Second, it functions to lower cellular ATP levels. H_2O_2-exposed cells lose as much as 75–80% of their ATP content within minutes of exposure (64). The mechanism directly responsible for ATP loss in H_2O_2-exposed cells is not fully understood. One thing is clear: The drop in ATP is not, in itself, cytotoxic to cells in the short term because the drop still occurs in H_2O_2-exposed cells that have been pretreated with oxidant inhibitors and iron chelators and are resistant to injury (64). Further, ATP depletion occurs in response to other stresses that are not directly cytotoxic (65–67). Rather, it appears that the rapid catabolism of ATP following H2O2 exposure leads to the accumulation of downstream purine metabolites, including xanthine and hypoxanthine. These metabolites, which are undetectable in control cells, serve as substrate for the xanthine dehydrogenase/xanthine oxidase (XD/XO) enzyme. XD/XO is responsible for the conversion of xanthine and hypoxanthine to uric acid (57). When it functions as a dehydrogenase, NAD is the electron acceptor. However, when the enzyme functions as an oxidase, molecular oxygen is the electron acceptor and this reaction generates O_2^-. Thus, the breakdown of ATP makes substrate available for an enzyme reaction that is known to be substrate limited and that has the potential to generate O_2^-.

While the two forms of the XD/XO enzyme are interconvertable, proteolytic cleavage of the enzyme results in the enzyme permanently functioning as an oxidase. In resting endothelial cells, the majority (80%) of the enzyme is in the XD form, but upon exposure to activated neutrophils, the ratio of XD to XO is reversed. Studies by Phan et al. have shown that conversion is the result of cleavage by neutrophil elastase (57,68). Thus, exposure of endothelial cells to activated neutrophils results in the activation of an enzyme for O_2^- production at the same time as

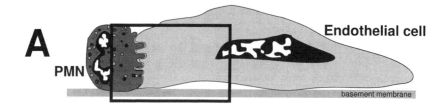

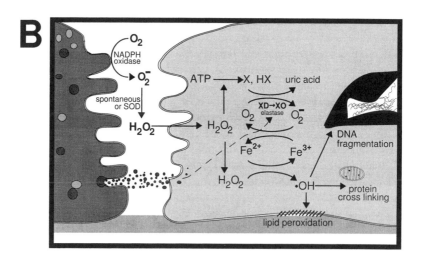

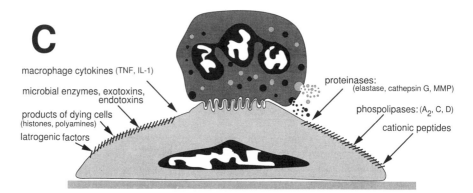

substrate for the enzyme is becoming available. It should be noted that leukocyte elastase is not the only method for converting XD to XO. A number of inflammatory cytokines including tumor necrosis factor-α (TNF-α), the C5a complement chemotactic peptide, and the N-formyl chemotactic peptides have also been shown to accomplish the same goal (69). In any event, the end result is that the neutrophil provides the substrate (H_2O_2) for radical generation and, at the same time, induces the target cell, itself, to produce O_2^- to serve as a reducing equivalent.

These data strongly suggest that the target endothelial cell is the source of O_2^- necessary for the cytotoxicity reaction. Other data suggest that the target endothelial cells are also the source of the iron (56). Low-molecular-weight iron chelators that cross cell membranes provide substantial protection against injury when target endothelial cells are treated and then washed. In contrast, pretreatment of neutrophils with these same agents does not interfere with their subsequent ability to kill endothelial cells. Likewise, treatment of endothelial cells with high-molecular-weight iron chelators that do not easily cross cell membranes does not protect. Thus, it appears that the target cells are the source of both the iron and O_2^- used in the cytotoxicity process. Of interest, it appears that iron availability is the limiting factor in intracellular $\cdot OH$ generation. This is based on the finding that as iron levels fall, so does sensitivity to oxidant injury (70), while oxidant injury increases when cells are supplemented with iron under conditions in which it can gain entry into the cell (70,71). A schematic view of endothelial cell injury by activated neutrophils is presented in Figure 6 (part B). A more detailed overview of neutrophil-endothelial cell interactions leading to oxidant injury can be found in recent reviews (72,73).

Biochemical Targets in Oxidant Injury

What are the cellular targets in oxidant injury? This question is difficult to definitively address since highly reactive radicals such as $\cdot OH$ can interact with a number of cellular macromolecules. Lipids of the plasma membrane may be a particularly important target for $\cdot OH$ attack (74). Interaction of $\cdot OH$ with a molecule of unsaturated fatty acid leads to the formation of a lipid radical, which then interacts with molecular oxygen to form a lipid peroxide. This, in turn, spontaneously fragments to release a low-molecular-weight aldehyde and in the process generates a second lipid radical from a nearby unsaturated fatty acid. The process then repeats itself. Once initiated, therefore, the pathway is self-propagating. When sufficient damage to the plasma membrane occurs, basic biophysical properties of the membrane are altered. Enzymatic processes, transport functions, and ion control mechanisms are all compromised, leading ultimately to cell death.

FIG. 6. Schematic representation of events in leukocyte-mediated endothelial cell injury. (A) Leukocyte activation promotes adhesion to target endothelial cells. (B) Leukocyte activation results in organization of surface NADPH oxidase complex and formation of O_2^- and H_2O_2. Leukocyte H_2O_2 is metabolized within the target cell to the toxic $\cdot OH$. (C) Endothelial cells are exposed to a variety of other potentially injurious substances in conjunction with oxidants.

Membrane lipids are considered a likely target of radical damage because once the attack is initiated, it is self-propagating. However, lipids are not the only possible target. ·OH can cross-link proteins through formation of S-S bonds and cause DNA fragmentation (74). Protein inactivation can directly result in cell death, while DNA damage can result in inhibition of replication or reduction in protein synthesis. Either may be lethal. In summary, with all of the different possibilities, it is probably safe to say that the widespread nature of target molecules for .OH attack is what makes the ·OH so toxic.

Interaction Between Oxygen Radicals and Other Effector Molecules

While oxidants generated during acute inflammation are capable of lethally injuring cells by themselves, the inflammatory milieu contains a complex mix of potentially injurious chemicals. All of the neutrophil granule contents listed in Table 1 are present. Likewise, oxidants generated by macrophages at the site of injury as well as macrophage cytokines and growth factors (Table 2) can be found. Tissue debris and products released from dead and dying cells are also present in these lesions as well as, at least in cases of infectious etiology, microbial products. Do these agents contribute to the overall pattern of tissue injury observed in inflammatory lesions? Do they act alone or do they act in concert with oxidants? These questions have been addressed in terms of several effector molecules.

Leukocyte proteolytic enzymes, in particular, have been well studied and should serve as a model. Human neutrophils contain a variety of neutral proteinases. The two major serine proteinases are elastase and cathepsin G. Plasminogen activator is also present. Human neutrophils have significant amounts of two matrix metalloproteinases (e.g., a 92-kD gelatinase and an interstitial collagenase) (50). In the neutrophil, these enzymes are stored preformed in granules and released when the cells are exposed to activating stimuli. Macrophages are also a source of some of the same proteolytic enzymes. Macrophages are capable of synthesizing plasminogen activator. Macrophages express, among the metalloproteinases, a 92-kD gelatinase and an interstitial collagenase that is distinct from that of the neutrophil but similar or identical to its fibroblast counterpart (75). Blood monocytes express a low-molecular-weight metalloproteinase (matrilysin) (76), but this enzyme is downregulated as the cells differentiate. On the other hand, alveolar macrophages express another low-molecular-weight enzyme, referred to as metalloelastase, which is capable of cleaving elastin as well as multiple other substrates (77). In contrast to neutrophils, however, macrophages do not have significant amounts of elastase or cathepsin G.

Is there evidence to suggest a role for leukocyte proteinases in the acute inflammatory response? In vitro, stimulated neutrophils and isolated neutrophil proteinases can cause retraction and dislodgement of endothelial cells from a monolayer without killing the cells (51,52). Inhibiton of serine proteinase function prevents retraction and dislodgement of the cells, while metalloproteinase inhibition, that is, with TIMP-

2, does not. Endothelial cell retraction is associated with a loss of permeability barrier function. It has been suggested that endothelial cell retraction is all that is required for the plasma leak seen in acute lung inflammation. Leukocyte oxidants do not appear to play a direct role in endothelial cell retraction/dislodgement. However, oxidants can function in at least three ways to facilitate proteolytic enzyme action. First, myeloperoxidase-dependent oxidants (primarily hypochlorous acid) can facilitate proteolytic enzyme action by inactivating the major serine proteinase inhibitor, α1-antiproteinase. Second, leukocyte oxidants can activate matrix metalloproteinases, which in turn can proteolytically inactivate α1-antiproteinase (reviewed in 5). Finally, leukocyte oxidants can alter the structure of the extracellular matrix in such a manner as to make the matrix components more sensitive to proteolytic digestion (78–80). This, in turn, can alter the capacity of the matrix to support endothelial cell adhesion.

In addition to inducing endothelial cell retraction and dislodgement, neutrophil serine proteinases can also directly kill cells (58,81,82). However, cytotoxicity produced by isolated enzymes occurs after prolonged exposure to high concentrations of enzyme. Whether this has physiological relevance is difficult to know. Given the close contact that exists between activated neutrophils and their targets, a locally high concentration of enzyme could be achieved. Another consideration is that target cells exposed to activated neutrophils are exposed to granule enzymes in conjunction with leukocyte oxidants. As has already been discussed, one way in which neutrophil elastase can contribute to oxidant-induced cell injury is by inducing XD to XO conversion (58,68). Another possibility is that cells exposed to multiple, potentially injurious agents suffer lethal injury under conditions in which each agent alone would be nontoxic or produce repairable injury. For example, oxidant-exposed cells may be more adversely affected by exposure to proteolytic enzymes than control cells. In support of this, we conducted experiments in which endothelial cells were exposed to a sublytic concentration of H_2O_2 and then treated, along with control cells, with neutrophil elastase and neutrophil cathepsin G. Both enzymes were cytotoxic to oxidant-stressed cells at concentrations that had no effect on control cells (83). How this synergistic interaction is brought about at the molecular level is not fully understood. One could envision, for example, how an oxidant-stressed cell might be less able to repair proteolytic enzyme-induced damage to the cell membrane than a similarly exposed control cell. Alternatively, oxidant-exposed cell membranes may be more sensitive to proteolytic attack.

Neutrophil proteinases are not unique in their ability to injure oxidant-stressed cells. Studies by Ginsburg et al. (84) have shown that mammalian and bacterial phospholipases are also capable of producing lethal injury in cells that are concomitantly exposed to H_2O_2 under conditions in which these agents are nontoxic to control cells. Of interest in their studies, it was shown that streptococcal cells carrying membrane-bound streptolysin S could adhere tightly to endothelial cells without producing measurable damage to the cells. However, when the endothelial cells with bacteria attached were simultaneouly exposed to reagent H_2O_2, the combination of soluble peroxide and bound streptolysin S was cytotoxic (85).

Other neutrophil products that have potential for cytotoxicity are the low molecular weight cationic peptides termed "defensins" (86–88). Cationic moieties bind strongly to the surface of cells through electrostatic charge and dramatically alter virtually every cell surface phenomenon. In leukocytes, cationic moieties nonspecifically activate the oxidant burst and the exocytotic process (89). At the same time, these moieties dramatically increase adhesive tendencies of cells. Microbial particles with cationic peptides bound to them are readily phagocytosed by leukocytes, and when enough cationic charge is present, the microbial particles are phagocytosed by other cells (e.g., endothelial cells and fibroblasts) as well (85). At high enough concentration, cationic moieties are toxic. With such a variety of effects, it is not surprising that cationic moieties can interact with oxidants. It has been shown in this regard that low amounts of several different cationic peptides will stably bind to endothelial cells with no apparent effect. However, if the cells are then exposed to sublytic amounts of H_2O_2, they are rapidly lysed (84). These effects of cationic peptides are analogous to what is observed with proteinases and phospholipases. Thus, a wide variety of leukocyte agents, with widely differing activities (but all of which are membrane-active agents), can interact with oxidants to bring about lethal injury. The end result is that concentrations of H_2O_2 that would normally be nontoxic now become lethal. No doubt, the efficiency of microbial killing by leukocytes is greatly increased by the combinations of effector moieties present in conjunction with leukocyte oxidants. It appears, likewise, that tissue injury may also be increased in the same way.

Interaction of Oxidants with Macrophage Cytokines

Up to this point, we have been concerned with the interaction of oxidants and other effector molecules from the neutrophil or with those derived from microbial sources. Macrophages are also present at sites of inflammation. As described earlier, activated macrophages produce a number of different cytokines and growth factors in addition to their own oxidants and proteolytic enzymes. Certain macrophage cytokines such as TNF-α and interleukin-1 (IL-1) are essential for neutrophil-mediated injury by virtue of the fact that these cytokines upregulate endothelial cell adhesion structures for neutrophils (46). In addition, these same cytokines can influence the physiology of both neutrophils and their targets to increase injury. On the effector cell side, these cytokines act as "priming" agents (20,21). That is, they nonspecifically potentiate the respiratory burst induced by a number of different agonists. On the target cell side, they increase sensitivity to oxidant injury (90–94). The mechanism by which this occurs has not been fully elucidated. However, cytokines such as TNF-α and IL-1 also stimulate intracellular oxidant generation, in some cells at least (95,96). As already discussed, oxidant production by target cells may be an important component in the injury-producing pathway. Whether additional mechanisms exist remain to be determined. Part C of Figure 6 schematically depicts the contribution of various effector molecules to lethal injury in oxidant-stressed cells.

In summary, the delicate vascular structures found in the lung appear to be a prime target in acute lung inflammation. Injury to the vascular endothelium or to its underlying extracellular matrix, leading either to retraction and dislodgement of the capillary lining cells or to actual killing of these cells, results in the loss of barrier function. This, in turn, leads to the clinical and histological picture that typifies inflammatory lung disease. The prominent inflammatory cells in acute lung injury include both neutrophils and macrophages. Both cell types are capable of producing oxidants and other inflammatory mediators, and it is reasonable to suggest that both contribute to tissue injury. At the biochemical level, there is strong evidence to indicate that lethal cell injury is largely due to the action of leukoctye oxidants. However, as we have seen, oxidants do not function in a vacuum but in a microenvironment that contains numerous other molecules capable of producing cell and tissue injury. Thus, the actual inflammatory lesion is undoubtably the end result of a number of interactions between oxidants and other inflammatory effector molecules.

Other Cellular Targets of Oxidants

Although the foregoing discussion has centered almost entirely on endothelial cells, other types of cells are also injured in an oxidant-mediated fashion. In the lung, both interstitial fibroblasts and alveolar epithelial cells are killed by activated neutrophils (97,98). Cytotoxicity can be duplicated with reagent H_2O_2 and ameliorated with catalase, $\cdot OH$ scavengers, and iron chelators. In the kidney, mesangial cells and tubule epithelium are oxidant targets (81,99). Cells of the heart, liver, gut, and central nervous system have also been shown to suffer from oxidant injury in inflammation (100–102). Undoubtably, all cells are inherently sensitive to oxidant injury, though differences in levels of pro-oxidant and antioxidant factors determine relative sensitivity.

CHRONIC LUNG INJURY: EXTRAPOLATION FROM EVENTS IN ACUTE INJURY

Chronic lung inflammation demonstrates many of the same features as seen in the acute form of the disease. However, the inflammatory response is less intense than in the acute disease and evidence of repair is concomitantly seen. Repair may result in a tissue architecture that is minimally different from that of the preinjury state. Contrarily, the repair process may lead to fibrosis with its attendant consequences. When this is extensive, lung function is irreparably compromised. Histological and ultrastructural features of chronic lung inflammation are indicated as part of Figures 3 and 4.

Based on the discussions of oxidant production in response to asbestos/silicates (see earlier discussion) and the role of oxidants in acute inflammatory cell injury, it is reasonable to suggest that oxidants underlie cell injury in chronical inflammatory lung disease as well. Lung cell injury in asbestosis/silicosis can occur either through direct toxicity or indirectly, through activation of inflammatory cells. With respect to direct toxicity, virtually all of the cells in the lung have been shown to be deleteriously affected by exposure to asbestos and/or silicates in culture. These include alveolar macrophages, pulmonary epithelial cells, endothelial cells, fibroblasts, and mesothelial cells (103–113). Alveolar macrophages and pulmonary epithelial cells are directly exposed to inhaled particles. Both cell types can endocytose small particles and attempt to phagocytose larger ones. Studies with both cell types have shown that in the presence of antioxidant enzymes, iron chelators, and ·OH scavengers, uptake is reduced and toxicity is inhibited (111,113). In addition, exposure of lung epithelial cells to sublytic concentrations of asbestos fibers results in increased levels of copper-zinc and manganese SOD activity (114), a common response to oxidant stress. Since these in vitro experiments have been done with pure populations of cells (no leukocytes present), the implication is that oxidants must be generated either cell-free or within the target cells.

Asbestos fibers and silicates can induce oxygen radicals generation in the absence of leukocytes, and cell injury can occur under these conditions. Does this then suggest that the chronic lung diseases produced by exposure to these agents does not involve inflammatory cells? Not necessarily. Inflammatory cells, both macrophages and neutrophils, are seen in the lower respiratory tract in association with chronic inflammation. It is not unreasonable to suggest, based on the high level of oxidant production by these cells when activated, that they contribute to cell injury. Again, while direct in vivo proof is difficult to obtain, in vitro studies support this. Specifically, it has been shown that asbestos-activated neutrophils are able to injure pulmonary cells (111,112). As with other cell injury models, injury involves both detachment of viable cells from the monolayer, and cell killing. Injury appears to be primarily oxidant mediated, based on the use of inhibitors. What makes these findings of interest is that neutrophil activation and neutrophil-induced injury occur under conditions in which the asbestos fibers alone are unable to injure the target cells and where unactivated neutrophils by themselves (no asbestos fibers present) are not cytotoxic. Thus, even if asbestos fibers can cause lung parenchymal cell injury directly, injury from asbestos-stimulated inflammatory cells is likely to be a more efficient process.

SUMMARY AND CONCLUSIONS

In summary, lung fibrosis constitutes one of the major long-term health consequences of exposure to asbestos and various other mineral dusts. While the pathophysiology of the disease is not fully understood, both chronic inflammation and inappropriate wound healing are involved. Understanding of both processes is required to get an overall picture of the disease process. The focus of this review has been on mechanisms by which asbestos and mineral dusts initiate the inflammatory response. The following general statements can be supported.

1. Inhalation of appropriate-sized asbestos particles and silica crystals results in

lodgement of the minerals in the terminal airways. Here the particles can be taken up by resident cells including alveolar macrophages and pulmonary epithelial cells. After extended exposure, asbestos fibers can also be found in interstitial macrophages, interstitial fibroblasts, and lung capillary endothelial cells. When neutrophils are found in the interstitial and alveolar spaces, they also have phagocytosed particles within them.

2. The mechanism by which asbestos fibers are taken up by cells is not fully understood, though active phagocytosis appears to be involved. Coating of the mineral fibers with proteins in the bronchoalveolar fluid (particularly IgG) enhances phagocytosis, suggesting a role for Fc receptors. From the cell standpoint, it appears that the mineral fibers are treated like other foreign bodies. There is evidence that oxygen radicals play a role in mineral uptake.

3. Ingestion of asbestos and silicates by lung cells results in cell injury. While all of the mechanisms by which injury can occur have not been fully explored, experimental evidence suggests that injury may occur as a direct consequence of mineral dust injestion or may occur as a result of inflammatory cell activation. In either case, generation of oxygen radicals is involved.

4. There are two possible ways in which oxygen radicals can be generated in the presence of asbestos fibers and silica particles. One involves the particles themselves serving as the catalyst. These minerals are uniquely suited for this purpose since they contain a large amount of surface iron. In aqueous buffers, mineral oxides are covered with surface hydroxyl groups. Silanol groups (-Si-OH) bind ferric iron to produce a silicon-oxygen-iron coordination complex. The iron in the complex serves to catalyze single electron transfer reactions. There is substantial evidence that in the presence of H_2O_2, asbestos surface iron can catalyze its reduction to $\cdot OH$. There is additional evidence, though less complete, to suggest that asbestos surface iron can catalyze electron transfer to molecular oxygen to form O_2^-. Following subsequent spontaneous reduction to H_2O_2 and asbestos iron-catalzyed reduction to $\cdot OH$, this would result in the completely cell-free generation of a radical capable of producing cell injury.

5. A second (and probably the most important) source of oxygen radicals is the inflammatory cells of the host. Asbestos fibers and silicate crystals activate inflammatory cells in a similar manner to other particulate stimuli. Given the fact that the activating stimuli (i.e., the mineral dusts) have iron on their surface in a form that is capable of mediating electron transfer, the fibers themselves can promote conversion of host-generated oxidants (O_2^- and H_2O_2) into the highly toxic $\cdot OH$. It should be noted in this regard that ingestion of fibers by potential target cells ensures that when these cells are exposed to activated inflammatory cells, they will have sufficient transition iron within them to catalzye $\cdot OH$ production.

Thus, while asbestos fibers and related mineral dusts do not initiate a rapid acute inflammatory response such as seen in ARDS, they have the capacity, by virtue of chemical and macromolecular structure, to maintain the inflammatory system in a state of chronic activation. This and with the host's attempt to limit and repair the damage constitute the main pathophysiological events that in susceptible individuals result in the onset of pulmonary fibrosis.

REFERENCES

1. Phan SH, Thrall RS. *Pulmonary Fibrosis*, Vol. 80. Phan SH, Thrall RS, eds. New York: Marcel Dekker, 1995.
2. Fridovich I. The biology of oxygen radicals. *Science*, 209:875–880, 1978.
3. Halliwell B. Reactive oxygen species in living systems: Source, biochemistry, and role in human disease. *Am. J. Med.* 92 (suppl. 3C):14S–22S, 1992.
4. Clark RA. The human neutrophil respiratory burst oxidase. *J. Infect. Dis.* 161:1140–1147, 1990.
5. Weiss SJ. Tissue destruction by neutrophils. *N. Engl. J. Med.* 320:365–375, 1989.
6. Remick DG, DeForge LE. Cytokines and Pulmonary Fibrosis. In: Phan, SH and Thrall, RS, eds., *Pulmonary Fibrosis*, pp. 599–644. New York, Marcel Dekker, 1995.
7. Haber F, Weiss J. The catalytic decomposition of hydrogen peroxide by iron. *Proc. R. Soc. Ser. A*, 147:332–351, 1934.
8. Halliwell B, Gutteridge JMC. Oxygen toxicity, oxygen radicals, transition metals and disease. *Biochem. J.* 219:1–11, 1984.
9. Stadtman ES, Berlett BS, Chock PB. Manganese-dependent disproportionation of hydrogen peroxide in bicarbonate buffer. *Proc. Natl. Acad. Sci. (USA)* 87:384–390, 1990.
10. Varani J, Ginsburg I, Gibbs DF, Mukhopadhyay P, Sulavik, Johnson KJ, Weinberg JM, Ryan US, Ward PA. Hydrogen peroxide-induced cell and tissue injury: protective effects of Mn^{2+}. *Inflammation* 15:291–301, 1991.
11. Varani J, Fligiel SEG, Till GO, Kunkel RG, Ryan US, Ward PA. Pulmonary endothelial cell killing by human neutrophils: Possible involvement of hydroxyl radical. *Lab. Invest.* 53:656–661, 1985.
12. Perkins RC, Scheule RK, Holian A. In vitro bioactivity of asbestos for the human alveolar macrophage and its modification by IgG. *Am. J. Respir. Cell Mol. Biol.* 4:532–537, 1991.
13. Scheule RK, Holian A. Modification of asbestos bioactivity for the alveolar macrophage by selective protein adsorption. *Am. J. Respir. Cell Mol. Biol.* 2:441–448, 1990.
14. Ginsburg I. Cationic polyelectrolytes, potent opsonic agents which activate the respiratory burst in leukocytes. *Free Radical Res. Commun.* 8:11–16, 1989.
15. Moy JN, Gleich GJ, Thomas LL. Noncytotoxic activation of neutrophils by eosinophil granule major basic protein: Effect on superoxide anion generation and lysosomal enzyme release. *J. Immunol.* 145:2626–2632, 1990.
16. Oseas RS, Allen J, Yang HH, Baehner RI, Boxer LA. Rabbit cationic protein enhances leukocyte adhesiveness. *Immunology* 33:523–526, 1981.
17. Warren JS, Ward PA, Johnson KJ, Ginsberg I. Modulation of acute immune complex-mediated tissue injury by the presence of polyanionic substances *Amer. J. Patho.* 128:67–77, 1987.
18. Geffner JR, Trevani AS, Schatner M, Malchiodi E, Lopez DH, Lazzari M, Isturiz MA. Activation of human neutrophils and monocytes induced by immune complexes prepared with cationized antibodies and antigens. *Clin. Immunol. Immunopathol.* 69:9–15, 1993.
19. Cantin A, Dubois F, Begin R. Lung exposure to mineral dust enhances the capacity of lung inflammatory cells to release superoxide. *J. Leuko. Biol.* 43:299–303, 1988.
20. Larrick JW, Graham D, Toy K, Lin LS, Senyk G, Fendly BM. Recombinant tumor necrosis factor causes activation of human granulocytes. *Blood* 69:640–647, 1987.
21. Shalaby MR, Aggarwal BB, Rindernecht E, Svedersky LP, Finkle BS, Palladino MA. Activation of human polymorphonuclear neutrophil functions by γ-interferon and tumor necrosis factor. *J. Immunol* 135:2069–2074, 1985.
22. Kennedy TP, Dodson R, Rao NV, Ky H, Hopkins C, Baser M, Tolley E, Hoidal JR. Dusts causing pneumoconiosis generate ·OH and produce hemolysis by acting as fenton catalysts. *Arch. Biochem. Biophys.* 269:359–364, 1990.
23. Hodgson AA. Chemistry and physics of asbestos. In: Michaels H, Chissick SS, eds. *Asbestos*, Vol 1. New York: Wiley, 1979;67–114.
24. Zussman J. *The Crystal Structures of Amphibole and Serpentine Minerals*. Gaithersburg, MD: National Bureau of Standards Special Publication 506, 1978.

25. DeWaele JK, Adams FC. The surface characterization of modified chrysotile asbestos. *Scanning Electron Microsc.* 2:209–228, 1988.
26. Harrington JS. Chemical studies of asbestos. *Ann. NY Acad. Sci.* 132:1–47, 1965.
27. Pooley FD. Mineralogy of asbestos: The physical and chemical properties of the dusts they form. *Semin. Oncol.* 8:243–249, 1981.
28. Kamp DW, Graceffa P, Pryor WA, Weitzman SA. The role of free radicals in asbestos-induced diseases. *Free Radical Biol. Med.* 12:293–315, 1992.
29. Lund LG, Aust AE. Iron mobilization from asbestos by chelators and ascorbic acid. *Arch. Biochem. Biophys.* 278:60–64, 1990.
30. Weitzman SA, Graceffa P. Asbestos catalyzes hydroxyl and superoxide radical generation from hydrogen peroxide. *Arch. Biochem. Biophys.* 228:373–376, 1984.
31. Eberhardt MK, Roman-Franco AA, Quiles MR. Asbestos-induced decomposition of hydrogen peroxide. *Environ. Res.* 37:287–292, 1985.
32. Zalma R, Bonneau L, Guignard J, Pezerate H. Formation of oxy-radicals by oxygen reduction arising from the surface activity of asbestos. *Can. J. Chem.* 65:2338–3241, 1987.
33. Zalma R, Bonneau L, Guignard J, Pezerat H. Production of hydroxyl radicals by iron in solid compounds. *Toxicol. Environ. Chem.* 13:171–181, 1987.
34. Pezerate H, Zalma R, Guignard J, Jaurand MC. Production of oxygen radicals by the reduction of oxygen arising from the surface activity of mineral fibers. In: Bignon J, Peto J, Seracci R, eds., *Non-occupational Exposure to Mineral Fibers.* Lyon, France: IARC Scientific Publications, 1989;100–111.
35. Pryor WA, Hales BJ, Premovic PI, Church DF. The radicals in cigarette tar: The nature and suggested physiological implications. *Science* 220:425–427, 1983.
36. Cosgrove JP, Borish ET, Church DF, Pryor WA. The metal-mediated formation of hydroxyl radicals by aqueous extracts of cigarette tar. *Biochem. Biophys. Res. Commun.* 132:390–396, 1985.
37. Pryor WA, Prie DG, Church DF. Electron-spin resonance study of maintream and sidestream cigarette smoke: Nature of the free radicals in gas-phase smoke and in cigarette tar. *Environ. Health Perspect.* 47:345–355, 1983.
38. Pryor WA, Tamura M, Dooley MM, Premovic I, Hales BJ. Reactive oxy-radicals from cigarette smoke and their physiological effects. In: Greenwald R, Cohen G, eds., *Oxy-radicals and Their Scavenger Systems: Cellular and Medical Aspects.* New York, Elsevier, 1983;185–192.
39. Pryor WA, Uehara K, Church DF. The chemistry and biochemistry of the radicals in cigarette smoke: ESR evidence for the binding of the tar radical to DNA and polynucleotides. In: Bors W, Saran M, Tait D, eds., *Oxygen Radicals in Chemistry and Biology.* Berlin, Germany: Walter de Gruyter, 1984;193–201.
40. Pryor WA, Tamura M, Church DF. ESR spin trapping study of the radicals produced by NOx/ olefin reactions: A mechanism for the production of the apparently long-lived radicals in gas-phase cigarette smoke. *J. Am. Chem. Soc.* 106:5073–5079, 1984.
41. Till GO, Johnson KJ, Kunkel R, Ward PA. Intravascular activation of complement and acute lung injury. Dependency on neutrophils and toxic oxygen metabolites. *J. Clin. Invest.* 69:1126–1135, 1982.
42. Johnson KJ, Ward PA. Acute immunologic pulmonary alveolitis. *J. Clin Invest.* 54:349–357, 1974.
43. Johnson KJ, Wilson BS, Till GO, Ward PA. Acute lung injury in rat caused by immunoglobulin A immune complexes. *J. Clin. Invest.* 74:358–369, 1984.
44. Johnson KJ, Ward PA. Role of oxygen metabolites in immune complex injury of lung. *J. Immunol.* 126:2365–2369, 1981.
45. Johnson KJ, Ward PA, Kunkel RG, Wilson BS. Mediation of IgA induced lung injury in the rat. Role of macrophages and reactive oxygen products. *Lab. Invest.* 54:499–506, 1986.
46. Ward PA, Mulligan MS, Vaporciyan AA. Endothelial and leukocytic adhesion molecules in the pathogenesis of acute pulmonary injury. *Thrombosis Haemostasis* 70:155–157, 1993.
47. Johnson KJ, Rehan A, Ward PA. The role of oxygen radicals in kidney disease. In: Halliwell I, ed., *Oxygen Radicals and Tissue Injury: Proc. Upjohn Symp.* Bethesda, MD: FASEB Publications, 1988;115–121.
48. Simpson PJ, Fantone JC, Lunchessi BR. Myocardial ischemia and reperfusion Injury. Oxygen radicals and the role of the neutrophil. In: Halliwell I, ed., *Oxygen Radicals and Tissue Injury: Proc. Upjohn Symp.* Bethesda, MD: FASEB Publications, 1988;63–77.
49. Kelbanoff SJ, Clark RA, eds. *The Neutrophil: Function and Clinical Disorders.* New York: North Holland, 1978:74–75.

50. Mulligan MS, Desrochers PE, Chinnaiyan AM, Gibbs DF, Varani J, Johnson KJ, Weiss SJ. In vivo suppression of immune complex-induced alveolitis by secretory leukoproteinase inhibitor and tissue inhibitor of metalloproteinase-2. *Proc. Natl. Acad. Sci. (USA)* 90:11523–11527, 1993.

51. Harlan JM, Killen PD, Harker LA, Striker GE, Wright DG. Neutrophil mediated endothelial injury in vitro: Mechanisms of cell detachment. *J. Clin. Invest.* 68:1394–1399, 1981.

52. Harlan JM, Schwartz BR, Reidy MA, Schwartz SM, Ochs HD, Harker LA. Activated neutrophils disrupt endothelial monolayer integrity by an oxygen radical-independent mechanism. *Lab. Invest.* 52:141–150, 1985.

53. Sacks T, Moldow CF, Craddock PR, Bowers TK, Jacob HA. Oxygen radicals mediate endothelial cell damage by complement-stimulated granulocytes: An in vitro model of immune complex vasculitis. *J. Clin. Invest.* 61:1161–1167, 1978.

54. Weiss SJ, Young J, LoBuglio AF, Slivka A, Nimeh NF. Role of hydrogen peroxide in neutrophil-mediated destruction of cultured endothelial cells. *J. Clin. Invest.* 68:714–720, 1981.

55. Martin WJ. Neutrophils kill pulmonary endothelial cells by a hydrogen peroxide-dependent pathway: An in vitro model of neutrophil-mediated lung injury. *Am. Rev. Res. Dis.* 130:209–213, 1984.

56. Gannon DE, Varani J, Phan SH, Ward JH, Kaplan J, Till GO, Simon RH, Ryan US, Ward PA. Source of iron in neutrophil-mediated killing of endothelial cells *Lab. Invest.* 57:37–44, 1987.

57. Phan SH, Gannon DE, Varani J, Ryan US, Ward PA. Xanthine oxidase activity in rat pulmonary artery endothelial cells and its modulation by activated neutrophils. *Am. J. Pathol.* 134:1201–1211, 1989.

58. Rodell TC, Cheronis JC, Ohnemus CL, Piermattaei DJ, Repine JE. Xanthine oxidase mediates elastase induced injury to isolated lungs and endothelium *J. Appl. Physiol.* 63:2159–2163, 1987.

59. Terada LS, Guidot DM, Leff JA, Willingham IR, Hanley ME, Piermattei D, Repine JE. Hypoxia injures endothelial cells by increasing endogenous xanthine oxidase activity. *Proc. Natl. Acad. Sci. (USA)* 89:3362–3366, 1992.

60. Arnaout MA, Lanier LL, Faller DV. Relative contribution of the leukocyte molecules MO-1, LFA-1 and P-150.95 (leu M5) in adhesion of granulocytes and monocytes to vascular endothelium is tissue and stimulus-specific. *J. Cell Physiol.* 137:305–309, 1988.

61. Wencel ML, Morganroth ML, Schoeneich SO, Gannon DE, Varani J, Todd RF, Ryan US, Boxer LA. Cytoplasts and MO-1 deficient neutrophils pretreated with plasma and LPS induce lung injury. *Am. J. Physiol.* 256:H751–H759, 1989.

62. Marlin SD, Springer TA. Purified intercellular adhesion molecule-1 (ICAM-1) is a ligand for lymphocyte function-associated antigen-1 (LFA-1). *Cell* 51:813–819, 1987.

63. Mulligan MS, Varani J, Warren JS, Till GO, Smith CW, Anderson DC, Todd RF III, Ward PA. Roles of rats in integrin neutrophils in complement and oxygen radical mediated acute inflammatory reactions. *J. Immunol.* 148:1847–1857, 1992.

64. Varani J, Phan SH, Gibbs DF, Ryan US, Ward PA. H_2O_2-mediated cytotoxicity of rat pulmonary endothelial cells; Changes in adenosine triphosphate and purine products and effects of protective interventions. *Lab. Invest.* 63:683–689, 1990.

65. Jennings RB, Hawkings HK, Lowe JE, Hill ML, Klotman S, Reimer KA. Relationship between high energy phosphate and lethal injury in myocardial ischemia in dogs. *Am. J. Pathol.* 92:187–93, 1977.

66. Li Q, Huhl CM, Altschuld RA, Stokes BT. Energy depletion-repletion and calcium transients in single cardiomyocytes. *Am J. Physiol.* 257:427–434, 1989.

67. Kane AB, Petrovich DR, Stern RO, Farber JL. ATP depletion and loss of cell integrity in anoxic heptocytes and silica-treated P388D, macrophages. *Am. J. Physiol.* 249:256–262, 1985.

68. Phan SH, Gannon DE, Ward PA, Karmiol S. Mechanism of neutrophil-induced xanthine dehydrogenase to xanthine oxidase conversion in endothelial cells: Evidence for a role for elastase. *Am. J. Respir. Cell Mol. Biol.* 6:270–278, 1992.

69. Friedl HP, Till GO, Ryan US, Ward PA. Mediator-induced activation of xanthine oxidase in endothelial cells. *FASEB J.* 3:2512–2518, 1989.

70. Varani J, Dame MK, Gibbs DF, Taylor CG, Weinberg JM, Shayevitz J, Ward PA. Human umbilical vein endothelial cell killing by activated neutrophils. Loss of sensitivity to injury is accompanied by decreased iron content during in vitro culture and is restored with exogenous iron. *Lab. Invest.* 66:708–712, 1992.

71. Balla G, Vercellotti GM, Eaton JW, Jacob HS. Iron-loading of endothelial cells augments oxygen damage. *J. Lab Clin. Med.* 116:546–550, 1990.

72. Varani J, Ward PA. Mechanisms of neutrophil-dependent and neutrophil-independent endothelial cell injury. *Biol. Signals* 3:1–14, 1994.

73. Varani J, Ward PA. Mechanisms of endothelial cell injury in acute inflammation. *Shock* 2:311–319, 1994.
74. Farber JL, Kyle ME, Coleman JB. Biology of disease: Mechanisms of cell injury by activated oxygen species. *Lab. Invest.* 62:670–679, 1990.
75. Welgus HG, Campbell EJ, Zvi B-S, Senior RM, Teitelbaum SL. Human alveolar macrophages produce a fibroblast-like collagenase and collagenase inhibitor *J. Clin. Invest.* 76:219–224, 1985.
76. Busiek DF, Ross FP, McDonnell S, Murphy G, Matrisian LM, Welgus HG. The matrix metalloprotease matrilysin (PUMP) is expressed in developing human mononuclear phagocytes. *J. Biol. Chem.* 267:9087–9092, 1992.
77. Shapiro SD, Griffin GL, Gilbert DJ, Jenkins NA, Copeland NG, Welgus HG, Senior RM, Ley TJ. Molecular cloning, chromosomal localization, and bacterial expression of a murine macrophage metalloelastase. *J. Biol. Chem.* 267:4664–4671, 1992.
78. Vissers MCM, Winterbourn CC. The effect of oxidants on neutrophil-mediated degradation of glomerular basement membrane collagen. *Biochim. Biophys. Acta* 889:277–286, 1986.
79. McGowan SE, Murray JJ. Direct effects of neutrophil oxidants on elastase-induced extracellular matrix proteolysis. *Am. Rev. Respir. Dis.* 135:1286–1293, 1987.
80. Burkhardt H, Rehkope E, Kasten M, Rauls S, Heimann P. Interaction of polymorphonuclear leukocytes with cartilage in vitro: Catabolic effects of serine proteinases and oxygen radicals. *Scand. J. Rheumatol.* 17:183–195, 1988.
81. Varani J, Taylor CG, Riser B, Shumaker DK, Yeh K-Y, Dame M, Gibbs DF, Todd RF, Dumler F, Bromberg J, Killen PD. Mesangial cell killing by leukocytes: Role of leukocyte oxidants and proteolytic enzymes. *Kidney Int.* 42:1169–1177, 1992.
82. Guthrie LA, Johnson RB, Henson PM, Worthen GS. Neutrophil-mediated injury to endothelial cells: Enhancement by endotoxin and essential role of neutrophil elastase. *J. Clin. Invest.* 77:1233–1240, 1986.
83. Varani J, Ginburg I, Schuger L, Gibbs D, Bromberg J, Johnson KJ, Ryan US, Ward PA. Endothelial cell killing by neutrophils: Synergistic interaction of oxygen products and proteases. *Am. J. Pathol.* 135:435–438, 1989.
84. Ginsburg I, Gibbs DF, Schuger L, Johnson KJ, Ryan US, Ward PA, Varani J. Vascular endothelial cell killing by combination of membrane-active agents and hydrogen peroxide. *Free Radical Biol. Med.* 7:369–374, 1988.
85. Ginsburg I, Varani J. Interaction of viable group A streptococci and hydrogen peroxide in killing of vascular endothelial cells. *Free Radical Biol. Med.* 14:495–500, 1993.
86. Selsted ME, Szklorek D, Lehrer RI. Purification and antimicrobial activity of antimicrobial peptides of rabbit granulocytes. *Infect. Immun.* 45:150–159, 1984.
87. Ganz T. Extracellular release of antimicrobial defenses by human polymorphonuclear leukocytes. *Infect. Immun.* 56:568–574, 1987.
88. Weiss J, Victor M, Elsbach P. Role of charge and hydrophobic interactions in the action of bactericidal and permeability-increasing protein of neutrophils on gram negative bacteria. *J. Clin. Invest.* 71:540–548, 1983.
89. Ginsburg I. Cationic polyelectrolytes, a new look at their possible roles as opsonins, as stimulators of the respiratory burst in leukocytes, in bacteriolysis and as modulators of immune complex disease. *Inflammation* 11:489–515, 1987.
90. Leung DYM, Geha KS, Newburger JW, Burns JC, Fiers W, Lapierre LA, Pober JS. Two monokines, interleukin-1 and tumor necrosis factor, render cultured endothelial cells susceptible to lysis by antibodies circulating during Kawasaki syndrome *J. Exp Med.* 164:1958–1962, 1986.
91. Sato N, Goto T, Haranaka K, Satomi N, Sawasaki Y. Actions of tumor necrosis factor on cultured vascular endothelial cells: Morphologic modulation, growth inhibition and cytotoxicity. *J. Natl. Cancer Inst.* 76:1113–1117, 1986.
92. Schuger L, Varani J, Marks RM, Kunkel SL, Johnson KJ, Ward PA. Cytotoxicity of tumor necrosis factor-alpha for human umbilical vein endothelial cells. *Lab. Invest.* 61:62–67, 1989.
93. Varani J, Bendelow MJ, Sealey D, Gannon D, Ryan US, Kunkel SL, Ward PA. TNF-α induced susceptibility of endothelial cells to neutrophil-mediated killing. *Lab. Invest.* 59:292298, 1988.
94. Slungaard A, Vercellotti GM, Walker G, Nelson RD, Jacob HS. Tumor necrosis factor a/cachectin stimulates eosinophil oxidant production and toxicity toward human endothelium. *J. Exp. Med.* 171:2025–2041, 1990.
95. Matsubara T, Ziff M. Increased superoxide anion release from human endothelial cells in response to cytokines. *J. Immunol.* 137:3295–3298, 1986.

96. Radeke HH, Meier B, Topley N, Floge J, Habermehl GG, Resch K. Interleukin 1α and tumor necrosis factor-α induce oxygen radical production in mesangial cells. *Kidney Int.* 37:767–775, 1990.
97. Simon RH, Edwards JA, Reza MM, Kunkel RG. Injury to rat pulmonary alveolar epithelial cells by H_2O_2: Dependence on phenotype and catalase. *Amer. J. Physiol.* 1991;260:L318–L325.
98. Simon RH, DeHart PD, Todd RF III. Neutrophil-induced injury of rat pulmonary alveolar epithelial cells. *J. Clin. Invest.* 78:1373–1386, 1986.
99. Andreoli SP, McAtter JA. Reactive oxygen molecule mediated injury in endothelial and renal tubular epithelial cells in vitro. *Kidney Int.* 38:785–794, 1990.
100. Starke PE, Farber JL. Ferric iron and superoxide ions are required for the killing of cultured hepatocytes by hydrogen peroxide. *J. Biol. Chem.* 260:10099–10104, 1985.
101. Werns SW, Shea MJ, Driscoll EM, Cohen C, Abrans GD, Pitt B, Lucchesi BR. The independent effects of oxygen radical scavengers on canine infarct size. *Circ. Res.* 56:895–898, 1985.
102. McCord JM. Oxygen-derived free radicals in post-ischemic tissue injury. *N. Engl. J. Med.* 312:159–163, 1985.
103. Gabrielson EW, Rosen GM, Grafstrom RC, Strauss KE, Harris CC. Studies on the role of oxygen radicals in asbestos-induced cytopathology of cultured human lung mesothelial cells. *Carcinogenesis* 7:1161–1164, 1986.
104. Lemaire I. Characterization of the bronchoalveolar cellular response in experimental asbestosis: Different reactions depending on the fibrogenic potential. *Am. Rev. Respir. Dis.* 131:144–149, 1985.
105. Brody AR, Hill LH, Adkins B. Chrysolite asbestos inhalation in rats: Deposition pattern and reaction of alveolar epithelium and pulmonary macrophages *Am. Rev. Respir. Dis.* 123:670–679, 1981.
106. Pinkerton KE, Pratt PC, Brody AR, Crapo JE. Fiber localization and its relationship to lung reaction in rats after chronic inhalation of chrysolite asbestos. *Am. J. Pathol.* 117:484–493, 1984.
107. Gellert AR, Langford JA, Winter RJD, Uthayakumar S, Sinhag G, Rudd RM. Asbestosis: Assessment by bronchoalveolar lavage and measurement of pulmonary epithelial permeability. *Thorax* 40:508–514, 1985.
108. Jaurand MC, Kaplan H, Thiollet J, Pinchon MC, Bernardin JF, Bignon J. Phagocytosis of chrysotile fibers by pleural mesothelial cells in culture. *Am. J. Pathol.* 94:529–538, 1979.
109. Garcia JGN, Dodson RF, Callahan KS. Effect of environmental particulates on cultured human and bovine endothelium: Cellular injury via an oxidant-dependent pathway. *Lab. Invest.* 61:53–61, 1989.
110. Goodglick LA, Kane AB. Cytotoxicity of long and short crocidolite asbestos fibers in vitro and in vivo. *Cancer Res.* 50:5153–5163, 1990.
111. Gracie JGN, Gray LD, Dodson RF, Callahan KS. Asbestos-induced endothelial cell activation and injury: Demonstration of fiber phagocytosis and oxidant-dependent toxicity. *Am. Rev. Respir. Dis.* 138:958–964, 1988.
112. Amp DWG, Dunne M, Weitzman SA, Dunn MM. The interaction of asbestos and neutrophils injures cultured human pulmonary epithelial cells: Role of hydrogen peroxide. *J. Lab. Clin. Med.* 114:604–612, 1989.
113. Hobson J, Wright JL, Churg A. Active oxygen species mediate asbestos fiber uptake by tracheal epithelial cells. *FASEB J.* 4:3135–3139, 1990.
114. Mossman BT, Marsh JP, Shatos MA. Alteration of superoxide dismutase activity in tracheal epithelial cells by asbestos and inhibition of cytoxicity by antioxidants. *Lab. Invest.* 54:204–212, 1986.

PART IV

Molecular and Cellular Aspects of
Free-Radical Toxicity

Free Radical Toxicology
Edited by K. B. Wallace
Copyright © 1997 Taylor & Francis

16

Free-Radical-Mediated Alterations of Gene Expression by Xenobiotics

Cynthia R. Timblin, Yvonne M. W. Janssen,
and Brooke T. Mossman

*Department of Pathology, University of Vermont College of Medicine,
Burlington, Vermont, USA*

INTRODUCTION

A number of toxic agents can cause generation of free radicals either spontaneously, through metabolic pathways, and/or after interaction with cells. Cellular production of free radicals by agents may involve both direct interactions with macromolecules or indirect mechanisms involving a number of signaling cascades. At low doses of xenobiotics, free-radical reactions that may be deleterious are quelled by compensatory increases in antioxidant defenses by target cells of disease and/or cells of the immune system (1–3). Extracellular fluids such as serum, blood, and lavage fluids also contain a number of naturally occurring antioxidants, such as ceruloplasmin, ascorbate, extracellular superoxide dismutase (ECSOD), bilirubin, etc., which may quench free radical reactions before they affect cells (4–6). However, when the ratio of oxidative stress to antioxidant status becomes disproportional, alterations in gene expression and disease develop.

Although a number of xenobiotics generate free radicals, a direct and causal link between free radicals and the development of disease has been demonstrated in only a few animal models. These studies have focused on use of transgenic mice overexpressing antioxidant enzymes (7–9) and administration of antioxidants to rodents (reviewed in 6). Transfection of cells in vitro with antioxidant enzymes or addition of antioxidants to medium has also been helpful in determining whether cell injury is modified by agents such as paraquat, ionizing radiation, asbestos, and hyperoxia (10–13), but the relationship of cytotoxicity to disease is questionable.

Multiple pathways of production of free radicals by xenobiotics are depicted in Figure 1 for a typical target cell of free radical injury, an epithelial cell of the respiratory tract. This schema is provided to orient the reader to the complex nature of free-radical generation by xenobiotics, mechanisms of cell interaction with free

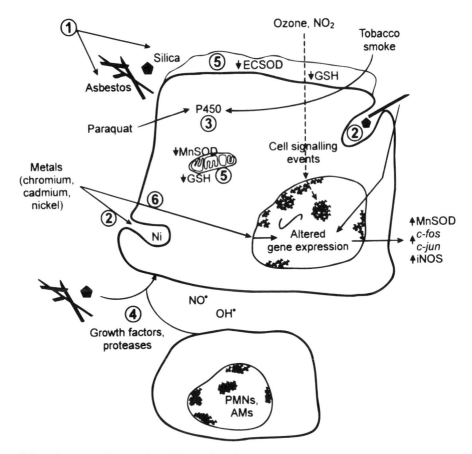

FIG. 1. Pathways of generation of free radicals by xenobiotics. The numbers denote processes occurring after exposure of epithelial cells of the lung to inhaled oxidants: (1) catalytic generation due to physicochemical composition; (2) partial or complete phagocytosis; (3) stimulation of P-450 or other metabolic pathways; (4) elicitation of an immune response (PMN, polymorphonuclear leukocyte; AM, alveolar macrophage; NO·, nitric oxide; OH·, hydroxyl radical); (5) depletion of antioxidant status (Mn-SOD, manganese-containing superoxide dismutase; GSH, glutathione; ECSOD, extracellular superoxide dismutase); (6) oxidative modifications of DNA, RNA, or proteins (iNOS, inducible nitric oxide synthase; NO_2, nitrogen dioxide).

radicals, and xenobiotic agents affecting lung that are associated with the causation of disease. It is clear that many inhaled pathogenic agents (tobacco smoke, silica, asbestos) may catalytically drive free-radical reactions either extracellularly or intracellularly due to their inherent chemical composition. For example, the amphibole type of asbestos, crocidolite $[Na_2(Fe^{3+})_2(Fe^{2+})_3Si_8O_{22}(OH_2)]$, has a high iron content, which generates OH· from H_2O_2 by a modified Haber–Weiss or Fenton reaction (14–16). Moreover, iron can be mobilized from fibers after their uptake by cells (17). Inhaled oxidant gases such as ozone may spontaneously produce free radicals that may affect lung lining fluids but may never enter cells directly because of rapid quenching or decomposition (18). Other agents including asbestos and chemicals in cigarette smoke may activate enzymatic metabolic pathways such as cytochrome P-450, resulting in oxidative stress (19), whereas particulates, such as crystalline nickel bisulfide and mineral dusts, are not metabolized, but may be phagocytized by cells and cause an oxidative burst (20,21). These reactions may be intrinsic to the recruitment of alveolar macrophages, neutrophils, and other cells of the immune system and the development of inflammation. Lastly, many xenobiotics may deplete antioxidant enzymes or glutathione stores, thus altering the redox status of the cell and making it more susceptible to oxidant-induced effects (22–24). These pathways may involve oxidative modification of DNA, RNA, and proteins.

Since other chapters in this volume cover selected examples of free-radical-mediated tissue damage including injury to lung as well as signal transduction cascades induced by free radicals, this chapter focuses on alterations in gene expression by xenobiotics that can be related to either the pathogenesis and/or hallmarks of the disease process. These include cell injury, proliferation, and the processes of fibrogenesis and carcinogenesis. Some information on gene expression related to antioxidant defense mechanisms also is discussed.

METALS

Exposure and Disease

Exposure to metal compounds in the workplace or domestic settings can give rise to a variety of acute syndromes as well as chronic diseases (25). A number of factors govern metal-induced cellular and organ effects. For instance, the type of metal, the chemical form, route of exposure, and mechanisms of uptake and excretion are all variables that modulate metal-induced cellular effects (25–29). Coexposure to various metals or occurrence of additional metal species also can enhance or antagonize metal toxicity. For instance, it has been demonstrated that zinc can antagonize the toxicity caused by exposure to cadmium (27), whereas magnesium antagonizes nickel-induced toxicity (29). This antagonistic action results from competition of zinc and magnesium with binding sites for cadmium or nickel, respectively, that are present on key proteins or enzymes. Thus, cellular or tissue concentrations of these essential trace elements are critical in determination of the ultimate toxic effects of metals.

A wide variety of pathological effects is observed following metal exposure. For instance, in occupationally exposed populations a number of cancers and disorders of the respiratory system are observed, as well as pathologies in other organs. Exposure to nickel is associated with nasal cavity, lung, kidney, stomach, and pharyngeal cancers. Other pathological effects of nickel exposure include dermatitis and asthma-like attacks (29). Limited evidence exists for a carcinogenic effect of cadmium (27). However, cadmium exposure has been causally linked to development of chronic respiratory disease including chronic bronchitis, progressive massive fibrosis, and alveolar damage (27). Although metals such as chromium and iron are essential to normal cellular function, excessive exposure can also cause disease (17,25,26). Occupational exposure to chromium is linked to allergic dermatitis and respiratory and nasal cancer. Iron overload is associated with development of cirrhosis, hepatocellular carcinoma, and colorectal tumors.

Although a number of metals appear to cause toxicity as a result of their unique interaction with specific proteins to deregulate their normal function, considerable evidence suggests that free radicals may participate in metal-induced damage (26). Some metals appear to catalyze free-radical formation in redox-cycling reactions (i.e., iron, chromium). Other metal compounds (i.e., cadmium) cause oxidant stress due to their ability to interact with protein thiols, changing the redox state of the cell. Studies employing antioxidant compounds have demonstrated that these agents can ameliorate metal-induced damage to macromolecules, therefore confirming that free radicals may be key players in metal-induced damage to cells or tissues (25,26).

Metals and Gene Expression

Upon exposure to metal compounds, target cells may respond by reprogramming expression of genes with differing functions. The classes of genes induced may dictate the fate of the cell. Metal-induced damage, cell death, growth arrest, and/or cell proliferation are distinct events that occur after exposure to a number of metabolic stresses and require activation of signal transduction cascades and upregulation of regulatory genes that may be important in adaptation and defense (3).

The exact mechanisms of gene activation by metals and consequent alterations in cell function are unclear. An increasing body of evidence suggests that free radicals may be involved in the reprogramming of gene expression triggered by metals (26). In this respect, some genes induced by a variety of metal compounds encode proteins with antioxidant functions. Upregulation of metallothionein, hemeoxygenase, or manganese-containing superoxide dismutase (Mn-SOD) is though to be indicative of oxidative stress. Proteins encoded by these genes have antioxidant or metal binding functions, thereby limiting the formation of free radical reactions or conditions of oxidant stress.

Cadmium

The metal cadmium has served as a model compound to examine alterations in expression of stress-responsive genes that can also occur after exposure to other metal compounds or free radicals. Exposure to cadmium causes upregulation of a variety of genes that include antioxidant proteins, stress proteins indicative of protein toxicity, or proto-oncogenes (27). For instance, striking increases in gene expression of metallothionein have been observed following exposure to cadmium in a variety of cell systems or tissues. Specific metal-regulatory transcription factors (MTF) (30) that bind to metal-responsive promoter elements (MRE) control the upregulation of metallothionein genes (31). It is believed that metallothionein, a sulfhydryl molecule with a high affinity for cadmium binding, prevents cadmium from interacting with macromolecules that may trigger genotoxic and carcinogenic effects of cadmium (25,27). Testicular cells, target cells of cadmium-induced tumors in rodents, show a relative lack of induction of metallothionein, which may contribute to the carcinogenic process (32). Increased expression of metallothionein observed in other cells or organs plays an important role in the cellular defense system against cadmium toxicity (27,33).

Hemeoxygenase is an enzyme that catalyzes breakdown of heme to biliverdin. Subsequent action of biliverdin reductase converts biliverdin to bilirubin, a protein with antioxidant properties. Thus activation of hemeoxygenase represents a protective mechanism against free radicals by reducing heme pools, which can provide iron for Fenton reactions (34). Investigation of hemeoxygenase mRNA levels has demonstrated that agents that generate free radicals or deplete glutathione pools induce hemeoxygenase efficiently (35). Thus, increased mRNA levels of hemeoxygenase are indicative of an oxidant stress response. Studies in our laboratory employing rat lung epithelial cells have revealed that exposure to 10 μM cadmium induces mRNA levels of hemeoxygenase after 1, 2, 4, and 16 h of exposure (Figure 2). In addition, exposure of rats to cadmium aerosols causes increases in mRNA and protein levels of metallothionein in type II epithelial cells (33). These data indicate that epithelial cells of the lung are capable of mounting an oxidant stress response following exposure to cadmium. However, other cell types of the lung may be more sensitive to the toxicity of cadmium. For example, cadmium causes progressive alveolar fibrosis in rats, which is preceded by an inflammatory response (36). Moreover, gene expression studies in lung have revealed upregulation of the inflammatory gene cathepsin L, a marker gene of macrophage activation, after exposure to cadmium (36). Furthermore, exposure of inflammatory cells (i.e., neutrophils) to cadmium in vitro results in increased mRNA levels of the inflammatory gene interleukin-8 (IL-8), which are accompanied by increased production of superoxide

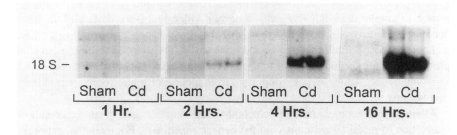

FIG. 2. Upregulation of mRNA levels of hemeoxygenase in rat lung epithelial cells exposed to cadmium (Cd). Rat lung epithelial cells were exposed to 10 μM of $CdCl_2$ for 1, 2, 4, or 16 h and harvested for extraction of RNA (22). Northern blot analysis was performed using a hemeoxygenase cDNA probe (34). Note the increases in hemeoxygenase mRNA levels in cadmium-exposed cells that are apparent at the early time points and become more pronounced after 16 h of exposure.

(O_2^-) (37). Preexposure to the antioxidant and glutathione precursor N-acetyl-L cysteine prevents cadmium-induced expression of IL-8 or release of O_2^- (37), suggesting that cadmium-induced oxidant stress may be involved in upregulation of inflammatory genes that may contribute to cadmium-induced lung damage.

In cadmium-exposed rat lungs, increased expression of procollagen alpha 1-(I) and -(III) are observed (36). These molecular changes correlate with an almost complete filling of the alveolar spaces with fibroblasts and collagen, a hallmark of progressive pulmonary fibrosis (36). These data indicate that the fibroblast is a major target cell cadmium-induced lung disease in the rat.

A number of other genes induced by cadmium appear to reflect proteotoxicity. For instance, induction of heat-shock genes (HSP60, 68, and 70) is observed after exposure to cadmium in a variety of cell types (38–42). Induction of HSP70 by cadmium is modulated by glutathione levels, suggesting a role for free radicals in upregulation of this gene (38). Increases in HSP70 mRNA are mediated by increased binding of the heat-shock factor activator protein to the heat-shock DNA regulatory element (HSE) that is present in the promoter region of the HSP70 gene (40). In addition, dissociation of the negative regulator constitutive HSE-binding factor (CHBF) that normally is bound to the HSE is triggered by cadmium (42). Both of these events are responsible for upregulation of HSP70 mRNA levels. Induction of HSP68 by cadmium is observed under conditions where general protein synthesis in the cell is already shut down, indicating preferential induction of HSP by cadmium (41). The exact roles of HSPs are unclear, but appear to involve chaperoning of damaged proteins to specific sites within the cell (43).

A novel stress-induced protein was isolated in mouse peritoneal macrophages following exposure to cadmium or other oxidative or sulfhydryl-reactive compounds (44). This protein, designated macrophage 23-kD stress protein, MSP23, has homology to the antioxidant, alkylhydroperoxide reductase. These results further indicate that free radicals may be involved in the cadmium-mediated induction of stress proteins.

The signaling pathways that are induced by cadmium upstream of alterations in gene expression are unclear. Studies investigating cadmium-induced hypertrophic responses employing NRK-49F cells, a normal kidney rat fibroblast cell line, have demonstrated increases in mRNA levels of the early response genes, c-*fos*, c-*jun*, and c-*myc* (45,46). Inhibitors of protein kinase C (PKC) abolished cadmium-induced proto-oncogene expression, suggesting an involvement of PKC in cadmium-induced signaling events, which may be important in induction of hypertrophy or proliferation (45,46).

Alterations in gene expression induced by cadmium can also occur as a result of interaction of metal compounds with the genetic machinery. For example, exposure to cadmium causes formation of a number of alterations in DNA that include single-strand breaks, DNA protein cross-links, and lesions that lead to frameshift mutations (27). DNA damage by cadmium also triggers increased mRNA levels of O_6-methyl-guanine DNA methyltransferase in hepatoma cells (47). This DNA repair enzyme is induced by a variety of environmental stresses that induce DNA strand breaks, including agents that are free radical generators, and is involved in protection against genotoxic agents.

Nickel

A number of other molecular events are observed after exposure to selective metal compounds that ultimately lead to alterations in gene expression. For instance, crystalline nickel compounds, once taken up by cells, can enter the nucleus and bind to specific regions in heterochromatin. Protein–DNA cross-links then occurs that ultimately lead to decondensation of chromatin and loss of genetic information (20,25,29,48). In addition, changes in chromatin structure also can lead to alterations in patterns of DNA methylation. Increased DNA methylation patterns can result in silencing of genes in an inherited, irreversible fashion (49). Some of the known consequences of nickel interactions with chromatin include inactivation of a senescence gene and cell transformation (48). Examples of gene silencing or altered functions of gene products caused by nickel are thrombospondin (50) and the retinoblastoma protein (51), proteins involved in inhibition of angiogenesis and endothelial cell migration (50) and cell cycle regulation (51), respectively.

Chromium

Chromium compounds can damage DNA through mechanisms that may involve free radicals (25,26,28). Moreover, chromium, due to its ability to bind to DNA and regulatory enzymes, can decrease the fidelity of DNA polymerase during replication and increases its processivity (52). In addition, synthesis of mRNA occurs in vitro by nonspecific initiation when chromium is bound to DNA. A number of studies that employ different cell systems have demonstrated that chromium alters the expression of a number of hormonally or chemically inducible genes such as metallothionein (53) and phosphoenolpyruvate carboxykinase (PEPCK) (54).

Metals and Gene Regulation

Table 1 summarizes a number of alterations in gene expression observed following exposure of cells to metals. In some cases, metal-induced oxidant stress may be involved as indicated by the function of the gene product (i.e., MnSOD) and/or similarities in induction patterns triggered with use of free radical generating systems. Some genes that are affected by metals encode DNA repair enzymes (47), antioxidant proteins (31,33–35), or stress proteins (38–42) that signal protein damage. Limited studies in whole animals also provide evidence for metal-induced activation of inflammatory cascades producing oxidants, a feature of many metal-induced diseases (36,37). However, studies are needed in vitro to provide insight into cell signaling

TABLE 1. *Classes of genes induced by metal compounds*

Antioxidant proteins:	(MnSOD)
	Heme oxygenase
	Metallothionein
Inflammatory proteins:	Cathepsin-L
	Interleukin-8
Proteins involved in proliferation:	c-Fos
	c-Jun
	c-Myc
Proteins in tissue remodeling:	Procollagen alpha-1 (I)
	Procollagen alpha-1 (III)
Stress proteins:	HSP60
	HSP68
	HSP70
	Macrophage 23-kD stress protein (MSP23)
DNA repair enzymes:	O_6-Methylguanine DNA methyltransferase

Note. A number of genes encoding proteins with different functions are upregulated after exposure to selected metal compounds. Most studies on gene expression have utilized cadmium. However, since a number of these genes are induced by oxidants it is conceivable that a number of metal compounds that cause oxidative stress also upregulate expression of these genes.

cascades that are triggered by metal compounds and how alterations in gene expression may be involved in disease.

PARAQUAT

Metabolic Activation and Toxicity

Free radicals generated by a diverse group of exogenous chemical agents are linked to the pathogenesis of various lung diseases. Many of these cytotoxic and/or carcinogenic chemicals require activation by cellular metabolic pathways in order to mediate their toxic effects. Individual cells in the lung (i.e., Clara cells, bronchial and alveolar epithelial cells) contain the cytochrome P-450 monooxygenase system that functions in the detoxification of drugs and xenobiotics (55). In the process of detoxification, many chemicals are converted into a more toxic and reactive form than the parent compound. These reactive forms can mutate DNA, thereby activating protooncogenes or inactivating tumor suppressor genes, and interact with components of signaling cascades leading to alterations in gene expression. Reactive intermediates are the mediators of the cytotoxic effects of many pulmonary toxicants including paraquat and certain components in tobacco smoke.

Paraquat (1,1'-dimethyl-4,4'-bipyridinium), a commonly used herbicide, produces lung damage even when administered by routes in which exposure of the lung is secondary (56). Clinical features of paraquat poisoning include pulmonary edema and fibrosis (57). Pathologically, disease development is divided into two distinct phases: the destructive phase and the proliferative phase (57). The destructive phase is characterized by loss of type I and type II epithelial cells, infiltration of inflammatory cells, and the development of hemorraghic pulmonary edema. The proliferative phase is characterized by proliferation of fibroblasts, excessive collagen deposition, loss of lung function, and the development of fibrosis.

The toxicity of paraquat is mediated through the production of free radicals via cyclic reduction–oxidation reactions (56,57). Paraquat is actively imported by pneumocytes and metabolized by NADPH cytochrome P-450 reductase to a reduced form, the monocation radical ($PQ^{\cdot+}$) (56,58,59) (Figure 3). Reaction of the paraquat radical with molecular oxygen generates O_2^- and regenerates paraquat (PQ^{2+}), which can be reduced again. Subsequent reactions of O_2^- leads to the formation of H_2O_2 and generation of the highly reactive OH, which can react with a number of cellular macromolecules including lipids, nucleic acids, and proteins (56,60,61). Another aspect of the toxicity of paraquat is the depletion of cellular NADPH (56,57). NADPH is consumed by the reduction of paraquat and other cellular enzyme systems that serve to detoxify O_2^-. Depletion of cellular reducing equivalents changes the redox status of the cell, promoting conditions of oxidative stress and leading to changes in transcription factor activation and gene expression (62,63).

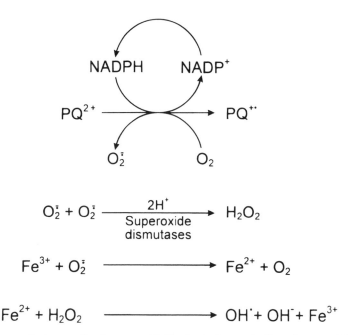

FIG. 3. Free radical generation by paraquat. Single-electron reduction of paraquat (PQ^+) by NADPH-dependent cytochrome P-450 produces the paraquat radical ($PQ^{\cdot+}$). Spontaneous reaction of $PQ^{\cdot+}$ with molecular oxygen (O_2) regenerates paraquat, which can undergo repeated cycles of reduction–oxidation (redox cycle). Dismutation of superoxide (O_2^-) by superoxide dismutases generates hydrogen peroxide (H_2O_2). Subsequent reactions with iron (Fe^{3+}) can convert O_2^- and H_2O_2 to the very reactive hydroxyl radical (OH').

Importance of Free Radicals

The importance of reactive oxygen intermediates in the pathogenesis of paraquat-induced disease is emphasized in studies examining the role of antioxidant enzymes. Studies in vitro using established cell lines demonstrate that exposure to paraquat results in an increase in activity of two antioxidant enzymes, MnSOD and copper-zinc-containing superoxide dismutase (CuZnSOD) (64). Furthermore, induction of MnSOD activity by the cytokine tumor necrosis factor-α (TNFα) protects cells from the toxic effects of paraquat (65). A direct link between induction of SOD activity and resistance to paraquat was demonstrated in experiments in which cells that overexpress SOD from a transfected plasmid were shown to be more resistant to cytotoxicity when exposed to paraquat (64). Studies in animal models demonstrate increased amounts of a second radical-scavenging protein, metallothionein, in the lungs of animals exposed to paraquat (66).

Induction of SODs, enzymes, and other free-radical scavengers is thought to be one mechanism by which cells eliminate reactive oxygen species and ameliorate toxicity induced by paraquat. Production of free radicals in excess of antioxidant defenses may lead to cytotoxicity and cell death or aberrant gene expression, unregulated cell proliferation, and development of disease. The precise mechanism by which paraquat-induced free radicals mediate cell death or induce the proliferation of pulmonary fibroblasts is not known. However, many of the endpoints of paraquat-induced toxicity (i.e., cell death or increased cell proliferation) are also seen in other models of free-radical-mediated lung disease and thus are likely to occur through similar mechanisms.

Tobacco Smoke

Tobacco smoke, which is implicated in the development of both malignant (lung cancer) and nonmalignant (chronic bronchitis and emphysema) lung disease, contains a complex mixture of smoke-borne free radicals and metabolizable aromatic hydrocarbons that mediate oxidative damage to cells and tissues (67). Considerable evidence links the production of free radicals to the toxicity and pathogenicity of tobacco smoke (67,68). A number of sources of free radicals occur in tobacco smoke (67). Oxygen- and carbon-centered free radicals are generated during the combustion of tobacco, but these species are thought to be too reactive and short-lived to be of biological consequence in the absence of further reactions with other smoke constituents. Reaction of nitrogen oxides with other components in smoke to form more reactive intermediates is postulated to be another mechanism of generation of free radicals (67). Polycyclic aromatic hydrocarbons (PAH) present in tobacco smoke are another source of oxidants. These compounds are metabolized by cytochrome P-450 enzyme systems and consequently are an intracellular source of free radicals (69). In addition to smoke-derived free radicals, components of tobacco smoke elicit an inflammatory response, and the release of reactive oxygen species from these cell types (i.e., neutrophils, macrophages) can contribute to the disease process (70).

The chemical complexity of tobacco smoke makes it extremely difficult to define the precise molecular mechanisms involved in the toxicology and pathogenicity of smoke-induced diseases. As described earlier, a number of components in tobacco smoke or their metabolic conversion by cellular pathways create an environment of oxidative stress. In vitro studies using aqueous fractions of tobacco smoke or isolated components of smoke and established cell lines have provided some insight into molecular responses triggered by smoke. Exposure of cells to water-soluble tobacco smoke fractions leads to increased expression of the gene encoding hemeoxygenase, a small, cytoplasmic protein that indirectly acts as an antioxidant (71,72). Increased gene expression correlates with increased amounts of hemeoxygenase protein, suggesting a functional role for hemeoxygenase in antioxidant defense against smoke-induced oxidative stress. As is observed with a number of chemicals that induce hemeoxygenase, the mechanism of smoke-induced hemeoxygenase gene expression is linked to the redox status of the cell. Cells exposed to tobacco smoke are depleted of the free-radical scavenger glutathione, and stabilization of glutathione pools with exogenous cysteine blocks induction of hemeoxygenase gene expression (71). Tobacco smoke also induces transcription of the protooncogene c-*fos* and increases the amount of Fos protein in cells (72). As early response genes such as c-*fos* are involved in the regulation of cell proliferation, increased transcription and translation of proliferation-related genes in response to tobacco smoke may be one mechanism contributing to carcinogenesis.

AH-Receptor Genes

One of the best characterized examples of tobacco smoke-induced alterations of gene expression is the induction of Ah-receptor-regulated (aryl hydrocarbon receptor) genes by polycyclic aromatic hydrocarbons (PAH). PAHs are potent promutagens and procarcinogens that are oxidized by cytochrome P-450 into reactive intermediates that can cause oxidative DNA damage and initiation of mutagenic events responsible for tumor initiation and development (69,73,74). PAHs are ligands for the Ah-receptor, and thus, the Ah-receptor and its activities are directly linked to the toxicological and carcinogenic effects of these compounds (69,75). In its inactive form, the Ah-receptor is complexed in the cytoplasm with specific proteins that maintain the receptor in its ligand binding conformation (Figure 4). Upon ligand binding, the Ah-receptor dissociates from its cytoplasmic partners and dimerizes with a second protein called ARNT (Ah-receptor-nuclear-translocator), which translocates to the nucleus and binds to specific DNA sequences located in the promoter region of Ah-receptor-responsive genes. This then activates gene transcription (69,75). Thus, the Ah-receptor functions as a ligand-activated transcription factor. Genes that are regulated by the Ah-receptor are divided into two classes: (1) drug (xenobiotic) metabolizing enzymes [i.e., cytochrome P-450, glutathione *S*-transferase Ya subunit, UDP-glucuronosyltransferase, NADP(H):oxidoreductase], and (2) gene products that regulate cell differentiation and proliferation (TGFα and -β,

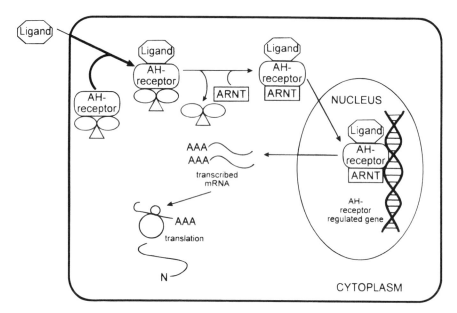

FIG. 4. Ah-receptor-mediated induction of gene transcription. The Ah-receptor is complexed in the cytoplasm to specific proteins that maintain the receptor in its ligand binding conformation. Upon ligand binding (e.g., PAHs), the Ah-receptor dissociates from its cytoplasmic partners and complexes with the translocator protein ARNT. The Ah-receptor/ARNT complex translocates to the nucleus, binds specifically to defined DNA sequence elements located in the promoter region of Ah-receptor-regulated genes, and activates gene transcription. Newly transcribed mRNAs are translated into proteins that mediate various cellular events.

c-*fos*, c-*jun*) (69,75). Many of these Ah-receptor-regulated genes have fundamental roles in normal cell physiology, but aberrant regulation of their expression may be a mechanism of the toxic or carcinogenic effect of PAHs.

TCDD (2,3,7,8-Tetrachlorodibenzo-*p*-dioxin)

Many of the studies on regulation of Ah-receptor activity and gene transcription have employed TCDD (2,3,7,8-tetrachlorodibenzo-*p*-dioxin) as the inducing ligand. TCDD is a halogenated aromatic hydrocarbon produced as a by-product during the synthesis of the herbicide 2,4,5-trichlorophenoxyacetic acid (2,4,5-T) (56). TCDD is a potent inducer of cytochrome P-450 gene transcription and a number of other genes regulated by the Ah-receptor (76). In contrast to PAHs, TCDD is not oxidized by cytochrome P-450 and consequently does not act as a mutagen, but mediates its effects through epigenetic mechanisms (56,77). Exposure of cells in vitro to TCDD results in increased steady-state mRNA levels of the protooncogenes c-*jun* and c-*fos*, and increased DNA-binding activity of the transcription factor AP-1 (77). Early response c-*jun* and c-*fos* genes that encode subunits of AP-1 are important components of the regulatory system controlling cell proliferation. Aberrant expression of these genes may be one mechanism by which TCDD and related compounds (i.e., PAHs) mediate their carcinogenic effects.

TCDD-induced transcriptional activation is thought to be mediated by reactive oxygen species. A number of in vitro studies have demonstrated that activation of the AH-receptor by TCDD induces transcription of the gene encoding cytochrome P-450, *CYP1A1* (69,76,78). Cytochrome P-450 has been shown to catalyze the oxidative degradation of arachidonic acid, a major membrane phospholipid, a process that generates free radicals and alters the redox status of the cell (79,80). *N*-Acetyl-L-cysteine can block TCDD-induced gene transcription, suggesting that excessive production of oxidants is a likely mechanism of TCDD-dependent transcriptional activation (80).

In summary, the production of excessive amounts of free radicals by cellular metabolic pathways is a key component in the development of chemically induced lung disease by paraquat and tobacco smoke. Metabolic conversion of chemical agents generates reactive intermediates that can interact with various cellular macromolecules. The cell responds to intracellular changes in redox status by activating cellular defense systems. Toxic agents such as paraquat and PAHs also elicit increased production of antioxidant defense enzymes that function to eliminate free radicals. Excessive production of reactive molecules that can occur during redox cycling (i.e., by paraquat) or following activation of metabolizing enzymes (i.e., tobacco smoke) may overwhelm antioxidant defenses and lead to free radical-mediated cytotoxicity and cell death. Free radicals also mediate the aberrant induction of genes involved in the regulation of cell proliferation (62). Unregulated cell proliferation is a hallmark of carcinogenesis and critical to the disease process (81,82).

OXIDANT GASES

Exposure and Lung Disease

The human lung can encounter a number of distinct reactive gases. For instance, in urban areas where formation of photochemical smog occurs, exposure to ozone, nitrogen dioxide, organic intermediates, and other reactive gases is an unavoidable result (83,84). Inhalation of these gases can lead to a variety of pulmonary disorders such as inflammatory diseases, bronchitis, edema, airway hypersensitivity, pulmonary fibrosis, and, potentially, lung cancers (83,84).

Free Radicals and Gene Expression

Various free-radical species occur in oxidant gases. Furthermore, a number of chemical reactions occur upon interaction of these reactive species with other reactive intermediates in extracellular lining fluid or cells (83,84). In addition, pulmonary target cells exposed to ozone respond with increases in release of nitric oxide

(NO) and H_2O_2, causing formation of additional free radical species (85,86). The complexity of these reactions makes evaluation of the critical free-radical species important in disease difficult.

The mechanisms by which free radicals in oxidant gases (or their reactive metabolites) damage the lung are unclear. In animal studies and cells in vitro, expression of a number of genes is upregulated in response to oxidant gases. These genes encode proteins with antioxidant properties, inflammatory mediators, and proteins involved in tissue remodeling and secretion of mucin.

Ozone

Ozone has been used as a model oxidant gas to study alterations in gene expression and mechanisms of disease. Exposure to ozone or other gases causes acute damage to the airway epithelium, characterized by denudation of bronchial epithelial cells followed by compensatory proliferation and an inflammatory response (83). Examination of inflammatory cascades has revealed upregulation of a number of genes that are involved in generation of the inflammatory response. For instance, inhalation of ozone or sulfur dioxide causes increases in MIP-2 mRNA levels in tracheal or whole-lung homogenates (87,88). This chemokine mediates recruitment of neutrophils to the site of cell damage. Increases in mRNA levels of TNF and interleukin-1 occur in macrophages from ozone-exposed rats (85). Increased expression of the inducible form of nitric oxide synthase, also is observed in type II epithelial cells obtained from rat lung exposed to ozone (85,86). This is accompanied by increases in nitric oxide release, as well as release of H_2O_2 and reactive oxygen metabolites with an important function in clearance of inhaled pathogens. However, these reactive species also have the ability to modify expression of a wide variety of genes on their own.

The transcription factor nuclear factor kappa B (NF-κB) controls the expression of a number of inflammatory genes, including MIP-2 and nitric oxide synthase, and may thus be critical in regulation of the inflammatory response (89,90). Examination of human bronchial epithelial cells has demonstrated that pyrogallol, a chemical-generating system of oxidants, activates NF-κB and is accompanied by increased expression of nitric oxide synthase mRNA levels (91). These findings, as well as research in other model systems, corroborate the role of NF-κB in the inflammatory response that occurs in lung after exposure to oxidant gases.

As mentioned previously, upregulation of antioxidant proteins following an oxidative insult may protect cells or tissues from excessive damage. Increased expression of mRNA levels of the antioxidants CuZnSOD, catalase, and glutathione peroxidase occurs in ozone-exposed rat lungs (92). Accompanying increases in enzymatic activities that are observed may serve to protect the lung tissue from ozone-induced toxicity. Increases in mRNA and activity of MnSOD by endotoxin, without affecting activities of the other antioxidant enzymes, resulted in protection against ozone-induced lipid peroxidation and lung edema, suggesting that this antioxidant enzyme may be important in protection against oxidant-induced lung damage (93).

Bronchitis is one of the pulmonary disorders that occurs after inhalation of oxidant gas. Proliferation of mucous (goblet) cells and hypersecretion of mucus characterize the transformation of control airway epithelium to a mucus-cell metaplasia phenotype (94). This phenotype is induced by ozone and sulfur dioxide and is accompanied by increased mRNA levels of the mucin gene (95). Thus, early increases in gene expression of mucin in airways may signal development of bronchitis.

To study mechanisms of airway remodeling that occur after exposure to ozone, mRNA levels of fibronectin, type 1 collagen, and alpha 1(I) procollagen were measured in rat lungs. Increases in mRNA levels of these genes were apparent after exposure to ozone (96,97). In situ hybridization studies revealed focal increases in alpha 1 (I) procollagen in the lung parenchyma at the septal tips and the bronchiolar–alveolar duct junctions (97). The products of these genes contribute to pulmonary fibrosis, another endpoint of oxidant-gas-induced lung disease.

In summary, several lung disorders occur after exposure to oxidant gases. The development of these diseases in animal models is accompanied by increases in expression of a number of genes that appear to reflect these events. Increased mRNA levels of inflammatory mediators, mucin, and extracellular matrix constituents therefore appear to be indicative of oxidant-gas-induced lung disease.

ASBESTOS AND SILICA

Disease Causation After Inhalation of Minerals

Mineral dusts such as asbestos and silica are associated with the development of fibrotic pulmonary disease (98–100). The pathogenicity and the development of lung disease are dependent on both the chemical composition and the physical properties of the individual mineral dusts inhaled. Asbestos, a family of mineral silicate fibers, is subdivided into two major classes: serpentine, of which chrysotile is the only type, and amphibole, which includes crocidolite, amosite, tremolite, anthophyllite, and actinolite (98,99). These fibers differ in their physical and chemical composition, factors that may be important in the pathogenicity of each fiber type. Chrysotile is a curly, less durable fiber that often occurs in bundles. In contrast, amphiboles are needle-like and more durable in lung. A number of nonfibrous silica particulates (such as Minusil-5, quartz, and cristobalite) occur naturally or as contaminants with other minerals. These various polymorphs also differ in their ability to cause lung disease (101).

Inhalation of asbestos fibers or silica particles is associated with the development of asbestosis or silicosis, respectively (98,100). In addition, exposure to asbestos is linked to the development of bronchogenic carcinoma and malignant mesothelioma (98). Common features of mineral dust-induced diseases are chronic inflammation and unregulated proliferation of target cells of the lung and/or pleura (81,82,98,99,102). Development of pulmonary fibrosis is characterized by excessive collagen deposition, progressive lung stiffening, impaired gas exchange, disability, and death. Asbestos-induced lung cancer (bronchogenic carcinoma) originates in tracheobronchial epithelial cells or alveolar epithelial cells, whereas malignant meso-thelioma is a fatal tumor arising from mesothelial cells or mesenchymal cells of the pleura, pericardium, and peritoneum. Mesothelioma and possibly bronchogenic carcinoma are more prevalent in workers exposed to crocidolite asbestos due to its high iron content and persistence in the lung (98,99).

Minerals and Free Radicals

The mechanisms of mineral dust-induced diseases are not clearly understood. Many mineral dust-induced biologic effects appear to be mediated by the production of reactive oxygen species (103–105). These free radicals are liberated from redox reactions catalyzed directly on the surface of asbestos fibers or silica particles. Alternatively, release of reactive oxygen intermediates from inflammatory cells is observed during the inflammatory response that is triggered in lungs by mineral dusts. For instance, in animal models of asbestos-induced disease, asbestos fibers are phagocytized by alveolar macrophages and neutrophils (21,106). Phagocytosis of asbestos fibers by these cells and target cells of disease both in vivo and in vitro induces a respiratory burst and release of reactive oxygen species. Longer fibers, which are not completely engulfed by phagocytic cells, result in "frustrated phagocy-tosis" and may serve as chronic stimuli for release of reactive oxygen intermediates from phagocytes. The release of cytokines such as TNF and interleukin-1 from alveolar macrophages and other cell types during the inflammatory response may also contribute to oxidative injury by asbestos or silica (107,108).

Generation of free radicals through redox reactions catalyzed by iron may also be important in mineral dust-induced disease. Iron present on the surface of asbestos fibers or on silica particles after adsorption can drive the formation of OH· from O_2^- and H_2O_2 (14,16,109). The amount of free radicals produced is directly related to the iron content of the mineral dust. Pretreatment of asbestos (15,106,110,111) or silica (109) with iron chelators ameliorates the cytotoxic effects of these minerals on cells, implicating iron in the process of free-radical generation. Therefore, the pathogenicity of different types of mineral dusts may be linked to their iron content.

The importance of oxygen free-radicals in the pathogenesis of asbestos or silica-induced disease is further highlighted by studies performed in vitro and in vivo. Studies in vitro using cultures of pulmonary target cells have demonstrated that asbestos-induced cytotoxicity can be ameliorated by concomitant exposure to antiox-idants (112). In animal models, administration of polyethylene glycol-conjugated catalase, a scavenger of reactive oxygen intermediates, during inhalation of asbestos ameliorates pulmonary toxicity, inflammation, and the development of asbestosis (102). Thus, the importance of free radicals in asbestos-induced disease is firmly established. However, it is not clearly understood how asbestos and free radicals interact with cells at the molecular level to cause alterations in cell growth or how these pathways lead to development of disease.

Gene Expression Studies

Considerable evidence links free radicals to asbestos-induced expression of genes involved in antioxidant defense and cell proliferation. In rodent models of pulmonary fibrosis, inhalation of high concentrations (7–10 mg/m^3 air) of asbestos or silica causes inflammation and development of fibrosis, which is associated with increased steady-state mRNA levels of genes encoding the antioxidant enzymes MnSOD, CuZnSOD, and glutathione peroxidase (113,114). Moreover, the induction of MnSOD, mRNA and protein levels correlates directly with the extent of the inflammatory response triggered by minerals. Furthermore, development of disease in inhalation models is also associated with increased steady-state mRNA levels of the proliferation-associated genes, c-*jun*, and the gene encoding ornithine decarboxylase (ODC) (114). c-*jun* is a member of a multigene family that is transiently induced in response to a variety of stimuli and encodes subunits (Jun homodimers or Jun/Fos heterodimers) of the transcription factor AP-1, discussed previously. ODC is an essential enzyme in the biosynthesis of polyamines required for cell proliferation (115). In contrast to crocidolite, exposure to chrysotile asbestos elicits significantly increased steady-state mRNA levels only for MnSOD (but not proliferation-related genes) highlighting the importance of fiber composition and geometry in changes in gene expression (116).

Model systems employing cultures of rodent tracheal epithelial and pleural mesothelial cells have been used to examine the cellular and molecular events triggered by asbestos-generated free radicals. In pleural mesothelial cells, exposure to crocidolite asbestos causes increased expression of the antioxidants MnSOD and hemeoxygenase (22). Both crocidolite and chrysotile asbestos cause dose-dependent and persistent increases in the expression of c-*fos* and c-*jun* in pleural mesothelial cells, and c-*jun* expression in tracheal epithelial cells (117). In tracheal epithelial cells, exposure to crocidolite asbestos directly activates AP-1-dependent gene transcription (118). Unregulated expression of the protooncogene c-*jun* can lead to aberrant proliferation and transformation of a number of different cell types (62). For example, tracheal epithelial cells transiently transfected with a plasmid that overexpresses c-*jun* leads to increased proliferation and enhanced ability of these cells to grow in soft agar, an indication of cellular transformation (118). Persistent induction of early response genes (i.e., c-*jun*), may be one mechanism by which asbestos induces chronic cell proliferation and changes in cell phenotype indicative of neoplastic transformation.

Considerable evidence indicates that the redox status of cells may be important in the control of transcription factor activation and expression of a number of genes. For example, the transcription factors AP-1 (62) and NF-κB (63,119,120) appear to be modulated by the redox status of cells. The transcription factor NF-κB also regulates the transcription of a number of genes involved in cell proliferation and inflammation (89). It has been shown that binding of AP-1 (62) or NF-κB (121) to their respective regulatory sequences is abolished by oxidation (121). Critical cysteine residues within the proteins can be affected by oxidation and mediate this redox regulation. A number of model systems that involve oxidant stress have demonstrated

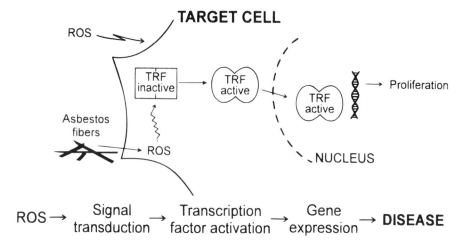

FIG. 5. Model for asbestos induced cell proliferation and disease development. Reactive oxygen intermediates (O_2^-, OH·) generated by exposure to asbestos mediate activation of signaling pathways leading to transcription factor activation and transcription of proliferation-related genes. Chronic stimulation of cell proliferation leads to fixation of genetic damage and eventually the selection of neoplastic cells.

increases in NF-κB (120) and Fos and Jun (AP-1) DNA binding activity (122). Thus, oxidants may activate signaling cascades leading to activation of AP-1 and NF-κB.

Rodent pleural mesothelial cells exposed to crocidolite asbestos are depleted of total cellular glutathione, indicating a change in the redox status of the cell (22,123). Modulation of glutathione levels in these cells appears to control c-*fos* and c-*jun* gene expression. For example, induction of c-*fos* and c-*jun* in these cells by asbestos is blocked by *N*-acetyl-L-cysteine (NAC), a glutathione precursor, and amplified by pretreatment with buthionine sulfoximine (BSO), which depletes glutathione pools (22). Exposure of rodent tracheal epithelial cells to crocidolite asbestos also induces NF-κB DNA-binding activity and NF-κB-dependent gene expression (123). This DNA-binding activity is significantly decreased by preexposure to NAC. These data suggest that oxidants or alterations in redox status caused by asbestos may contribute to activation of the transcription factors AP-1 and NF-κB.

A working model of asbestos-induced disease is the persistent stimulation by asbestos fibers and free radicals of cell signaling cascades leading to activation of transcription factors and regulated genes (Figure 5). These events may be triggered by oxidants catalyzed directly on the fiber surface or during phagocytosis by inflammatory and/or resident cells of the lung. Chronic stimulation of proliferation-related genes may lead to unregulated cell proliferation and facilitate the fixation of genetic damage into the genome.

SUMMARY

Xenobiotic agents generating free radicals through either their metabolism or other pathways induce gene expression through a number of signaling pathways and interaction with transcription factors. It is likely that multiple pathways are involved with complex agents such as asbestos and crystalline silica, which may both interact with the surface of cells and be internalized, thus acting as a continuous source of intracellular free radicals. Certain transcription factors, such as NF-κB, are particularly oxidant sensitive in terms of induction, suggesting that oxidants produced by xenobiotics are directly involved. The increased expression of a number of genes with common transcription factor binding sites in their promoter regions is observed with a number of agents. For example, promoter regions of the Mn-SOD gene and the gene encoding ODC have AP-1 sites. Thus an oxidant stress may induce multiple genes with diverse functions. Recent studies also suggest that transcription factors may act cooperatively or competitively in DNA binding and regulation. Unraveling the complex signaling pathways and transcription factors involved in various oxidant stresses is critical to an understanding of the pathogenesis of diseases induced by oxidants and therapeutic approaches.

ACKNOWLEDGMENTS

The authors wish to thank Judy Kessler and Tony Quinn for providing the illustrations, Bernie Ravenelle for assistance in preparing the manuscript, and Timothy R. Quinlan for helpful suggestions.

REFERENCES

1. Quinlan T, Spivack S, Mossman BT. Regulation of antioxidant enzymes in lung after oxidant injury. *Environ Health Perspect* 1994;102:79–87.
2. Quinlan TR, Marsh JP, Janssen YMW, Borm PA, Mossman BT. Oxygen radicals and asbestos-mediated disease. *Environ Health Perspect* 1994;102:107–110.
3. Janssen YMW, Borm PJA, Van Houten B, Mossman BT. Cell and tissue responses to oxidative damage. *Lab Invest* 1993;69:261–274.
4. Frei B, Stocker R, Ames BN. Antioxidant defenses and lipid peroxidation in human blood plasma. *Proc Natl Acad Sci USA* 1988;85:9748–9752.
5. Frei B, England L, Ames BN. Ascorbate is an outstanding antioxidant in human blood plasma. *Proc Natl Acad Sci USA* 1989;86:6377–6381.
6. Heffner JE, Repine JE. Pulmonary strategies of antioxidant defense. *Am Rev Respir Dis* 1989; 140:531–554.
7. Wispe J, Warner B, Clark J, Dey CR, Newman J, Glasser SW, Crapo JD, Chang LY, Whitsett JA. Human Mn-superoxide dismutase in pulmonary epithelial cells of transgenic mice confers protection from oxygen injury. *J Biol Chem* 1992;267:23937–23941.
8. White C, Nguyen D-D, Suzuki K, Taniguchi N, Rusakow LS, Avraham KB, Groner Y. Expression of manganese superoxide dismutase is not altered in transgenic mice with elevated level of copper-zinc superoxide dismutase. *Free Radical Biol Med* 1993;15:629–636.
9. Mossman BT, Mason R, McDonald J, Gail D. Advances in molecular genetics, transgenic models and gene therapy for the study of pulmonary diseases. *Am J Respir Crit Care Med* 1995;151:2065–2069.

10. Mossman BT, Surinrut P, Brinton BT, Marsh JP, Heintz NH, Lindau-Shepard B, Shaffer JB. Transfection of a manganese-containing superoxide dismutase gene into hamster tracheal epithelial cells ameliorates asbestos-mediated cytotoxicity. *Free Radical Biol Med* 1996;21:125–131.

11. Lindau-Shepard B, Shaffer JB, Del Vecchio PJ. Overexpression of manganous superoxide dismutase (MnSOD) in pulmonary endothelial cells confers resistance to hyperoxia. *J Cell Physiol* 1994;161:237–242.

12. Hirose K, Longo D, Oppenheim J, Matsushima K. Overexpression of mitochondrial manganese superoxide dismutase promotes the survival of tumor cells exposed to interleukin-1, tumor necrosis factor, selected anticancer drugs, and ionizing radiation. *FASEB J* 1993;7:361–368.

13. Bagley AC, Krall J, Lynch RE. Superoxide mediates the toxicity of paraquat for Chinese hamster ovary cells. *Proc Natl Acad Sci USA* 1986;83:3189–3193.

14. Weitzman SA, Graceffa P. Asbestos catalyzes hydroxyl and superoxide radical generation from hydrogen peroxide. *Arch Biochem Biophys* 1984;228:373–376.

15. Weitzman S, Weitberg A. Asbestos-catalyzed lipid peroxidation and its inhibition by desferrioxamine. *Biochem J* 1985;225:259–262.

16. Gulumian M, Van Wyk JA. Hydroxyl radical production in the presence of fibers by a Fenton-type reaction. *Chem Biol Interact* 1987;62:89–97.

17. Lund LG, Aust AE. Iron-catalyzed reactions may be responsible for the biochemical and biological effects of asbestos. *BioFactors* 1991;3:83–89.

18. Pryor WA. How far does ozone penetrate into the pulmonary air/tissue boundary before it reacts? *Free Radical Biol Med* 1992;12:83–88.

19. Graceffa P, Weitzman S. Asbestos catalyzes the formation of the 6-oxobenzo[a]pyrene radical from 6-hydroxybenzo[a]pryrene. *Arch Biochem Biophys* 1987;253:481–484.

20. Costa M. Perspectives on the mechanism of nickel carcinogenesis gained from models of in vitro carcinogenesis. *Environ Health Perspect* 1989;81:63–76.

21. Hansen K, Mossman BT. Generation of superoxide (O_2^-) from alveolar macrophages exposed to asbestiform and nonfribrous particles. *Cancer Res* 1987;47:1681–1686.

22. Janssen YMW, Heintz NH, Mossman BT. Induction of c-*fos* and c-*jun* proto-oncogene by asbestos is ameliorated by *N*-acetyl-L-cysteine in mesothelial cells. *Cancer Res* 1995;55:2085–2089.

23. Boehme DS, Maples KR, Henderson RF. Glutathione release by pulmonary alveolar macrophages in response to particles in vitro. *Toxicol Lett* 1992;60:53–60.

24. Bergelson S, Pinkus R, Daniel V. Intracellular glutathione levels regulated Fos/Jun induction and activation of glutathione *S*-transferase gene expression. *Cancer Res* 1994;54:36–40.

25. Workshop Report from the Division of Research Grants, National Institutes of Health. Metal Carcinogenesis—A Chemical Pathology Study Section Workshop. *Cancer Res* 1992;52:4058–4063.

26. Stohs SJ, Bagchi D. Oxidative mechanisms in the toxicity of metal ions. *Free Radical Biol Med* 1995;18:321–336.

27. Waalkes MP, Coogan TP, Barter RA. Toxicological principles of metal carcinogenesis with special emphasis on cadmium. *Crit Rev Toxicol* 1992;22:175–201.

28. Cohen MD, Kargacin B, Klein CB, Costa M. Mechanisms of chromium carcinogenicity and toxicity. *Crit Rev Toxicol* 1993;23:255–281.

29. Costa M. Molecular mechanisms of nickel carcinogenesis. *Annu Rev Parmacol Toxicol* 1991; 31:321–327.

30. Brugnera E, Georgiev O, Radtke F, Heuchel R, Baker E, Sutherland GR, Schaffner W. Cloning, chromosomal mapping and characterization of the human metal-regulatory transcription factor MTF-1. *Nucleic Acids Res* 1994;22:3167–3173.

31. Dalton T, Palmiter RD, Andrews GK. Transcriptional induction of the mouse metallothionein-1 gene in hydrogen peroxide-treated Hepa cells involves a composite major late transcription factor/antioxidant response element and metal response promoter elements. *Nucleic Acids Res* 1994;22:5016–5023.

32. Shiraishi N, Hochadel JF, Coogan TP, Koropatnick J, Waalkes MP. Sensitivity to cadmium-induced genotoxicity in rat testicular cells is associated with minimal expression of the metallothionein gene. *Toxicol Appl Pharmacol* 1995;130:229–236.

33. Hart BA, Gong Q, Eneman JD, Durieux-Lu CC. In vivo expression of metallothionein in rat alveolar macrophages and type II epithelial cells following repeated cadmium aerosol exposures. *Toxicol Appl Pharmacol* 1995;133:82–90.

34. Keyse SM, Tyrell RM. Heme oxygenase is the major 32-kDa stress protein induced in human

skin fibroblasts by UVA radiation, hydrogen peroxide, and sodium arsenite. *Proc Natl Acad Sci USA* 1989;86:99–103.

35. Keyse SM, Applegate LA, Tromvoukis Y, Tyrrell RM. Oxidant stress leads to transcriptional activation of the human heme oxygenase gene in cultured skin fibroblasts. *Mol Cell Biol* 1990;10:4967–4969.

36. Frankel FR, Steeger JR, Damiano VV, Sohn M, Oppenheim D, Weinbaum G. Induction of unilateral pulmonary fibrosis in the rat by cadmium chloride. *Am J Respir Cell Mol Biol* 1991;5:385–394.

37. Horiguchi H, Mukaida N, Okamoto S, Teranishi H, Kasuya M, Matsushima K. Cadmium induces interleukin-8 production in human peripheral blood mononuclear cells with the concomitant generation of superoxide radicals. *Lymphokine Cytokine Res* 1993;12:421–428.

38. Abe T, Konishi T, Katoh T, Hirano H, Matsukuma K, Kashimura M, Higashi K. Induction of heat shock 70 mRNA by cadmium is mediated by glutathione suppressive and non-suppressive triggers. *Biochim Biophys Acta* 1994;1201:29–36.

39. Hiranuma K, Hirata K, Abe T, Hirano T, Matsuno K, Hirano H, Suzuki K. Induction of mitochondrial chaperonin, hsp60, by cadmium in human hepatoma cells. *Biochem Biophys Res Commun* 1993;194:531–536.

40. Liu RY, Corry PM, Lee YJ. Regulation of chemical stress-induced hsp70 gene expression in murine L929 cells. *J Cell Sci* 1994;107:2209–2214.

41. Ovelgonne JH, Souren JE, Wiegant FA, Van Wijk R. Relationship between cadmium-induced expression of heatshock genes, inhibition of protein synthesis and cell death. *Toxicology* 1995;99:19–30.

42. Liu RY, Corry PM, Lee YJ. Potential involvement of a constitutive heat shock element binding factor in the regulation of chemical stress-induced hsp70 gene expression. *Mol Cell Biochem* 1995;144:27–34.

43. Hightower LE. Heat shock, stress proteins, chaperones, and proteotoxicity. *Cell* 1991;66:191–197.

44. Ishii T, Yamada M, Sato H, et al. Cloning and characterization of a 23-kDa stress-induced mouse peritoneal macrophage protein. *J Biol Chem* 1993;268:18633–18636.

45. Tang N, Enger MD. Cadmium induces hypertrophy accompanied by increased myc mRNA accumulation in NRK-49F cells. *Cell Biol Toxicol* 1991;7:401–411.

46. Tang N, Enger MD. Cd(2+)induced c-myc mRNA accumulation in NRK-49F cells is blocked by the protein kinase inhibitor H7 but not by HA1004, indicating that protein kinase C is a mediator of the response. *Toxicology* 1993;81:155–164.

47. Fritz G, Kaina B. Stress factors affecting expression of O_6-methylguanine-DNA methyltransferase mRNA in rat hepatoma cells. *Biochim Biophys Acta* 1992;1171:35–40.

48. Sen P, Conway K, Costa M. Comparison of the localization of chromosome damage induced by calcium chromate and nickel compounds. *Cancer Res* 1987;47:2142–2147.

49. Lee YW, Klein CB, Kargacin B, Salnikow K, Kitahara J, Dowjat K, Zhitkovich A, Christie NT, Costa M. Carcinogenic nickel silences gene express in by chromatin condensation and DNA methylation: A new model for epigenetic carcinogens. *Mol Cell Biol* 1995;15:2547–2557.

50. Salnikow K, Cosentino S, Klein C, Costa M. Loss of thrombospondin transcriptional activity in nickel-transformed cells. *Mol Cell Biol* 1994;14:851–858.

51. Lin X, Dowjat WK, Costa M. Nickel-induced transformation of human cells causes loss of the phosphorylation of the retinoblastoma protein. *Cancer Res* 1994;54:2751–2754.

52. Snow ET, Xu L-S. Chromium (III) bound to DNA templates promotes increased polymerase processivity and decreased fidelity during replication in vitro. *Biochemistry* 1991;30:11238–11245.

53. Alcedo JA, Misra M, Hamilton JW, Wetterhahn KE. The genotoxic carcinogen chromium (VI) alters the metal-inducible expression but not the basal expression of the metallothionein gene *in vivo*. *Carcinogenesis* 1994;15:1089–1092.

54. McCaffrey J, Wolf CM, Hamilton JW. Effects of the genotoxic carcinogen chromium(VI) on basal and hormone-inducible phosphoenolpyruvate carboxykinase gene expression in vivo: correlation with glucocorticoid- and developmentally regulated expression. *Mol Carcinogen* 1994;10:189–198.

55. Boyd MR. Metabolic activation and lung toxicity: A basis for cell-selective pulmonary damage by foreign chemicals. *Environ Health Perspect* 1984;55:47–51.

56. Doull J, Klaassen CD, Amdur MO, eds. *Toxicology: The Basic Science of Poisons*. 2nd ed. New York: MacMillan.

57. Goldfrank LR, Flomenbaum NE, Lewin NA, Weisman RS, Howland MA, Goffman RS, eds. *Toxicologic Emergencies*. 5th ed. Norwalk, CT: Appleton & Lange.

58. Rose MS, Smith LL, Wyatt I. Evidence for energy-dependent accumulation of paraquat into rat lung. *Nature* 1974;252:314–315.

59. Horton JK, Brigelius R, Mason RP, Bend JR. Paraquat uptake into freshly isolated rabbit lung epithelial cells and its reduction to the paraquat radical under anaerobic conditions. *Mol Pharmacol* 1986;29:484–488.

60. Farrington JA, Ebert M, Land EJ, Fletcher K. Bipyridylium quaternary salts and related compounds. V. Pulse radiolysis studies of the reaction of paraquat radical with oxygen. Implications for the mode of action of bipyridyl herbicides. *Biochim Biophys Acta* 1973;314:372–381.

61. Bus JS, Gibson JE. Paraquat: Model for oxidant-initiated toxicity. *Environ Health Perspect* 1984;55:37–46.

62. Angel P, Karin M. The role of Jun, Fos and the AP-1 complex in cell-proliferation and transformation. *Biochim Biophys Acta* 1991;1072:129–157.

63. Hayashi T, Ueno Y, Okamoto T. Oxidoreductive regulation of nuclear factor κ B. Involvement of a cellular reducing catalyst thioredoxin. *J Biol Chem* 1993;268:11380–11388.

64. Krall J, Bagley AC, Mullenbach GT, Hallewell RA, Lynch RE. Superoxide mediates the toxicity of paraquat for cultured mammalian cells. *J Biol Chem* 1988;263:1910–1914.

65. Warner BB, Burhans MS, Clark JC, Wispe JR. Tumor necrosis factor-α increases Mn-SOD expression: Protection against oxidant injury. *Am J Physiol* 1991;260:L296–L301.

66. Sato M. Dose-dependent increases in metallothionein synthesis in the lung and liver of paraquat-treated rats. *Toxicol Appl Pharmacol* 1991;107:98–105.

67. Church DF, Pryor WA. Free-radical chemistry of cigarette smoke and its toxicological implications. *Environ Health Perspect* 1985;64:111–126.

68. Frei B, Forte TM, Ames BN, Cross CE. Gas phase oxidants of cigarette smoke induce lipid peroxidation and changes in lipoprotein properties in human blood plasma. *Biochem J* 1991;277:133–138.

69. Hankinson O. The aryl hydrocarbon receptor complex. *Annu Rev Pharmacol Toxicol* 1995;35:307–340.

70. Hunninghake GW, Crystal RG. Cigarette smoking and lung destruction. Accumulation of neutrophils in the lungs of cigarette smokers. *Am Rev Respir Dis* 1983;128:833–838.

71. Müller T, Gebel S. Heme oxygenase expression in Swiss 3T3 cells following exposure to aqueous cigarette smoke fractions. *Carcinogenesis* 1994;15:67–72.

72. Müller T. Expression of c-*fos* in quiescent Swiss 3T3 cells exposed to aqueous cigarette smoke fractions. *Cancer Res* 1995;55:1927–1932.

73. Goldstein JA, Faletto MB. Advances in mechanisms of activation and deactivation of environmental chemicals. *Environ Health Perspect* 1993;100:169–176.

74. Jerina DM, Chadha A, Cheh AM, Schurdak ME, Wood AW, Sayer JM. Covalent bonding of bay-region diol epoxides to nucleic acids. *Adv Exp Med Biol* 1991;283:533–553.

75. Okey AB, Riddick DS, Harper PA. Molecular biology of the aromatic hydrocarbon (dioxin) receptor. *Trends Pharmacol Sci* 1994;15:226–232.

76. Vanden Heuvel JP, Clark GC, Kohn MC, et al. Dioxin-responsive genes: Examination of dose-response relationships using quantitative reverse transcriptase-polymerase chain reaction. *Cancer Res* 1994;54:62–68.

77. Puga A, Nebert DW, Carrier F. Dioxin induces expression of c-*fos* and c-*jun* proto-oncogenes and a large increase in transcription factor AP-1. *DNA Cell Biol* 1992;11:269–281.

78. Vanden Heuvel JP, Lucier G. Environmental toxicology of polychlorinated dibenzo-*p*-dioxins and polychlorinated dibenzofurans. *Environ Health Perspect* 1993;100:189–200.

79. Rifkind AB, Gannon M, Gross SS. Arachidonic acid metabolism by dioxin-induced cytochrome P-450: A new hypothesis on the role of P-450 in dioxin toxicity. *Biochem Biophys Res Commun* 1990;172:1180–1188.

80. Yao Y, Hoffer A, Chang C, Puga A. Dioxin activates HIV-1 gene expression by an oxidative stress pathway requiring a functional cytochrome P450 CYP1A1 enzyme. *Environ Health Perspect* 1995;103:366–371.

81. Ames BN, Gold LS. Too many rodent carcinogens: Mitogenesis increases mutagenesis. *Science* 1990;249:970–971.

82. Preston-Martin S, Pike MC, Ross RK, Jones PA, Henderson BE. Increased cell division as a cause of human cancer. *Cancer Res* 1990;50:415–7421.

83. Mustafa MG. Biochemical basis of ozone toxicity. *Free Radical Biol Med* 1990;9:245–265.

84. Gaston B, Drazen JM, Loscalzo J, Stamler JS. The biology of nitrogen oxides in the airways. *Am J Respir Crit Care Med* 1994;149:538–551.
85. Laskin DL, Pendino KJ, Punjabi CJ, Rodriguez del Valle M, Laskin JD. Pulmonary and hepatic effects of inhaled ozone in rats. *Environ Health Perspect* 1994;102(Suppl 10):61–64.
86. Punjabi CJ, Laskin JD, Pendino KJ, Goller NL, Durham SK, Laskin DL. Production of nitric oxide in rat type II pneumocytes: Increased expression of inducible nitric oxide synthase following inhalation of a pulmonary irritant. *Am J Respir Cell Mol Biol* 1994;11:165–172.
87. Driscoll KE, Simpson L, Carter J, Hassenbein D, Leikauf GD. Ozone inhalation stimulates expression of a neutrophil chemotactic protein, macrophage inflammatory protein 2. *Toxicol Appl Pharmacol* 1993;119:306–309.
88. Farone A, Huang S, Paulauskis J, Kobzik L. Airway neutrophilia and chemokine mRNA expression in sulfur dioxide-induced bronchitis. *Am J Respir Cell Mol Biol* 1995;12:345–350.
89. Liou HC, Baltimore D. Regulation of the NF-κB/rel transcription factor and IκB inhibitor system. *Curr Opin Cell Biol* 1993;5:477–487.
90. Xie Q, Kashiwabara Y, Nathan C. Robe of transcription factor NF-κB/Rel in induction of nitric oxide synthase. *J Biol Chem* 1994;269:4705–4708.
91. Adcock IM, Brown CR, Kwon O, Barnes PJ. Oxidative stress induces NF kappa B DNA binding and inducible NOS mRNA in human epithelial cells. *Biochem Biophys Res Commun* 1994; 199:1518–1524.
92. Rahman I-U, Clerch LB, Massaro D. Rat lung antioxidant enzyme induction by ozone. *Am J Physiol* 1991;260:L412–L418.
93. Rahman I-U, Massaro D. Endotoxin treatment protects rats against ozone-induced lung edema: With evidence for the role of manganese superoxide dismutase. *Toxicol Appl Pharmacol* 1992;113:13–18.
94. Harkema JR, Hotchkiss JA. Ozone- and endotoxin-induced mucous cell metaplasias in rat airway epithelium: Novel animal models to study toxicant-induced epithelial transformation in airways. *Toxicol Lett* 1993;68:251–263.
95. Jany B. Molecular cloning of human respiratory tract mucin and studies of mucin gene expression in tracheobronchial epithelium of the rat. *Pneumologie* 1993;47:479–487.
96. Choi AM, Elbon CL, Bruce SA, Bassett DJ. Messenger RNA levels of lung extracellular matrix proteins during ozone exposure. *Lung* 1994;172:15–30.
97. Armstrong LC, Watkins K, Pinkerton KE, Last JA. Collagen mRNA content and distribution in the lungs of rats exposed to ozone. *Am J Respir Cell Mol Biol* 1994;11:25–34.
98. Mossman BT, Gee JBL. Asbestos-related diseases. *N Engl J Med* 1989;320:1721–1730.
99. Mossman BT, Bignon J, Corn M, Seaton A, Gee JBL. Asbestos: Scientific developments and implications for public policy. *Science* 1990;247:294–301.
100. Craighead JE, Kleinerman J, Abraham JL, Gibbs AR, Green F, Harley RA, Ruettner JR, Vallyathan NV, Juliano EB. Diseases associated with exposure to silica and nonfibrous silicate minerals. *Arch Pathol Lab Med* 1988;112:673–720.
101. Absher MP, Trombley L, Hemenway DR, Mickey RM, Leslie KO. Biphasic cellular and tissue response of rat lungs after eight-day aerosol exposure to the silicon dioxide cristobalite. *Am J Pathol* 1989;134:1243–51.
102. Mossman BT, Marsh JP, Sesko A, Hill S, Shatos MA, Doherty J, Petruska J, Adler KB, Hemenway D, Mickey R, Vacek P, Kagan E.. Inhibition of lung infury, inflammation, and interstitial pulmonary fibrosis by poly-ethylene glycol-conjugated catalase in a rapid inhalation model of asbestosis. *Am Rev Respir Dis* 1990;141:1266–1271.
103. Kamp DW, Gracefa P, Pryor W, Weitzman S. The role of free radicals in asbestos-induced diseases. *Free Radic Biol Med* 1992;12:293–315.
104. Mossman BT, Marsh JP, Shatos MA, Doherty J, Gilbert R, Hill S. Implication of active oxygen species as second messengers of asbestos toxicity. *Drug Chem Toxicol* 1987;10:157–165.
105. Mossman BT, Jimenez LA, BeruBe K, Quinlan T, Janssen YMW. Possible mechanisms of crystalline silica-induced lung disease. *Appl Occup Environ Hyg* 1995;10:1115–1117.
106. Shatos MA, Doherty JM, Marsh JP, Mossman BT. Prevention of asbestos-induced cell death in rat lung fibroblasts and alveolar macrophages by scavengers of active oxygen species. *Environ Res* 1987;44:103–116.
107. Driscoll KE, Strzelecki J, Hassenbein D, Janssen YMW, Marsh J, Oberdorster, Ilossman BT. Tumor necrosis factor (TNF): Evidence for the role of TNF in increased expression of manganese superoxide dismutase after inhalation of mineral dusts. *Ann Occup Hyg* 1994;38:375–382.

108. Piguet PF, Collart MA, Grau GE, Sappino AP, Vassalli P. Requirement of tumour necrosis factor for the development of silica-induced pulmonary fibrosis. *Nature* 1990;344:245–247.
109. Kennedy TP, Dodson R, Rao NV, Ky H, Hopkins C, Baser M, Tolley E, Hoidal JR. Dusts causing pneumoconiosis generate ·OH and produce hemolysis by acting as Fenton catalysts. *Arch Biochem Biophys* 1989;269:359–364.
110. Kamp DW, Israbian VA, Preusen SE, Zhang CX, Weitzman SA. Asbestos causes DNA strand breaks in cultured pulmonary epithelial cells: Role of iron-catalyzed free radicals. *Am J Physiol. (Lung Cell Mol Physiol)* 1995;12:L471–L480.
111. Hardy JA, Aust AE. The effect of iron binding on the ability of crocidolite asbestos to catalyze DNA single-strand breaks. *Carcinogenesis* 1995;16:319–325.
112. Mossman BT, Marsh JP. Evidence supporting a role for active oxygen species in asbestos-induced toxicity and lung disease. *Environ Health Perspect* 1989;81:91–94.
113. Janssen YMW, Marsh JP, Absher MP, Hemenway D, Vacek PM, Leslie KO, Borm PJ, Mossman BT. Expression of antioxidant enzymes in rat lungs after inhalation of asbestos or silica. *J Biol Chem* 1992;267:10625–10630.
114. Quinlan TR, Marsh JP, Janssen YMW, Leslie KO, Hemenway D, Vacek P, Mossman BT. Dose-responsive increases in pulmonary fibrosis after inhalation of asbestos. *Am J Respir Crit Care Med* 1994;150:200–206.
115. Pegg AE. Polyamine metabolism and its importance in neoplastic growth and as a target for chemotherapy. *Cancer Res* 1988;48:759–774.
116. Quinlan TR, BeruBe KA, Marsh JP, Janssen YTM, Taishi P, Leslie KD, Hemenway D, O'Shaughnessy PT, Vacek P, Mossman BT. Patterns of inflammation, cell proliferation, and related gene expression in lung after inhalation of chrysotile asbestos. *Am J Pathol* 1995;147:728–739.
117. Heintz NH, Janssen YM, Mossman BT. Persistent induction of c-*fos* and c-*jun* expression by asbestos. *Proc Natl Acad Sci* 1993;90:3299–3303.
118. Timblin CR, Janssen YMW, Mossman BT. Transcriptional activation of the proto-oncogene c-*jun* by asbestos and H_2O_2 is directly related to increased proliferation and transformation of tracheal epithelial cells. *Cancer Res* 1995;55:2723–2726.
119. Galter D, Sabine MIHM, Dröge W. Distinct effects of glutathione disulphide on the nuclear transcription factors κB and the activator protein-1. *Eur J Biochem* 1994;221:639–648.
120. Meyer M, Caselmann WH, Schüter V, Schreck R, Hofschneider PH, Baeuerle P. Hepatitis B virus transactivator MHBs': Activation of NF-κB, selective inhibition by antioxidants and integral membrane localization. *EMBO J* 1992;11:2991–3001.
121. Staal FJT, Roederer M, Herzenberg LA, Herzenberg LA. Intracellular thiols regulate activation of nuclear factor kappa B and transcription of human immunodeficiency virus. *Proc Natl Acad Sci USA* 1990;87:9943–9947.
122. Devary Y, Gottlieb RA, Smeal T, Karin M. The mammalian ultraviolet response is triggered by activation of Src tyrosine kinases. *Cell* 1992;71:1081–1091.
123. Janssen YMW, Barchowsy A, Treadwell M, Driscoll KE, Mossman BT. Asbestos induces nuclear factor κB (NfκB) DNA-binding activity and NF-κB-dependent gene expression in tracheal epithelial cells. *Proc Natl Acad Sci USA* 1995;92:8458–8462.

Free Radical Toxicology
Edited by K. B. Wallace
Copyright © 1997 Taylor & Francis

17

Free-Radical-Induced Changes in Cell Signal Transduction

George E. N. Kass

School of Biological Sciences, University of Surrey, Guildford, Surrey, United Kingdom

INTRODUCTION

Cells in multicellular organisms are continuously exposed to messages sent from neighboring or more distantly located cells that inform them whether to remain unchanged or whether to change status or function through processes of differentiation, proliferation, or even self-destruction. Overall, such changes are to the benefit of the organism as a whole. These messages are conveyed to their target cells by means of specific signaling molecules known as hormones, neurotransmitters, growth factors, or cytokines. Signaling molecules can be proteins, small peptides, amino acids, nucleotides, retinoids, fatty acid derivatives, and even gases such as nitric oxide and carbon monoxide. Target cells are identified by means of specific proteins called receptors. These receptors may be located within the cell, as is the case for steroid hormone receptors, or at the surface of the cell, as for growth factors or neurotransmitters. The function of the receptor is to relay the message carried by its specific signaling molecule to a range of proteins that will alter metabolism and gene expression within the target cell in order to modify or maintain its phenotype (Figure 1). Alternatively, they may transiently alter the levels of low-molecular-weight molecules or ions, such as cyclic adenosine monophosphate (cAMP), cyclic guanosine monophosphate (cGMP), and Ca^{2+}, that act as so-called second messengers. In general, the coupling between most receptors and their final metabolic and genetic targets involves a self-amplifying cascade of protein kinases and phosphatases, as well as second messengers that very often cross-talk with other signaling pathways or even receptors through the generation of new signaling molecules (1).

While alterations in cellular differentiation or proliferation are traditionally viewed as associated with endogenous signaling molecules, it is now becoming increasingly clear that the very same changes can be elicited under a number of circumstances by compounds foreign to the organism, such as drugs, environmental pollutants,

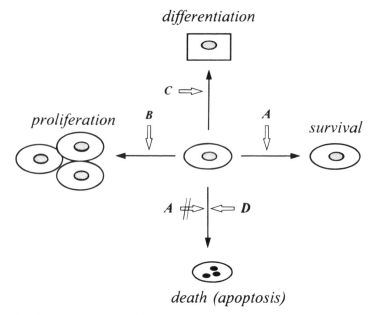

differentiation

proliferation   B   A   *survival*

A   ⇏ | ⇐ D

death (apoptosis)

FIG. 1. Signaling molecules control the behavior of cells. Each cell displays a set of receptors that allow it to respond to different signals. A survival signal (A) is often required, otherwise the cell may die by apoptosis. Death may also be elicited by specific "death" signals (D), whereas signals B and C will stimulate the cell to divide or to differentiate.

heavy metals, and products derived from microorganisms. Many of these compounds are either free radicals or generate free radicals during cellular metabolism.

FREE RADICALS AND CELL PROLIFERATION, DIFFERENTIATION, AND DEATH

Free Radicals and Biological Systems

Living organisms are unavoidably exposed to free radicals of various chemical and biological origins (2). The sources of these chemically highly reactive species may be from physiological production, as a consequence of "leaky" metabolic pathways such as the mitochondrial electron transport chain, or from formation by specialized enzymes including NADPH oxidase and NO synthase. Alternatively, they are produced accidentally (or intentionally) from exposure to ionizing radiation, transition metals, or xenobiotics that are bioactivated to yield free-radical species.

The study of the interaction of free radicals with living organisms has traditionally focused on the cytotoxicity that results from their high chemical reactivity toward many cellular components (2–6). The targets for free radicals include the cell's antioxidant and free-radical scavenging group of molecules (e.g., glutathione, ascorbate, vitamin E), unsaturated fatty acids of cellular membrane lipids and phospholipids, nucleic acids, and cysteine and tyrosine residues on proteins.

The mechanisms by which free radicals kill cells have been extensively studied over the past decades, and the current consensus is that free radicals, by virtue of their direct or indirect interaction with oxygen to form oxygen-based radicals such as superoxide anion (O_2^-) and hydroxyl radicals (OH·), damage the target cell by inducing a condition of oxidative stress. Injury from free radicals is usually highly acute and typically leads to necrotic forms of cell death. Cell death may result from (a) the loss of cell membrane integrity following radical-initiated lipid peroxidation, (b) impaired protein functioning resulting in imbalance in ionic and particularly intracellular Ca^{2+} homeostasis, (c) the loss of cellular energy supply, and (d) DNA damage leading to the destruction of the cell's genetic material (for recent reviews on this topic see, e.g., refs 2,4,7,8). In contrast, levels of free radicals that are below the threshold for cytotoxicity can have very diverse effects, such as inducing cell proliferation, differentiation, or programmed cell death by apoptosis.

The scope of this review is to summarize briefly our current understanding of the interaction of free radicals with cellular signaling pathways and how this plays an important role in the cellular modifications caused by free radicals. One particular free radical, NO, has recently attracted a great deal of attention because of its identity as endothelium-derived relaxing factor (EDRF) (9). Enhanced synthesis of NO may occur during free-radical-mediated cell injury in response to increases in cytosolic free Ca^{2+} concentration ($[Ca^{2+}]_i$) or induction of the inducible form of NO synthase, and NO is well known to be toxic to cells both in vivo and in vitro. However, because it belongs to the class of signaling molecules, NO is not further discussed here, and several specialized reviews may be consulted elsewhere (see, e.g., refs. 9–12).

Free Radicals and Cell Proliferation

A large body of evidence has shown that the addition of superoxide or hydrogen peroxide to cells will stimulate cell proliferation in vitro. For example, hamster BHK-21 fibroblasts (13), human fibroblasts (14), smooth muscle cells (15,16), and rat insulinoma RINm5F cells (17) all respond to added oxygen free radicals, the pro-oxidant H_2O_2, or following exposure to redox-cycling quinones with increased rates of DNA replication and cell division. An important point to consider here is that these effects are only observed at very low concentrations of radicals or peroxide, and the dose-response curve is typically biphasic with inhibition of growth and cell death occurring at high doses (13,17). Although all direct evidence for the stimulation of proliferation by oxygen free radicals has been obtained under in vitro conditions, the same phenomenon may well underlie the well-known action of oxygen-derived free radicals and pro-oxidants as tumor promoters (18–20).

In contrast to their cell proliferative action, free radicals can also induce a transient growth arrest response, depending on the cell type and free-radical experimental system used. The latter response is particularly characteristic of ionizing and UV irradiation (21), and is believed to provide time for DNA repair before allowing the cell to enter S phase.

Free Radicals and Cell Differentiation

Less is known about the effect free radicals have on the state of cellular differentiation. Sohal et al. (22) hypothesized that oxidative stress as a result of increased radical generation will accelerate the rate of cell differentiation and that this may be linked to the phenomenon of aging (23). Support for this theory is provided by the observation that mouse neuroblastoma cells will differentiate when grown under high oxygen tension (24). Similarly, human skin and lung fibroblasts (25), AF8 and SJ-N-KP neuroblastoma cells (26), and NG108-15 neuroblastoma-glioma hybrid cells (27) could be induced to differentiate based on both morphological and biochemical criteria by exposure to ionizing radiation. Work by Nishihira et al. (28) has shown that superoxide radicals can enhance the differentiation of rat monocytic c-WRT-LR leukemia cells to macrophage-like cells in the presence of platelet-activating factor, and Kobayashi et al. (29) found that superoxide radicals caused c-WRT-7 leukemia cells to differentiate to macrophage-like cells. Likewise, the hydroxyl radical has been implicated in the differentiation of HL-60 cells to macrophage-like cells by a protein kinase C activating phorbol ester (30).

Free Radicals and Programmed Cell Death by Apoptosis

The elimination of cells in an organisms can occur in two distinct ways: necrosis, resulting from accidental injury and characterized by extensive damage to membranes, organelles and other cellular constituents, and apoptosis, which involves a "programmed cell death" pathway with characteristic changes in cell shape and chromatin integrity (31,32). Apoptosis plays a major role in the shaping of organs during embryogenesis, maintenance of tissue homeostasis, and elimination of "unwanted" cells such as cancerous cells, virally infected cells, and autoreactive T lymphocytes.

Although traditionally viewed as a physiological form of cell death, evidence is now strongly showing that chemical-induced toxicity, and particularly injury caused by free radicals (33,34) and many anticancer drugs (35), can be mediated by apoptosis as well as necrosis. Probably one of the best documented examples of free-radical-induced apoptosis is that caused by ultraviolet light and various types of ionizing radiation (31,36–40). Further examples of radical-mediated apoptosis include the induction of apoptosis in RINm5F insulinoma and FL5.12 B-lymphocyte precursor cells by redox-cycling quinones (17,41) and apoptotic death of lymphoid cells (HL-60, U937, Daudi, Molt-4), bovine aortic endothelial cells, LLC-PK1 renal tubular epithelial cells, FL5.12 B-lymphocyte precursor cells, and embryonal carcinoma cells by direct addition of H_2O_2 (39,41–44). Further, albeit indirect, evidence for radicals causing apoptosis stems from the protective effects by a range of natural and synthetic antioxidants, transition metal ion chelators, and spin traps (45,46) or by modulating endogenous levels of superoxide dismutase (47,48). Interestingly, several antioxidants also appear to block or delay apoptosis elicited by glucocorticoids, the endoplasmic reticulum Ca^{2+}-ATPase inhibitor thapsigargin, or growth factor or cytokine deprivation (41,45–47). Since the latter treatments are not anticipated to generate free radicals or conditions of oxidative stress directly, a role for free radicals and oxidative stress in the process of apoptosis may be indicated. This possibility would certainly be in line with the proposal that a redox imbalance underlies the loss of CD4[+] T lymphocytes by apoptosis in HIV-infected patients (49,50).

Mechanisms Involved in the Cellular Effects of Free Radicals

There is substantial evidence supporting the contention that the alterations in cell proliferation, differentiation, and engagement of apoptosis elicited by free radicals are mediated by cell signaling events. As becomes evident later in this chapter, most evidence to date implicates protein phosphorylation, phospholipid metabolism, second-messenger formation, transcription factor function, and gene expression as targets for free radicals. However, in view of the complexity that characterizes the network of pathways linking receptor activation to alterations in gene expression and changes in cell phenotype, our understanding of many of the cellular effects of free radicals is still very fragmentary.

FREE RADICALS AND PROTEIN PHOSPHORYLATION AND DEPHOSPHORYLATION PROCESSES

Protein Serine and Threonine Kinases

Among the many protein kinases that phosphorylate their protein targets on specific serine and threonine residues, protein kinase C is probably the best characterized with regard to the modulation of its activity by free radicals. Protein kinase C exists as a family of many isoforms, with the "conventional" ones (α, βI, βII, γ) being activated by Ca^{2+} and diacylglycerol (Figure 2), while the regulation and function of the "novel" (δ, ϵ, η, θ, and μ) and atypical isoforms (ζ, ι) are more complex and less well understood (51,52).

In 1989, our laboratory and two other laboratories independently reported that low levels of free radicals and oxidative stress activate protein kinase C (53–55). Using isolated hepatocytes challenged with sublethal concentrations of redox-cycling quinones we found that protein kinase C activity in the presence of Ca^{2+} and diacylglycerol was increased severalfold (53). The dose-response relationship between protein kinase C activation and oxidative stress was biphasic, and cytotoxic levels of free radicals were found to inhibit the enzyme rapidly. The increase in

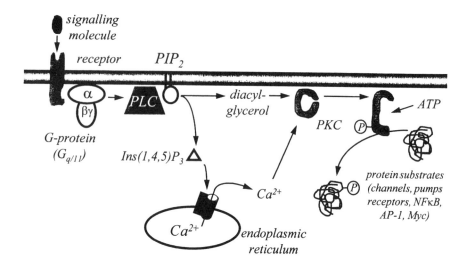

FIG. 2. Schematic illustration of the phospholipase C-linked pathways involved in protein kinase C signaling. The binding of a signaling molecule to its receptor triggers, through a trimeric GTP-binding protein (G-protein) or tyrosine phosphorylation (not shown), the activation of a phosphatidylinositol 4,5-bisphosphate (PIP$_2$)-specific phospholipase C (PLC) that hydrolyzes PIP$_2$ to generate two second messengers, inositol 1,4,5-trisphosphate [Ins(1,4,5)P$_3$] and diacylglycerol. Ins(1,4,5)P$_3$ binds a specific intracellular receptor to mobilize Ca^{2+}. Protein kinase C (PKC) becomes then activated through its binding to diacylglycerol and Ca^{2+}, and phosphorylates protein substrates as well as itself (autophosphorylation).

protein kinase C activity was not only fully reversible by thiol-reducing agents but could also be achieved by incubating partially purified brain protein kinase C with oxidized glutathione (GSSG), demonstrating that the activation of protein kinase C by oxygen-radical-generating quinones was due to oxidative stress and subsequent thiol oxidation of the protein kinase C enzyme. A similar activation of protein kinase C was found to occur in several other in vitro and in an in vivo experimental system (Table 1). In apparent contrast, Gopalakrishna and Anderson (55) reported that different regimens of oxidative treatment of purified protein kinase C led to the inactivation of the regulatory domain, thereby rendering the enzyme cofactor independent. We observed a similar effect when we used highly purified rat brain protein kinase C (in contrast to partially purified enzyme) together with a GSSG/GSH redox buffer (SK Duddy, GEN Kass, and HF Gilbert, unpublished observations). Interestingly, a loss of cofactor dependency was also observed when intact cells were treated with the thiol-modifying agent N-ethylmaleimide (53), raising the possibility that other thiol group(s), probably on the regulatory domain of the enzyme, may be involved in the abrogation of the requirement for Ca^{2+} and diacylglycerol, whereas mild oxidative stress only alters those thiol residue(s) controlling the enzyme's phosphorylation activity. It is likely that the latter residue(s) are found on the kinase domain of the enzyme. Whether the difference between the effects of

TABLE 1. *Activation of protein kinase C by free radicals and pro-oxidants*

Cell type or source of PKC	Radical-generating system or pro-oxidant	Effect on protein kinase C activity	Reference
Rat hepatocytes	Redox-cycling quinones	Increase in cofactor dependent activity[a]	53
Mouse epidermal JB6 cells	Redox-cycling quinone, xanthine/xanthine oxidase	Increase in cofactor-dependent activity	54
Human HL-60 myeloid cells	X-irradiation	Increase in cofactor-dependent activity	143
Pig pulmonary artery endothelial cells	Nitrogen dioxide	Increase in cofactor-dependent activity	164
Rat liver (in vivo)	Carbon tetrachloride	Increase in cofactor-dependent activity	165
A7r5 smooth muscle cells	Hydrogen peroxide	Increase in cofactor-dependent activity	16
Jurkat T cells	Hydrogen peroxide	Increase in cofactor-dependent and -independent activities	166
C6 glioma and B16 melanoma cells	Hydrogen peroxide	Increase in cofactor-independent activity	55
Purified rat brain PKC	Hydrogen peroxide + Fe^{2+}	Increase in cofactor-dependent and -independent activities	167
UC11MG astrocytoma cells	Hydrogen peroxide	Increase of in situ phosphorylation of MARCKS[b]	168
Swiss 3T3 fibroblasts	Doxorubicin	Increase of in situ phosphorylation of MARCKS[b]	169
Human B lymphocyte precursor cells	γ-Irradiation	Increase in kinase activity	72

[a] Activity in the presence of Ca^{2+}, diacylglycerol, and phosphatidylserine.
[b] MARCKS, myristoylated alanine-rich C kinase substrate protein.

free radicals and pro-oxidants observed in cells as compared to the direct effects on purified enzyme reflects differential accessibility of critical cysteine residue(s) as a result of the subcellular localization of protein kinase C (53,55) or whether ancillary cellular proteins or factors are involved remains to be answered. Similarly, the question of the isoform specificity of the modification by free radicals has not yet been addressed. In view of protein kinase C's well-known role in proliferation and tumor promotion, it is tempting to speculate that oxidative activation of protein kinase C contributes to the tumor-promoting property of free radicals (18–20).

The activity of several other serine/threonine protein kinases (Table 2) has also been found to become increased during the exposure of mammalian cells to free radicals. Larsson and Cerutti (56) reported that mouse epidermal JB6 cells responded to oxygen derived free radicals by increased S6 kinase activity. These authors presented experimental support that the mechanism of free-radical-mediated S6 kinase activation was mediated by an increase in $[Ca^{2+}]_i$ and Ca^{2+}/calmodulin-dependent kinase activity, but it is presently unclear which form of S6 kinase

TABLE 2. *Partial list of protein kinases subject to activation by free radicals and pro-oxidants*

Protein kinase	Amino acid specificity	Target cells	Radical-generating system or pro-oxidant	Reference
Protein kinase C	Serine/threonine	Hepatocytes, B, T lymphocytes, mouse epidermal cells, etc.	Redox-cycling quinones, xanthine oxidase, irradiation	53–55, 72, 143,164–169
pp90[rsk] S6 kinase	Serine/threonine	Mouse epidermal, HL-60 cells	Xanthine oxidase, irradiation	56,57
ERK1 and ERK2	Serine/threonine, tyrosine	NIH-3T3 fibroblasts, neutrophils	Irradiation, H_2O_2 diamide	59,60
MEK	Serine/threonine, tyrosine	Neutrophils	H_2O_2 diamide	60
SAP kinase	Serine/threonine, tyrosine	U-937, kidney epithelial cells	UV, ionizing irradiation, ischemia/ reperfusion	61–63
Insulin receptor	Tyrosine	Adipocytes, hepatoma cells	H_2O_2	66–68
Epidermal growth factor receptor	Tyrosine	Human squamous and epidermal carcinoma cells	H_2O_2, UV irradiation	80,85
p56[lck]	Tyrosine	B and T lymphocytes	Irradiation, H_2O_2	71,77
p53/p56[lyn]	Tyrosine	HL-60	irradiation	73
p72[syk]	Tyrosine	B lymphocytes	H_2O_2	75
ZAP-70	Tyrosine	T lymphocytes	H_2O_2	76
Ltk	Tyrosine	Transfected COS cells	Diamide	170

(pp70[S6K] or pp90[rsk]) was the target in that study. Another study performed to examine the effects of γ-irradiation on U937 lymphoid cell S6 kinase activity found that only pp90[rsk] but not pp70[S6K] was activated (57).

More recent evidence also points to the response by the mitogen-activated protein (MAP) kinase pathways in the effects of free radicals. MAP kinase pathways include the extracellular signal-regulated kinase (ERK) pathways 1 and 2, which act as a convergence point for signals emerging from protein kinase C via G-proteins and from receptor protein tyrosine kinases via Ras and Raf-1. ERKs are therefore an important signal transduction link between the plasma membrane and the nucleus (58). Stevenson et al. (59) demonstrated that x-irradiation and hydrogen peroxide treatment of NIH-3T3 fibroblasts led to the activation of ERK1 and ERK2. This was shown to result in T-cell-specific factor (p62[TCF]) phosphorylation and subsequent activation of the serum response factor-serum response element p62[TCF] complex on the c-*fos* promoter (59). Similarly, hydrogen peroxide and the pro-oxidant diamide activate ERKs in neutrophils, and this appears to be due to the upstream stimulation of MEK (mitogen-activated protein kinase or extracellular signal-regulated kinase; see Figure 3) (60).

Other serine/threonine protein kinases that are targeted by free radicals and that

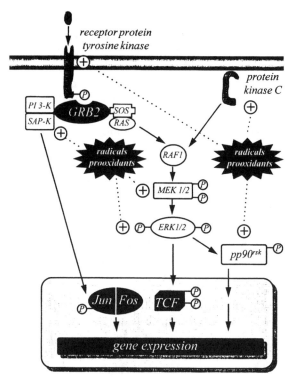

FIG. 3. Free radicals and pro-oxidants can stimulate mitogen-activated protein (MAP) kinase pathways. MAP kinases are the convergence point for many signals arising from stimulation of tyrosine kinase-linked as well as PLC-linked receptors. Many of the steps involved can be modulated by free radicals including the tyrosine kinase-linked receptor, extracellular signal-regulated protein kinase (ERK) or its upstream kinase (MEK), the stress-activated protein kinases (SAP-K), pp90rsk, and protein kinase C.

are also members of the MAP kinase family are the recently identified stress-activated protein (SAP) kinases that preferentially phosphorylate the c-Jun NH_2-terminal activation domain (61,62). SAP kinases are reported to be activated by ischemia and reperfusion injury (63), ultraviolet (UV), and ionizing irradiation (61,62,64). The latter appears to require the binding of SAP kinases to SH2/SH3-containing adapter protein Grb2 and the p85α subunit of phosphoinositide 3-kinase (64). SAP kinases may therefore play a major role in the response of mammalian cells to irradiation by phosphorylating *c-jun* and consequently augmenting AP-1 transcriptional activity (discussed later).

Protein Tyrosine Kinases

The first indication that free radicals could modulate protein tyrosine kinase activities stems from the observation that conditions of oxidative stress can mimic the cellular effects of insulin, an activator of a receptor with intrinsic tyrosine kinase activity (65). Indeed, it was subsequently shown that hydrogen peroxide stimulates tyrosine phosphorylation of the insulin receptor and other proteins (66–68) through stimulation of its tyrosine kinase activity (66,67). Using redox-active quinones, Chan et al. (69) observed that oxygen-derived free radicals similarly activated tyrosine phosphorylation in rat hepatocytes, possibly through insulin receptor activation.

Recently, major progress in our understanding of the interaction between free radicals and protein tyrosine kinases has been made (see Table 2). Thus, exposure of B-lymphocyte precursor cells to low doses of γ-irradiation has been shown to result within minutes in the phosphorylation of several proteins on tyrosine residues (70). Most importantly, the doses of irradiation found to stimulate tyrosine phosphorylation also caused cell death by apoptosis, and the prevention of tyrosine phosphorylation by genistein prevented apoptosis (70). Similarly, the phosphatase inhibitor orthovanadate augmented tyrosine phosphorylation as well as sensitizing the cells to radiation-induced apoptosis. These findings suggest that lymphocyte cell death as a result of radiation therapy is causally linked to the activation of one or more signaling pathways involving tyrosine phosphorylation.

Enhanced protein phosphorylation may result from either activation of protein kinases or inhibition of protein phosphatase activity (discussed later), or from a combination of both effects. In the case of B-lymphocyte irradiation, no detectable change in protein tyrosine phosphatase activity could be detected, suggesting that enhanced tyrosine kinase activity was involved. However, the identity and number of protein tyrosine kinases mediating the effects of γ-irradiation are still unclear. Uckun et al. (70) observed no activation of the Src-related kinases $p59^{fyn}$, $p53/p56^{lyn}$, $p55^{blk}$, or $p56^{lck}$, although Waddick et al. (71) reported an early but transient activation of $p56^{lck}$ (Figure 4). Subsequently, evidence was provided that irradiation-mediated activation of protein kinase C in B-lymphocyte precursor cells (Table 1) involves an upstream tyrosine kinase regulated phosphorylation step (72). Similarly, HL-60 lymphoid cells responded to ionizing irradiation by an activation of $p53/p56^{lyn}$ with only little changes in $p59^{fyn}$, $p56^{lck}$, and $pp60^{c-src}$ activity (73). Interestingly, $p53/p56^{lyn}$ was found to bind to $p34^{cdc2}$ in irradiated cells (73). Because of the pivotal role of the latter in the G2-M transition in the cell cycle, the interaction between $p53/p56^{lyn}$ and $p34^{cdc2}$ may be responsible for the cell cycle arrest and possibly apoptosis observed in mammalian cells in response to ionizing radiation (74).

Several studies have used H_2O_2 as a free-radical-generating agent to investigate protein tyrosine kinases. It is often difficult to distinguish between the oxidative effects of H_2O_2 (and also of organic peroxides) and those resulting from free-radical formation, and this may explain some of the differences between ionizing irradiation and direct peroxide application in the reported effects on protein kinases. Ledbetter and co-workers (75) found that exposure of B-lymphocytic precursor cells to H_2O_2 resulted in the activation of $p72^{syk}$ but had no effect on $p59^{fyn}$, $p53/p56^{lyn}$, or $p56^{lck}$,

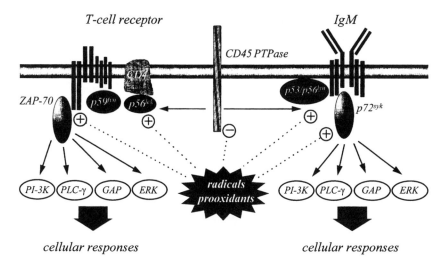

FIG. 4. Ilustration of the different tyrosine protein kinase and phosphatase enzyme cascades that are targeted by free radicals and pro-oxidants in B and T lymphocytes. The left-hand side depicts the components of the T-cell receptor and the right-hand side the B-cell receptor (IgM). Signaling through these receptors activates a number of effector enzymes, including phosphoinositide 3-kinase (PI-3K), phospholipase C-γ (PLC-γ), GTPase activating protein (GAP), and extracellular signal-regulated protein kinase (ERK).

the latter being in contrast to the effects of ionizing radiation. The activation of Syk tyrosine kinase appears to be the primary target for H_2O_2, and is believed to be responsible for the increase in $[Ca^{2+}]_i$ observed in these cells after treatment with the peroxide. The major targets for H_2O_2 in T-lymphocytes were found to be ZAP-70 (76) and p56^{lck} (77,78), and the responsiveness of ZAP-70 to H_2O_2 required the presence of T-cell receptor ζ and ε chains. Detailed analysis of the p56^{lck} protein revealed that H_2O_2 and the pro-oxidant diamide induce the autophosphorylation of Tyr-394 and Tyr-505 (77–79). Phosphorylation of this residue is involved in the activation of p56^{lck} by H_2O_2 but is believed to be mediated by an H_2O_2-sensitive yet unidentified protein tyrosine kinase distinct from p56^{lck} itself (79). Another protein tyrosine kinase that is a target for H_2O_2 is epidermal growth factor (EGF) receptor (80). This receptor responds to the pro-oxidant by enhanced autophosphorylation of Tyr-1,173 residue, which is also phosphorylated on activation of the receptor by its natural ligand.

An additional source of free radicals reported to have a marked effect on protein tyrosine phosphorylation is UV irradiation (Table 2). Ledbetter's laboratory showed that UVB and UVC, but not UVA, induced tyrosine phosphorylation in B and T lymphocytes, leading in the latter case to an increase in $[Ca^{2+}]_i$ as a result of ZAP-70 and phospholipase C-γ1 activation (76,81). The EGF receptor also becomes activated following irradiation of mammalian cells with UVB and UVC. Activation of the EGF receptor is thought to be responsible for the activation of gene expression through a downstream cascade involving Ras, Raf-1, ERKs, and TCF (Figure 3) (82–85).

Protein Phosphatases

A number of protein phosphatases, mainly protein tyrosine phosphatases, have been shown to be targeted by free radicals. Unlike protein kinases, most, if not all, protein phosphatases examined are inhibited on exposure of mammalian cells to doses of free radicals or pro-oxidants found to stimulate cellular protein phosphorylation.

Several studies, utilizing phosphorylated synthetic substrates such as poly-(Glu, Tyr) or p-nitrophenol phosphate, showed that free-radical generation through menadione or H_2O_2 treatment of a number of different cell types inhibits total cellular protein tyrosine phosphatase activity (68,74,86,87). The identity of most target protein tyrosine phosphatases is still unclear, with the exception in T lymphocytes and HL-60 cells of CD45 (60,78,88) and in HER 14 fibroblasts of a phosphatase acting on the EGF receptor (89). Interestingly, γ-irradiation of B-lymphocyte precursors was without effect on total protein tyrosine phosphatase activity (70). Protein serine/threonine phosphatases have also been studied for their interaction with free radicals and pro-oxidants, and it was found that the activity of protein phosphatase 2A (but not protein phosphatase 1) was diminished in H_2O_2-treated T lymphocytes (88). In contrast, using purified enzyme incubated with H_2O_2, Zor et al. (90) showed that only the activity of protein phosphatase 2B (calcineurin) but not that of protein phosphatases 2A and 1 was inhibited by this in vitro treatment. Interestingly, Wagner and Mutus (91) observed that the modification of only one or two selective thiol groups on protein phosphatase 2B resulted in a transient, up to 10-fold increase in enzyme activity when the purified enzyme was titrated with thiol-modifying Ellman's reagent. Further modification of the remaining thiol groups inhibited the enzyme's activity. Whether a similar activation of protein phosphatase 2B can occur in an intact cellular environment remains to be determined.

As pointed out earlier, alterations in protein phosphorylation are the result of changes in the balance between kinase or phosphatase activities. Although protein serine/threonine and in particular tyrosine phosphatase activities are often inhibited under conditions where cellular protein phosphorylation is augmented, the stimulatory effect of the kinases generally predominates and the inhibition of phosphatase activity therefore only enhances target protein phosphorylation. Thus, protein kinases are generally regarded as the major regulators of the cellular effects of free radicals and pro-oxidants.

Mechanisms of Free-Radical-Mediated Activation of Protein Kinases and Inactivation of Protein Phosphatases

As suggested previously (53), some common structural features shared by kinases, in particular the location of groups of cysteines near positively charged amino acids, which renders their thiol groups particularly susceptible to modification, may predispose them to oxidative activation. In contrast, protein phosphatases are usually inactivated by free radicals and pro-oxidants. A common feature of the cellular effects of free radicals and pro-oxidants is that they induce oxidative stress and alter the cellular redox balance. Indeed, thiol-modifying agents such as $HgCl_2$ or phenylarsine oxide have been known to trigger cell signaling through protein kinase activation and protein phosphatase inhibition in manners analogous to natural ligands or free radicals (92–96). Consequently, a common mechanism that underlies the cellular phenotypic changes caused by free radicals through protein phosphorylation most likely involves alterations in the thiol redox balance of selective protein kinases and phosphatases.

FREE RADICALS AND SECOND-MESSENGER GENERATION

In addition to altering cellular protein phosphorylation status, free radicals have also been shown to cause changes in second-messenger levels. These effects of free radicals may be caused through the activation of phospholipases or adenylyl and guanylyl cyclases. Free radicals are also capable of altering Ca^{2+} signaling by modulating Ca^{2+} homeostatic and mobilization processes in cells.

Phospholipases

It has been known for many years that acute and lethal free-radical injury to cells can lead to enhanced phospholipid turnover (97–99). There is also evidence that low, nontoxic levels of free radicals can modulate phospholipase activity. For example, it is well known that platelet aggregation can be enhanced by micromolar doses of H_2O_2 or superoxide anion (100,101), probably through hydroxyl radical formation (102). The target for free radicals here is phospholipase A_2 (103,104), which upon activation leads to enhanced arachidonate release and its further metabolism to endoperoxides and thromboxanes. The latter step was also reported to be activated by H_2O_2 through stimulation of cyclooxygenase activity (104). The effect of free radicals on phospholipase A_2 activity may not be direct. Thus, in platelets phospholipase A_2 activation appears to be mediated by the Na^+/H^+ antiporter (102), and in other tissues such as Kupffer cells, vascular smooth muscle cells, or keratinocytes by Ca^{2+}, protein kinase C, or EGF receptor and ERKs, respectively (83,105,106).

Another phospholipase targeted by free radicals is the phosphatidylinositol 4,5-bisphosphate-specific phospholipase C that mediates $Ins(1,4,5)P_3$ and diacylglycerol formation (Figure 2). Several reports have documented an increase in $Ins(1,4,5)P_3$ levels on exposure of mammalian cells to free radicals, including endothelial cells (107), melanocytes (108), and B and T lymphocytes (72,78,81,88). As discussed earlier, the protein tyrosine kinase coupled phospholipase C-γ is activated by free radicals through an upstream phosphorylation event that in lymphocytes appears to be mediated by ZAP-70 and p72[syk] (75,76). In contrast, the mechanism of activation of the

G-protein-coupled form of phospholipase C (phospholipase C-β) remains obscure, although there is some evidence for a possible role of the radical-induced lipid peroxidation breakdown product 4-hydroxynonenal in this process (109). Recently, it has been shown that phospholipase D, which metabolizes phospholipids to phosphatidate, is also activated by H_2O_2 in endothelial cells (110) and NIH 3T3 fibroblasts (111). The mechanism of activation as well as its cellular consequences remain unclear.

Adenylyl and Guanylyl Cyclases

Both adenylyl and guanylyl cyclases are affected by free radicals and pro-oxidants. For example, H_2O_2, at micromolar levels, enhances forskolin-stimulated adenylyl cyclase in murine A10 smooth muscle cells (112). Free radicals derived from H_2O_2 rather than H_2O_2 itself appeared responsible for the enhancement of cAMP formation, and the stimulation was completely impaired by inhibitors of protein tyrosine kinase activity. The latter findings suggest that adenylyl cyclase activation is mediated by an upstream free-radical-stimulated tyrosine phosphorylation event.

Guanylyl cyclase is a major effector of NO action and is responsible for the vasodilator action of this free-radical signaling molecule through the formation of cGMP from GTP (9). Pro-oxidants and thiol oxidizing agents can also activate this enzyme in intact platelets through formation of a protein-glutathione mixed disulfide (113). Strikingly, the concentration of H_2O_2 that was necessary to activate cGMP formation was higher than the concentrations mediating platelet activation through phospholipase A_2 (discussed earlier) and, as expected from the known inhibitory function of cGMP in platelets, H_2O_2 at these higher concentrations antagonized ADP-mediated aggregation (114).

Ca^{2+} Signaling

The divalent cation Ca^{2+} has been the focus of much research on the mechanisms of free-radical-mediated acute lethal injury. This is because there is considerable evidence showing that conditions of oxidative stress cause a general perturbation of intracellular Ca^{2+} homeostasis leading to a sustained and pathological increase in $[Ca^{2+}]_i$. The latter in turn results in the activation of numerous Ca^{2+}-stimulated catabolic processes mediated by phospholipases, proteases and endonucleases. The role of Ca^{2+} in toxicity has been extensively reviewed in several recent publications (7,8) and is not further discussed here as it lies outside the scope of this review.

Intracellular Ca^{2+} signals require the coordinate action of multiple Ca^{2+}-translocating enzymes (primarily Ca^{2+}-ATPases) and signaling molecules and second messengers [mainly Ins(1,4,5)P$_3$] (Figure 5). The Ca^{2+}-translocating ATPases ensure that $[Ca^{2+}]_i$ is maintained at around 0.1 μM against an extracellular Ca^{2+} concentration in the millimolar range by pumping Ca^{2+} across the plasma membrane out of the cell and active sequestration by intracellular organelles (115,116). Additionally, the major portion of Ca^{2+} in the cytosolic compartment is not free but bound to both soluble

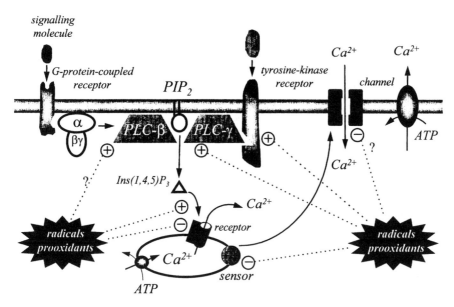

FIG. 5. Effect of free radicals and pro-oxidants on Ca^{2+} signaling. Ca^{2+} release from an intracellular store is caused by Ins(1,4,5)P$_3$, which is released following the activation of phospholipase C-β or -γ. Ca^{2+} release from this pool is accompanied by the opening of specific Ca^{2+} channels in the plasma membrane of the cell through a still poorly understood mechanism. Free radicals have been found to target nearly every single step of the signal transduction pathways acting on Ca^{2+}, and can therefore stimulate or inhibit them, depending on the dose or target cell.

cytosolic proteins and membrane surfaces. Intracellular Ca^{2+} signaling is achieved upon the transient release of the cation from a discrete pool localized in a subdomain of the endoplasmic reticulum (116), and possibly the nucleus (117), followed by the opening of Ca^{2+} channels in the plasma membrane to allow the entry of extracellular Ca^{2+} (118,119). The release of Ca^{2+} from intracellular pool is mainly triggered by the second messenger Ins(1,4,5)P$_3$ derived from plasma membrane phosphatidylinositol 4,5-bisphosphate by the action of phospholipases C-β and -γ (120,121). Ins(1,4,5)P$_3$ in turn binds to a transmembrane channel-linked receptor and enables the release of stored Ca^{2+}. This initial intracellular pool-based mobilization is then rapidly followed by plasma membrane Ca^{2+} channel opening through a complex mechanism depending on a putative messenger sensing the filling state of the Ins(1,4,5)P$_3$-sensitive Ca^{2+} store (118,119,122). From this interaction between Ca^{2+} release from internal pools and entry across the plasma membrane results a complex pattern of cytosolic Ca^{2+} waves (also often referred to as Ca^{2+} oscillations).

Free radicals and pro-oxidants have been found to target most of the components of the Ca^{2+} signaling machinery. Work from the laboratory of Thomas has shown that the pro-oxidant and free-radical-generating organic peroxide, *t*-butyl hydroperoxide, can generate in rat hepatocytes Ca^{2+} waves that are virtually identical to those caused by true Ca^{2+}-mobilizing signaling molecules that activate cells through

Ins(1,4,5)P$_3$ generation (123). Likewise the subcellular locus from where the waves originate as well as their progress after *t*-butyl hydroperoxide treatment were found to be indistinguishable from Ca^{2+} waves following α_1-adrenergic receptor agonist treatment. However, the free-radical-mediated phenomenon occurred in the absence of inositol phosphate formation (123). Investigation of the mechanism underlying peroxide-induced Ca^{2+} waves revealed that the oxidative stress generated by *t*-butyl hydroperoxide leads to an increase in the sensitivity of the Ins(1,4,5)P$_3$ receptor for Ins(1,4,5)P$_3$ through a thiol oxidation process (123–126) on the receptor protein (127). Indeed, it has been known for several years that thiol-modifying agents such as thimerosal can elicit Ca^{2+} waves in several cell types (128,129). Likewise, H$_2$O$_2$ induces Ca^{2+} signals in endothelial cells (130,131) and in B and T lymphocytes (75,76). Larsson and Cerutti (56) reported that superoxide anion at concentrations activating S6 kinase also elevates [Ca^{2+}]$_i$. UV irradiation increases [Ca^{2+}]$_i$ in T lymphocytes (76), while γ-irradiation of T lymphocytes or thymocytes has no or little effect on [Ca^{2+}]$_i$ (40,132). Unfortunately, the vast majority of studies on the effects of free radicals on [Ca^{2+}]$_i$ are based on [Ca^{2+}]$_i$ measurements in whole cell populations and thus do not allow us to draw any conclusions as to whether the radicals produce Ca^{2+} waves similar to those seen in response to Ins(1,4,5)P$_3$-generating signaling molecules. Furthermore, the mechanism of Ca^{2+} signaling caused by free radicals (in contrast to the pathological [Ca^{2+}]$_i$ elevation during cytotoxic injury) is usually obscure except in the case of lymphocytes, where it has been associated with an elevation of Ins(1,4,5)P$_3$ as a result of phospholipase C-γ activation through ZAP-70 and p72^{syk} (75,76).

A rather different effect on Ca^{2+} signaling is observed in endothelial cells treated with *t*-butyl hydroperoxide. In this cell type, the peroxide does not produce changes in [Ca^{2+}]$_i$ on its own but instead selectively blocks Ca^{2+} entry through Ca^{2+} channels following Ins(1,4,5)P$_3$-mediated Ca^{2+} store release by the agonist bradykinin (133). This effect of *t*-butyl hydroperoxide on Ca^{2+} signaling was identified as specifically targeting the store-dependent Ca^{2+} entry pathway (134); however, the effect occurs at doses resulting in rapid cell death. Inhibition of Ca^{2+} signaling also occurred in hepatocytes treated with the redox-active quinone menadione, and was reported to be due to inhibition of Ins(1,4,5)P$_3$-receptor function. However the effect of menadione appeared to be mediated by adduct formation on critical thiol group(s) of the Ins(1,4,5)P$_3$-receptor protein rather than through a process involving free radicals (135,136). Likewise, an alteration in T-lymphocyte redox balance through a selective decrease in intracellular GSH content by buthionine sulfoximine treatment results in compromised Ca^{2+} signaling through the T-cell receptor. Here, a decrease in GSH was found to produce an inhibition of [Ca^{2+}]$_i$ increase as a result of impaired phospholipase C-γ activation by the T-cell receptor (137).

MODULATION OF TRANSCRIPTION FACTOR ACTION AND GENE EXPRESSION BY FREE RADICALS

A hallmark of most signaling pathways is that the message is directed through the cells down to the nucleus, where selective alterations in gene transcription and expression take place. It is these changes that are considered responsible for the phenotypic effects caused by signaling molecules, and it is therefore not surprising that free radicals have been found to also modulate gene transcription in numerous cell types and experimental systems.

A comprehensive discussion of the effects of free radicals on gene expression is found in chapter 16 of this volume, and I only briefly summarize this topic here. Free radicals, like signaling molecules, can regulate gene expression through the activation or repression of selective transcription factors, such as activator protein-1 (AP-1), nuclear transcription factor κB (NFκB), and T-cell-specific factor-1α (TCF-1α). The modulation of transcription factor activity has been found to be mediated either through direct modification of the transcription factor or via activation or inhibition of an upstream signaling pathway. Thus, the activation of NFκB by H_2O_2 (138,139), UV (76,140), and ionizing irradiation (72) is well established and has been linked to the transcription of a number of immediate-early genes, including c-*fos* and c-*jun* (141–146). Likewise, AP-1 has been found to become activated following UV irradiation of HeLa cells (82,84).

While many of the effects of free radicals on transcription factors and gene expression are the result of upstream activating signals mediated by, for example, protein kinase C (143,145), receptor-linked tyrosine kinases (84), Src-type protein tyrosine kinases (73,75,76), or Ca^{2+} signals (146), the ability of free radicals to produce DNA damage directly and indirectly (2) also has important consequences to transcription factor activity and gene expression. Datta et al. (147) reported that the genes encoding for *cdc2*, *cdc25*, and cyclins A and B are downregulated following ionizing irradiation of U-937 cells. Likewise, G_1 and G_2 cell cycle arrests as a result of DNA damage from free radicals is mediated by the *GADD*, *MyD*, and *p21*[WAF1/Cip1] gene products (148–150). In particular, the transcriptional activation of GADD45 and WAF1/Cip1 appears pivotal in the cell cycle delay observed after DNA damage (153), and this is effected by the DNA-damage-sensing transcription factor p53 (150–152). AP-1 activity may also be regulated by DNA damage as shown by Xanthoudakis et al. (153), who identified the AP-1 activating protein Ref-1 as a DNA repair enzyme. Recent evidence in fact points to the existence of a complex network of DNA-damage-sensing protein kinases and other downstream kinases that transduce the DNA damage signal to DNA repair and cell cycle control genes and proteins (154).

CONCLUSIONS AND FUTURE PERSPECTIVES

Clearly free radicals should not only be viewed as a class of very reactive agents whose biological effects are restricted to acute lethal cell death. Instead they can have very subtle perturbing effects on cell function. It is probably these more complex effects that are at the basis of many of the human diseases such as atherosclerosis, aging, neurodegenerative diseases, and cancer that are often attributed to free radicals. As I have briefly summarized in this review, many components of signaling pathways appear to be susceptible to modulation by free radicals, some displaying either enhanced or impaired activity to a physiological stimulus, while others become spontaneously active, thereby bypassing normal receptor control mechanisms. Although it could be argued that the targeting of cell signaling by free radicals may produce a distorted signal in the target cell or may activate a wrong signal at the wrong time, there is evidence that some of the signals may be beneficial to the cell. An example for this would be the cell cycle arrest imposed on the cell following free-radical-mediated DNA strand breaks to allow the cell to correctly repair the damage before progressing to DNA replication (82). Free radicals may in fact be utilized as an integral component of some signaling pathways. There is compelling evidence for this in the downstream signaling events elicited by tumor necrosis factor α receptor (155). A further aspect to consider in this context is that free radicals may modulate cell signaling in an indirect way by modifying or creating new signaling molecules, such as 4-hydroxynonenal (109,156,157), oxidized low-density lipoproteins (158) or 8-epi-prostaglandin $F_{2\alpha}$, a free-radical-catalyzed oxidation product of arachidonic acid (159).

An emerging picture is that the targeting of a cell's signaling machinery is highly dependent on the dose of free radicals and that many pathways respond in a biphasic mode, with activation often followed by inhibition. The latter has been clearly shown for protein kinase C (53) and NFκB (50), as examples (Figure 6). Such a complex dose-response relationship is also reflected in the complexity of the responses of cells to free radicals, as shown by the work of Dypbukt et al. (17), who reported that the same insulinoma cell line responds to low doses of free radicals by stimulation of cell proliferation, to intermediate doses by apoptosis, and finally to higher doses by necrosis. This complex pattern of behavior appeared to be mediated by differential effects of the free radicals on protein kinase C activity (17). A future challenge will be to elucidate the signaling targets of free radicals that cause cells to enter prolifera-

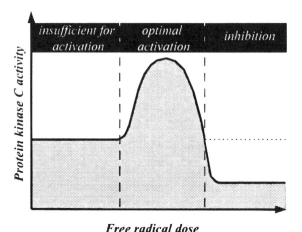

Free radical dose

FIG. 6. Dose-response relationship for the activation of protein kinase C by free radicals and pro-oxidants.

tion and to distinguish them from the signals responsible for cell differentiation or apoptosis. An even greater challenge will be to extrapolate our understanding of what happens under in vitro conditions to the in vivo situation.

Interestingly, the use of antioxidants has revealed that some diseases involve a previously unsuspected imbalance in cellular redox and possibly free-radical generation. This seems to be the case with HIV-infected patients, who have a characteristic decrease in plasma and T-lymphocyte GSH levels (50,160). Since this has been linked to enhanced viral replication and expression (136,161), there may be potential benefits in the treatment of AIDS with the antioxidant and GSH precursor *N*-acetylcysteine (162,163). However, in addition to the use of antioxidants, it is expected that the ability of free radicals to act through signal transduction pathways may open new avenues for selective therapeutic interventions. A proper understanding of the molecular events underlying the effects of free radicals on cell signaling becomes therefore of prime importance.

REFERENCES

1. Schöfl C, Prank K, Brabant G. Mechanisms of cellular information processing. *Trends Endocrinol Metab* 1994;5:53–59.
2. Halliwell B, Gutteridge JMC. *Free Radicals in Biology and Medicine.* 2nd ed. Oxford: Oxford University Press; 1989.
3. Halliwell B, Gutteridge JMC. Role of free radicals and catalytic metal ions in human disease: An overview. *Methods Enzymol* 1990;186:1–85.
4. Kass GEN, Nicotera P, Orrenius S. Calcium-modulated cellular effects of oxidants. In: Cochrane CG, Gimbrone MA, Jr., eds. *Biological Oxidants: Generation and Injurious Consequences.* San Diego: Academic Press; 1992:133–156.
5. Sies H. Strategies of antioxidant defense. *Eur J Biochem* 1993;215:213–219.
6. Halliwell B. Free radicals, antioxidants, and human disease: Curiosity, cause, or consequence? *Lancet* 1994;344:721–724.
7. Nicotera P, Bellomo G, Orrenius S. Calcium-mediated mechanisms in chemically induced cell death. *Annu Rev Pharmacol Toxicol* 1992;32:449–470.
8. Trump BF, Berezesky IK. Calcium-mediated cell injury and cell death. *FASEB J* 1995;9:219–228.
9. Moncada S, Palmer RMJ, Higgs EA. Nitric oxide: Physiology, pathophysiology and pharmacology. *Pharmacol Rev* 1991;43:109–142.
10. Nathan C. Nitric oxide as a secretory product of mammalian cells. *FASEB J* 1992;6:3051–3064.
11. Gross SS, Wolin MS. Nitric oxide: Pathophysiological mechanisms. *Annu Rev Physiol* 1995; 57:737–769.
12. Zhang J, Snyder SH. Nitric oxide in the nervous-system. *Annu Rev Pharmacol Toxicol* 1995; 35:213–233.
13. Burdon RH, Alliangana D, Gill V. Hydrogen-peroxide and the proliferation of BHK-21-cells. *Free Radical Res* 1995;23:471–486.
14. Murrell GA, Francis MJ, Bromley L. Modulation of fibroblast proliferation by oxygen free radicals. *Biochem J* 1990;265:659–665.
15. Gallagher DL, Betteridge LJ, Patel MK, Schachter M. Effect of oxidants on vascular smooth muscle proliferation. *Biochem Soc Trans* 1993;21:98S.
16. Stäuble B, Boscoboinik D, Tasinato A, Azzi A. Modulation of activator protein-1 (AP-1) transcription factor and protein kinase C by hydrogen peroxide and D-α-tocopherol in vascular smooth muscle cells. *Eur J Biochem* 1994;226:393–402.
17. Dypbukt JM, Ankarkrona M, Burkitt M, Sjöholm Å, Ström K, Orrenius S, Nicotera P. Different pro-oxidant levels stimulate growth, trigger apoptosis, or produce necrosis of insulin-secreting RINm5F cells: The role of intracellular polyamines. *J Biol Chem* 1994;269:30553–30560.

18. Slaga TJ, Klein-Szanto AJP, Triplett LL, Yotti LP, Trosko JE. Skin tumor-promoting activity of benzoyl peroxide, a widely used free radical-generating compound. *Science* 1981;213:1023–1025.
19. Cerutti PA. Pro-oxidant states and tumor promotion. *Science* 1985;227:375–381.
20. Troll W, Wiesner R. The role of oxygen radicals as a possible mechanism of tumor promotion. *Annu Rev Pharmacol Toxicol* 1985;25:509–528.
21. Maity A, McKenna WG, Muschel RJ. The molecular basis for cell cycle delays following ionizing radiation: A review. *Radiother Oncol* 1994;31:1–13.
22. Sohal RS, Allen RG, Nations C. Oxygen free radicals play a role in cellular differentiation: An hypothesis. *J Free Radical Biol Med* 1986;2:175–181.
23. Sohal RS, Dubey A. Mitochondrial oxidative damage, hydrogen-peroxide release, and aging. *Free Radical Biol Med* 1994;16:621–626.
24. Erkell LJ. Differentiation of mouse neuroblastoma cells under increased oxygen tension. *Exp Cell Biol* 1980;48:374–380.
25. Rodemann HP, Peterson HP, Schwenke K, von Wangenheim KH. Terminal differentiation of human fibroblasts is induced by radiation. *Scanning Microsc* 1991;5:1135–1143.
26. Rocchi P, Ferreri AM, Simone G, et al. Gamma-radiation-induced differentiation on human neuro-blastoma-cells in culture. *Anticancer Res* 1993;13:419–422.
27. Sugihara M, Fujita Y, Enomoto KI, Maeno T, Ishida T. Induction of differentiation by radiation and hyperthermia in neuroblastoma-glioma hybrid-cells. *Cell Biochem Function* 1994;12:137–142.
28. Nishihira J, Ishibashi T, Takeichi N, Sakamoto W, Nakamura M. A role for oxygen radicals in rat monocytic leukemia cell differentiation under stimulation with platelet-activating factor. *Biochim Biophys Acta* 1994;1220:286–290.
29. Kobayashi M, Nishihara J, Fujii Y, Maeda H, Hosokawa M, Takeichi N. Involvement of oxygen radicals in the differentiation of rat myelomonocytic leukemia cells in vitro and in vivo. *Leuk Res* 1994;18:199–203.
30. Yang KD, Shaio MF. Hydroxyl radicals as an early signal involved in phorbol ester-induced monocytic differentiation of HL60 cells. *Biochem Biophys Res Commun* 1994;200:1650–1657.
31. Kerr JFR, Searle J, Harmon BV, Bishop CJ. Apoptosis. In: Potten CS, ed. *Perspectives on Mammalian Cell Death.* Oxford: Oxford University Press; 1987:93–128.
32. Arends MJ, Wyllie AH. Apoptosis: Mechanisms and roles in pathology. *Int Rev Exp Pathol* 1991;32:223–254.
33. Buttke TM, Sandstrom PA. Oxidative stress as a mediator of apoptosis. *Immunol Today* 1994;15:7–10.
34. Sarafian TA, Bredesen DE. Is apoptosis mediated by reactive oxygen species? *Free Radical Res* 1994;21:1–8.
35. Hickman JA. Apoptosis induced by anticancer drugs. *Cancer Metastasis Rev* 1992;11:121–139.
36. Montagna W, Wilson JW. A cytologic study of the intestinal epithelium of the mouse after total-body X-irradiation. *J Natl Cancer Inst* 1955;15:1703–1736.
37. Hugon J, Borgers M. Ultrastructural and cytochemical studies on karyolytic bodies in the epithelium of the duodenal crypts of whole body X-irradiated mice. *Lab Invest* 1966;15:1528–1543.
38. Servomaa K, Rytömaa T. UV light and ionizing radiations cause programmed death of rat chloroleu-kaemia cells by inducing retropositions of a mobile DNA element (L1Rn). *Int J Radiat Biol* 1990;57:331–343.
39. Lennon SV, Martin SJ, Cotter TG. Dose-dependent induction of apoptosis in human tumour cell lines by widely diverging stimuli. *Cell Prolif* 1991;24:203–214.
40. Zhivotovsky B, Nicotera P, Bellomo G, Hanson K, Orrenius S. Ca^{2+} and endonuclease activation in radiation-induced lymphoid cell death. *Exp Cell Res* 1993;207:163–170.
41. Hockenbery DM, Oltvai ZN, Yin XM, Milliman CL, Korsmeyer SJ. Bcl-2 functions in an antioxidant pathway to prevent apoptosis. *Cell* 1993;75:241–251.
42. Gramzinski RA, Parchment RE, Pierce GB. Evidence linking programmed cell death in the blastocyst to polyamine oxidation. *Differentiation* 1990;43:59–65.
43. Ueda N, Shah SV. Endonuclease-induced DNA damage and cell death in oxidant injury to renal tubular epithelial cells. *J Clin Invest* 1992;90:2593–2597.
44. de Bono DP, Yang WD. Exposure to low concentrations of hydrogen peroxide causes delayed endothelial cell death and inhibits proliferation of surviving cells. *Atherosclerosis* 1995; 114:235–245.
45. Wolfe JT, Ross D, Cohen GM. A role for metals and free radicals in the induction of apoptosis in thymocytes. *FEBS Lett* 1994;352:58–62.

46. Slater AFG, Nobel CSI, Maellaro E, Bustamante J, Kimland M, Orrenius S. Nitrone spin traps and a nitroxide antioxidant inhibit a common pathway of thymocyte apoptosis. *Biochem J* 1995;306:771–778.
47. Greenlund LJS, Deckwerth TL, Johnson EM Jr. Superoxide dismutase delays neuronal apoptosis: A role for reactive oxygen species in programmed neuronal death. *Neuron* 1995;14:303–315.
48. Wong GHW. Protective roles of cytokines against radiation: Induction of mitochondrial MnSOD. *Biochim Biophys Acta* 1995;1271:205–209.
49. Roederer M, Staal FJT, Anderson M, Rabin R, Raju PA, Herzenberg L, Herzenberg LA. Disregulation of leukocyte glutathione in AIDS. *Ann N Y Acad Sci* 1993;677:113–125.
50. Dröge W, Schulze-Osthoff K, Mihm S, Galter D, Schenk H, Eck H-P, Roth S, Omünder H. Functions of glutathione and glutathione disulfide in immunology and immunopathology. *FASEB J* 1994;8:1131–1138.
51. Buchner K. Protein kinase C in the transduction of signals toward and within the cell nucleus. *Eur J Biochem* 1995;228:211–221.
52. Nishizuka Y. Protein kinase C and lipid signaling for sustained cellular responses. *FASEB J* 1995;9:484–496.
53. Kass GEN, Duddy SK, Orrenius S. Activation of hepatocyte protein kinase C by redox-cycling quinones. *Biochem J* 1989;260:499–507.
54. Larsson R, Cerutti P. Translocation and enhancement of phosphotransferase activity of protein kinase C following exposure in mouse epidermal cells to oxidants. *Cancer Res* 1989;49:5627–5632.
55. Gopalakrishna R, Anderson WB. Ca^{2+}- and phospholipid-independent activation of protein kinase C by selective oxidative modification of the regulatory domain. *Proc Natl Acad Sci USA* 1989;86:6758–6762.
56. Larsson R, Cerutti P. Oxidants induce phosphorylation of ribosomal protein S6. *J Biol Chem* 1988;263:17452–17458.
57. Kharbanda S, Saleem A, Shafman T, Emoto Y, Weichselbaum R, Kufe D. Activation of the pp90[rsk] and mitogen-activated serine/threonine protein kinases by ionizing radiation. *Proc Natl Acad Sci USA* 1994;91:5415–5420.
58. Hunter T. Protein kinases and phosphatases: The yin and yang of protein phosphorylation and signaling. *Cell* 1995;80:225–236.
59. Stevenson MA, Pollock SS, Coleman CN, Calderwood SK. X-irradiation, phorbol esters, and H_2O_2 stimulate mitogen-activated protein kinase activity in NIH-3T3 cells through the formation of reactive oxygen intermediates. *Cancer Res* 1994;54:12–15.
60. Fialkow L, Chan CK, Rotin D, Grinstein S, Downey GP. Activation of the mitogen-activated protein kinase signaling pathway in neutrophils: Role of oxidants. *J Biol Chem* 1994;269:31234–31242.
61. Kyriakis JM, Banerjee P, Nikolakaki E, Dai TA, Rubie EA, Ahmed MF, Avruch J, Woodgett JR. The stress-activated protein-kinase subfamily of c-jun kinases. *Nature* 1994;369:156–160.
62. Derijard B, Hibi M, Wu IH, Barrett T, Su B, Deng TL, Karin M, Davis RJ. Jnk—A protein-kinase stimulated by UV-light and Ha-ras that binds and phosphorylates the c-Jun activation domain. *Cell* 1994;76:1025–1037.
63. Pombo CM, Bonventre JV, Avruch J, Woodgett JR, Kyriakis JM, Force T. The stress-activated protein kinases are major c-Jun amino-terminal kinases activated by ischemia and reperfusion. *J Biol Chem* 1994;269:26546–26551.
64. Kharbanda S, Saleem A, Shafman T, Emoto Y, Taneja J, Rubin E, Weichelbaum R, Woodgett J, Avruch J, Kyriakis J, Kufe D. Ionizing radiation stimulates a Grb2-mediated association of the stress-activated protein-kinase with phosphatidylinositol 3-kinase. *J Biol Chem* 1995; 270:18871–18874.
65. May JM, de Haën C. The insulin-like effect of hydrogen peroxide on pathways of lipid synthesis in rat adipocytes. *J Biol Chem* 1979;254:9017–9021.
66. Hayes GR, Lockwood DH. Role of insulin receptor phosphorylation in the insulinomimetic effects of hydrogen peroxide. *Proc Natl Acad Sci USA* 1987;84:8115–8119.
67. Koshio O, Akanuma Y, Kasuga M. Hydrogen peroxide stimulates tyrosine phosphorylation of the insulin receptor and its tyrosine kinase activity in intact cells. *Biochem J* 1988;250:95–101.
68. Heffetz D, Bushkin I, Dror R, Zick Y. The insulinomimetic agents H_2O_2 and vanadate stimulate protein tyrosine phosphorylation in intact cells. *J Biol Chem* 1990;265:2896–2902.
69. Chan TM, Chen E, Tatoyan A, Shargill NS, Pleta M, Hochstein P. Stimulation of tyrosine-specific protein phosphorylation in the rat liver plasma membrane by oxygen radicals. *Biochem Biophys Res Commun* 1986;139:439–445.

70. Uckun FM, Tuel-Ahlgren L, Song CW, Waddick K, Myers DE, Kirihara J, Ledbetter JA, Schieven GL. Ionizing radiation stimulates unidentified tyrosine-specific protein kinases in human B-lymphocyte precursors, triggering apoptosis and clonogenic cell death. *Proc Natl Acad Sci USA* 1992;89:9005–9009.

71. Waddick KG, Chae HP, Tuel-Ahlgren LM, Jarvis LJ, Dibirdik I, Myers DE, Uckun FM. Engagement of the CD19 receptor on human B-lineage leukemia cells activates LCK tyrosine kinase and facilitates radiation-induced apoptosis. *Radiat Res* 1993;136:313–319.

72. Uckun FM, Schieven GL, Tuel-Ahlgren LM, Dibirdik I, Myers DE, Ledbetter JA, Song CW. Tyrosine phosphorylation is a mandatory proximal step in radiation-induced activation of the protein kinase C signaling pathway in human B-lymphocyte precursors. *Proc Natl Acad Sci USA* 1993;90:252–256.

73. Kharbanda S, Yuan Z-M, Rubin E, Weichselbaum R, Kufe D. Activation of Src-like p56/p53[lyn] tyrosine kinase by ionizing radiation. *J Biol Chem* 1994;269:20739–20743.

74. Juan C-C, Wu FY-H. Vitamin K3 inhibits growth of human hepatoma HepG2 cells by decreasing activities of both p34[cdc2] kinase and phosphatase. *Biochem Biophys Res Commun* 1993;190:907–913.

75. Schieven GL, Kirihara JM, Burg DL, Geahlen RL, Ledbetter JA. p72[syk] tyrosine kinase is activated by oxidizing conditions that induce lymphocyte tyrosine phosphorylation and Ca^{2+} signals. *J Biol Chem* 1993;268:16688–16692.

76. Schieven GL, Mittler RS, Nadler SG, Kirihara JM, Bolen JB, Kanner SB, Ledbetter JA. ZAP-70 tyrosine kinase, CD45, and T cell receptor involvement in UV- and H_2O_2-induced T cell signal transduction. *J Biol Chem* 1994;269:20718–20726.

77. Nakamura K, Hori T, Sato N, Sugie K, Kawakami T, Yodoi J. Redox regulation of a src family protein tyrosine kinase p56[lck] in T cells. *Oncogene* 1993;8:3133–3139.

78. Secrist JP, Burns LA, Karnitz L, Koretzky GA, Abraham RT. Stimulatory effects of the protein tyrosine phosphatase inhibitor, pervanadate, on T-cell activation events. *J Biol Chem* 1993;268:5886–5893.

79. Hardwick JS, Sefton BM. Activation of the Lck tryosine protein kinase by hydrogen peroxide requires the phosphorylation of Tyr-394. *Proc Natl Acad Sci USA* 1995;92:4527–4531.

80. Gamou S, Shimizu N. Hydrogen peroxide preferentially enhances the tyrosine phosphorylation of epidermal growth factor receptor. *FEBS Lett* 1995;357:161–164.

81. Schieven GL, Kirihara JM, Gilliland LK, Uckun FM, Ledbetter JA. Ultraviolet radiation rapidly induces tyrosine phosphorylation and calcium signaling in lymphocytes. *Mol Biol Cell* 1993; 4:523–530.

82. Devary Y, Gottlieb RA, Smeal T, Karin M. The mammalian ultraviolet response is triggered by activation of Src tyrosine kinases. *Cell* 1992;71:1081–1091.

83. Miller CC, Hale P, Pentland AP. Ultraviolet B injury increases prostaglandin synthesis through a tyrosine kinase-dependent pathway. Evidence for UVB-induced epidermal growth factor receptor activation. *J Biol Chem* 1994;269:3529–3533.

84. Sachsenmaier C, Radler Pohl A, Zinck R, Nordheim A, Herrlich P, Rahmsdorf HJ. Involvement of growth factor receptors in the mammalian UVC response. *Cell* 1994;78:963–972.

85. Warmuth I, Harth Y, Matsui MS, Wang N, DeLeo VA. Ultraviolet radiation induces phosphorylation of the epidermal growth factor receptor. *Cancer Res* 1994;54:374–376.

86. Hecht D, Zick Y. Selective inhibition of protein tyrosine phosphatase activities by H_2O_2 and vanadate in vitro. *Biochem Biophys Res Commun* 1992;188:773–779.

87. Sullivan SG, Chiu DT, Errasfa M, Wang JM, Qi JS, Stern A. Effects of H_2O_2 on protein tyrosine phosphatase activity in HER14 cells. *Free Radical Biol Med* 1994;16:399–403.

88. Whisler RL, Goyette MA, Grants IS, Newhouse YG. Sublethal levels of oxidant stress stimulate multiple serine/threonine kinases and suppress protein phosphatases in Jurkat T cells. *Arch Biochem Biophys* 1995;319:23–35.

89. Monteiro HP, Ivaschenko Y, Fischer R, Stern A. Inhibition of protein tyrosine phosphatase activity by diamide is reversed by epidermal growth factor in fibroblasts. *FEBS Lett* 1991;295:146–148.

90. Zor U, Ferber E, Gergely P, Szucs K, Dombradi V, Goldman R. Reactive oxygen species mediate phorbol ester-regulated tyrosine phosphorylation and phospholipase A_2 activation: Potentiation by vanadate. *Biochem J* 1993;295:879–888.

91. Wagner J, Mutus B. Transient activation of calcineurin during thiol modification. *Sec Mess Phosphoprot* 1995;13:199–215.

92. Garcia Morales P, Minami Y, Luong E, Klausner RD, Samelson LE. Tyrosine phosphorylation in

T cells is regulated by phosphatase activity: Studies with phenylarsine oxide. *Proc Natl Acad Sci USA* 1990;87:9255–9259.

93. van Belzen N, Rijken PJ, Verkleij AJ, Boonstra J. Sulfhydryl reagents alter epidermal growth factor receptor affinity and association with the cytoskeleton. *J Receptor Res* 1991;11:919–940.

94. Kanner SB, Kavanagh TJ, Grossmann A, et al. Sulfhydryl oxidation down-regulates T-cell signaling and inhibits tyrosine phosphorylation of phospholipase Cγ1. *Proc Natl Acad Sci USA* 1992; 89:300–304.

95. Rahman SM, Pu MY, Hamaguchi M, Iwamoto T, Isobe K, Nakashima I. Redox-linked ligand-independent cell surface triggering for extensive protein tyrosine phosphorylation. *FEBS Lett* 1993;317:35–38.

96. Nakashima I, Pu MY, Nishizaki A, Rosila I,m Ma L, Katano Y, Ohkusu K, Rahman SM, Isobe K, Hanaguchi M. Redox mechanism as alternative to ligand binding for receptor activation delivering disregulated cellular signals. *J Immunol* 1994;152:1064–1071.

97. Chien KR, Pfau RG, Farber JL. Ischemic myocardic injury: Prevention by chloropromazine of an accelerated phospholipid degradation and associated membrane dysfunction. *Am J Pathol* 1979;97:505–530.

98. Farber JL, Young EE. Accelerated phospholipid degradation in anoxic rat hepatocytes. *Arch Biochem Biophys* 1981;221:312–320.

99. Glende EA Jr., Pushpendran KC. Activation of phospholipase A$_2$ by carbon tetrachloride in isolated rat hepatocytes. *Biochem Pharmacol* 1986;35:3301–3307.

100. Handin RL, Karabin R, Boxer GJ. Enhancement of platelet function by superoxide anion. *J Clin Invest* 1977;59:959–965.

101. Del Principe D, Menichelli A, De Matteis W, Di Corpo ML, Di Giulio S, Finazzi-Agro A. Hydrogen peroxide has a role in the aggregation of human platelets. *FEBS Lett* 1985;185:142–146.

102. Iuliano L, Pedersen JZ, Pratico D, Rotilio G, Violi F. Role of hydroxyl radicals in the activation of human platelets. *Eur J Biochem* 1994;221:695–704.

103. Hashizume T, Yamaguchi H, Kawamoto A, Tamura A, Sato T, Fujii T. Lipid peroxide makes rabbit platelet hyperaggregable to agonists through phospholipase A$_2$ activation. *Arch Biochem Biophys* 1991;289:47–52.

104. Hecker G, Utz J, Kupferschmidt RJ, Ullrich V. Low levels of hydrogen peroxide enhance platelet aggregation by cyclooxygenase activation. *Eicosanoids* 1991;4:107–113.

105. Llopis J, Farrell GC, Duddy SK, Kass GEN, Gahm A, Orrenius S. Eicosanoids released following inhibition of the endoplasmic reticulum Ca^{2+} pump stimulate Ca^{2+} efflux in the perfused rat liver. *Biochem Pharmacol* 1993;45:2209–2214.

106. Rao GN, Runge MS, Alexander RW. Hydrogen peroxide activation of cytosolic phospholipase A$_2$ in vascular smooth muscle cells. *Biochim Biophys Acta* 1995;1265:67–72.

107. Shasby MD, Yorek M, Shasby SS. Exogenous oxidants initiate hydrolysis of endothelial cell insitol phospholipids. *Blood* 1988;72:491–499.

108. Carsberg CJ, Ohanian J, Friedmann PS. Ultraviolet radiation stimulates a biphasic pattern of 1,2-diacylglycerol formation in cultured human melanocytes and keratinocytes by activation of phospholipases C and D. *Biochem J* 1995;305:471–477.

109. Rossi MA, Di Mauro C, Esterbauer H, Fidale F, Dianzani MU. Activation of phosphoinositide-specific phospholipase C of rat neutrophils by the chemotactic aldehydes 4-hydroxy-2,3-*trans*-nonenal and 4-hydroxy-2,3-*trans*-octenal. *Cell Biochem Function* 1994;12:275–280.

110. Natarajan V, Taher MM, Roehm B, Parinandi NL, Schmid HH, Kiss Z, Garcia JG. Activation of endothelial cell phospholipase D by hydrogen peroxide and fatty acid hydroperoxide. *J Biol Chem* 1993;268:930–937.

111. Kiss Z, Anderson WH. Hydrogen peroxide regulates phospholipase D-mediated hydrolysis of phosphatidylethanolamine and phosphatidylcholine by different mechanisms in NIH 3T3 fibroblasts. *Arch Biochem Biophys* 1994;311:430–436.

112. Tan CM, Xenoyannis S, Feldman RD. Oxidant stress enhances adenylyl-cyclase activation. *Circ Res* 1995;77:710–717.

113. Wu XB, Brüne B, von Appen F, Ullrich V. Reversible activation of soluble guanylate cyclase by oxidizing agents. *Arch Biochem Biophys* 1992;294:75–82.

114. Ambrosio G, Golino P, Pascucci I, Rosolowsky M, Campbell WB, DeClerck F, Tritto I, Chiariello M. Modulation of platelet function by reactive oxygen metabolites. *Am J Physiol* 1994;267:H308–H318.

115. Carafoli E. Intracellular calcium homeostasis. *Annu Rev Biochem* 1987;56:395–433.

116. Pozzan T, Rizzuto R, Volpe P, Meldolesi J. Molecular and cellular physiology of intracellular calcium stores. *Physiol Rev* 1994;74:595–636.
117. Nicotera P, Orrenius S, Nilsson T, Berggren PO. An inositol 1,4,5-trisphosphate-sensitive Ca^{2+} pool in liver nuclei. *Proc Natl Acad Sci USA* 1990;87:6858–6862.
118. Llopis J, Kass GEN, Gahm A, Orrenius S. Evidence for two pathways of receptor-mediated Ca^{2+} entry in hepatocytes. *Biochem J* 1992;284:243–247.
119. Putney JWJ, Bird GS. The inositol phosphate-calcium signaling system in nonexcitable cells. *Endocr Rev* 1993;14:610–631.
120. Divecha N, Irvine RF. Phospholipid signaling. *Cell* 1995;80:269–278.
121. Clapham DE. Calcium signaling. *Cell* 1995;80:259–268.
122. Fasolato C, Innocenti B, Pozzan T. Receptor-activated Ca^{2+} influx: How many mechanisms for how many channels? *Trends Pharmacol Sci* 1994;15:77–83.
123. Rooney TA, Renard DC, Sass EJ, Thomas AP. Oscillatory cytosolic calcium waves independent of stimulated inositol 1,4,5-trisphosphate formation in hepatocytes. *J Biol Chem* 1991; 266:12272–12282.
124. Missiaen L, Taylor CW, Berridge MJ. Spontaneous calcium release from inositol trisphosphate-sensitive calcium stores. *Nature* 1991;352:241–244.
125. Renard DC, Seitz MB, Thomas AP. Oxidized glutathione causes sensitization of calcium release to inositol 1,4,5-trisphosphate in permeabilized hepatocytes. *Biochem J* 1992;284:507–512.
126. Bird GS, Burgess GM, Putney JWJ. Sulfhydryl reagents and cAMP-dependent kinase increase the sensitivity of the inositol 1,4,5-trisphosphate receptor in hepatocytes. *J Biol Chem* 1993; 268:17917–17923.
127. Kaplin AI, Ferris CD, Voglmaier SM, Snyder SH. Purified reconstituted inositol 1,4,5-trisphosphate receptors. Thiol reagents act directly on receptor protein. *J Biol Chem* 1994;269:28972–28978.
128. Swann K. Thimerosal causes calcium oscillations and sensitizes calcium-induced calcium release in unfertilized hamster eggs. *FEBS Lett* 1991;278:175–178.
129. Thorn P, Brady P, Llopis J, Gallacher DV, Petersen OH. Cytosolic Ca^{2+} spikes evoked by the thiol reagent thimerosal in both intact and internally perfused single pancreatic acinar cells. *Pflugers Arch* 1992;422:173–178.
130. Vercellotti GM, Severson SP, Duane P, Moldow CF. Hydrogen peroxide alters signal transduction in human endothelial cells. *J Lab Clin Med* 1991;117:15–24.
131. Doan TN, Gentry DL, Taylor AA, Elliott SJ. Hydrogen peroxide activates agonist-sensitive Ca^{2+}-flux pathways in canine venous endothelial cells. *Biochem J* 1994;297:209–215.
132. Hallahan DE, Bleakman D, Virudachalam S, Lee D, Gordina D, Kufe DW, Weichselbaum RR. The role of intracellular calcium in the cellular response to ionizing radiation. *Radiat Res* 1994;138:392–400.
133. Elliott SJ, Doan TN. Oxidant stress inhibits the store-dependent Ca^{2+}-influx pathway of vascular endothelial cells. *Biochem J* 1993;292:385–393.
134. Elliott SJ, Eskin SG, Schilling WP. Effect of *t*-butyl-hydroperoxide on bradykinin-stimulated changes in cytosolic calcium in vascular endothelial cells. *J Biol Chem* 1989;264:3806–3810.
135. Pruijn FB, Sibeijn JP, Bast A. Changes in inositol-1,4,5-trisphosphate binding to hepatic plasma membranes caused by temperature, *N*-ethylmaleimide and menadione. *Biochem Pharmacol* 1990;40:1947–1952.
136. Pruijn FB, Sibeijn JP, Bast A. Menadione inhibits the α_1-adrenergic receptor-mediated increase in cytosolic free calcium concentration in hepatocytes by inhibiting inositol 1,4,5-trisphosphate-dependent release of calcium from intracellular stores. *Biochem Pharmacol* 1991;42:1977–1986.
137. Staal FJ, Anderson MT, Staal GE, Herzenberg LA, Gitler C. Redox regulation of signal transduction: tyrosine phosphorylation and calcium influx. *Proc Natl Acad Sci USA* 1994;91:3619–3622.
138. Schreck R, Rieber P, Baeuerle PA. Reactive oxygen intermediates as apparently widely used messengers in the activation of the NF-κB transcription factor and HIV-1. *EMBO J* 1991; 10:2247–2258.
139. Flescher E, Ledbetter JA, Schieven GL, Vela Roch N, Fossum D, Dang H, Ogawa N, Talal N. Longitudinal exposure of human T lymphocytes to weak oxidative stress suppresses transmembrane and nuclear signal transduction. *J Immunol* 1994;153:4880–4889.
140. Devary Y, Rosette C, DiDonato JA, Karin M. NF-κB activation by ultraviolet light not dependent on a nuclear signal. *Science* 1993;261:1442–1445.
141. Crawford D, Zbinden I, Amstad P, Cerutti P. Oxidant stress induces the proto-oncogenes c-fos and c-myc in mouse epidermal cells. *Oncogene* 1988;3:27–32.

142. Sherman ML, Datta R, Hallahan DE, Weichselbaum RR, Kufe DW. Ionizing radiation regulates expression of the c-jun protooncogene. *Proc Natl Acad Sci USA* 1990;87:5663–5666.
143. Hallahan DE, Sukhatme VP, Sherman ML, Virudachalam S, Kufe D, Weichselbaum RR. Protein kinase C mediates x-ray inducibility of nuclear signal transducers EGR1 and JUN. *Proc Natl Acad Sci USA* 1991;88:2156–2160.
144. Nose K, Shibanuma M, Kikuchi K, Kageyama H, Sakiyama S, Kuroki T. Transcriptional activation of early-response genes by hydrogen peroxide in a mouse osteoblastic cell line. *Eur J Biochem* 1991;201:99–106.
145. Datta R, Hallahan DE, Kharbanda SM, Rubin E, Sherman ML, Huberman E, Weichselbaum RR, Kufe DW. Involvement of reactive oxygen intermediates in the induction of c-jun gene transcription by ionizing radiation. *Biochemistry* 1992;31:8300–8306.
146. Maki A, Berezesky IK, Fargnoli J, Holbrook NJ, Trump BF. Role of $[Ca^{2+}]_i$ in induction of *c-fos*, *c-jun*, and *c-myc* mRNA in rat PTE after oxidative stress. *FASEB J* 1992;6:919–924.
147. Datta R, Hass R, Gunji H, Weichselbaum R, Kufe D. Down-regulation of cell cycle control genes by ionizing radiation. *Cell Growth Differ* 1992;3:637–644.
148. Zhan Q, Lord KA, Alamo IJ, Hollander MC, Currier F, Ron D, Kohn KW, Hoffman B, Liebermann DA, Fornace AJJ. The gadd and MyD genes define a novel set of mammalian genes encoding acidic proteins that synergistically suppress cell growth. *Mol Cell Biol* 1994;14:2361–2371.
149. Gujuluva CN, Baek JH, Shin KH, Cherrick HM, Park NH. Effect of UV-irradiation on cell cycle, viability and the expression of p53, gadd153 and gadd45 genes in normal and HPV-immortalized human oral keratinocytes. *Oncogene* 1994;9:1819–1827.
150. Namba H, Hara T, Tukazaki T, Migita K, Ishikawa N, Ito K, Nagataki S, Yamashita S. Radiation-induced G1 arrest is selectively mediated by the p53-WAF1/Cip1 pathway in human thyroid cells. *Cancer Res* 1995;55:2075–2080.
151. Smith ML, Chen IT, Zhan Q, Bae I, Chen CY, Gilmer TM, Kastan MB, O'Connor PM, Fornace AJJ. Interaction of the p53-regulated protein Gadd45 with proliferating cell nuclear antigen. *Science* 1994;266:1376–1380.
152. Zhan Q, Bae I, Kastan MB, Fornace AJJ. The p53-dependent γ-ray response of GADD45. *Cancer Res* 1994;54:2755–2760.
153. Xanthoudakis S, Miao G, Wang F, Pan YC, Curran T. Redox activation of Fos-Jun DNA binding activity is mediated by a DNA repair enzyme. *EMBO J* 1992;11:3323–3335.
154. Gottlieb TM, Jackson SP. Protein kinases and DNA damage. *Trends Biochem Sci* 1994;19:500–503.
155. Schulze-Osthoff K, Beyaert R, Vandevoorde V, Haegeman G, Fiers W. Depletion of the mitochondrial electron transport abrogates the cytotoxic and gene-inductive effects of TNF. *EMBO J* 1993;12:3095–3104.
156. Barrera G, Di Mauro C, Muraca R, Ferrero D, Cavalli G, Fazio VM, Paradisi L, Dianzani MU. Induction of differentiation in human HL-60 cells by 4-hydroxynonenal, a product of lipid peroxidation. *Exp Cell Res* 1991;197:148–152.
157. Fazio VM, Barrera G, Martinotti S, Farace MG, Giglioni B, Frati L, Manzari V, Dianzani MU. 4-Hydroxynonenal, a product of cellular lipid peroxidation, which modulates c-myc and globin gene expression in K562 erythroleukemic cells. *Cancer Res* 1992;52:4866–4871.
158. Escargueil Blanc I, Salvayre R, Negre Salvayre A. Necrosis and apoptosis induced by oxidized low density lipoproteins occur through two calcium-dependent pathways in lymphoblastoid cells. *FASEB J* 1994;8:1075–1080.
159. Yin K, Halushka PV, Yan YT, Wong PY. Antiaggregatory activity of 8-epi-prostaglandin $F_{2α}$ and other F-series prostanoids and their binding to thromboxane A_2/prostaglandin H_2 receptors in human platelets. *J Pharmacol Exp Ther* 1994;270:1192–1196.
160. Staal FJ, Roederer M, Israelski DM, Bubp J, Mole LA, McShane D, Deresinski SC, Ross W, Sussman H, Raju PA. Intracellular glutathione levels in T cell subsets decrease in HIV-infected individuals. *AIDS Res Hum Retroviruses* 1992;8:305–311.
161. Staal FJ, Roederer M, Herzenberg LA. Intracellular thiols regulate activation of nuclear factor κB and transcription of human immunodeficiency virus. *Proc Natl Acad Sci USA* 1990;87:9943–9947.
162. Dröge W, Eck HP, Mihm S. HIV-induced cysteine deficiency and T-cell dysfunction-A rationale for treatment with *N*-acetylcysteine. *Immunol Today* 1992;13:211–214.
163. Roederer M, Staal FJ, Ela SW, Herzenberg LA. *N*-Acetylcysteine: Potential for AIDS therapy. *Pharmacology* 1993;46:121–129.
164. Patel JM, Sekharam KM, Block ER. Oxidant and angiotensin II-induced subcellular translocation of protein kinase C in pulmonary artery endothelial cells. *J Biochem Toxicol* 1992;7:117–123.

165. Pronzato MA, Domenicotti C, Rosso E, et al. Modulation of rat liver protein kinase C during "in vivo" CCl₄-induced oxidative stress. *Biochem Biophys Res Commun* 1993;194:635–641.
166. Whisler RL, Newhouse YG, Beiqing L, Karanfilov BK, Goyette MA, Hackshaw KV. Regulation of protein kinase enzymatic activity in Jurkat T cells during oxidative stress uncoupled from protein tyrosine kinases: Role of oxidative changes in protein kinase activation requirements and generation of second messengers. *Lymphokine Cytokine Res* 1994;13:399–410.
167. Palumbo EJ, Sweatt JD, Chen S-J, Klann E. Oxidation-induced persistent activation of protein kinase C in hippocampal homogenates. *Biochem Biophys Res Commun* 1992;187:1439–1445.
168. Brawn KM, Chiou WJ, Leach KL. Oxidant-induced activation of protein kinase C in UC11MG cells. *Free Radical Res* 1995;22:23–37.
169. Lanzi C, Gambetta RA, Perego P, Banfi P, Franzi A, Guazzoni L, Zunino F. Protein kinase C activation by anthracyclines in Swiss 3T3 cells. *Int J Cancer* 1991;47:136–142.
170. Bauskin AR, Alkalay I, Ben-Neriah Y. Redox regulation of a protein tyrosine kinase in the endoplasmic reticulum. *Cell* 1991;66:685–696.

Free Radical Toxicology
Edited by K. B. Wallace
Copyright © 1997 Taylor & Francis

18

Free-Radical Oxygen-Induced Changes in Chemical Carcinogenesis

James E. Klaunig, Yong Xu, Stephen Bachowski, and Jiazhong Jiang

Division of Toxicology, Department of Pharmacology and Toxicology, Indiana University School of Medicine, Indianapolis, Indiana, USA

Reactive oxygen species are generated in cells during normal cell metabolism and in turn participate in the regulation of cell growth, enzymatic reactions and eicosanoid metabolism (1). Several human chronic disease states, including cancer, have been associated with oxidative stress produced through either an increase in free-radical generation and/or a decrease in antioxidants in the target cells and tissues (1,2). A role for reactive oxygen in cancer induction and formation is well supported by human epidemiological studies. Antioxidants, which reduce reactive oxygen species, have also been shown to provide protection against cancer development (3,4). In contrast, excessive intake of transition metals such as iron, which facilitate the production of free radicals in cells and tissue, appear to enhance cancer formation (5,6).

The carcinogenic process by chemicals appears to be a multistage process definable by at least three stages: initiation, promotion and progression (Figure 1). The initiation stage involves the production of a nonlethal, heritable mutation in cells by interaction of a chemical with DNA. This mutation may provide a growth advantage to the cell. The stage of tumor promotion is an epigenetic process that specifically targets the initiated cells. This stage produces the clonal expansion of the initiated cell population. The stage of progression results in the development of benign and malignant neoplastic lesions (7).

Increasing evidence has implicated a role for oxidative stress in all three stages of the carcinogenic process. The elucidation of specific cellular effects of reactive oxygen species in each of the three stages is important for cancer therapy and prevention in humans. The subsequent discussion focuses on the potential molecular mechanisms and cellular responses underlying the effects of reactive oxygen species during the carcinogenesis process.

REACTIVE OXYGEN GENERATION BY CARCINOGENS

Xenobiotics with either complete carcinogenic properties or selective tumor-promoting or tumor-initiating properties exist in the human environment and are

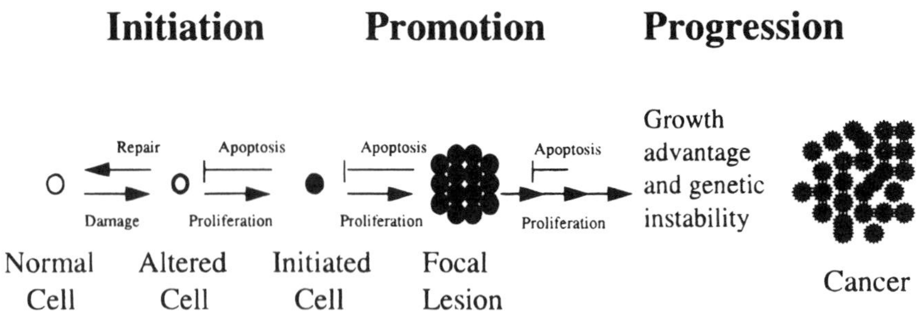

Initiation   Promotion   Progression

FIG. 1. The process of chemical carcinogenesis.

responsible for human cancer formation. Xenobiotics can generate reactive oxygen species when they enter cells, by metabolizing directly to primary radical intermediates or by activating endogenous sources of reactive oxygen species (1). The evidence that these chemicals generate reactive oxygen suggests a relationship between reactive oxygen species generation and the carcinogenic properties of chemicals (Table 1).

The formation of reactive oxygen species has been indirectly demonstrated by the induction of both lipid and DNA oxidative damage in animals treated with

TABLE 1. *Xenobiotics and oxyradical effects in chemical carcinogenesis*

Chemicals	Experimental models	Oxyradical or effects	Reference
Genotoxic			
N-nitroso compounds	murine	MDA oh8dG	8–10
BaP	mice	oh8dG	12
AFB-1	rats	oh8dG	11
Heterocyclic amines	in vitro	·OH	14
MMC and 2-acetylaminofluorene	in vitro	·OH etc.	10,13
Nongenotoxic			
Chlorinated compounds (TCDD, dieldrin, DTT, lindane)	murine & in vitro	Lipid peroxid, superoxide ion, etc.	140,148,149
Radiation	in vitro and in vivo	DNA damage	10,150
Phenobarbital	murine	·OH, oh8dG, lipid peroxid.	119,141,148
Metal (nickel, BrCl, chromium, Fe-NTA iodobenzene)	murine	·OH, oh8dG, MDA, NO	151–154
Peroxisome prolif. (DEHP, WY-14,643, clofibrate, ciprofibrate, PFDA)	murine	·OH, oh8dG, etc.	10,18,19, 155,156
CCl₄		Trichloromethyl peroxyl radical	121
Phorbol ester (TPA, PMA)	cells, murine	·OH, oh8dG	157
Quinones	V79 cells	oh8dG	158

chemical carcinogens (8–12). Since reactive oxygen compounds induce pathophysio-logical changes that produce abnormal cell growth, the interaction of the genetic effects and oxidative effects of carcinogens should be considered in determining the basis for their carcinogenic action. This is supported in part by the association between the mutagenic properties of complete carcinogens and their ability to generate reactive oxygen species. Mutagens such as mitomycin C can generate reactive oxygen species in vitro (13). Similarly, Sato and co-workers (14) reported a direct relationship between reactive oxygen species generation and the mutagenic potential of heterocyclic amines. Hepatocarcinogenic heterocyclic amines generate reactive oxygen species when activated with purified hepatic P-450 reductase. The degree of reactive oxygen species generation for each heterocyclic amine examined correlated with its mutagenic potential in the Ames test.

While the formation of reactive oxygen species by complete carcinogens has been associated with the initiation stage of the cancer process, much more evidence exists for a role of oxygen radical generation during tumor promotion. Many of the tumor-promoting agents have been shown to produce oxidative stress in their target cells. These compounds include peroxisome proliferators, chlorinated compounds, radia-tion, metal ions, barbiturates, and phorbol esters (Table 1). All of these compounds also have the capability to induce replicative DNA synthesis in both normal and preneoplastic target tissues (Table 2). The induction of DNA synthesis is important for the selective clonal expansion of the initiated cell population and may impart additional mutations on the target cell during the induced rapid cell proliferation. Oxidative stress and/or reactive oxygen species formation may be important in mediating the cell proliferation and DNA synthesis induction by tumor-promoting compounds. Studies with the hepatic tumor promoter dieldrin provide support for this premise. Dieldrin is a selective liver tumor promoter in mice but not in rats. A species-specific effect of dieldrin in inducing DNA synthesis in mice (but not in

TABLE 2. DNA S-phase synthesis and oxidative stress induced by hepatocarcinogens in animals

Chemicals	DNA synthesis (reference)	Oxidative damage or reactive oxygen species generation (reference)
WY14,643	134,159	19
DEHP	132,159	18
Nafenopin	133	139
Clofibrate	134	18
2-Nitropropane	160	163
TCDD	137	140,151
DDT	136	138
Lead nitrate	123	143
Carbon tetrachloride	123	142
Ethylene dibromide	123	143
Trichloroethylene	161	164
Furan	162	165
Dieldrin	135	166

rats) was found (15). Correlatively, a pronounced increase of DNA oxidative damage (8-hydroxy-2'-deoxyguanosine, 8·ohdG) and lipid peroxidation was found solely in mouse hepatocytes but not in rat hepatocytes following dieldrin treatment (166). The addition of the antioxidant vitamin E with the dieldrin treatment prevented the DNA synthesis induction, as well as the formation of the oh8dG and the lipid peroxidation. In addition, cotreatment of the antioxidant vitamin E with dieldrin prevented the dieldrin-induced selective clonal expansion in preneoplastic mouse liver focal lesions (16). These studies suggest a possible role for oxidative stress induction by tumor promoters during the promotion phase of carcinogenesis.

REACTIVE OXYGEN GENERATION THROUGH ENZYME ACTIVITY

Reactive oxygen species generated from cellular organelles (in particular the endoplasmic reticulum, peroxisomes and mitochondria) constitute a major source of oxygen radicals produced in cells (Figure 2). Enzymes in these organelles, such as NADPH cytochrome P-450 reductase, heme-containing enzymes, and enzymes in the peroxisomal fatty acid beta-oxidation pathway (fatty acyl CoA oxidase), appear to be directly responsible for oxygen species generation. The reactive oxygen-generating ability of chemical carcinogens (Table 1) may be related to the induction of these enzymes in the organelles. Peroxisome proliferators are a well-studied

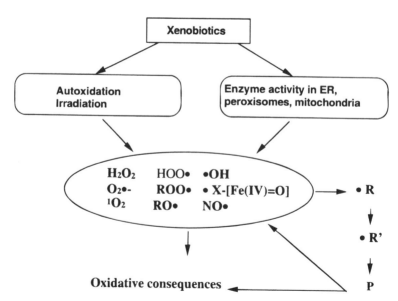

FIG. 2. Generation of reactive oxygen species by xenobiotics in cells. H_2O_2, hydrogen peroxide; HOO·; perhydroxyl radical; ·OH, hydroxyl radical; O_2^-, superoxide radical; ROO·, peroxyl radical; RO·, alkoxyl radical; $^1O_2$, singlet oxygen; ·X−[Fe(IV)=O], ferryl heme protein radical; ·R → ·R' → P, long-range effects of free-radical migration.

example. Peroxisomes are major sites of oxygen utilization where molecular oxygen is used to remove hydrogen from organic substrates. An end product of this reaction is hydrogen peroxide. Typically, catalase, which is present in the peroxisomes, reduces the hydrogen peroxide to water. Certain xenobiotics (peroxisome proliferators) are able to induce an increase in the number and size of peroxisomes in the cell. When this occurs, enzymes responsible for beta-oxidation of fatty acids in peroxisomes are increased 20- to 30-fold while catalase activity are increased only twofold (17). Thus, more hydrogen peroxide is produced than can be scavenged by the catalase. It has been suggested that hydrogen peroxide can in turn "leak" from these peroxisomes. This additional hydrogen peroxide causes an oxidative stress in the cell. The excess production of hydrogen peroxide in the cells has been demonstrated with a number of peroxisome proliferating compounds including DEHP, [4-chloro-6-(2,3-xylidino)-2-pyrimidinylthio]acetic acid (WY-14,643), and clofibrate (18,19).

The induction of cytochrome P-450 enzymes may also contribute to reactive oxygen species generation by xenobiotics. P-450 enzymes found in the endoplasmic reticulum can generate free oxygen radicals in the process of normal cellular metabolism. Reactive oxygen could therefore be generated both from the direct metabolism of xenobiotics by the P-450 enzyme system and through the indirect action of P-450 enzymes themselves. The oxidative stress status in cells will depend on the activity and quantity of the P-450 enzymes. An association between the ability of xenobiotics, in particular tumor promoters, to induce P-450 enzymes and to induce cancer has been proposed (20). Cancer induction, therefore, may be due in part to the chronic induction of P-450 enzymes with the resultant production of reactive oxygen. Exposure of rodents to the hepatic tumor promoters dieldrin and phenobarbital provides support for this suggestion. Fourteen- and fourfold increases in the activity of P-450 2B were observed in hepatic microsomes of mice and rats, respectively, exposed to dieldrin and a 112- and 584-fold increase in mice and rats, respectively, exposed to phenobarbital. Reactive oxygen generation (as measured by DMPO spin trap) of these same microsomes showed a pattern correlative between oxygen radical formation and P-450 2B induction (Figure 3). Auclair and co-workers (21) found a similar correlation between increased superoxide anion generation, oxygen uptake, and increased P-450 enzyme activity in microsomes from phenobarbital-treated rats. These findings suggest a link between the generation of reactive oxygen by tumor-promoting compounds and induction of P-450 enzymes.

MOLECULAR CONSEQUENCES OF REACTIVE OXYGEN

Oxidative stress induced by chemical carcinogens can cause the damage to critical cellular macromolecules leading to chemical carcinogenesis (Figure 4). The DNA, lipid, and protein components of the cell are targets of reactive oxygen species generated by chemical carcinogens. Damage to these cell components by oxygen radicals may result in functional and/or structural modification of nucleic acids,

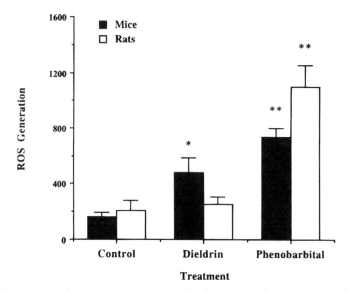

FIG. 3. Comparison of reactive oxygen generation by the hepatic microsomes of mice and rats exposed to dieldrin and phenobarbital. Significance; *p < .05, p < .01 by ANOVA test, compared to hepatic microsomes in animals with normal diet (control). The hepatic microsomes of B6C3F1 mice and F344 rats were isolated 1 wk after being exposed to NIH-07 diet or the diets containing 10 ppm dieldrin or 500 ppm phenobarbital. Compared to control mice and rats, 14- and 4-fold increases in the activity of P-450 2B were observed in hepatic microsomes of mice and rats, respectively, exposed to dieldrin and a 112- and 584-fold increase in mice and rats exposed to phenobarbital. Reactive oxygen species (ROS) generation was measured in an in vitro system contained 0.5 mg microsome protein, 2 mM NADPH, 5 U glucose-6-phosphate dehydrogenase, 40 mM DMPO adjusted to 250 μl with 0.25 M sucrose–0.5 mM glucose–TKM buffer, pH 7.4. Reaction was started after adding microsome. After incubation at 35°C for 30 min, the reaction mixture was passed through a 0.45 μm Durapore filter unit (Ultrafree-MC, Millipore) and immediately analyzed in HPLC-EC. Two 8 × 100 mm Waters Nova-Pak C18 columns, 4 μm, in a Radial-Pak cartridge with an extension kit protected by a Nova-Pak C18 Guard-Pak insert were eluted with an 18% aqueous MeOH:acetonitrile (13:8) containing 50 mM sodium citrate and 50 mM sodium acetate (pH5.1) at 1.0 ml/min flow rate. A CC-5/LC-4C ameperometer detector from BAS System (West Lafayette, IN) was set at +0.6 V potential and 0.1 filter.

protein, membrane, and enzymes. Damage that is extensive enough may result in cell death. Sublethal effects of reactive oxygen can produce DNA damage and initiate changes in enzymes or receptor activity, modification of membrane fluidity, and damage to second-message pathways and gene expression. All of these toxic endpoints have been reported in studies involving the chemical induction of cancer.

DNA Oxidative Damage

Oxidative DNA damage, in particular the formation of DNA hydroxyl adducts and DNA malonedialdehyde adducts, may be important in chemical carcinogenesis

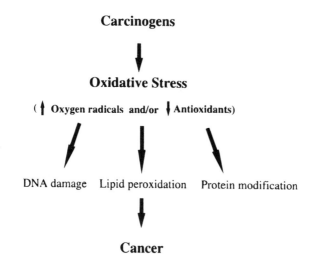

FIG. 4. Oxidative-stress-induced damage of intracellular macromolecules.

(22–24). The formation of oxidative DNA adducts can interfere with normal cell growth control by producing genetic mutations and/or altering normal gene expression.

Facilitation of oxidative DNA damage by metal ions, in particular copper, has been demonstrated (7). Copper can interact directly with guanine/cytosine sites of DNA bases and may serve to stimulate formation of hydroxyl radicals from other reactive oxygen species through Fenton or Haber-Weiss reactions (25). The location of copper ions at the guanine and cytosine base sites may help explain why most of the oxidative DNA damage appears to occur at these bases (7,26). An increase of G to T mutations in human cancers has been demonstrated in a suppressor gene, the p53 gene (27,28). Mutation of the p53 gene (29) and oh8dG formation (12) following benzo[a]pyrene and hepatitis B virus exposure in mice has been found, suggesting a link between the induction of oxidative stress and specific gene mutation (30). Four different pathways by which oxidative DNA damage leads to mutations have been suggested, including (1) chemical modification of nucleotide moieties in DNA causing alteration in their hydrogen bonding or "coding" specificity; (2) a damage-dedicated exacerbation of polymerase-specific hot spots; (3) a damage-induced conformational change in the DNA templates that prevent accurate replication by DNA polymerases; and (4) the induction of a DNA polymerase conformation that is error prone (31).

In addition to gene mutation, oxidative DNA damage appears to participate in other DNA-altering pathways. One such mechanism, DNA hypomethylation, has received increased interest recently (32). Hypomethylation of the c-raf gene is associated with sensitivity of mice strains to chemical carcinogens (33). Similarly, hypomethylation of Ha-ras and Ki-ras may be an epigenetic mechanism for facilitating their aberrant expression in tumors (34). An interrelationship between oxidative DNA damage and DNA hypomethylation has been implicated in chemically induced carcinogenesis (32). In rats fed a choline-deficient diet, hypomethylation of CCGG sites within several genes (c-myc, c-fos, c-Ha-ras) that are involved in growth regulation was seen resulting in the alteration of mRNA levels of these genes (35). The DNA hypomethylation status is also correlated with increased lipid peroxidation (36) and oh8dG formation (37). In addition, cells from patients with the genetic disease Bloom's syndrome (an autosomal recessive disorder characterized by high incidence of cancer at an early age) displayed both increased hypomethylation and increased oxidative stress that were linked with increased DNA damage in these cells (38). Studies by Turk and co-workers (39) have shown an association between oh8dG formation and DNA hypomethylation. These investigators noted that with increased formation of oh8dG a decrease in the ability of DNA methyltransferase to methylate a target cytosine one or two nucleotides 5' away from oh8dG site was seen. Thus, the formation of DNA oxidative adducts and DNA hypomethylation appear to be interrelated and are frequently seen in cells undergoing oxidative stress. The induction of DNA damage by reactive oxygen species may produce nonrepairable alterations to the cell, potentially impacting on the initiation and promotion stages of the cancer process. Modification of the hypomethylation state of the DNA by reactive oxygen may alter gene regulation, resulting in the selective growth advantage to the initiated cell population during the tumor promotion phase of carcinogenesis.

Lipid Peroxidation

Polyunsaturated fatty acids (PUFA) in cells are easily oxidized by oxygen free radicals to form carbon-centered lipid peroxyl radicals and lipid hydroperoxides. Lipid peroxyl radicals can further propagate peroxidation chain reactions by removing a hydrogen atom from a nearby PUFA. This in turn can generate a molecule of malondialdehyde (MDA) and other breakdown products. The lipid radicals may diffuse into the membrane, thereby spreading lesion. The formation of these lipid radicals can affect the structural and functional integrity of cell membranes, resulting in a loss of cellular homeostasis and modified cellular function. Membrane damage can also result in the modification of ion transport systems and loss of gap junctional intercellular communication, both of which are stimulators of cell growth.

The initiation of lipid peroxidation results in at least three changes in cells: (1) spreading oxidative damage in cells by chain reactions and oxidation of proteins (1); (2) forming adducts with DNA such as DNA-MDA (24) that might result in gene mutations and cancer (40); and (3) changing membrane structure resulting in the modification of signaling pathways or cell death. All of these changes to lipid may contribute to modification of growth control and potentially could participate in the promotion stage of cancer.

Protein Modification

Proteins are easily attacked by reactive oxygen species and free-radical intermediates of lipid peroxidation. The formed protein radicals can be rapidly transferred to other sites within the protein infrastructure. Amino acids with thiol functional groups are particularly susceptible to reactive oxygen species. Since thiol groups are important in maintaining protein structure and enzyme activity, modification of this group can change both structure and function for the protein. This reactive oxygen-protein interaction can increase protein function. This is seen with the induction of guanylate cyclase enzyme activity by oxidative stress, which in turn increases cGMP, which can stimulate the activity of specific protein kinases (41). In contrast, a decrease in protein function can occur. Oxidative stress has been shown to reduce calcium-dependent ATPase enzyme activity (42).

Structural damage by reactive oxygen to the membrane transport proteins can alter ionic homeostasis, leading to modification of intercellular calcium and potassium concentrations. Changes in these ions can in turn modify intracellular signaling pathways. Structural protein damage may also modify membrane-associated receptor proteins and gap junction proteins, resulting in changes in intercellular signaling pathways. With extreme structural protein damage, reactive oxygen species may produce loss of primary, secondary, or tertiary protein structure, thus allowing the protein to be targeted for subsequent attack by macrooxyproteinases leading to membrane proteolysis (43). Protein oxidative damage can therefore result in alterations of either cell structure or cell function through both direct and indirect mechanisms, which in turn may modify normal growth control of the target tissue.

EFFECTS OF REACTIVE OXYGEN ON INTERCELLULAR AND INTRACELLULAR SIGNALING PATHWAYS

Cancer-causing chemicals and particularly tumor-promoting compounds may elicit their cellular effects through activation and modulation of several signaling pathways (Figure 5). Experimental evidence has directly showed the influence of reactive oxygen species on multiple signaling pathways of intercellular calcium, protein kinase C, nitric oxide, gap junction intercellular communication, and transcription factors (44).

Calcium

Calcium is an important signaling factor responsible for regulating a wide range of cellular processes (45) including cell proliferation and cell differentiation (46). Oxidative stress has been reported to increase intracellular calcium through structural modification of the plasma membrane, resulting in an influx of calcium from extracellular sources (47). Intracellular calcium levels may also be increased by the release of calcium from intracellular stores by the stimulation of reactive oxygen (48,49).

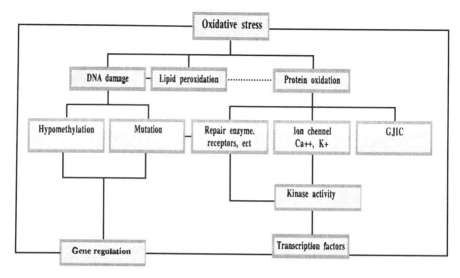

FIG. 5. Effects of oxidative stress on gene regulation.

Increases in intracellular calcium concentrations can produce several effects. Increased intracellular calcium can activate quiescent cells, inducing DNA synthesis and cell proliferation. Increased intracellular calcium may also induce terminal differentiation and programmed cell death (apoptosis) of senescent cells, resulting in a disturbance of normal tissue homeostasis (46). In both of these scenarios, calcium may selectively allow the initiated cell population to expand during the tumor promotion process through selective growth of the initiated cells and selective death or differentiation of the normal surrounding noninitiated cells.

The increase of intracellular calcium stimulated by reactive oxygen species has been suggested to be an important first step to other cellular changes (50). The induction of c-*fos*, c-*jun*, and c-*myc* by increased intercellular calcium in rat proximal tubular epithelium after oxidative stress has been demonstrated (51). DNA strand breakage and poly-ADP ribosylation can also be mediated by changes in intracellular calcium following oxidative stress (52). Since the change in chromatin structure results in c-*fos* activation (53) and the activation of protein kinase C increases c-*jun* expression (54), the DNA damage and protein kinase C activity may be a second tier of cellular changes produced by an increase in intercellular calcium following cellular oxidative stress.

Protein Kinase C

Protein kinase C (PKC) is a family of closely related lipid-dependent and diacyglycerol-activated isoenzymes known to play an important role in the signal transduction pathways involved in hormone release, mitogenesis, and tumor promotion.

Studies have indicated that the sustained activation or inhibition of PKC activity may play a critical role in the regulation of cellular growth including cell proliferation, differentiation, and tumorigenesis. PKC is responsible for multiple drug resistance that is involved in metastasis of cancer where an increase in PKC activity correlates with increased resistance and metastatic potential (55). Reactive oxygen species have been shown to mediate activation of PKC in cells (56,57). The mechanism of PKC activation by oxidative stress may be through increases in intracellular calcium concentrations. PKC activity is potentiated by increased intracellular calcium concentrations induced via oxidative stress (58). TCDD, a liver tumor promoter, causes a modification in the growth factor response through receptor modification that is linked to PKC activation (59). Similarly, the hepatic tumor-promoting effects of chlorinated hydrocarbons have been linked to activation of PKC (60). The role that PKC plays in the tumor promotion process appears to be compound specific. In rat hepatocytes activation and translocation of PKC from soluble to particulate cell fractions was seen following 12-O-tetradecanoylphorbol 13-acetate (TPA) treatment but was not detected with phenobarbital (61,62). Both TPA and phenobarbital have been shown to induce oxidative stress in cells. This chemical-specific effect on PKC activation may be related to the extent and amount of sulfhydryl oxidation of the PKC protein. While low levels of reactive oxygen species may induce the PKC activity, greater oxidative stress may inhibit PKC activation. This is supported by the fact that with mild oxidation of the PKC molecule by hydrogen peroxide, PKC is activated. As the hydrogen peroxide concentration increased and the oxidation of the PKC protein increased, a decrease in PKC activity was seen. Similarly, the liver tumor promoter carbon tetrachloride, a known inducer of oxidative stress, increased the activity of PKC in a dose-responsive matter at low concentrations but reduced PKC activity at high doses (63,64).

Gap Junction Intercellular Communication

Inhibition of gap junction intercellular communication (GJIC) by tumor-promoting carcinogens has been proposed as a mechanism by which initiated preneoplastic cells may escape the growth control of normal surrounding cells, allowing the preneoplastic cell to selectively proliferate (65,66). Gap junctions are cellular organelles located in the plasma membrane that allow for the passive transfer of low-molecular-weight materials (1 kD or less) between the cytoplasm of adjacent cells (67). A function of gap junctional communication appears to be the exchange of low-molecular-weight growth-regulating substances between adjacent cells (67). A role for gap junctional intercellular communication in the growth inhibition of neoplastically transformed cells by adjacent normal cells has been demonstrated (68). Gap junctional intercellular communication has been shown to be inhibited by most tumor promoters in a variety of cultured cells (66). The exact mechanism by which xenobiotics may regulate gap junctional intercellular communication is unknown, but previous work has shown that oxidative stress can downregulate the communication and that tumor promoter inhibition can be prevented by antioxidants (69–71). The mechanism by which reactive oxygen species inhibit gap junctional intercellular communication may be mediated through direct oxidative damage to membrane lipids and proteins resulting in the alteration of the membrane structure. On the other hand, intracellular calcium accumulation that activates PKC results in the downregulation of gap junctional intercellular communication by phosphorylation of gap junction protein. Additionally, decreased gene expression of the gap junction protein may be modified by oxidative stress to the cell.

Nitric Oxide

· One of the best examples of a reactive oxygen functioning as a second messenger or signaling molecule is nitric oxide (NO). NO is reported to participate in the physiology or pathophysiology of every organ system (72). Exposure to elevated NO in cells could have potential genotoxic effects through several mechanisms that involve reaction with oxygen, including the formation of carcinogenic N-nitroso compounds, direct deamination of DNA bases, and oxidation of DNA after formation of peroxynitrite and/or hydroxyl radicals (73). NO has also been demonstrated to produce gene mutations in vitro (74) and may play a role in the regulation of cytochrome P-450 activity (75). During chronic infection, NO is continually released by macrophages (76). This sustained release of NO has been proposed to be a factor in cancer induction (77). A number of tumor promoters can activate macrophages (78–81), which can potentially release NO. Similar activation of NO by macrophages has also been implemented after partial hepatectomy, suggesting a role for NO in the induction of cell division and DNA synthesis (82). Finally, the complete chemical carcinogens 2-nitropropane (83) and cigarette smoking (84) have been reported to stimulate NO generation.

Transcription Factors

Activation of transcription factors is an important signaling pathway by which reactive oxygen may regulate gene expression. Transcription factors are low-molecular-weight proteins that can bind with promoter regions of genes and thus regulate gene expression. Transcription factor activation is involved in the development, growth, and aging of cells (85). Subcellular localization from the cytoplasm to the nucleus is the first step of transcription factor activation (86). Reactive oxygen is believed to be involved in the regulation, as can be seen with the activation of nuclear factor κ-B (NF-κB) and activator protein-1 (AP-1) by direct oxidation and phosphorylation.

NF-κB is a heterodimer consisting of a 50-kD and a 65-kD subunit. The activity of the NF-κB dimer is controlled by an inhibitory subunit IκB. In nonstimulated cells NF-κB stays in the cytoplasm. It migrates into the nucleus only after the removal of the inhibitory factor IκB (87). Oxidative stress can stimulate the removal of IκB from NF-κB heterodimer to activate this transcription factor (88,89). AP-1 is another transcription factor that binds to the sequence of phorbol ester responsive element in the promoter regions of several genes (90). AP-1 is also a dimer of a protein complex joined by c-*fos*, c-*jun*, *jun*-B, and *jun*-D in a leucine zipper. External stimuli can cause either transcriptional regulation or posttranslational regulation of AP-1 (44). Reactive oxygen can induce PKC activity that activates preexisting c-*jun*, resulting in AP-1 activation (54). Ultraviolet (UV) radiation, a proven free-radical producer, has been shown to increase the mRNA for c-*jun* (91). It is possible that the redox state of the cell may act as a second-messenger system in the modulation these transcription factors (54,92).

The direct relationship between the exposure to chemical carcinogens and the activation of the transcription factors has been reported. Carbon tetrachloride administration to rats induced a pronounced dose- and time-dependent increase in the expression of the AP-1 dimer, c-*fos* and c-*jun*, in liver (93). Since the same activation pattern of carbon tetrachloride appears for PKC activity (64), the induction of AP-1 by carbon tetrachloride may be the result of PKC activation. Similarly, 2,3,7,8-tetrachlorodibenzo-*p*-dioxin (TCDD), which can induce oxidative stress in cells, rapidly increased calcium influx and elevated membrane-bound PKC in hepatoma cells. These changes then produced an induction of the immediate early proto-oncogenes c-*fos*, *jun*-B, c-*jun*, and *jun*-D, and an increase in AP-1 activity. While the induction of these changes by TCDD was slower than that seen with phorbol esters, the magnitude of the effects caused by both treatments was similar (94). AP-1 binding activity was also shown to be increased by the tumor promoter phorbol 12-myristate 13-acetate (TPA) in HeLa cells (95) and the tumor promoter phenobarbital in HepG2 hepatoma cells (96). NF-κB activation was increased in cultured cells by the metal carcinogen chromium (97). In our laboratory, an increased DNA binding activity of NF-κB in nucleus was observed in livers of mice treated with the tumor promoter dieldrin. Interestingly, coadministration of vitamin E and dieldrin decreased NF-κB activity to control levels. Since dieldrin-induced oxidative stress was also found in the livers of these mice, dieldrin-induced reactive oxygen may be responsible for this activation of NF-κB.

EFFECT OF REACTIVE OXYGEN ON THE REGULATION OF CELL GROWTH

The oxidative modification of signaling pathways, as discussed earlier, contributes to the effects of reactive oxygen species on gene regulation in cells (Figure 5). Hypomethylation, damage of chromatin structure, alteration of ion channels, PKC activation, and breakdown products of lipid peroxidation (1) are involved in the regulation of genes, resulting in abnormal cell growth. A direct and immediate cellular response of oxidative stress may be the induction and interaction of transcription factors with DNA. The activation of AP-1 may be achieved by increased intracellular calcium and PKC activity in oxidative stress status (51,98). AP-1 is also induced by Michael reaction-centered compounds (i.e., double bound with electron-withdrawing groups) (99) and by depletion of glutathione (100). NF-kB has been activated by photosensitization-generated oxidative DNA damage (101).

The activation of transcription factors may induce the transcription of a battery of genes. In bacteria at least nine genes are controlled by a single regulator protein, oxyR (102). The oxyR activation has been demonstrated to be directly and reversibly regulated by oxidation (103). In both *Drosophila* and mouse 3T6 fibroblasts, hydrogen peroxide can activate protein binding to the DNA heat-shock regulatory element (104). Reactive oxygen species generated by xenobiotics can work as second messengers to regulate gene expression by activating NF-kB in eukaryotic cells (105,106). Furthermore, the activation of AP-1 has been associated with the expression of glutathione *S*-transferase (96,100,107), collagenase (108), quinone reductase (96), and calcium-activated neutral protease (93). Both transcription factors are related to the activation of c-myc gene (109,110), which is important in regulation of cell growth.

The induction of oxidative stress may be directly involved in the regulation of cell growth. Oxidants have been found to induce the expression of c-*fos* and c-*myc* genes in liver cells (109). Since c-*myc*, c-*fos*, and c-*jun* genes are also expressed during liver regeneration (111,112), a linkage between the induction of oxidative stress and these important cell growth genes may be present. The c-*jun* gene expression in preneoplastic liver foci has been examined by Nakano and co-workers (113). They found that nearly all preneoplastic liver foci expressed c-*jun* and that c-*jun* expression correlated with expression of glutathione *S*-transferase. The c-*fos* protein has been shown to induce cellular transformation (114). The activation of the transcription factor NF-kB is also necessary for tumor growth and metastasis (115) and is responsible for the expression of intercellular adhesion molecules that are linked to metastasis of cancer cells (116).

ROLE OF REACTIVE OXYGEN IN THE THREE STAGES
OF CARCINOGENIC PROCESS

Reactive oxygen can directly or indirectly cause functional and/or structural alterations in cells that may lead to carcinogenesis. Reactive oxygen species may act via different mechanisms in the three stages of chemical carcinogenesis: initiation, promotion, and progression (Figure 6).

Role of Oxidative Stress in Initiation Stage

The formation of cancer is a multistage process definable by at least three steps: initiation, promotion, and progression (Figure 1). The first step of this process, the initiation stage, involves the production of a nonlethal, heritable mutation in the target cell. After interaction of the target cell with a DNA-damaging carcinogen (a genotoxic carcinogen), one of three consequences may occur. The damage to the

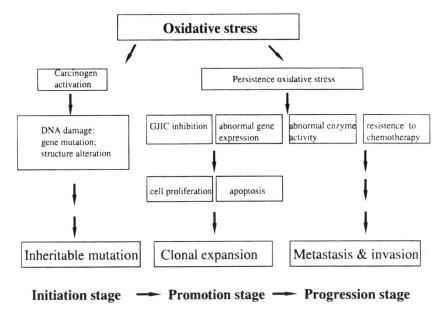

FIG. 6. Effects of oxidative stress in all stages of chemical carcinogenesis.

cell and the cellular DNA may be repaired, returning the altered cell to its normal state. The injury to the cell, however, may be too severe and not compatible with survival, resulting in cell death. Alternately, the damage may produce a mutation that is compatible with cell survival and results in the formation of an initiated cell. This mutation may provide a growth advantage to the cell. However, in most cases the initiated cell remains under the growth control of the surrounding normal cells. For the mutation to be set and the initiated cell formed, a round of DNA synthesis must occur to "lock in" the mutation. Chemical carcinogens that function at this stage of the cancer process have been referred to as initiators.

The metabolic activation of a chemical carcinogen to an electrophilic, DNA-damaging moiety, is a necessary step for this stage. Reactive oxygen species are believed to mediate the activation of such carcinogens via hydroperoxide-dependent oxidation that can be mediated by peroxyl radicals. This has been shown to occur with aflatoxin B1, aromatic amines, and polycyclic aromatic hydrocarbon dihydrodiols (2). Reactive oxygen species or their by-product of lipid peroxidation, MDA, can also directly react with DNA to form oxidative DNA adducts. G to T mutations in the p53 gene (29) caused by 8·ohdG formation following benzo[a]pyrene (BaP) treatment is one such example (12). Complete carcinogens have also been shown to generate reactive oxygen species in vivo. This is supported by the generation of superoxide and hydrogen peroxide by 3-methylcholanthrene (3MC) and BaP and also formation of 8·ohdG and MDA by aflatoxin B1, BaP and nitrosamines (8–42,117,118). The presence of carcinogen-DNA adducts and oxidative DNA adducts generated by chemical carcinogens suggests an interactive role of reactive oxygen species in initiation. Reactive oxygen species, therefore, can have multiple effects during the initiation stage of carcinogenesis by mediating carcinogen activation, by causing DNA damage, and also by interfering in DNA repair.

Role of Oxidative Stress in Promotion Stage

Tumor promotion involves the selective clonal expansion of the initiated cell population. Promotion appears to be an epigenetic process occurring specifically in the initiated cell population and therefore does not involve the acquisition of additional mutations to the initiated cell. The events of this stage are reversible with removal of the promoting pressure. The resulting focal lesion produced by the clonal expansion of the initiated cell is considered preneoplastic and is still under normal growth control of the normal surrounding tissue. A number of chemicals that produce their effects specifically at this stage of the cancer process have been identified and labeled as tumor promoters. Tumor promoters comprise a diverse group of chemical compounds including hormones, pesticides, chlorinated organics, pharmaceuticals, etc. Unlike initiators, tumor promoters are for the most part tissue and target specific. Chemicals that function at this stage selectively stimulate the proliferation of the initiate cell population while producing terminal differentiation in normal surrounding cells. Oxidative stress may function at this stage by selectively inducing gene transcription and control of apoptosis and cell proliferation in preneoplastic foci.

Reactive oxygen species have been proven to be specifically generated in initiated cell populations such as preneoplastic foci in liver. Chen and co-workers (131) suggested that expression of specific forms of cytochrome P-450 within preneoplastic foci may be an important factor in the rate of cell proliferation and gamma-glutamyl transpeptidase (GGT) expression in this foci. Since reactive oxygen species generation is associated with P-450 enzyme induction, oxidative stress may be produced in initiated cells, starting the growth expansion of these initiated cells. Higher levels of reactive oxygen species have been found in preneoplastic nodules of rat liver than in the surrounding normal tissue. After phenobarbital treatment a increase in oxidative stress was noted in these nodules (119). Other additional sources of reactive oxygen species in preneoplastic foci may be from the oxidation of glutathione by GGT, an enzyme at higher concentration in enzyme-altered foci in livers (120). The accumulation of neutrophils following topical application of tumor promoters in skin may also be a source of reactive oxygen species (2). The potential multiple sources of reactive oxygen species produced by tumor promoters may present a persistent stress to initiated cells that results in physiological and pathophysiological changes allowing for their selective growth.

Oxidative stress will also trigger many signaling pathways as noted earlier. These include (1) hypomethylation resulting from oh8dG formation, (2) accumulation of intracellular calcium by the alternation of membrane structure and function resulting from lipid and protein oxidative damage, (3) PKC activation triggered by calcium and protein oxidation, and (4) inhibition of GJIC regulated by PKC and membrane oxidation. Carbon tetrachloride, dieldrin, and phenobarbital have all been shown to modify one or more of these pathways. Carbon tetrachloride, a hepatic carcinogen in both mice and rats, is metabolized by cytochrome P-450 to yield the trichloromethyl radical, which can then react with molecular oxygen to form the trichloromethylpero-xyl radical (121). The effect of carbon tetrachloride can be prevented by the P-450 inhibitor SKF-525A (122). Carbon tetrachloride produced an increase in intracellular calcium that appeared to activate PKC in the liver (64). The activation of AP-1 by PKC has also been reported in rat liver treated with carbon tetrachloride (93). This may account for the increased hepatic DNA S-phase synthesis (123). The selective induction of hepatic cytochrome P-450 enzymes by dieldrin in mice also appears to be linked to reactive oxygen species generation in hepatocytes, which results in the formation of oh8dG and MDA, inhibition of gap junctional intercellular communication, and activation of NF-kB. Similarly, phenobarbital enhances the formation of reactive oxygen species in foci (119).

Another mechanism by which reactive oxygen species may regulate tumor growth is by enhancing specific gene expression in initiated cells by either increasing DNA synthesis or decreasing apoptosis (124,125). The pro-oncogenes of c-*myc*, c-*fos*, and c-*jun* are positive regulators of the cell cycle that drive cells from the G1 phase into the S phase. In contrast, p53, a negative growth regulator, arrests cells in the G1 phase. During cell proliferation, p53 may induce apoptosis to eliminate the cells that bypass the G1-S phase checkpoint (126). All of the preceding genes can be activated by oxidative stress in cells. The activation of p53 protects cells from death by UV irradiation (127). However, persistent oxidative stress in cells caused by tumor promoters may result in DNA oxidative damage and mutation. Oxidative damage to the p53 gene results in uncontrolled growth and is related to tumorigenesis. This connection between cell proliferation and cancer has been reviewed by several investigators and serves as the basis for a carcinogenicity model relating cellular dynamics to tumor response (128–131). A direct relationship between oxidative stress induction and stimulation of DNA S-phase synthesis by tumor promoters is showed in Table 2. The peroxisome proliferators di(2-ethylhexyl)phthalate (DEHP), nafenopin, and clofibrate all induce DNA synthesis in F344 rats (132–134). The barbiturate phenobarbital has been shown to induce DNA S-phase synthesis in both mice and rats (135). The inorganic compound lead nitrate induced S-phase synthesis in male Wistar rats (123). Chlorinated compounds, such as carbon tetrachloride, ethylene dibromide, DDT, and TCDD, produce an early increase in DNA S-phase synthesis (123,136,137). Interestingly, all of these compounds have been associated with changes in the oxidative stress level within the liver. Lipid peroxidation has been observed with DEHP, clofibrate and DDT in rats (18,138). Nafenopin increased conjugated dienes in rats and TCDD produced superoxide anion formation in mice (139,140). Likewise phenobarbital has been shown to decrease hepatic vitamin E levels, while carbon tetrachloride increased urinary MDA (141,142). Finally, Ledda-Columbano et al. (143) showed that lead nitrate and ethylene dibromide increased expression of tumor necrosis factor-α (TNF-α). TNF-α has itself been shown to promote free-radical formation. Thus, an association of these carcinogens in induction of cell proliferation and the induction of oxidative stress appears to be present. This correlation is further supported by a positive correlation between oh8dG formation and cell proliferation in the livers of mice exposed to pentachlorophenol (144).

Role of Oxidative Stress in Progression Stage

Tumor progression is the least understood of the three stages. Tumor progression represents the biological changes in the initiated, clonally expanded cell population from a preneoplastic stage to a neoplasm (7). This transformation involves the acquisition of additional mutations and genetic damage. With increased DNA damage benign neoplasm can progress to malignant neoplasia. The progression stage is exemplified by the loss of normal growth control, resulting in either expansion growth (benign neoplasm) or invasive growth (malignant neoplasm) of the neoplastic cell population.

Oxidative stress may play a role in tumor progression through induction of uncontrolled growth, genomic instability, chemotherapy resistance, invasion, and metastasis. Tumor cells continually undergo high and persistent oxidative stress (evidenced by higher oh8dG levels in carcinomas than normal tissues) (145). This persistent oxidative stress is not high enough to cause cell death, since tumor cells have a decreased sensitivity to oxidative stress as a result of increased membrane and DNA resistance to oxidants and higher levels of antioxidants (145,146). Persistent alteration of signaling pathways by oxidative stress that will trigger the expression of oncogenes also occurs in the progression stage. Activation of NF-κB activation has also been seen during tumor progression. Inhibition of NF-κB inhibited the development of tumors and caused tumor regression in mice (115). Enhanced DNA damage, such as modified bases and strand breaks, may lead to further mutation and chromosomal aberrations. A heritable genetic lesion may be produced in a benign tumor and lead to further transformation to the malignant state. The cancer cells emerging from the multiple steps of a carcinogenic process with inactivated or deleted tumor-suppresser genes and/or activated oncogenes are less dependent than normal cells on external growth factors. These cells are also less dependent on calcium-mediated second-messenger external calcium to proliferate and/or differentiate (46). Antioxidant levels induced by persistent oxidative stress in cancer cells appear to increase the chemotherapy resistance of these cells. Protein oxidative damage in tumor cells inhibits protease inhibitors and facilitates tumor invasion (145). Oxidative-stress-activated NF-κB can modify the expression of cell adhesion molecules such as E-cadherin, intercellular adhesion molecule 1, and vascular adhesion molecule 1, resulting in an increase in metastasis (116). Chronic inflammation not only releases reactive oxygen species but also enhances the attachment of cancer cells to vascular endothelial cells, facilitating an increase in metastasis growth (116,147). Oxidative stress, therefore, can further enhance the inheritable genetic alterations from tumor cells to cancer cells and may be responsible for many of the characteristics of malignancy, including chemotherapy-resistance, invasion, and metastasis.

SUMMARY

Oxidative stress participates in the formation and growth of cancer cells. Many chemical carcinogens induce oxidative stress in target cells, which correlates with the ability of the compound to induce P-450, peroxisomal, or other enzyme activity. The production of oxidative stress by chemical carcinogens results in damage to critical cellular macromolecules including DNA, lipid, and protein. Oxidative stress also modify intercellular and intracellular signaling pathways involving calcium, PKC activity, gap junctional intercellular communication, nitric oxide, and transcription factors. The cellular structural and functional modification produced by oxidative stress can result in cell death if severe enough or can modify normal gene function. All of these changes can influence cell growth and cell death. The production of oxidative stress, therefore, can result in cellular changes that have input in every stage of the cancer process.

REFERENCES

1. Rice-Evans C and Burdon R (1993). Free radical-lipid interactions and their pathological consequences. *Prog. Lipid Res.* 32(1):71–110.
2. Trush MA and Kensler TW (1991). An overview of the relationship between oxidative stress and chemical carcinogenesis. *Free Radical Biol. Med.* 10:201–209.
3. Ames BN (1983). Dietary carcinogens and anticarcinogens. Oxygen radicals and degenerative diseases. *Science.* 221(4617):1256–64
4. Willet WC and MacMahon B (1984). Diet and cancer—An overview. *N. Engl. J. Med.* 310(10):633–638.
5. Nelson RL (1992). Dietary iron and colorectal cancer risk. *Free Radical Biol. Med.* 12:161–168.
6. Stevens RG and Nerishi K (1992). Iron and oxidative damage in human cancer. In *Biological Consequences of Oxidative Stress: Implications for Cardiovascular Disease and Carcinogenesis,* eds. L Spatz and AD Bloom, pp. 138–161. New York: Oxford University Press.
7. Guyton KZ and Kensler TW (1993). Oxidative mechanisms in carcinogenesis. [Review] *Br. Med. Bull.* 49(3). 523–44.
8. Bartsch H, Hietanen E and Malaveille C, (1988). Carcinogenic nitreactive oxygen speciesamine: Free radical aspects of their action. *Free Rad. Biol. Med.* 7:637–644.
9. Chung F-L and Xu Y (1992). Increased 8-oxydeoxyguanosine levels in lung DNA of A/J mice and F344 rats treated with the tobacco-specific nitreactive oxygen speciesamine 4-(methylnitreactive oxygen speciesamine)-1-(3-pyridyl)-1-butanone. *Carcinogenesis* 13:1269–1272.
10. Srinivasan S and Glauert P (1990). Formation of 5-hydroxymethyl-2'-deoxyuridine in hepatic DNA of rats treated with γ-irradiation, diethylnitrosamine, 2-acetylaminofluorene or the peroxisome proliferator ciprofibrate. *Carcinogenesis* 11:2021–2024.
11. Shen H-M, Ong CN, Lee BL and Shi CY (1995). Aflatoxin B1-induced 8-hydroxydeoxyguanosine formation in rat hepatic DNA. *Carcinogenesis* 16(2):419–422.
12. Mauthe RJ, Cook VM, Coffing SL and Baird WM (1995). Exposure of mammalian cell cultures to benzo[a]pyrene and light results in oxidative DNA damage as measured by 8-hydroxydeoxyguanosine formation. *Carcinogenesis* 16(1):133–137.
13. Komiyama T, Kikuchi T and Sugiura Y (1982). Generation of hydroxyl radical by anticancer quinone drugs, carbazilquinone, mitomycin C, aclacinomycin A and adriamycin, in the presence of NADPH-cytochrome P-450 reductase. *Biochem. Pharmacol.* 31(22):3651–6.

14. Sato K, Akaike T, Kojima Y, Ando M, Nagao M and Maeda H (1992). Evidence of direct generation of oxygen free radicals from heterocyclic amines by NADPH/Cytochrome P-450 reductase in vitro. *Jpn J. Cancer Res.* 83(11):1204–1209.

15. Kolaja KL, Stevenson DE, Johnson JT, Walborg EF and Klaunig JE (1995). Hepatic effects of dieldrin and phenobarbital in male B6C3F1 mice and Fisher 344 rats: Species selective induction of DNA synthesis. In: *Progress in Clinical and Biological Research*, Vol. 391, *Growth Factors and Tumor Promotion*, eds. RM McClaim et al., pp. 397–408. New York: Wiley-Liss.

16. Kolaja KL, Stevenson DE, Johnson JT, Walborg EF Jr. and Klaunig JE (1996). Subchronic effects of dieldrin and phenobarbital on hepatic DNA synthesis in mice and rats. *Fundam. Appl. Toxicol.* 29(2):219–228.

17. Rao MS and Reddy JK (1991). An overview of peroxisome proliferator-induced hepatocarcinogenesis. *Environ. Health Perspect.* 93:205–209.

18. Tamura H, Lida T, Watanabe T and Suga T (1990). Long term effects of hypolipidaemic peroxisome proliferator administration on hepatic hydrogen peroxide metabolism in rats. *Carcinogenesis* 11:445–450.

19. Wada N, Marsman DS and Popp JA (1992). Dose related effects of hepatocarcinogen Wy 14,623 on peroxisomes and cell replication. *Fundam. Appl. Toxicol.* 18:149–154.

20. Lubet RA, Nims RW, Ward JM, Rice JM and Diwan BA (1989). Induction of cytochrome P-450 and its relationship to liver tumor promotion. *J. Am. Coll. Toxicol.* 8(2):259–268.

21. Auclair C, de Prost D and Hakim J (1978). Superoxide anion production by liver micreactive oxygen speciesomes from phenobarbital treated rat. *Biochem. Pharmacol.* 27: 355–358.

22. Breimer LH (1990). Molecular mechanisms of oxygen radical carcinogenesis and mutagenesis: The role of DNA base damage. *Mo. Carcinogen.* 3:188–197.

23. Floyd RA (1990). The role of 8-hydroxyguanine in carcinogenesis. *Carcinogenesis* 11(9): 1447–1450.

24. Chaudhary AK, Nokubo M, Marnett LJ and Blair IA (1994). Analysis of the malondialdehyde-2′-deoxyguanosine adduct in rat liver DNA by gas chromatography/electron capture negative chemical ionization mass spectrometry. *Biol. Mass Spectrom.* 23:457–464.

25. Pezzano H and Podo F. (1980) Structure of binary complexes of mono- and polynucleotides with metal ions of the first transition group. *Chem. Rev.* 80:365–399.

26. Cheng KC, Cahill DS, Kasa H, Nishimura S and Loeb LA (1992). 8-Hydroxyguanine, an abundant form of oxidative DNA damage, causes G-T and A-C substitutions. *J. Biol. Chem.* 267:166–172.

27. Hollstein M, Sidransky D, Vogelstein B and Harris CC (1991). p53 mutations in human cancers. [Review] *Science.* 253(5015):49–53.

28. Bressac B, Kew M, Wands J and Ozturk M (1991). Selective G to T mutations of p53 gene in hepatocellular carcinoma from southern Africa [see comments]. *Nature* 350(6317):429–431.

29. Ruggeri B, Dirado M, Zhang SY, Bauer B, Goodrow T and Klein-Szanto AJ (1993). Benzo(a)pyrene-induced murine skin rumors exhibit frequent and characteristic G to T mutations in the p53 gene. *Proc. Natl. Acd. Sci. USA.* 90(3):1013–1017.

30. Scorsone KA, Zhou YZ, Butel JS and Slagle BL (1992). p53 mutation cluster at codon 249 in hepatitis B virus-positive hepatocellular carcinomas from China. *Cancer Res.* 52(6):1635–1638.

31. Feig DI, Reid TM and Loeb LA (1994). Reactive oxygen species in tumorigenesis. [Review]. *Cancer Res.* 54(7 Suppl). 1890s–1894s.

32. Wainfan E and Poirier LA (1992). Methyl groups in carcinogen effects on DNA methylation and gene expression. *Cancer Res.* 52:2071s–2077s.

33. Ray JS, Harbison ML, McClain RM and Goodman JI (1994). Alterations in the methylation status and expression of the raf oncogene in phenobarbital-induced and spontaneous B6C3F1 mouse liver tumors. *Mol. Carcinogen.* 9(3):155–166.

34. Vorce RL and Goodman JI (1989). Hypomethylation of ras oncogenes in chemically induced and spontaneous B6C3F1 mouse liver tumors. *Mol. Toxicol.* 2(2):99–116.

35. Christman JK, Sheikhnejad G, Dizik M, Abileah S and Wainfan E (1993). Division of Molecular Biology, Michigan Cancer Foundation, Detroit. Reversibility of changes in nucleic acid methylation and gene expression induced in rat liver by severe dietary methyl deficiency. *Carcinogenesis* 14(4):551–557.

36. Rushmore TH, Ghazarian DM, Subrahmanyan V, Farber E and Ghoshal AK (1987). Probable free radical effects on rat liver nuclei during early hepatocarcinogenesis with a choline-devoid low methionine diet. *Cancer Res.* 47(24 Pt 1):6731–6740.

37. Hinrichsen LI, Floyd RA and Sudilovsky O (1990). Is 8-hydroxydeoxyquanosine a mediator of carcinogenesis by a choline-devoid diet in the rat liver? *Carcinogenesis* 11(10):1879–1881

38. Nicotera TM (1991). Molecular and biochemical aspects of Bloom's syndrome. *Cancer Genetics and Cytogenetics.* 53(1):1–13.

39. Turk PW, Laayoun A, Smith SS and Weitzman SA (1995). DNA adduct 8-hydoxyl-2'-deoxyguanosine (8-hydoxyguanosine) affects function of human DNA methyltransferase. *Carcinogenesis* 16:1253–1255.

40. Mukai FH and Goldstein BD (1976). Mutagenicity of malonaldehyde, a decomposition product of peroxidized polyunsaturated fatty acids. *Science.* 191(4229):868–869.

41. White AA, Crawford KM, Patt CS and Lad PJ (1976). Activation of soluble guanylate cylase from rat lung by incubation or by hydrogen peroxide. *J. Biol. Chem.* 251(23):7304–7312.

42. Bellomo G, Mirabelli F, Richelmi P and Orrenius S (1983). Critical role of sulfhydryl groups(s) in the ATP-dependent Ca^{2+} sequestration by the plasma membrane fraction from rat liver. *FEBS Lett.* 163:136–139.

43. Davies KJA (1986). Intracellular proteolytic systems may function as secondary antioxidants defenses: An hypothesis. *J. Free Radical Biol. Med.* 9:155–173.

44. Kerr LD, Inoue J and Verma IM (1992). Signal transduction: The nuclear target. *Curr. Opin. Cell Biol.* 4(3):496–501.

45. Berridge MJ (1994). The biology and medicine of calcium signalling. [Review] *Mol. Cell. Endocrinol.* 98(2):119–124.

46. Whitfield JF (1992). Calcium signals and cancer. *Crit. Rev. Oncogen.* 3:55–90.

47. Harman AW and Maxwell MJ (1995). An evaluation of the role of calcium in cell injury. [Review] *Annu. Rev. Pharmacol. Toxicol.* 35:129–44.

48. Dreher D and Junod AF (1995). Differential effects of superoxide, hydrogen peroxide, and hydroxyl radical on intracellular calcium in human endothelial cells. *J. Cell. Physiol.* 162(1):147–153.

49. Persoon-Rothert M, Egas-Kenniphaas JM, van der Valk-Kokshoorn EJ, Buys JP and van der Laarse A (1994). Oxidative stress-induced perturbations of calcium homeostasis and cell death in cultured myocytes: role of extracellular calcium. *Mol. Cell. Biochem.* 136(1):1–9.

50. Gerutti P (1989). Pathophysiological mechanisms of active oxygen. *Mutat. Res.* 214:81–88.

51. Maki A, Berezsky IK, Fargnoli J, Holbrook NJ and Trump BF (1992). Role of (Ca2+)i in induction of c-fos, c-jun, and c-myc mRNA in rat PTE after oxidative stress. *FASEB J.* 6(3):919–924.

52. Muehlematter D, Larrson R and Cerutti P (1980). Active oxygen induced DNA strand breakage and poly ADP-ribosylation in promotable and non-promotable JB6 mouse epidermal cells. *Carcinogenesis* 9:239–245.

53. Stewart AF, Herrera RE and Nordheim A (1990). Rapid induction of c-fos transcription reveals quantitative linkage of RNA polymerase II and topoisomerase I enzyme activities. *Cell.* 60:141–149.

54. Meyer M, Pahl HL and Baeuerle PA (1994). Regulation of the transcription factors NFkB and AP-1 by redox changes. *Chem. Biol. Interact.* 91(2–3):91–100.

55. Blobe GC, Obeid LM and Hannun YA (1994). Regulation of protein kinase C and role in cancer biology. [Review] *Cancer Metastasis Rev.* 13(3–4):411–31.

56. Larsson R and Cerutti P (1989). Translocation and enhancement of phosphotransferase activity of protein kinase C following exposure in mouse epidermal cells to oxidants. *Cancer Res.* 49:5627–5632.

57. Brawn MK, Chiou WJ and Leach KL (1995). Oxidant-induced activation of protein kinase C in UC11MG cells. *Free Radical Res.* 22(1):23–37.

58. Jones D, Thor M, Smith M, Jewell S and Orrenius S (1983). Inhibition of ATP dependent microsomal Ca2+ sequestion during oxidative stress and its prevention by glutathione. *J. Biol. Chem.* 258:6390–6393.

59. Zorn NE, Russell DH, Buckley AR and Sauro MD (1995). Alterations in splenocyte protein kinase C (PKC) activity by 2,3,7,8-tetrachlorodibenzo-*p*-dioxin in vivo. *Toxicol. Lett.* 78(2):93–100.

60. Kass GEN, Duddy SK and Orrenius S (1989). Alterations of hepatocyte protein kinase C by redox-cycling quinones. *Biochem. J.* 260:499–507.

61. Jirtle RL and Meyer SA (1991). Liver tumor promotion: Effect of phenobarbital on EGF and protein kinase C signal transduction and transforming growth factor-beta 1 expression. *Digest. Dis. Sci.* 36(5):659–68.

62. Brockenbrough JS, Meyer SA, Li CX and Jirtle RL (1991). Reversible and phorbol ester-specific defect of protein kinase C translocation in hepatocytes isolated from phenobarbital-treated rats. *Cancer Res.* 51(1):130–6.

63. Gopalakrishna R and Anderson WB (1989). Ca^{2+} and phospholipid-independent activation of protein kinase C by selective oxidative modification of the regulatory domain. *Proc. Natl. Acad. Sci. USA* 86:6758–6762.

64. Pronzato AA, Domenicotti C, Rosso E, Bellocchio A, Patrone M, Marinari UM, Melloni E and Poli G (1993). Modulation of rat liver protein kinase C during in vivo CCl_4-induced oxidative stress. *Biochem. BioPhys. Res. Commun.* 194(2):635–641.

65. Klaunig JE (1991). Alterations in intercellular communication during the stage of promotion. *Proc. of Soc. Exp. Biol. Med.* 198:688–692.

66. Klaunig JE, Ruch RJ, Hampton JA, Weghorst CM and Hartnett JA (1990). *Gap-Junctional Intercellular Communication and Murine Hepatic Carcinogenesis. Mouse Liver Carcinogenesis: Mechanisms and Species Comparisons*, pp. 277–291. New York: Alan R. Liss.

67. Loewenstein WR (1979). Junctional intercellular communication and the control of growth. *Biochim. Biophys. Acta.* 560:1–65.

68. Esinduy CB, Chang CC, Trosko JE and Ruch RJ (1995). In vitro growth inhibition of neoplastically transformed cells by non-transformed cells: Requirement for gap junctional intercellular communication. *Carcinogenesis* 16(4):915–921.

69. Ruch RJ and Klaunig JE (1988). Kinetics of phenobarbital inhibition of intercellular communication in mouse hepatocytes. *Cancer Res.* 48(9):2519–23

70. Cerutti PA (1991). Oxidant stress and carcinogenesis. *Eur. J. Clin. Invest.* 21:1–5.

71. Troll W and Wiesner R (1985). The role of oxygen radicals as a possible mechanism of tumor promotion. *Annu. Rev. Pharmacol. Toxicol.* 25:509–528.

72. Nathan C. (1992) Nitric oxide as a secretory product of mammalian cells. *FASEB J.* 6:3051–3064.

73. Liu RH and Hotchkiss JH (1995). Potential genotoxicity of chronically elevated nitric oxide: a review. [Review] *Mutat. Res.* 339(2):73–89.

74. Routledge MN. (1993) Mutations induced by saturated aqueous nitric oxide in the pSP189 supF gene in human Ad293 and E. coli MBM7070 cells. *Carcinogenesis* 14(7):1251–1254.

75. Wink DA, Osawa Y, Darbyshire JF, Jones CR, Eshenaur SC and Nims RW (1993). Inhibition of cytochromes P-450 by nitric oxide and a nitric oxide-releasing agent. *Arch. Biochem. Biophys.* 300:115–123.

76. Nathan CF and Tsunawake S (1986). Secretion of toxic oxygen products by macrophages: regulatory cytokines and their effects on the oxidase. *Ciba Foundation Symp.* 118:211–230.

77. Ohshima H and Bartsch H (1994) Chronic infections and inflammatory processes as cancer risk factors: possible role of nitric oxide in carcinogenesis. *Mutat. Res.* 305(2). 253–264.

78. ElSisi AED, Earnest DL and Sipes IG (1992). Vitamin A potentiation of carbon tetrachloride hepatotoxicity: role of liver macrophages and active oxygen species. *Toxicol. Appl. Pharmacol.* 119:295–301.

79. Laskin DL and Pilaro A (1986). Potential role of activated macrophages in acetaminophen hepatotoxicity. I. Isolation and characterization of activated macrophages from rat liver. *Toxicol. Appl. Pharmacol.* 86:204–215.

80. Laskin DL, Robertson FM, Pilaro AM and Laskin JD (1988). Activation of liver macrophages following phenobarbital treatment of rats. *Hepatology* 8:1051–1055.

81. Shiratori Y, Takikawa H, Kawase T and Sugimoto T (1986). Superoxide anion generating capacity and lysosomal enzyme activities of Kupffer cells in galactosamine-induced hepatitis. *Gastroenterol. Jpn.* 21:135–144.

82. Katsumoto F, Miyazaki K and Nakayama F. (1989). Stimulation of DNA synthesis in hepatocytes by Kupffer cells after partial hepatectomy. *Hepatology.* 9(3):405–410.

83. Bors W, Michel C, Dalke C, Stettmaier K, Saran M and Andrae U (1993). Radical intermediates during the oxidation of nitropropanes. The formation of NO_2 from 2-nitropropane, its reactivity with nucleosides, and implications for the genotoxicity of 2-nitropropane. *Chem. Res. Toxicol.* 6(3):302–9.

84. Deliconstantinos G, Villiotou V and Stavrides JC (1994). Scavenging effects of hemoglobin and related heme containing compounds on nitric oxide, reactive oxidants and carcinogenic volatile nitreactive oxygen speciesocompounds of cigarette smoke. A new method for protection against the dangerous cigarette constituents. *Anticancer Res.* 14(6B):2717–2726.

85. Vellanoweth RL, Suprakar, PC and Roy AK (1994). Biology of disease transcription factors in development, growth, and aging. *Lab. Invest.* 70:784–799.

86. Whiteside ST and Goodbourn S (1993). Signal transduction and nuclear targeting: regulation of transcription factor activity by subcellular localization. *J. Cell Sci.* 104:949–955.

87. Grimm S and Baeuerle PA (1993). The inducible transcription factor NF-kB: Structure-function relationship of its protein subunits. *Biochem. J.* 290:297–308
88. Baeuerle PA and Baltimore D (1988). IkB: A specific inhibitor of the NF-kB transcription factor. *Science.* 242:540–546.
89. Schreck R, Rieber P and Baeuerle PA (1991). Reactive oxygen intermediates as apparently widely used messengers in the activation of the NF-kB transcription factor and HIV-1. *EMBO J.* 10:2247–2258
90. Radler-Pohl A, Gebel S, Sachsenmaier C, Kinig H, Kramer M, Oehler T, Streile M, Ponta H, Rapp U, Rahmsdorf HJ, Cato ACB, Angel P and Herrlich P (1993). The activation and activity control of AP-1 (Fos/Jun). *Ann. NY Acad. Sci.* 684:127–148.
91. Devary Y, Gottlieb RA, Lau LF and Karin M (1991). Rapid and preferential activation of the c-jun gene during the mammalian UV response. *Mol. Cell. Biol.* 11:2804–2811.
92. Jabbar SA, Hoffbrand AV and Wickremasinghe RG (1994) Redox reagents and staureactive oxygen speciesporine inhibit stimulation of the transcription regulation NF-kB following tumor necrosis factor treatment of chronic B-leukaemia cells. *Leukemia Res.* 18:523–530
93. Zawaski K, Greubele A, Kaplan D, Reddy S, Mortensen A and Novak RF (1993). Evidence for enhanced expression of c-Fos, c-Jun and the Ca2+ activated neutral protease in rat liver following carbon tetrachloride administration. *Biochem. Biophys. Res. Commun.* 197(2):585–590.
94. Puga A, Nebert DW and Carrier F (1992). Dioxin induces expression of c-fos and c-jun proto-oncogenes and a large increase in transcription factor AP-1. *DNA Cell Biol.* 11(4):269–81.
95. Schenk H (1994). Distinct effects of thioredoxin and antioxidants on the activation of transcription factors NF-kB and AP-1. *Proc. Natl. Acad. Sci. USA* 91:1672–1676
96. Pinkus R, Bergelson S, Daniel V. (1993). Phenobarbital induction of AP-1 binding activity mediate activation of glutathione S-trasferase and quinone reductase gene expression. *Biochem. J.* 290:637–640.
97. Ye J, Young HA, Mao Y, Shi X. (1995). Chromium(VI)-induced nuclear factor-kB activation in intact cells via free radical reactions. *Carcinogenesis* 16:2401–2405.
98. Moser GJ and Smart RC (1981). Hepatic tumor promoting chlorinated hydrocarbons stimulate protein kinase C activity. *Carcinogenesis* 10(5):851–856.
99. Talalay P, De Long MJ and Prochaska HJ (1988). Identification of a common chemical signal regulating the induction of enzymes that protect against chemical carcinogenesis. *Proc. Natl. Acad. Sci., USA.* 85:8261–8265.
100. Bergelson S, Pinkus R and Daniel V (1994). Intracellular glutathione levels regulate Fos/Jun induction and activation of glutathione S-transferase gene expression. *Cancer Res.* 54:36–41.
101. Legrand-Poels S, Bours V, Piret B, Pflaum M, Epe B, Rentier B and Piette J (1995). Transcription factor NF-kappa B is activated by photosensitization generating oxidative DNA damages. *J. Biol. Chem.* 270(12):6925–6934.
102. Cristman MF, Morgan RW, Jacobson FS and Ames BN (1985). Positive control of a regulon for defenses against oxidative stress and some heat-shock proteins in *Salmonella typhimurium.* *Cell.* 41:753–762.
103. Storz G, Tartaglia LA and Ames BN (1990). Transcriptional regulator of oxidative stress-inducible genes: direct activation by oxidation. *Science.* 248(4952):189–194.
104. Becker J, Mezger V, Courgeon AM and Best-Belpomme M (1990). Hydrogen peroxide activates immediate binding of a *Drosophila* factor to DNA heat-shock regulatory element in vivo and in vitro. *Eur. J. Biochem.* 189:553–558.
105. Lenardo M, Baltimore D (1989). NF-κB: A pleiotropic mediator of inducible and tissue specific gene control. *Cell* 58:227–229.
106. Pahl HL and Baeuerle PA (1994). Oxygen and the control of gene expression. [Review] *Bioessays* 16(7):497–502.
107. Friling RS, Bergelson S and Daniel V (1992). Two adjacent AP-1-like binding sites form the electrophile-responsive element of the murine glutathione S-transferase Ya subunit gene. *Proc. Natl. Acad. Sci. USA* 89:668–672.
108. Angel P and Karin M (1992). Specific members of the Jun protein family regulate collagenase expression in response to various extracellular stimuli. *Matrix Suppl.* 1:156–64.
109. Amstad P, Crawford D, Muehlematter D, Zbinden I, Larsson R and Cerutti P (1990). Oxidants stress induces the proto-oncogenes, C-fos and C-myc in mouse epidermal cells. *Bull. Cancer* 77(5):501–502.

110. la Rose FL, Pierce JW and Sonenshein GE (1994). Differential regulation of the c-myc oncogene promoter by the NFkB rel family of transcription factors. *Mol. Cell. Biol.* 14:1039–1044.

111. Sobczak J, Mechti N, Tournier MF, Blanchard JM and Duguet M (1989). c-myc and c-fos gene regulation during mouse liver regeneration. *Oncogene* 4(12):1503–1508.

112. Alcorn JA, Feitelberg SP and Brenner DA (1990). Transient induction of c-jun during hepatic regeneration. *Hepatology* 11:909–915.

113. Nakano N, Hatayama I, Satoh K, Suzuki S, Sato K and Tsuchida S (1994). c-Jun expression in single cells and preneoplastic foci induced by diethylnitrosamine in B6C3F1 mice: comparison with the expression of pi-class glutathione S-transferase. *Carcinogenesis* 15(9):1853–1857.

114. Miller AD, Curran T, Verma IM (1984). c-fos Protein can induce cellular transformation: A novel mechanism of activation a cellular oncogene. *Cell.* 36(1):51–60.

115. Higgins KA, Perez JR, Coleman TA, Dorshkind, K, McComas WA, Sarmiento UM, Rosen CA and Narayanan R (1993). Aintisense inhibition of the p65 subunit of NF-kappa B blocks tumorigenicity and causes tumor regression. *Proc. Natl. Acad. Sci. USA* 90(21):9901–9905.

116. Tozawa K, Sakurada S, Kohri K and Okamoto T (1995). Effects of anti-nuclear factor kappa B reagents in blocking adhesion of human cancer cells to vascular endothelial cells. *Cancer Res.* 55(18):4162–7

117. Frenkel K (1992). The role of active oxygen species in biological damage and the effect of some chemopreventive agents. *In Protease Inhibitors as Cancer Chemopreventive Agents*, eds. W Troll and AR Kennedy. New York: Plenum.

118. Frenkel K, Donahue JM and Banerjee S (1988). Benzo[a]pyrene-induced oxidative DNA damage: A possible mechanism for promotion by complete carcinogens. In *Oxy-radicals in Molecular Biology and Pathology*. UCLA Symposia on Molecular and Cellular Biology, New Series, Vol. 82, eds. P Cerutti, I Fridovich and J McCord, pp. 509–524. New York: Alan R. Liss.

119. Scholz W, Schutze K, Kunz W and Schwarz M (1990). Phenobarbital enhances the formation of reactive oxygen in neoplastic rat liver nodules. *Cancer Res.* 50(21):7015–7022.

120. Stark AA (1991). Oxidative metabolism of glutathione by gamma-glutamyl transpeptidase and peroxisome proliferation: The relevance to hepatocarcinogenesis. A hypothesis. *Mutagenesis.* 6:241–245.

121. Brattin WJ, Glende EA and Recknagel RO (1985). Pathological mechanisms in carbon tetrachloride hepatotoxicity. *J. Free Radicals Biol. Med.* 1:27–38.

122. Casini AF and Farber JL (1981). Dependence of the carbon-tetrachloride-induced death of cultured hepatocytes on the extracellular calcium concentration. *Am. J. Pathol.* 105:138–148.

123. Columbano A, Ledda-Columbano GM, Ennas MG, Curto M, Chelo A and Pani P (1987). Inability of mitogen-induced liver hyperplasia to support the induction of enzyme-altered islands induced by liver carcinogens. *Cancer Res.* 47:5557–5559.

124. Ames BN and Gold LS (1992). Animal cancer tests and cancer prevention. *Monogr. Natl. Cancer Inst.* 12:125–32.

125. Schulte-Hermann R, Timmermann-Trosiener I, Barthel G and Bursch W (1990). DNA synthesis, apoptosis, and phenotypic expression as determinants of growth of altered foci in rat liver during phenobarbital promotion. *Cancer Res.* 50:5127–5135.

126. Hermeking H and Eick D (1994). Mediation of c-Myc-induced apoptosis by p53. *Science.* 265(5181):2091–3.

127. Yuan J, Yeasky TM, Havre PA, and Glazer PM. (1995). Induction of p53 in mouse cells decreases mutagenesis by UV radiation. *Carcinogenesis* 16:2295–2300.

128. Butterworth BE and Goldsworthy TL (1991). The role of cell proliferation in multistage carcinogenesis. *Cell Proliferation* 198(2):683–687.

129. Cohen SM and Ellwein LB (1990). Proliferative and genotoxic cellular effects in 2-acetylaminofluorene bladder and liver carcinogenesis: Biological modeling of the ED01 Study. *Toxicol. Appl. Pharmacol.* 104:79–93.

130. Conolly RB, Reitz RH, Clewell III HJ and Andersen ME (1988). Pharmacokinetics, biochemical mechanism and mutation accumulation: a comprehensive model of chemical carcinogenesis. *Toxicol. Lett.* 43:189–200.

131. Chen ZY, Farin F, Omiecinski CJ and Eaton DL (1992). Association between growth stimulation by phenobarbital and expression of cytochromes P-450 1A1, 1A2, 2B1/2 and 3A1 in hepatic hyperplastic nodules in male F344 rats. *Carcinogenesis* 13:675–82.

132. Smith-Oliver T and Butterworth BE (1987). Correlation of the carcinogenic potential of di(2-

ethylhexyl)phthalate (DEHP) with induced hyperplasia rather than with genotoxic activity. *Mutat. Res.* 188:21–28.

133. Reddy JK and Rao MS (1977). Malignant tumors in rats fed nafenopin, a hepatic peroxisome proliferator. *J. Natl. Cancer Inst.* 59:1645–1650.

134. Reddy JK and Qureshi SA (1979). Tumorigenicity of the hypolipidaemic peroxisome proliferator ethyl-a-chlorophenoxy-isobutyrate (clofibrate) in rats. *Br. J. Cancer.* 40:476–482.

135. Stevenson DE, Kehrer JP, Kolaja KL, Walborg EF and Klaunig JE (1995). Effect of dietary antioxidants on dieldrin-induced hepatotoxicity in mice. *Toxicol. Lett.* 75(1-3):177–183.

136. Busser M-T and Lutz WK (1987). Stimulation of DNA synthesis in rat and mouse liver by various tumor promoters. *Carcinogenesis* 8(10):1433–1437.

137. Lucier GW, Tritscher A, Goldsworthy T, Foley J, Clark G, Goldstein J and Maronpot R (1991). Ovarian hormones enhance TCDD-mediated increases in cell proliferation and preneoplastic foci in a two stage model for rat heptocarcinogensis. *Cancer Res.* 51:1391–1397.

138. Barr SB, Pimente R, Simizu K, Azzalis LA, Costa IS and Junqueira BC (1994). Dose-dependent study of liver lipid peroxidation related parameters in rats treated with pp'-DDT. *Toxicol. Lett.* 79:33–38.

139. Lake BG, Evans JG, Walters DG and Price RJ (1991). Comparison of the hepatic effect of nafenopin, a peroxisome proliferator, in rats fed adequate or vitamin E- and selenium-deficient diets. *Hum. Exp. Toxicol.* 10:87–88.

140. Alsharif NZ, Lawson T and Stohs SJ (1994). 2,3,7,8-Tetrachlorodibenzo-*p*-dioxin is mediated by the aryl hydrocarbon (Ah) receptor complex. *Toxicology* 92(1–3):39–51.

141. Hendrich S, Krueger K, Chen HW and Cook L (1991). Phenobarbital increases rat hepatic preactive oxygen speciestaglandin F2alpha, glutathione *S*-transferase activity and oxidative stress. *Prostaglandins, Leukotrienes and Essential Fatty Acids* 42:45–50.

142. Bagchi M, Hassoun EA, Bagchi D and Stohs SJ (1993). Production of reactive oxygen species by peritoneal macrophages, hepatic mitochondria and micreactive oxygen speciesomes from endrin-treated rats. *Free Radical Biol. Med.* 14:149–155.

143. Ledda-Columbano GM, Columbano A, Cannas A, Simbula G, Okita K, Kayano K, Kubo Y, Katyal SL and Shinozuka H (1994). Dexamethasone inhibits induction of liver tumor necrosis factor-alpha mRNA and liver growth induced by lead nitrate and ethylene dibromide. *Am. J. Pathol.* 145(4):951–958.

144. Umemura T, Sai-Kato K, Takagi A, Hasegawa R and Kurokawa Y (1996). Oxidative DNA damage and cell proliferation in the livers of B6C3F1 mice exposed to pentachlorophenol in their diet. *Fundam. Appl. Toxicol.* 30:285–289.

145. Toyokuni S, Okamoto K, Yodoi J and Hiai H (1995). Persistent oxidative stress in cancer. *FEBS Lett.* 358:1–3.

146. Palozza P, Agostara G, Piccioni E and Bartoli GM (1994). Different role of lipid peroxidation in oxidative stress-induced lethal injury in normal and tumor thymocytes. *Arch. Biochem. Biophy.* 312(1):88–94.

147. Albelda SM (1993). Role of integrins and other cell adhesiomolecules in tumor progression and metastasis. [Review] *Lab. Invest.* 68(1):4–17.

148. Junqueira VB, Simizu K, Pimentel R, Azzalis LA, Barros SB, Koch O and Videla LA (1991). Effect of phenobarbital and 3-methylcholanthrene on the early oxidative component induced by lindane in rat liver. *Xenobiotica* 21(8):1053–1065.

149. Videla LA, Barros SB and Junqueira VB (1990). Lindane-induced liver oxidative stress. [Review]. *Free Radical Biol. Med.* 9(2):169–79.

150. Hagan U. (1989). Biochemical aspects of radiation biology. *Experientia* 45:7–12.

151. Bagchi M and Stohs SJ (1993). In vitro induction of reactive oxygen species by 2,3,7,8-tetrachlorodibenzo-*p*-dioxin, endrin, and lindane in rat peritoneal macrophages and hepatic mitochondria and micreactive oxygen speciesomes. *Free Radical Biol. Med.* 14:11–18.

152. Klein CB, Frenkel K and Costa M (1991). The role of oxidative processes in metal carcinogenesis. *Chem. Res. Toxicol.* 4:592–604.

153. Sai K, Umemura T, Takagi A, Hasegawa R and Kurokawa Y (1992). The protective role of glutathione, cysteine and vitamin C against oxidative DNA damage induced in rat kidney by potassium bromate. *Jpn J. Cancer Res.* 83(1):45–51.

154. Iqbal M, Giri U and Athar M (1995). Ferric nitrilotriacetate (Fe-NTA) is a potent hepatic tumor promoter and acts through the generation of oxidative stress. *Biochem. Biophys. Res. Commun.* 212:557–563.

155. Huang CY, Wilson MW, Lay LT, Chow CK, Robertson LW and Glauert HP (1994). Increased 8-

hydoxydeoxyguanosine in hepatic DNA of rats treated with the peroxisome proliferators ciprofibrate and perfluorodecanoic acid. *Cancer Lett.* 87(2):223–228.

156. Cattley RC and Glover SE (1993). Elevated 8-hydroxydeoxyguanosine in hepatic DNA of rats following exposure to peroxisome proliferators: relationship to carcinogenesis and nuclear localization. *Carcinogenesis* 14:2495–2499.

157. Witz G. (1991). Active oxygen species as factors in multistage carcinogensis. *Proc of Soc. of Exp. Bio. Med.* 198:675–682.

158. Dahlhaus M, Almstadt E, Henschke P, Luttgert S and Appel KE (1995). induction of 8-hydroxy-2-deoxyquanosine and single-strand breaks in DNA of V79 cells by tetrachloro-*p*-hydroquinone. *Mutat. Res.* 329:29–36.

159. Marsman DS, Cattley RC, Conway JG and Popp JA (1988) Relationship of hepatic peroxisome proliferation and replicative DNA synthesis to the hepatocarcinogenicity of the peroxisome proliferators di(2-ethylhexyl)phthalate (DEHP) and [4-chloro-6-(2,3-xylidino)-2-pyrimidinylthio]acetic acid (Wy14,643) in rats. *Cancer Res.* 48:6739–6744.

160. Cunningham ML, and Mathews HB. (1991). Relationship of hepatocarcinogenicity and hepatocellular proliferation induced by mitogenic noncarcinogens vs. carcinogens. II. 1– vs. 2-nitropropane. *Toxicol. Appl. Pharmacol.* 110:505–513.

161. Dees C, and Travis C. (1993). The mitogenic potential of trichloroethylene in B6C$_3$F$_1$ mice. *Toxicol. Lett.* 62:129–137.

162. Wilson DM, Goldsworthy TL, Popp JA and Butterworth BE (1992). Evaluation of genotoxicity, pathological lesions, and cell proliferation in livers of rats and mice treated with furan. *Environ. Mol. Mutagen.* 19:209–222.

163. Guo N, Conaway CC, Huyssain NS and Fiala ES (1990). Sex and organ differences of oxidative DNA and RNA damage due to treatment of Sprague-Dawley rats with acetoxime or 2-nitropropane. *Carcinogenesis* 11(9):1659–1662.

164. Kefalas V and Stacey NH (1989). Potentiation of carbon tetrachloride-induced lipid peroxidation by trichloroethylene in isolated rat hepatocytes: No role in enhanced toxicity. *Toxicol. Appl. Pharmacol.* 101:158–160.

165. Carfagna MA, Held SD, and Kedderis GL. (1993). Furan-induced cytolethality in isolated rat hepatocytes: Correspondence with in vivo dosimetry. *Toxicol. Appl. Pharmacol.* 123:265–273.

166. Bachowski S, Xu Y, Baker RK, Stevenson DE, Walborg EF and Klaunig JE (1995). The potential role of oxidative stress in nongenotoxic carcinogenesis in the mouse liver. In: *Growth Factors and Tumor Promotion, Implication for Risk Assessment,* eds. RM McClain et al., Progress in Clinical and Biological Research vol. 391, pp. 385–396. New York: Wiley-Liss.

Free Radical Toxicology
Edited by K. B. Wallace
Copyright © 1997 Taylor & Francis

19

Markers of Free-Radical-Mediated Tissue Injury: Tales of Caution and Woe

Mark D. Scott

Division of Experimental Pathology, Department of Pathology and Laboratory Medicine, Albany Medical College, Albany, New York, USA

John W. Eaton

Department of Pediatrics, Baylor College of Medicine, Houston, Texas, USA

PROLOGUE

On a soft and cloudless summer morning in southern Georgia, Marvin ("Skeeter") Phelps—driving his trusty 1969 Chevrolet pick-up truck—accidentally runs over one of the largest raccoons in Macon County. Forty-eight hours later, the dead raccoon is discovered by Clive Fairlamb, state forensic oxidologist, who is looking for cases of the dreaded oxidative encephalitis virus (OEV). Clive's roadside brain biopsy, upon later testing for malonyldialdehyde, shows signs of massive brain oxidation. Clive alerts the Communicable Diseases Center (CDC) in Atlanta, Georgia, that an epidemic of OEV is underway in Macon County. Eight months of investigation by an extraordinarily clever team of CDC scientists leads to the discovery of a tire print on the dead raccoon, suggesting vehicle—rather than virus—as cause of death.

There are two morals to this story:

1. Dead meat oxidizes.
2. Dead material that is oxidized did not necessarily die of oxidation.

INTRODUCTION

Partly for reasons implicit in the prologue, diagnosis of free-radical-mediated tissue injury is rarely possible. This is because cellular damage of any sort is liable to lead to incidental oxidation that does not necessarily indict oxidant damage in the etiology of the injury. Nonetheless, forensic oxidologists are now claiming that no fewer than 273 important diseases are clearly caused by oxidation reactions. In fact, the evidence for oxidant causality is only convincing in a very few cases.

Some of the parameters often measured by modern forensic oxidologists are shown in Figure 1. As denoted in this figure, a plethora of tools are available. However, as suggested by the prologue, investigators must carefully choose the appropriate test(s) for the (a) tissues being examined, (b) type of injury induced, and (c) mechanism by which the injury will be or has been administered. Based on these caveats, we first consider general assays relevant to a wide range of tissues and then discuss in slightly greater detail some of the newer, more specialized or more abused tools available to the forensic oxidologist.

GENERAL MEASURES OF OXIDANT STRESS

Consumption of Small "Consumable" Antioxidants

The concept of "oxidant stress" involves the idea that, although oxidation reactions may constantly occur, beyond a certain threshold cellular protective systems fail and products of unopposed oxidation accumulate. One obvious reflection of such

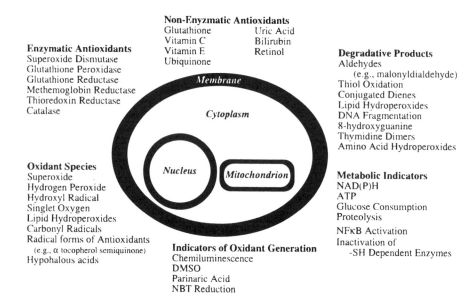

FIG. 1. Tools of the modern forensic oxidologist. Shown are some of the most commonly measured, and often abused, indicators of oxidative damage in cells.

stress is the net loss of small "consumable" antioxidants such as reduced glutathione (GSH), ascorbic acid, and vitamin E. Such loss will further predispose to oxidant damage inasmuch as experimental depletion of these antioxidants may profoundly sensitize cells to oxidant-mediated destruction. In some—but not all—circumstances, uncompensated oxidation will also lead to depletion of metabolic intermediates such as NAD(H), NADP(H), and ATP.

Measurements of cellular GSH concentration (1) are very simple, economical, and do, often, reflect the degree to which a cell or tissue has been oxidatively challenged. However, intracellular GSH is not a perfect predictor of oxidant sensitivity. For example, in many types of glucose-6-phosphate dehydrogenase (G-6-PD) deficiency (in which the ability of erythrocytes to reduce NADP to NADPH can be severely compromised), resting GSH levels may be near normal yet these red cells are exquisitely oxidant sensitive (2,3). Why? There may be several reasons for the enhanced sensitivity of G-6-PD-deficient cells. First, in G-6-PD deficiency it is the ability of the challenged red cell to *regenerate* GSH (by accelerating NADP reduction) that is compromised. Thus, steady-state GSH does not predict the response of these cells to oxidant challenge. Second, in erythrocytes and other cells, NADPH is not only important for the reduction of GSSG but also for the maintenance of catalase activity (4). Depending on the model system, decrements in catalase activity may cause greater oxidant sensitivity than loss of GSH (5). Third, GSH is not just an *anti*-oxidant. In the presence of ionic copper (6) or iron (7), GSH can drive metal-catalyzed oxidation reactions. This is also true of ascorbic acid, which, in the presence of transition metals, becomes more *pro-* than *anti*-oxidant.

Membrane-associated antioxidants such as α-tocopherol (vitamin E) and the ubiquinones (coenzyme Q) are at least as important as GSH (and NADPH) and may also be as schizophrenic. By and large, decrements in vitamin E are an accurate indicator of oxidative stress, and low membrane vitamin E does predispose to oxidative damage to membrane components, particularly, polyunsaturated fatty acids (8). However, as Stocker and colleagues have pointed out, vitamin E can also have pro-oxidant actions (9). This is particularly so if reducing agents such as vitamin C or ubiquinone are not present to "unload" the potentially reactive tocopherol semiquinone.

The consumption of metabolic cofactors has also been used as a measure of oxidant stress. Most often, the parameters measured have been total NAD(P)H and/ or ATP. As indicated earlier, NADPH is necessary for the maintenance of both hydrogen peroxide (H_2O_2) catabolizing pathways (GSH/glutathione peroxidase and catalase). Lowered NADPH will compromise the activities of both systems, leading to GSH depletion and an accumulation of inactive catalase (see Figure 2) (10). Therefore, direct measurement of NADP(H) may be desirable. However, this assay is relatively difficult to do and is fraught with complications (11). Furthermore, it has recently been observed that the amount of cellular NADPH tends to be underestimated since significant amounts are bound to NADPH-requiring proteins such as catalase.

Consequently it is often easier to measure other indicators of cellular oxidant

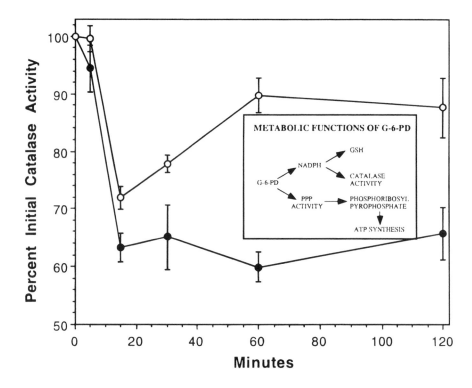

FIG. 2. Effect of H_2O_2 challenge on catalase activity in intact normal (○) and G6PD-deficient (●) erythrocytes. Shown is the percent change in catalase activity following challenge with 25 μM phenozine methosulfate over 2 h. Catalase activity in unchallenged samples showed no significant change from the initial value over the course of the experiment (values not shown). The values given represent the mean ± SD for a minimum of 3 independent experiments. Shown in the insert is the role that G-6-PD and NADPH play in H_2O_2 catabolism. Data modified from Scott et al. (11).

stress. Glucose consumption is closely coupled to NAD(P)H status and is easily measured. During compensated oxidant stress, glucose consumption increases and is diverted through the hexose monophosphate shunt (HMP, a diversion that is driven by the increased availability of NADP). A dramatic example of this oxidative activation of the HMP was the observation by Jacob and colleagues that glucose consumption increases nearly 30-fold in oxidant-stressed acatalasemic erythrocytes (an exaggeration of the normal response due to the absence of catalase-mediated clearance of H_2O_2) (12).

Although oxidant stress may often compromise cellular metabolism, decrements in intracellular ATP are by no means universally observed. It is true that certain clastogenic agents can cause ATP depletion (via activation of an NAD-consuming polyADP ribosylation of DNA-associated proteins) (13–15). However, decrements in cellular ATP are of limited usefulness as indicators of uncompensated oxidant stress.

Changes in Antioxidant Enzymes

Changes in the activity of several antioxidant enzymes have also been used as indirect measures of precedent oxidant stress. The induction of specific enzymes such as glutathione peroxidase, superoxide dismutase, and catalase has been observed in organisms as divergent as *Escherichia coli* and humans consequent to oxidant stress. For example, when *E. coli* are exposed to 100% O_2 there are ensuing increments in catalase (240%), peroxidase (1300%), and superoxide dismutase (130%) activity over a period of 24 h (16). Similarly, in the lungs of mice exposed to hyperbaric oxygen, there are increases in superoxide dismutase, glutathione peroxidase and catalase activity (17). Oxidant-induced *inactivation* of enzymes has also been a useful indicator of oxidant stress. One particularly interesting example of this is the H_2O_2-dependent inactivation of catalase by the broadleaf herbicide 3-amino-1,2,4-triazole. This test has been used since the early 1960s to estimate the in vivo and in vitro generation of H_2O_2 (18). Although an indirect measure, this method is thought to be an accurate reflection of H_2O_2 generation.

Detection of Oxidants

Perhaps the most convincing evidence of oxidant stress involves demonstration of the presence of increased amounts of oxidants per se. In general, these assays are based on the reaction of marker molecules with specific reactive oxygen species. Examples of these assays are: chemiluminescence (e.g., lucigenin for O_2^-), various electron spin resonance/electron paramagnetic resonance (ESR/EPR) probes, nitroblue tetrazolium reduction (O_2^-), cytochrome c reduction (O_2^-), 4-aminoantipyrine/peroxidase (H_2O_2), dimethyl sulfoxide (DMSO, ·OH radical), and the hydroxylation of phenols (·OH).

Chemiluminescence can be an extraordinarily sensitive method for the quantification of oxidant generation. The two most common agents used are lucigenin and luminol. Lucigenin (bis-*N*-methylacridinium nitrate) (19–21) readily crosses most membranes and is thought to be relatively specific for O_2^- with little interference by other species of activated oxygen (22). In contrast, luminol is thought to react with, and consequently reflect, oxidant species such as HOCl and H_2O_2 (23). Electron spin resonance (ESR), now more commonly referred to as electron paramagnetic resonance (EPR), when properly employed, permits the detection of specific reactive oxygen species via defined reactions with specific spin probes (24). Spin probes form relatively long-lived and stable radicals upon reaction with various radicals. Because of the increased longevity of these organic radicals, they can then be detected by the EPR instrument (25).

Luckily, for those of us with less well equipped laboratories, there are a number of non-EPR/chemiluminescence-based techniques for measuring reactive oxygen species. These include cytochrome c reduction, useful for both measuring O_2^- generation and in assaying superoxide dismutase (which, by dismuting O_2^-, inhibits O_2^- dependent cytochrome c reduction) (26). Quantitation of H_2O_2 is readily performed with a variety of techniques. These include, but are certainly not limited to, the aforementioned aminotriazole-mediated inactivation of catalase; the new spectrophotometric "FOX" assay, involving H_2O_2-dependent (chain) oxidation of ferrous to ferric iron which is then detected by xylenol orange (27); and the H_2O_2/peroxidase-mediated formation of a quinone-imine from 4-aminoantipyrine and phenol (28). One exceptionally sensitive procedure for H_2O_2 detection involves hematin- and H_2O_2-dependent conversion of dichlorofluorescein to the fluorescent dichlorofluorescein (29). While this latter procedure is sensitive down to 100 pmol of peroxide, some concerns as to its specificity exist. Indeed, as a general rule, all these procedures for peroxide detection are rather nonspecific and will detect, for example, organic hydroperoxides as well as H_2O_2. However, this deficiency is easily corrected by the assay of control samples containing catalase (or glutathione peroxidase/GSH).

In comparison to the detection of O_2^- and H_2O_2, measurement of hydroxyl radical ($\cdot$OH) is more of a problem. This is because free $\cdot$OH (if present at all) is extraordinarily reactive and evanescent (30). Furthermore, we lack enzymes that will specifically react with $\cdot$OH, and all so-called $\cdot$OH scavengers must compete with every other organic component in the system. As a result, in biological systems, one cannot really quantitate $\cdot$OH. There are, however, a number of procedures for detecting the presence of $\cdot$OH. These include the generation of methane or formaldehyde by reaction of $\cdot$OH with DMSO (31,32). Alternatively, the other product of $\cdot$H cleavage of DMSO, methanesulfinic acid, can also be quantitated spectrophotometrically (33). This latter technique may also be useful *in vivo*, as could the procedure for measuring OH-dependent generation of hydroxylated products (2,3- and 2,5-dihydroxybenzoate) of salicylic acid (2-hydroxybenzoic acid) (34).

Finally, not even a superficial discussion of detection techniques for oxidative species would be complete without mention of nitric oxide and peroxynitrite ($\cdot$NO and $\cdot$ONOO, respectively). Direct and indirect methods for detecting these radicals, as well as the biosynthesis these products, have been recently reviewed by Beckman (35). Over the last few years $\cdot$NO has emerged as an important mediator of oxidative injury. Perhaps one of the most important reactions of $\cdot$NO is reactivity with O_2^- to form $\cdot$ONOO. Because $\cdot$ONOO appears to be an important mediator of cellular injury, inclusion of SOD into the reaction mixture may have some ameliorating effects. Indeed, the facile reaction between O_2^- and $\cdot$NO may explain in part the biological necessity of SOD.

Unfortunately, while most of the above techniques are quite useful in well-defined in vitro systems, their utility is limited when applied either in vivo or even in isolated organs. This is because pathologically important oxidative tissue damage may be confined to certain cell types within a target tissue. For example, eosinophil peroxidase-mediated production of hypobromous acid may cause substantial damage to cardiac endothelial cells while having little effect on the bulk of the cardiac tissue (36). Therefore, measures of oxidation applied to the whole organ would likely reveal little oxidative damage to the *bulk* of the organ, although the damage to endothelium may have been lethal. Consequently, the forensic oxidative biochemist must have foreknowledge of the likely site of oxidative insult and choose an appropriate assay to measure damage at that site.

MEASURES OF LIPID PEROXIDATION

Maintenance of the integrity of cell and organelle membranes is crucial for cellular viability. Due to the presence of polyunsaturated fatty acids (PUFA) and the greatly elevated solubility of O_2 in lipid (O_2 is 30 times more soluble in lipid than aqueous solutions), membranes are particularly sensitive to oxidative attack. In addition, the generation of lipid radicals can also directly damage the protein and carbohydrate components of the membrane or change the membrane packing and fluidity to the extent that essential membrane proteins become nonfunctional.

As alluded to in the prologue, measurements of lipid peroxidation are probably the most often used, and abused, indicators of oxidant injury to biological material. Most commonly used assays are nonspecific measures of oxidative lipid degradation. Chief among these is the TBARS (thiobarbituric-acid-reactive substances) assay, often mistakenly called the malonyldialdehyde (MDA) assay (see Figure 3) (37). The most commonly cited reasons for the lack of specificity of the simple TBARS reaction are: (a) The majority of detected TBA-reactive material usually forms during heating of the sample (probably via metal-catalyzed reactions) rather than

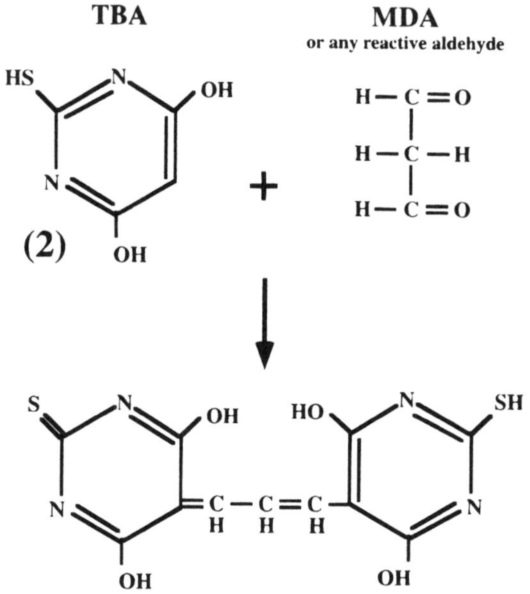

FIG. 3. Reaction between 2-thiobarbituric acid and malonyldialdehyde (MDA).

being present from the outset. (b) Actual malonyldialdehyde may represent only a small fraction of the detected oxidation products. (c) Even given this latter fact, TBA-reactive materials may themselves only reflect a small proportion of the oxidized products that form, for example, in a mixture of peroxidizing PUFA. (d) A variety of products not derived from PUFA oxidation—some not even derived from oxidative reactions—may react with thiobarbituric acid. For example, the TBARS assay readily detects products of oxidation of DNA, amino acids, and carbohydrates (38). Hence, this assay is neither overly sensitive nor specific because only a small fraction of the heterogeneous array of oxidatively generated aldehydes (which may derive from reactions with a number of target molecules) is available for reaction with TBA.

Nonetheless, this simple assay can yield useful information if the investigator is aware of these caveats and of the likely mechanism(s) of oxidative degradation in a particular experimental setting. The TBARS assay works best for homogeneous cellular suspensions and is less useful for whole-animal studies. Perhaps the primary deterrent to using the TBARS assay in whole animals is the fact that, to the extent that aldehydes are generated by lipid peroxidation, many of these are water soluble and readily lost from sites of generation. Furthermore, aldehyde/carbonyl-containing oxidative products are reactive with a number of biologic components and also may be metabolized by mitochondrial aldehyde dehydrogenase (39).

Reactive aldehydes are certainly not the only products of lipid peroxidation. Lipid peroxidation begins with the abstraction of an H from the hydrocarbon chain. This typically occurs at CH_2 groups adjacent to carbon-carbon double bonds. As a consequence of this H abstraction a resonance stabilized product—a conjugated diene—is formed. Conjugated dienes are readily quantified spectrophotometrically at 233 nm (40). However, while this method is easy to do, it is beset by multiple problems. In aerobic environments oxidized fatty acids containing conjugated dienes react rapidly with molecular oxygen to form peroxyl radicals, which may not be detected spectrophotometrically. Consequently, these studies are often done in the presence of O_2-free nitrogen. Furthermore, even in the absence of molecular oxygen, two conjugated dienes may react to form a cross-linked molecule that is also undetectable by the conjugated diene assay. In addition, complex mixtures of biological material contain many substances nonspecifically absorbing at 233 nm. Finally, at least one report indicates that much of the absorbing material may actually represent products of oxidized lipid:protein reactions that do not even contain the conjugated double bonds (41).

As just discussed, following abstraction of an H from the hydrocarbon chain, the resulting conjugated diene is most likely to react with molecular oxygen to form a peroxyl radical, also capable of abstracting an H from an additional lipid molecule. The resulting products are a lipid hydroperoxide (LOOH) and a new carbon-centered radical. The hydroperoxide is, in many ways, analogous to H_2O_2 in that it is relatively long-lived in the absence of redox-active metals such as Fe or Cu. Because of this longevity, lipid hydroperoxides can be excellent indicators of prior oxidant stress. Consequently a number of methods have been developed to measure their presence in lipids. Common to all of these methods, however, is the need to keep trace iron or copper from entering the assay system because these metals greatly accelerate the decomposition of the hydroperoxides. One of the easiest methods of measuring lipid hydroperoxides actually takes advantage of this redox metal reactivity. The FOX (ferrous oxidation with xylenol orange) assay takes advantage of the reaction between ferrous iron (Fe^{2+}) and lipid hydroperoxides in an acidic milieu, which yields ferric iron (Fe^{3+}) (27,42). In the presence of xylenol orange (3,3'-bis[*N,N*-di(carboxymethyl)-aminomethyl]-*o*-cresolsulfone-phthalein), a chromophoric chelate forms that is measured at 560 nm. This assay has been reported to be sensitive to the picomole level and can be used in a variety of models. Dichlorofluorescein (DCF), used as a measure of H_2O_2 for a number of years, also readily reacts with LOOH. Consequently, the DCF-LOOH reaction has been modified to act as a sensitive measure of biologically generated LOOH (43).

Because of the numerous problems, artifacts, and lack of specificity and/or sensitivity associated with a number of the more easily done assays, several new assays for lipid peroxidation have been developed over the last 10 years. One of the more specific and sensitive of these is based on the use of parinaric acid (9,11,13,15-octadecatetraenoic acid; PnA), a fluorescent polyunsaturated fatty acid that readily inserts into membranes of intact cells (44). Following such insertion, the in situ peroxidation of this lipid probe can be followed by a loss of fluorescence (45). Previous studies have demonstrated that the rate of PnA oxidation is roughly comparable to that of arachidonic acid. This probe has been useful in providing real-time measurements of lipid peroxidation in a number of models (artificial bilayers of known composition, erythrocyte ghosts, intact cells, and lipoproteins). Additionally, the possibility exists for injection of PnA-labeled lipoproteins (or other small particles) into animals to measure at least some types of in vivo oxidation.

Gross changes in the major lipid classes of the membrane [phosphatidylcholine (PC), phosphatidylserine (PS), phosphatidylethanolamine (PE), and sphingomyelin (SM)] can also be of value in the analysis of oxidant damage (46,47). First, the proportion of the individual classes can be examined via one-dimensional thin-layer chromatography separation (48) and quantified according to Bartlett (49). Furthermore, analysis of the phospholipid asymmetry can be used. A number of previous studies have demonstrated that the phospholipid "flipase" (translocase) involved in the maintenance of lipid asymmetry is oxidant sensitive (50). Several relatively sensitive assays exist to measure the loss of lipid asymmetry (51). These include trinitrobenzenesulfonic acid (TNBS) and fluorescamine (52). TNBS is an impermeable dye that reacts with the aminophospholipid head groups (PE and PS), while fluorescamine is a membrane-permeable agent that reacts with primary amino groups. Changes in the membrane bilayer can also be seen using coagulation as an endpoint (53). This results from the fact that PS, which is normally only found in the inner leaflet of the bilayer, has very potent procoagulation activity. Consequently, loss of lipid asymmetry may enhance the coagulative effect of cells.

However, gross changes in the amounts or orientation of phospholipid classes are unlikely to be seen after most acute oxidant injury (though they may be more readily observed following chronic insult), and a more informative parameter is changes in the fatty acyl groups themselves. Membrane fatty acyl composition is relatively easily determined by gas chromatographic (GC) analysis (54) of cell lipid extracts (55). Using this technique it is possible to quantitate the loss of unsaturated fatty acyl groups such as arachidonic acid and, often, the appearance of the larger lipid and cholesterol oxidation products. A further refinement of GC analysis is the use of gas chromatography-mass spectrometry (GC-MS), which allows for a more exact determination of lipid breakdown products (56).

More recently, specific lipid breakdown products have been used as markers of oxidant damage as well as being of biologic interest in themselves. Phospholipids containing a polyunsaturated fatty acyl residue at the sn-2 position are common constituents of cellular membranes, and lipoprotein particles and are subject to oxidative attack. Oxidative modification and/or fragmentation of phosphatidylcholines generates potent inflammatory mediators that bind to the platelet-activating factor (PAF) receptor and mimic most of the biologic actions of PAF (57). Thus, oxidation either through inappropriate inflammatory processes, endogenous oxygen metabolism, or uptake of peroxidized lipids from the diet can all lead to inappropriate and unregulated generation of potent inflammatory mediators.

Other biologically generated compounds may also be of value in documenting chronic oxidant stress. Lipofuscin is a naturally occurring fluorescent intracellular pigment that is observed in many tissues and is typically ascribed to cellular aging (58). Interestingly this "aging pigment" is observed in organisms as diverse as cultured cells, fungi, *Drosophila*, nematodes, rats, and humans (59). Because of the inherent fluorescence of lipofuscin, it has been used as a purported measure of in vivo oxidant stress. However, the biochemical origins of lipofuscin are unknown (60). While organic extraction of lipofuscin yields fluorescent compounds similar to lipid peroxidation products, other studies suggest that proteins, carbohydrates, and DNA may also significantly contribute to the formation of lipofuscin. Regardless of its origin, a number of studies demonstrate that oxidative damage to cellular components over time is the important factor in the formation of lipofuscin.

In summary, a bewildering array of methods—many of them not even mentioned here—currently exists for the detection and quantification of lipid oxidation. These range from the insensitive and nonspecific TBARS assay to the highly specific GC-MS analysis of lipid extracts. The important thing to keep in mind is that, in the right circumstances, any one of these tests may suffice, while all of these procedures can produce artifactual results when applied inappropriately.

PROTEIN OXIDATION

Proteins, the other major component of biological membranes and the predominant intracellular material, are also subject to oxidative damage (Table 1). Gross indicators of compensated protein oxidation are increases in proteolysis and compensatory protein synthesis. Indeed, a positive correlation exists between rates of proteolysis

TABLE 1. *General markers of protein damage*

Thiol
    Protein thiol oxidation: loss of protein activity
    Thiol titration
    Thiol alkylation
    Thiol affinity chromatography
    ^{3}H-NEM-PAGE visualization of -SH

Nonthiol
    Carbonyls
    Oxidative deamination/decarboxylation events
    Proteolysis
    Oxidant damage to metalloproteins: loss of metal or metal-mediated functions
    Special cases: hemoglobin, myoglobin, cytochromes
    Oxidant cross-linking of proteins
    Oxidant scission of proteins

and protein synthesis and the intracellular generation of reactive oxygen species (ROS) (61). At the protein level, oxidant-mediated protein damage may be detected by oxidized sulfhydryl groups, intra- and intermolecular cross-linking, modification of amino acid residues, and protein degradation (62). These products may arise as a consequence of direct damage by reactive oxygen species or via secondary radicals. Indeed, it is important to note that integral and extrinsic membrane proteins may be more likely damaged by secondary lipid radicals (e.g., alkoxy radicals) than by direct attack from oxygen radicals (63). Because of the wide diversity of assays available to assess protein damage, we only briefly discuss some of the newer, more specialized, or more commonly abused tools of the forensic oxidologist.

In general, ·OH-mediated attack appears to be the primary mechanism of oxidant damage to proteins (64). The elevated production of O_2^-/HO_2^- has virtually no effect on protein degradation, though these radicals have been reported to result in enzyme inactivation (most likely by oxidation of essential sulfhydryl groups) (65). H_2O_2, while not directly capable of initiating protein degradation, can produce conformational changes that result in an enhanced susceptibility to enzymatic degradation (66). Furthermore, H_2O_2, in the presence of micromolar concentrations of redox-active metals, can cause substantial enzyme inactivation and protein degradation. This damage appears to result from the metal-catalyzed Haber-Weiss reaction with ensuing generation of ·OH (67). Interestingly, direct ·OH-mediated protein degradation is dependent on the inclusion of O_2 in the reaction mixture; in the absence of O_2, protein cross-linking is the predominant form of damage. Oxygen may be necessary for the generation of carbonyl radicals, with a consequent increase in the ratio of protein degradation to protein cross-linking (68).

While proteins are an important target of ROS, direct measurements of oxidized proteins, as opposed to lipid oxidation, are less commonly employed. In part this may derive from the often active proteolytic system of cells; oxidatively damaged proteins are rapidly proteolyzed in normal cells consequently destroying the evidence (69). However, based on loss of enzymatic activity, a number of proteins have been identified that are particularly sensitive to oxidation (70). Historically, the loss of enzymatic activity has been a primary, though indirect, tool in the measurement of protein oxidation. A second method of historical preference has been the generation of TCA-soluble fragments, usually secondary to proteolytic degradation (71). However, in complex systems these assays do not provide any specificity as to the target of the oxidative insult.

More specific and informative methods have subsequently been developed. Oxidatively produced protein-based carbonyl groups (C=O) have been used as an easily measured and relatively stable reflection of protein oxidation. Using compounds that directly react with the carbonyl groups it is possible to approximate the degree of oxidation relative to a nonoxidized control (72). Similarly, a number of early studies demonstrated the importance of protein thiols in governing enzymatic activity, and these studies further demonstrated that oxidation of these thiols often preceded loss of enzymatic activity. Consequently, a number of assays measuring thiol oxidation were developed. These vary from gross measures of thiol oxidation (thiol titration) to more specific measures of thiol loss (^{3}H-NEM-PAGE visualization of -SH).

Thiol titration is the most common measure of protein thiol oxidation (73). This assay lacks specificity and simply represents a global change in cell thiol status. While a useful measure for heavily oxidized cells, subtle, yet crucial oxidative events can be easily missed. This same complaint is true for a number of other assays which measure gross changes in thiol status (e.g., thiol alkylation, thiol affinity chromatography) (74,75). However, because of the potential importance of thiol oxidation to the forensic oxidologist, some attempts have been made to measure specific changes in thiol oxidation. Among these methods is the direct visualization of reduced thiol groups.

Alterations in membrane proteins and reactive thiol groups (i.e., reduced thiols) can be directly examined using ^{3}H-NEM labeled membranes and either urea-triton (76,77), or sodium dodecyl sulfate (SDS) (78) polyacrylamide gel electrophoresis (PAGE) (79). For example, labeling of red cell membranes with ^{3}H-NEM prior to electrophoresis allows the subsequent visualization and quantitation of both protein and thiol changes following oxidant stress (Figure 4). The membrane reactive thiol group distribution is examined by autoradiography following urea-triton or SDS gel electrophoresis as previously described (80). The relative protein and reactive thiol group concentrations can then be determined by densitometry with protein and reactive thiol concentrations expressed as percentage of the total membrane extractable protein (membrane-specific and skeletal proteins).

Finally, in addition to assays applicable to a large variety of cells, tissues, or organisms, specialized cells may have assays applicable only to that cell. A case in point is the erythrocyte. Within this cell over 95% of the total protein is represented by a single species, hemoglobin. Oxidation of hemoglobin has proven to be an excellent marker of oxidant damage (81,82). As shown in Figure 5, oxidation of hemoglobin is accompanied by a spectral shift that can mathematically be quantitated to determine the concentration of various oxidized products of oxyhemoglobin (83).

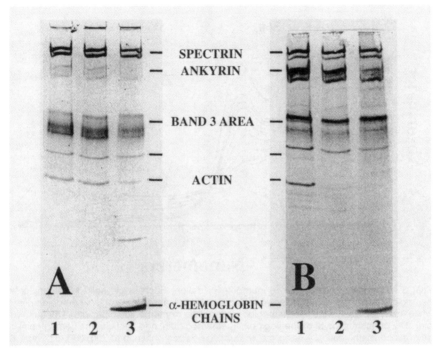

FIG. 4. ^{3}H-NEM-PAGE visualization of reactive thiol groups in erythrocyte membranes. Protein (A) and reactive thiol (B) distribution of normal (1), control-resealed (2), and unpaired α-hemoglobin chain loaded (3) erythrocytes following urea-triton polyacrylamide gel electrophoresis (78). Membrane ghosts were prepared and electrophoresed as described in Scott et al. (80,83). Samples shown are after 20 h of incubation at 37°C. Loss of reactive R-SH in cells loaded with α-hemoglobin chains probably results from release of heme/iron from the unstable α-chains.

In summary, an almost endless list of methods exists by which protein oxidation can be estimated. As with all the systems examined in this chapter, they range from nonspecific indicators of oxidation (e.g., proteolysis) to highly specific assays of specific proteins. With regard to the more general indicators of oxidation, assay sensitivity may be lacking and substantial, perhaps fatal, oxidative injury may occur prior to its detection. In contrast, when using highly specific measures (e.g., loss of activity of a specific enzyme) one may be examining the wrong indicator of injury. Thus, to repeat, one must carefully choose the appropriate assays for the oxidant used and the model system being examined.

DNA OXIDATION

DNA damage is commonly associated with oxidative challenge and the initiation of mutagenesis, carcinogenesis and apoptosis (Figure 6). Because of the wide diversity of assays available to assess DNA damage, as well as our own ignorance of

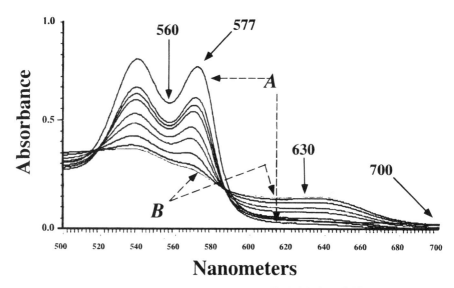

FIG. 5. Example of hemoglobin undergoing oxidation. Each black, solid line represents a hemoglobin scan done at a different time point. Line A denotes the initial hemoglobin scan, while line B represents the final hemoglobin scan (little oxyhemoglobin but lots of methemoglobin). The concentration of oxyhemoglobin, methemoglobin, and hemichrome hemoglobins are determined mathematically using the absorbance values obtained at 700, 630, 577, and 560 nm (8,84).

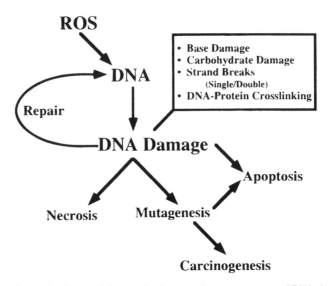

FIG. 6. General scheme of the mechanisms and consequences of DNA damage.

most of these techniques, we only briefly discuss some of the more generally used detection techniques.

The source of the initiating oxidants can be either endogenous or exogenous, but several general rules can be observed. Direct DNA damage by the O_2^- radical appears to be very rare (84). Indeed, in models in which DNA damage has been detected in response to O_2^- challenge, it was found that catalase, ·OH-scavengers, and certain metal chelators (e.g., desferrioxamine) as well as superoxide dismutase (SOD) were protective (85). These data indicate that O_2^- cannot directly damage DNA, but rather must be involved in the production of H_2O_2 and/or ·OH, which subsequently are responsible for the DNA damage. Similarly, damage by H_2O_2, a known mutagen in both prokaryotic (86–88) and eukaryotic (89) organisms, and by lipid hydroperoxides is also thought to be mediated by ·OH generation. Thus, DNA damage in response to either O_2^- or H_2O_2 appears to be mediated via the redox-metal-mediated production of ·OH (90,91). More recently, peroxynitrite (·ONOO) has also been implicated in DNA damage in reactions involving both the bases and the sugar moieties. DNA damage may also be initiated by secondary radicals arising from oxidative damage to the nuclear proteins and/or lipids (92). Finally, evidence of DNA damage may also be found outside of the nucleus. Depletion of NAD(H) is likely if there is extensive oxidant damage to DNA. As shown by a number of studies, ADP polyribosylation of DNA-associated proteins (a reaction which uses NAD as initial substrate) can cause profound depletion of NAD, an absolutely necessary cofactor in cellular metabolism (93,94).

·OH attack on DNA generally appears to be by a direct reaction with the sugar moieties or by an addition reaction with either purine or pyrimidine bases (95). Direct ·OH attack on the deoxyribose backbone results in cleavage of the sugar and the generation of a number of sugar fragments (e.g., 2'-deoxyguanosine-5'-aldehyde) that react with thiobarbituric acid (TBA) (39). Thus, if purified DNA is being examined, sugar damage can easily be assayed for using the previously mentioned TBARS assay. However, this reaction is of limited, if any, usefulness in more complex mixtures.

Other simple, but insensitive, methods for detecting DNA damage measure strand scission. In bacteria (e.g., *Escherichia coli*) plasmids serve as sensitive targets of DNA damage (96). The conversion of supercoiled to linear plasmid DNA can be readily quantified on agarose gels. Similarly, in eukaryotic organisms, double-strand breaks (hence DNA fragmentation) can also be observed using agarose gels. In contrast to the double-strand scissions, single-strand breaks are slightly harder to detect (97).

While these assays are suitable for either purified DNA or cultured cells, they are difficult to use in whole-animal studies. Consequently, newer methods have been developed to estimate DNA injury. These methods are based on the tendency for ·OH to undergo addition reactions with purine or pyrimidine bases (98). Often the products of this reaction are stable, with the modified bases being excised by repair enzymes. The excised bases are subsequently excreted from the cell/organism. This chemistry has been exploited by Bruce Ames and others to develop noninvasive assays for DNA damage that are suitable for long-term in vivo studies. In general these methods use high-performance liquid chromatography (HPLC) or mass spectroscopy to measure the hydroxylation products of DNA (99–101). Among the more commonly assayed products of oxidative DNA damage are 8-oxo-7,8-dihydro-2'-deoxyguanosine (102) and thymidine glycol (99). However, it is important to note that a number of these products may also arise from normal metabolic activity and from metabolism of bacterial flora. Therefore, appropriate controls must always be done.

Thus, indicators of DNA damage range from gross measurements of injury such as single- or double-strand breaks (DNA fragmentation, plasmid linearization) to specific measures of base damage. These assays are predominantly based on the known chemistry of reactions between ·OH-like radicals and DNA. It is important to remember that the chemical injury induced is dependent on the oxidant species, the availability of redox-active metals (i.e., Fe and Cu), the repair capacity of the cell, and, invariably, a host of other factors. Because of the importance of DNA damage in mutagenesis and carcinogenesis, accurate methodologies to detect these injuries will be of increasing importance.

SUMMARY

Much of what we know regarding free-radical-mediated injury has been gained using very imprecise assays and circumstantial evidence. This is not meant to imply that this information is wrong, but rather that it must be critically evaluated and confirmed using additional methodologies. Indeed, when appropriately used even very crude (e.g., TBARS) assays can and do provide valuable information to the forensic oxidologist. However, as can be gleaned from the preceding discussion, several general rules of caution can be generated. First and foremost, be sure the assay used is capable of measuring the kinds of injury likely occurring. Assays for cytostolic protein oxidation are not appropriate if one is using a lipophilic oxidant. Second, it is important that the investigator use multiple types of assays to assure the validity of results. While the measurement of conjugated dienes is simple, fast, and cheap, it should be coupled with other assays of lipid oxidation such as TBARS, parinaric acid, or gas chromatographic analysis. Third, it is essential that one choose an assay of appropriate sensitivity and reproducibility. DNA scission in response to H_2O_2 may yield some results, but it is likely a gross underestimate of the actual damage to the DNA.

REFERENCES

1. Beutler, E. (1984). Glutathione. In: *Red Cell Metabolism: A Manual of Biochemical Methods*, 3 ed. Grune & Stratton, Orlando, FL pgs. 131–134.
2. Beutler, E., Robson, M. Buttenwieser. E. (1957). The mechanism of glutathione destruction and protection in drug-sensitive erythrocytes. In vitro studies. *J. Clin. Invest.*, 36:617–628.

3. Eaton, JW, and Brewer, GJ (1974). Pentose phosphate metabolism. In: *The Red Blood Cell* (Surgenor, DM, Ed) pp. 435–471, Academic Press, New York.
4. Scott, MD, Zuo, L., Lubin, BH, and Chiu, DT-Y (1991). NADPH, not glutathione, status modulates oxidant susceptibility of hemoglobin in normal and glucose-6-phosphate dehydrogenase deficient erythrocytes. *Blood*, 77:2059–2064.
5. Scott, MD, Lubin, BH, Zuo, L., and Kuypers, FA (1991). Erythrocyte defense against H_2O_2: Preeminent importance of catalase. *J. Lab. Clin. Med.*, 118:7–16.
6. Paller, MS, and Eaton, JW, (1995) Hazards of antioxidant combinations containing superoxide dismutase. *Free Rad. Biol. Med.*, 18:883–890.
7. Scott, MD, and Eaton, JW (1995). Thalassemic erythrocytes: Cellular suicide arising from iron and glutathione-dependent oxidation reactions? *Br. J. Haem.*, 91:811–819.
8. van den Berg, JJM, Kuypers, FA, Roelofsen, B., and Op den Kamp, JAF, (1990) The cooperative action of vitamins E and C in the protection against peroxidation of parinaric acid in human erythrocyte membranes. *Chem. Phys. Lipids*, 53:309–320.
9. Bowry, VW, Ingold, KU, and Stocker, R. (1992). Vitamin E in human low-density lipoprotein. When and how this antioxidant becomes a pro-oxidant. *Biochem. J.*, 288:341–344.
10. Scott, MD, Wagner, TC, and Chiu, DT-Y (1993). Catalase activity and oxidant susceptibility in glucose-6-phosphate dehydrogenase deficient erythrocytes. *Biochim. Biophys. Acta*, 1181:163–168.
11. Wagner, TC, and Scott, MD (1994). Single extraction method for the spectrophotometric quantification of oxidized and reduced pyridine nucleotides in erythrocytes. *Anal. Biochem.*, 222:417–426.
12. Jacob, HS, Ingbar, SH, and Jandl, JH (1965). Oxidative hemolysis and erythrocyte metabolism in hereditary acatalasia. *J. Clin. Invest.*, 44:1187–1199.
13. Schraufstatter, IU, Hyslop, PA, Hinshaw, DB, Spragg, RG, Sklar, LA, and Cochrane, CG, (1986) Hydrogen peroxide-induced injury of cells and its prevention by inhibitors of poly(ADP-ribose) polymerase. *Proc. Natl. Acad. Sci. USA*, 83:4908–4912.
14. Schraufstatter, IU, Hinshaw, DB, Hyslop, PA, Spragg, RG, and Cochrane, CG. (1996). Oxidant injury of cells. (1986) DNA strand-breaks activate polyadenosine diphosphate-ribose polymerase and lead to depletion of nicotinamide adenine dinucleotide. *J. Clin. Invest.*, 77:1312–1320.
15. Gille, JJ, van Berkel, CG, Mullaart, E., Vijg, J., and Joenje, H. (1989). Effects of lethal exposure to hypoxia and to hydrogen peroxide on NAD(H) and ATP pools in Chinese hamster ovary cells. *Mutation Res.* 214:89–96.
16. Hassan, HM, and Fridovich, I. (1977). Enzymatic defenses against the toxicity of oxygen and of streptonigrin in Escherichia coli. *J. Bacteriol.*, 129:1574–1583.
17. Kimball, RE, Reddy, K., Pierce, TH, Schwartz, LW, Mustafa, MG, and Cross, CE (1976). Oxygen toxicity: augmentation of antioxidant defense mechanisms in rat lung. *Am. J. Physiol.*, 230:1425–1431.
18. Margoliash, E., Novogrodsky, A., and Schejter, A. (1960) Irreversible reaction of 3-amino-1,2,4-triazole and related inhibitors with the protein of catalase. *Biochem. J.*, 74:339–348.
19. Cadenas, E. and Sies, H. (1985). Detection of singlet oxygen by low-level chemiluminescence. In: *Handbook of Methods for Oxygen Radical Research* (Greenwald, RA, Ed.), pp. 191–195, CRC Press: Boca Raton, FL.
20. Corbisier, P., Houbion, A., and Remacle, J. (1987). A new technique for highly sensitive detection of superoxide dismutase activity by chemiluminescence. *Anal. Biochem.*, 164:240–247.
21. Peters, TR, Tosk, JM, and Goulbourne, EAJ (1990). Lucigenin chemiluminescence as a probe for measuring reactive oxygen species production in Escherichia coli. *Anal. Biochem.*, 186:316–319.
22. Minkenberg, I. and Ferber, E. (1984). Lucigenin-dependent chemiluminescence as a new assay for NAD(P)H-oxidase activity in particulate fractions of human polymorphonuclear leukocytes. Escherichia coli cell inactivation by superoxide anion and hydrogen peroxide. *J. Immunol. Meth.*, 71:61–67.
23. Murphy, ME, and Sies, H. (1990). Visible-range low-level chemiluminescence in biological systems. *Meth. Enzymol.*, 186:595–611.
24. Rosen, GM, and Halpern, HJ (1990). Spin trapping biologically generated free radicals: Correlating formation with cellular injury. *Meth. Enzymol.*, 186:611–621.
25. Mason, RP, and Knecht, KT (1994). In vivo detection of radical adducts by electron spin resonance. *Meth. Enzymol.*, 233;112–117.
26. Fridovich, I. (1986). Cytochrome c. In: *CRC Handbook of Methods for Oxygen Radical Research* (Greenwald, RA, Ed.) pp. 213–215. CRC Press: Boca Raton, FL

27. Jiang, ZY, Hunt, JV, and Wolff, SP (1992). Ferrous ion oxidation in the presence of xylenol orange for detection of lipid hydroperoxide in low density lipoprotein. *Anal. Biochem.*, 202:384–389.
28. Green, MJ, and Hill, AO (1984). Chemistry of dioxygen. *Meth. Enzymol.*, 105:3–22.
29. Cathcart, R., Schwiers, E., and Ames, BN (1983). Detection of picomole levels of hydroperoxides using a fluorescent dichlorofluorescein assay. *Anal. Biochem.*, 134:111–116.
30. Winterbourn, CC (1987). The ability of scavengers to distinguish OH· production in the iron-catalyzed Haber-Weiss reaction: comparison of four assays for OH·. *Free Radical Biol. Med.*, 3:33–39.
31. Repine, JE, Eaton, JW, Anders, MW, Hoidal, JR, and Fox, RB (1979). Generation of hydroxyl radical by enzymes, chemicals, and human phagocytes in vitro. Detection using the anti-inflammatory agent, dimethyl sulfoxide. *J. Clin. Invest.* 64:1642–1651.
32. Klein, SM, Cohen, G., and Cederbaum, AI (1981). Production of formaldehyde during metabolism of dimethyl sulfoxide by hydroxyl radical generating systems. *Biochem.*, 20:6006–6012.
33. Babbs, CF and Steiner, MG (1990). Detection and quantitation of hydroxyl radical using dimethyl sulfoxide as molecular probe. *Meth. Enzymol.*, 186:137–147.
34. Puppo, A., and Halliwell, B. (1988). Formation of hydroxyl radicals from hydrogen peroxide in the presence of iron. Is haemoglobin a biological Fenton reagent? *Biochem. J.* 249:185–190.
35. Beckman, JS, Chen, J., Ischiropoulos, H. and Crow, JP (1994). Oxidative chemistry of peroxynitrite. *Meth. Enzymol.*, 233:229–240.
36. Slungaard, A., and Mahoney, JR (1991). Bromide-dependent toxicity of eosinophil peroxidase for endothelium and isolated working rat hearts: A model for eosinophilic endocarditis. *J. Exp. Med.*, 173:117–126.
37. Gutteridge, JMC (1982). Free-radicals damage to lipids, amino acids, carbohydrates and nucleic acids determined by thiobarbituric acid reactivity. *Int. J. Biochem* 14:649–653.
38. Halliwell, B., and Gutteridge, JMC (1981). Formation of a thiobarbituric-acid-reactive substance from deoxyribose in the presence of iron salts. *FEBS Lett.*, 128:347–351.
39. Halliwell, B. and Gutteridge, JMC (1989). *Free Radicals in Biology and Medicine*, 2nd Edition. p. 230, Clarendon Press, Oxford.
40. Rechnagel, RO, and Glende, EA (1984). Spectrophotometric detection of lipid conjugated dienes. *Meth. Enzymol.*, 105:331–337.
41. Dormandy, TL, and Wickens, DG (1987). The experimental and clinical pathology of diene conjugation. *Chem. Phys. Lipids*, 45:353–364.
42. Nourooz-Zadeh, J., Tajaddini, J., and Wolff, SP (1994). Measurement of plasma hydroperoxide concentrations by ferrous oxidation-xylenol orange assay in conjunction with triphenylphosphine. *Anal. Biochem.*, 220:403–409.
43. Cathcart, R., Schwiers, ES, and Ames, BN (1984). Detection of picomole levels of lipid hydroperoxides using a dichlorofluorescein fluorescent assay. *Meth. Enzymol.*, 105:352–358.
44. Kuypers, FA, van den Berg, JJM, Schalkwijk, C., Roelofsen, B., and Op den Kamp, JAF (1987). Parinaric acid as a sensitive fluorescent probe for the determination of lipid peroxidation. *Biochim. Biophys. Acta*, 921:266–274.
45. van den Berg, JJM (1994). Effects of oxidants and antioxidants evaluated using parinaric acid as a sensitive probe for oxidative stress. *Redox Report*, 1:11–21.
46. Deuticke, B., Heller, KB, and Haest, CWM (1987). Progressive oxidative membrane damage in erythrocytes after pulse treatment with t-butylhydroperoxide. *Biochim. Biophys. Acta*, 899:113–124.
47. Kuypers, FA, Chiu, DT-Y, Mohandas, N., Roelofsen, B., Op den Kamp, JAF, and Lubin, BH (1987). The molecular species composition of phosphatidylcholine affects cellular properties in normal and sickle erythrocytes. *Blood*, 70:1111–1118.
48. Skipski, VP, and Barclay, M. (1969). Thin layer chromatography of phospholipids. *Meth. Enzymol.* 14, 530–598.
49. Bartlett, GR (1959). Phosphorus assay in column chromatography. *J. Biol. Chem.*, 234:466–468.
50. Herrmann, A., and Devaux, PF (1990). Alteration of the aminophospholipid translocase activity during in vivo and artificial aging of human erythrocytes. *Biochim. Biophys. Acta*, 1027:41–46.
51. Lubin, B., Chiu, D., Bastacky, J., Roelofsen, B., and Van Deenen, LLM (1981). Abnormalities in membrane phospholipid organization in sickled erythrocytes. *J. Clin. Invest.*, 67:1643–1649.
52. Lubin, BH, Kuypers, FA, Chui, DT-Y, and Shohet, SB (1988). Analysis of red cell membrane lipids. In: *Methods in Hematology: Red Cell Membranes* (Shohet, SB, and Mohandas, N., Eds.) pp 171–202, Churchill Livingstone, New York.
53. Franck, PFH, Bevers, EM, Lubin, BH, Comfurius, P., Chiu, DT-Y, Op den Kamp, JAF, Zwaal,

RFA, van Deenen, LLM, and Roelofsen, B. (1985). Uncoupling of the membrane skeleton from the lipid bilayer. The cause of accelerated phospholipid flip-flop leading to an enhanced procoagulant activity of sickled cells. *J. Clin. Invest.*, 75:183–190.

54. Kuypers, FA, Abraham, S., Lubin, B., and Chiu, D. (1988). Diet-induced asymmetry of the phosphatidylcholine fatty acyl composition in rat erythrocyte membranes. *J. Lab. Clin. Med.*, 111:529–536.

55. Rose, HG, and Oklander, M. (1965). Improved method for the extraction of lipids from human erythrocytes. *J. Lipid Res.*, 6:428–431.

56. Carpenter, KL, Wilkins, GM, Fussell, B., Ballantine, JA, Taylor, SE, Mitchinson, MJ, and Leake, DS (1994). Production of oxidized lipids during modification of low-density lipoprotein by macrophages or copper. *Biochem. J.*, 304:625–633.

57. Zimmerman, GA, Prescott, SM, and McIntyre, TM (1995). Oxidatively fragmented phospholipids as inflammatory mediators: the dark side of polyunsaturated lipids. *J. Nutr.*, 125:1661S–1665S.

58. Thaw, HH, Collins, VP, and Brunk, UT (1984). Influence of oxygen tension, prooxidants and antioxidants on the formation of lipid peroxidation products (lipofuscin) in individual cultivated human glial cells. *Mech. Age Dev.* 24:211–223.

59. Tsuchida, M., Miura, T. and Aibara, K. (1987). Lipofuscin and lipofuscin-like substances. *Chem. Phys. Lipids* 44:297–325.

60. Eldred, GE, and Katz, ML (1989). The autofluorescent products of lipid peroxidation may not be lipofuscin-like. *Free Radical Biol. Med.*, 7:157–163.

61. Richards, DMC, Dean, RT, and Jessup, W. (1988). Membrane proteins are critical targets in free radical mediated cytolysis. *Biochim. Biophys. Acta*, 946:281–288.

62. Willson, RL (1983). Free radical repair mechanisms and the interactions of glutathione and vitamin C and E. In: *Radioprotectors and Anticarcinogens*, (Nygaard, OF, and Simic, MG Eds). pp. 1–22. Academic Press, New York.

63. Wolff, SP, and Dean, RT (1986). Fragmentation of proteins by free radicals and its effect on their susceptibility to enzymatic hydrolysis. *Biochem. J.*, 234:399–403.

64. Dean, RT, and Pollack, JK (1985). Endogenous free radical generation may influence proteolysis in mitochondria. *Biochem. Biophys. Res. Commun.*, 126:1082–1089.

65. Starke-Reed, PE, and Oliver, CN (1989). Protein oxidation and proteolysis during aging and oxidative stress. *Arch. Biochem. Biophys.*, 275:559–567.

66. Fligiel, SE, Lee, EC. McCoy, JP, Johnson, KJ, and Varani, J. (1984). Protein degradation following treatment with hydrogen peroxide. *Am. J. Path.* 115:418–425.

67. Graf, E., Mahoney, JR, Bryant, RG, and Eaton, JW (1984). Iron-catalyzed hydroxyl radical formation. Stringent requirement for free iron coordination site. *J. Biol. Chem.*, 259:3620–3624.

68. Garrison, WM (1968). Radiation chemistry of organo-nitrogen compounds. *Curr. Top. Radiat. Res.*, 4:43–94.

69. Wharton, SA, and Hipkiss, AR (1985). Degradation of peptides and proteins of different sizes by homogenates of human MRC5 lung fibroblasts. Aged cells have a decreased ability to degrade shortened proteins. *FEBS Lett.*, 184:249–253.

70. Zerez, CR, Hseih, JW, and Tanaka, KR (1987). Inhibition of red blood cell enzyme by hemin: a mechanism for hemolysis in hemoglobinopathies. *Trans. Assoc. Am. Phys.*, 100:329–338.

71. Salo, DC, Pacifici, RE, Lin, SW, Giulivi, C., and Davies, KJA (1990). Superoxide dismutase undergoes proteolysis and fragmentation following oxidative modification and inactivation. *J. Biol. Chem.*, 265:11919–11927.

72. Levine, RL, Garland, D., Oliver, CN, Amici, A., Climent, I., Lenz, A-G, Ahn, B-W, Shaltiel, S., and Stadtman, ER. (1990). Determination of carbonyl content in oxidatively modified proteins. *Meth. Enzymol.*, 186:464–478.

73. Zits, SV (1983). Determination of the blood thiol disulfide balance using the coulometric titration method. *Meth. Enzymol.*, 100:116–130.

74. Rank BH, Hebbel RP, Carlsson, J. (1984). Oxidation of membrane thiols in sickle erythrocytes. *Prog. Clin. Biol. Res.*, 165:473–477.

75. Laurell, CB, Thulin, E., and Bywater, RP (1977). Thiol-disulfide interchange chromatography using Sepharose-linked thiol compounds to separate plasma proteins. *Anal. Biochem.*, 81:336–345.

76. Rovera, G., Margarian, C., and Borun, TW (1978). Resolution of hemoglobin subunits by electrophoresis in acid urea polyacrylamide gels containing Triton X-100. *Anal. Biochem.*, 85:506–518.

77. Rouyer-Fessard, P., Lecomte, MC, Boivin, P., and Beuzard, Y. (1987). Separation of red cell membrane proteins by urea-triton-polyacrylamide gel electrophoresis in one- and two-dimensional systems. *Electrophoresis.* 8:476–481.

78. Laemmli, UK (1970). Cleavage of structural proteins by bacteriophage T4. *Nature*, 227:680–685.
79. Scott, MD, Rouyer-Fessard, P., Lubin, BH, and Beuzard, Y. (1990). Entrapment of purified α-hemoglobin chains in normal erythrocytes: A model for β thalassemia. *J. Biol. Chem.*, 265:17953–17959.
80. Bonner, WM, and Laskey, LA (1974). A film detection method for tritium-labelled proteins and nucleic acids in polyacrylamide gels. *Eur. J. Biochem.*, 46:83–88.
81. Minetti, M., Mallozzi, C., Scorza, G., Scott, MD, Kuypers, FA, and Lubin, BH (1993). Role of oxygen and carbon radicals in hemoglobin oxidation. *Arch. Biochem. Biophys.*, 302:233–244.
82. Scott, MD, van den Berg, JJM, Repka, T., Rouyer-Fessard, P., Hebbel, RP, Beuzard, Y., and Lubin, BH (1993). Effect of excess α-hemoglobin chains on cellular and membrane oxidation in model β thalassemic erythrocytes. *J. Clin. Invest.*, 91:1706–1712.
83. Winterbourn, CC (1990). Oxidative reactions of hemoglobin. *Meth. Enzymol.*, 186:256–272.
84. Ewing, D. and Jones, SR (1987). Superoxide removal and radiation protection in bacteria. *Arch. Biochem. Biophys.*, 254:53–62.
85. Aronovitch, J., Godinger, D., Samuni, A., and Czapski, G. (1987). Ascorbate oxidation and DNA scission catalyzed by iron and copper chelates. *Free Rad. Res. Comm.*, 2:241–258.
86. Ananthaswamy, HN, and Eisenstark, A. (1977). Repair of hydrogen peroxide-induced single strand breaks in Escherichia coli deoxyribonucleic acid. *J. Bacteriol.*, 130, 187–191.
87. Demple, B., Halbrook, J., and Linn, S. (1983). Escherichia coli xth mutants are hypersensitive to hydrogen peroxide. *J. Bacteriol.*, 153:1079–1082.
88. Imlay, J.A. and Linn, S. (1987) Mutagenesis and stress responses induced in Escherichia coli by hydrogen peroxide. *J. Bacteriol.*, 169:2967–2976.
89. Floyd, R.A. (1981) DNA-ferrous iron catalyze hydroxyl free radical formation from hydrogen peroxide. *Biochem. Biophys. Res. Commun.*, 99:1209–1215.
90. Mello Filho, A.C., Hoffmann, M.E. and Meneghini, R. (1984) Cell killing and DNA damage by hydrogen peroxide are mediated by intracellular iron. *Biochem. J.*, 218:273–275.
91. Repine, J.E., Fox, R.B., and Berger, E.M. (1981) Hydrogen peroxide kills Staphylococcus aureus by reacting with staphylococcal iron to form hydroxyl radical. *J. Biol. Chem.*, 256:7094–7096.
92. Park, J. and Floyd, R. (1992) Lipid peroxidation products mediate the formation of 8-hydroxydeoxy-guanosine in DNA. *Free Radical Biol. Med.*, 12:245–250.
93. Skidmore, C.J., Davies, M.I., Goodwin, P.M., Halldorsson, H., Lewis, P.J., Shall, S. and Zia'ee, A.A. (1979) The involvement of poly(ADP-ribose) polymerase in the degradation of NAD caused by gamma-radiation and N-methyl-N-nitrosourea. *Eur. J. Biochem.*, 101:135–142.
94. Sims, J.L., Berger, S.L., and Berger, N.A. (1983) Poly(ADP-ribose) polymerase inhibitors preserve nicotinamide adenine dinucleotide and adenosine 5′-triphosphate pools in DNA-damaged cells: mechanism of stimulation of unscheduled DNA synthesis. *Biochem.*, 22:5188–5191.
95. Cadet, J. (1994) DNA damage caused by oxidation, deamination, ultraviolet radiation and pho-toexcited psoralens. In: *DNA Adducts: Identification and Biological Significance* (Hemminki, K., Dipple, A., Shuker, D.G.E., Kadlubar, F.F., Segerback, D., and Bartsch, H. Eds.) pp. 245–276 IARC Scientific Publications.
96. Aronovitch, J., Samuni, A., Godinger, D., and Czapski, G. (1986) In vivo degradation of bacterial DNA by H_2O_2 and o-phenanthroline. In: *Superoxide Dismutase in Chemistry, Biology and Medicine* (Rotilio, G. Ed.) pp. 346–348. Elsevier Science Publishers,
97. Erixon, K., and Ahnstrom, G. (1979) Single-strand breaks in DNA during repair of UV-induced damage in normal human and xeroderma pigmentosum cells as determined by alkaline DNA unwinding and hydroxyapatite chromatography. *Mut. Res.* 59:257–271.
98. Cadet, J., Berger, M., Morin, B., Raoul, S., and Wagner, J.R. (1995) Oxidative damage to DNA. In: *Analysis of Free Radicals in Biological Systems* (Favier, A.E., Cadet, J., Kalyanaraman, B., Fontecave, M., Pierre, J.-L., Eds.), pp. 51–64. Birkhauser Verlag, Basel
99. Cathcart R, Schwiers E, Saul RL, and Ames BN. (1984). Thymine glycol and thymidine glycol in human and rat urine: A possible assay for oxidative DNA damage. *Proc. Natl. Acad. Sci. USA*, 81:5633–5637.
100. Richter, C., Park, J.-W., and Ames, B.N. (1988) Normal oxidative damage to mitochondrial and nuclear DNA is extensive. *Proc. Natl. Acad. Sci. USA*, 85:6465–6467.
101. von Sonntag, C. and Schuchmann, H.-P. (1990) Radical-mediated DNA damage in presence of oxygen. *Meth. Enzymol.*, 186:511–520.
102. Fraga, C.R., Shigenaga, M.K., Park, J.-W., Degan, P., and Ames, B.N. (1990) Oxidative damage to DNA during aging: 8-hydroxy-2′-deoxyguanosine in rat organ DNA and urine. *Proc. Natl. Acad. Sci. USA*, 87:4533–4537.

Subject Index

A

Acceptor molecule, 15
Acetaldehyde, 235
Acetaminophen (paracetamol)
  covalent bonding, 181–182
  cytotoxicity, 181
  hepatotoxicity, 180–182
  mitochondrial injury, 197–198
  nephrotoxicity, 188–190
Acetoxime, DNA oxidative damage and, 97
N-Acetyl-L-cysteine, 329–330
N-Acetyl-p-aminophenol. See Acetaminophen
N-Acetyl-p-benzoquinone imine. See NAPQI
N-Acetylprocainamide, 266
Activator protein-1 (AP-1)
  activation, 387–388
  DNA-binding activity, 336
  modulation
    by free radicals, 365
    by redox status, 341
  posttranslational regulation, 387
Acute lymphoblastic leukemia (ALL)
  immunologic characteristics, 254
  ionizing radiation and, 256
  therapy-related, 254
Acute myeloid leukemia (AML)
  chromosome abnormalities, 252–253, 263
  ionizing radiation and, 256
  therapy-related, 253
  tumor suppressor gene and, 269
Acute respiratory distress syndrome (ARDS),
    295, 296
Additive nomenclature, 3, 4
Adenyl, 362
Adriamycin. See Doxorubicin
Advanced glycosylation end products
    (AGEs), 79
Aflatoxin B₁, 99
Aging
  nDNA oxidative damage and, 89

protein carbonyl and, 81
ROS protein modification and, 71
Agranulocytosis
  chemically-induced, 255–256, 258
  description, 256
  drugs causing, 265–266
AH-receptor genes, 335–336, 336f
AH-receptor-nuclear-translocator (ARNT),
    335, 336f
Air pollution
  DNA oxidative damage and, 102
  lung disease and, 337
ALA (aminolevulinic acid), 100
Alcohol. See Ethanol
Alcohol dehydrogenase
  in ethanol catabolism, 236
  ethanol oxidation, 30
  NADH levels and, 33
Aldehyde dehydrogenase
  metabolization of lipid peroxidation
    products, 155
  mitochondrial NAD+-dependent, 236
Aldehyde oxidase, 236
Aldehyde oxide, radical production, 33
Aldehydes
  reactive, 53, 59–60
  α,β-unsaturated, 53
Alkenyl radicals, 53
Alkoxyl radicals
  hydroperoxide homolysis, 52–53
  reactivity, proximity to target and, 36
Alkyl peroxides, protein modification and, 71
Alkyl radicals, 53, 131
ALL. See Acute lymphoblastic leukemia
Alloxan, redox cycling, 26
Aluminum
  Alzheimer's disease and, 233
  neurotoxicity, 233–234
Alzheimer's disease
  aluminum and, 233